Animal Venoms—Curse or Cure?

Animal Venoms—Curse or Cure?

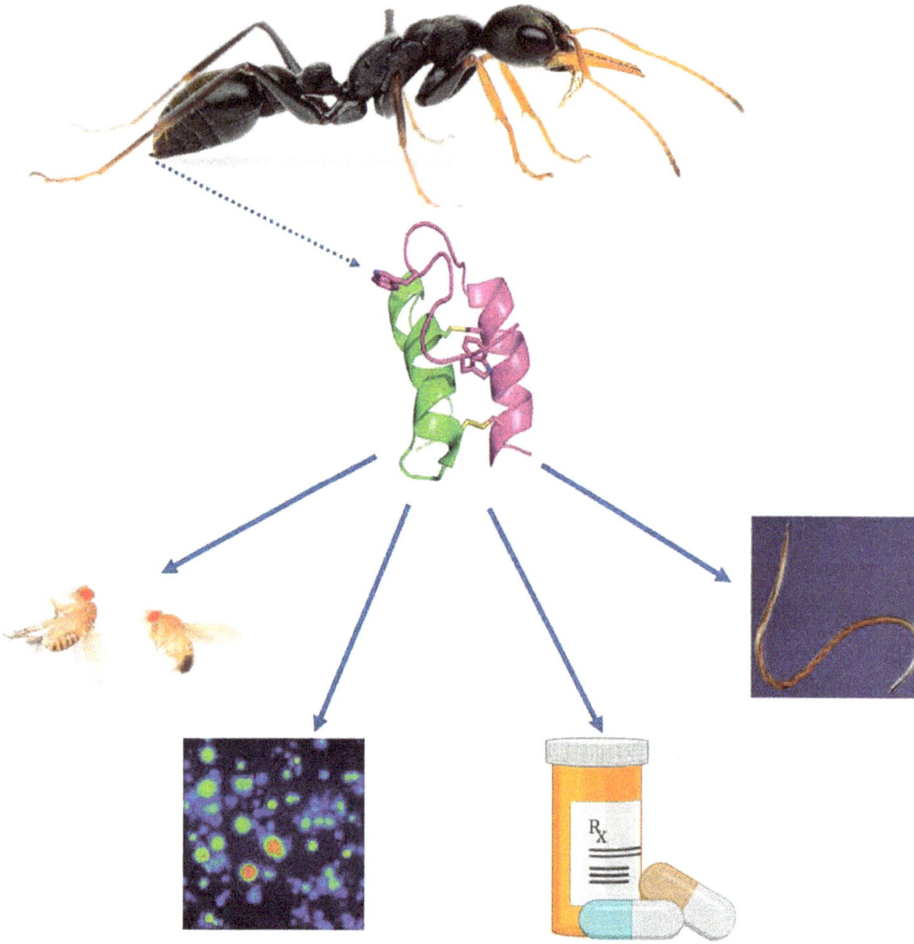

Animal Venoms and their potential applications: Image of *Myrmecia pilosula* adultworker ant courtesy of Alexander Wild (www.alexanderwild.com). Images of NMR structure of Δ-myrtoxin-Mp1a (=Mp1a) (adapted from Dekan et al. 2017, https://doi.org/10.1002/anie.201703360), intracellular calcium influxindicated by increased fluorescence in mouse dorsal root ganglia following the addition of 10 μM Mp1a and image of pill container all courtesy of Samantha A. Nixon. Image of female (left) and male (right) *Drosophila melanogaster* fruit flies courtesy of Shaodong Guo. Image of blood-filled adult female *Haemonchus contortus* nematodescourtesy of Philip Skuce.

Animal Venoms—Curse or Cure?

Editor

Volker Herzig

MDPI • Basel • Beijing • Wuhan • Barcelona • Belgrade • Manchester • Tokyo • Cluj • Tianjin

Editor
Volker Herzig
School of Science and
Engineering
University of the Sunshine Coast
Sippy Downs, QLD
Australia

Editorial Office
MDPI
St. Alban-Anlage 66
4052 Basel, Switzerland

This is a reprint of articles from the Special Issue published online in the open access journal *Biomedicines* (ISSN 2227-9059) (available at: www.mdpi.com/journal/biomedicines/special_issues/Venoms).

For citation purposes, cite each article independently as indicated on the article page online and as indicated below:

LastName, A.A.; LastName, B.B.; LastName, C.C. Article Title. *Journal Name* **Year**, *Volume Number*, Page Range.

ISBN 978-3-0365-1971-5 (Hbk)
ISBN 978-3-0365-1970-8 (PDF)

Cover image courtesy of Eivind A. B. Undheim.

Contents

About the Editor vii

Preface to "Animal Venoms—Curse or Cure?" ix

Volker Herzig
Animal Venoms—Curse or Cure?
Reprinted from: *Biomedicines* **2021**, *9*, 413, doi:10.3390/biomedicines9040413 1

Irina Gladkikh, Steve Peigneur, Oksana Sintsova, Ernesto Lopes Pinheiro-Junior, Anna Klimovich, Alexander Menshov, Anatoly Kalinovsky, Marina Isaeva, Margarita Monastyrnaya, Emma Kozlovskaya, Jan Tytgat and Elena Leychenko
Kunitz-Type Peptides from the Sea Anemone *Heteractis crispa* Demonstrate Potassium Channel Blocking and Anti-Inflammatory Activities
Reprinted from: *Biomedicines* **2020**, *8*, 473, doi:10.3390/biomedicines8110473 9

Sarah Lemke and Andreas Vilcinskas
European Medicinal Leeches—New Roles in Modern Medicine
Reprinted from: *Biomedicines* **2020**, *8*, 99, doi:10.3390/biomedicines8050099 27

Walden E. Bjørn-Yoshimoto, Iris Bea L. Ramiro, Mark Yandell, J. Michael McIntosh, Baldomero M. Olivera, Lars Ellgaard and Helena Safavi-Hemami
Curses or Cures: A Review of the Numerous Benefits Versus the Biosecurity Concerns of Conotoxin Research
Reprinted from: *Biomedicines* **2020**, *8*, 235, doi:10.3390/biomedicines8080235 39

David T. Wilson, Paramjit S. Bansal, David A. Carter, Irina Vetter, Annette Nicke, Sébastien Dutertre and Norelle L. Daly
Characterisation of a Novel A-Superfamily Conotoxin
Reprinted from: *Biomedicines* **2020**, *8*, 128, doi:10.3390/biomedicines8050128 61

Shirin Ahmadi, Julius M. Knerr, Lídia Argemi, Karla C. F. Bordon, Manuela B. Pucca, Felipe A. Cerni, Eliane C. Arantes, Figen Çalışkan and Andreas H. Laustsen
Scorpion Venom: Detriments and Benefits
Reprinted from: *Biomedicines* **2020**, *8*, 118, doi:10.3390/biomedicines8050118 71

Mathilde R. Israel, Thomas S. Dash, Stefanie N. Bothe, Samuel D. Robinson, Jennifer R. Deuis, David J. Craik, Angelika Lampert, Irina Vetter and Thomas Durek
Characterization of Synthetic Tf2 as a $Na_V1.3$ Selective Pharmacological Probe
Reprinted from: *Biomedicines* **2020**, *8*, 155, doi:10.3390/biomedicines8060155 103

Edward R. J. Evans, Lachlan McIntyre, Tobin D. Northfield, Norelle L. Daly and David T. Wilson
Small Molecules in the Venom of the Scorpion *Hormurus waigiensis*
Reprinted from: *Biomedicines* **2020**, *8*, 259, doi:10.3390/biomedicines8080259 117

Kathleen Yin, Jennifer R. Deuis, Zoltan Dekan, Ai-Hua Jin, Paul F. Alewood, Glenn F. King, Volker Herzig and Irina Vetter
Addition of K22 Converts Spider Venom Peptide Pme2a from an Activator to an Inhibitor of $Na_V1.7$
Reprinted from: *Biomedicines* **2020**, *8*, 37, doi:10.3390/biomedicines8020037 133

Andrea Seldeslachts, Steve Peigneur and Jan Tytgat
Caterpillar Venom: A Health Hazard of the 21st Century
Reprinted from: *Biomedicines* **2020**, *8*, 143, doi:10.3390/biomedicines8060143 . . . . **143**

Samantha A. Nixon, Zoltan Dekan, Samuel D. Robinson, Shaodong Guo, Irina Vetter, Andrew C. Kotze, Paul F. Alewood, Glenn F. King and Volker Herzig
It Takes Two: Dimerization Is Essential for the Broad-Spectrum Predatory and Defensive Activities of the Venom Peptide Mp1a from the Jack Jumper Ant *Myrmecia pilosula*
Reprinted from: *Biomedicines* **2020**, *8*, 185, doi:10.3390/biomedicines8070185 . . . . **171**

Xiaowei Zhou, Jie Xu, Ruimin Zhong, Chengbang Ma, Mei Zhou, Zhijian Cao, Xinping Xi, Chris Shaw, Tianbao Chen, Lei Wang and Hang Fai Kwok
Pharmacological Effects of a Novel Bradykinin-Related Peptide (RR-18) from the Skin Secretion of the Hejiang Frog (*Ordorrana hejiangensis*) on Smooth Muscle
Reprinted from: *Biomedicines* **2020**, *8*, 225, doi:10.3390/biomedicines8070225 . . . . **185**

Vladislav V. Babenko, Rustam H. Ziganshin, Christoph Weise, Igor Dyachenko, Elvira Shaykhutdinova, Arkady N. Murashev, Maxim Zhmak, Vladislav Starkov, Anh Ngoc Hoang, Victor Tsetlin and Yuri Utkin
Novel Bradykinin-Potentiating Peptides and Three-Finger Toxins from Viper Venom: Combined NGS Venom Gland Transcriptomics and Quantitative Venom Proteomics of the *Azemiops feae* Viper
Reprinted from: *Biomedicines* **2020**, *8*, 249, doi:10.3390/biomedicines8080249 . . . . **197**

Qing Liang, Tam Minh Huynh, Nicki Konstantakopoulos, Geoffrey K. Isbister and Wayne C. Hodgson
An Examination of the Neutralization of In Vitro Toxicity of Chinese Cobra (*Naja atra*) Venom by Different Antivenoms
Reprinted from: *Biomedicines* **2020**, *8*, 377, doi:10.3390/biomedicines8100377 . . . . **217**

Chunfang Xie, Laura-Oana Albulescu, Kristina B. M. Still, Julien Slagboom, Yumei Zhao, Zhengjin Jiang, Govert W. Somsen, Freek J. Vonk, Nicholas R. Casewell and Jeroen Kool
Varespladib Inhibits the Phospholipase A_2 and Coagulopathic Activities of Venom Components from Hemotoxic Snakes
Reprinted from: *Biomedicines* **2020**, *8*, 165, doi:10.3390/biomedicines8060165 . . . . **231**

Chunfang Xie, Laura-Oana Albulescu, Mátyás A. Bittenbinder, Govert W. Somsen, Freek J. Vonk, Nicholas R. Casewell and Jeroen Kool
Neutralizing Effects of Small Molecule Inhibitors and Metal Chelators on Coagulopathic *Viperinae* Snake Venom Toxins
Reprinted from: *Biomedicines* **2020**, *8*, 297, doi:10.3390/biomedicines8090297 . . . . **249**

Geoffrey K. Isbister, Nandita Mirajkar, Kellie Fakes, Simon G. A. Brown and Punnam Chander Veerati
Phospholipase A2 (PLA_2) as an Early Indicator of Envenomation in Australian Elapid Snakebites (ASP-27)
Reprinted from: *Biomedicines* **2020**, *8*, 459, doi:10.3390/biomedicines8110459 . . . . **265**

About the Editor

Associate Professor Volker Herzig

I was born in Germany, and even as a young boy, I was fascinated by the local spider fauna. As a teenager, I extended my interest to exotic spiders and kept several tarantula species as pets for many years in my parent's house. After finishing school, I studied Biology at the University of T übingen (Germany), finishing in 2001. The topic of my diploma thesis was the "Effects of state of nutrition, growth and sex on the quantity and composition of Phoneutria nigriventer (Keyserling, 1891) spider venom", which was based on research that I conducted in the lab of **Prof. Wagner F. dos Santos** during a 10-month stay at the University of Sao Paulo, Ribeirao Preto campus (Brazil).

I then continued as a PhD student in the lab of **Prof. Werner J. Schmidt** (topic: "The role of glutamate during expression of conditioned reward with consideration of the influence of the amygdala") at the University of T übingen and finished my PhD in 2004. With the support of several fellowships (DAAD, DFG and ARC), I undertook a 3-year stint as a postdoc in the lab of **Prof. Wayne C. Hodgson** at the Monash Venom Group, Monash University (Melbourne, Australia). From 2005 to 2008, I focussed my research on the venoms of Australian mygalomorph spiders.

In 2008, I joined the group of **Prof. Glenn F. King** at the Institute for Molecular Bioscience (IMB), The University of Queensland (Brisbane, Australia), where I stayed as a postdoc for almost 12 years. During this time, I diversified my venom and toxin research into other arthropods, including scorpions, assassin bugs, robber flies and ants. A major focus of my research comprised the identification and characterisation of novel arthropod toxins and their potential applications as bioinsecticides, antiparasitic compounds or treatments for pain, epilepsy and irritable bowel syndrome. During my time at the IMB, I also helped develop the ArachnoServer database on spider venom toxins, for which I am still acting as a curator of toxin records.

After receiving my ARC Future Fellowship in 2020, I joined the University of the Sunshine Coast (USC, Sippy Downs, Australia) as an associate professor to establish my own research group. The main interests of my current research at USC are the insecticidal and antiparasitic properties of arthropod venom components and their potential applications in agriculture, veterinary care and human medicine.

Preface to "Animal Venoms—Curse or Cure?"

This book is a compilation of all articles that have been published in the special issue of Biomedicines entitled Venoms–Curse or Cure?. It covers recent research and review articles on venoms, poisons and toxins from a taxonomically diverse selection of animals. With the broad range of toxin activities and their related molecular targets, this book is not only aimed at experimental and clinical toxinologists, but should also be of interest to related disciplines such as structural and molecular biology, ecology, evolution, genetics, physiology, pharmacology, and parasitology. Furthermore, some of the suggested potential applications of animal toxins such as molecular research tools, bioinsecticides or human and veterinary therapeutics are also reflected in this book. I would like to thank all authors, many of whom are leading researchers in their field, for their excellent contributions. I further hope the audience will not only find these articles both interesting and informative, but that some readers might gain inspirations leading to novel discoveries in this exciting field of research.

Volker Herzig
Editor

biomedicines

MDPI

Editorial

Animal Venoms—Curse or Cure?

Volker Herzig [1,2]

1 GeneCology Research Centre, University of the Sunshine Coast, Sippy Downs, QLD 4556, Australia; vherzig@usc.edu.au; Tel.: +61-7-5456-5382
2 School of Science, Technology and Engineering, University of the Sunshine Coast, Sippy Downs, QLD 4556, Australia

Abstract: An estimated 15% of animals are venomous, with representatives spread across the majority of animal lineages. Animals use venoms for various purposes, such as prey capture and predator deterrence. Humans have always been fascinated by venomous animals in a Janus-faced way. On the one hand, humans have a deeply rooted fear of venomous animals. This is boosted by their largely negative image in public media and the fact that snakes alone cause an annual global death toll in the hundreds of thousands, with even more people being left disabled or disfigured. Consequently, snake envenomation has recently been reclassified by the World Health Organization as a neglected tropical disease. On the other hand, there has been a growth in recent decades in the global scene of enthusiasts keeping venomous snakes, spiders, scorpions, and centipedes in captivity as pets. Recent scientific research has focussed on utilising animal venoms and toxins for the benefit of humanity in the form of molecular research tools, novel diagnostics and therapeutics, biopesticides, or anti-parasitic treatments. Continued research into developing efficient and safe antivenoms and promising discoveries of beneficial effects of animal toxins is further tipping the scales in favour of the "cure" rather than the "curse" prospect of venoms.

Keywords: venom; toxin; toxicity; lethality; envenomation; antivenom; venoms to drugs; therapeutics; biopesticide; anti-parasitic

check for updates

Citation: Herzig, V. Animal Venoms—Curse or Cure? *Biomedicines* **2021**, *9*, 413. https://doi.org/10.3390/biomedicines9040413

Received: 1 April 2021
Accepted: 9 April 2021
Published: 12 April 2021

Publisher's Note: MDPI stays neutral with regard to jurisdictional claims in published maps and institutional affiliations.

1. Introduction to Venomous Animals and Their Venoms

With an estimated 220,000 species or 15% of the global animal biodiversity being venomous [1], the majority of all animal lineages (57.5%) actually contain venomous representatives (Figure 1). Venom usage has convergently evolved in many animal lineages, and a recent estimate for arthropods, which are by far the most speciose venomous animals, suggested that venom systems have independently evolved in at least 19 lineages or even 29 times, if secretions that facilitate hemolymph or blood-feeding parasitism are also accounted for [2–4]. In comparison, flight (which, like venom, is also a trait that can endow animals with an evolutionary advantage but that comes at a high energetic cost) has convergently evolved only four times in the animal kingdom (i.e., in birds, bats, insects, and pterosaurs) [5]. Thus, with the exceptional abundance of independent evolutionary origins of animal venoms comes a vast diversity of venom system anatomies and venom application strategies. Direct injection into prey or predators has been realised via modified fang-like extremities (spiders, centipedes, crustaceans), antennae (beetles), pincers (pseudoscorpions), modified teeth (snakes), beaks (octopuses), stingers (scorpions), modified ovipositors (hymenopterans), proboscis (flies and bugs), barbs (fish), spurs (monotremes), hairs (caterpillars), harpoons (cone snails), and nematocysts (jellyfish, sea anemones). Even external application by spraying (snakes, scorpions, ants) [6–8] or release of toxins into the surrounding aqueous environment (cone snails) have also been reported [9]. Poisonous (i.e., lacking a morphological structure for direct venom delivery) amphibians have glands for the secretion of their toxins in order to deter predators when being ingested [10]. However, while the delivery strategies might differ between poisonous and venomous animals, the main purpose of animal poisons and venoms is to cause physiological changes that incapacitate or deter the targeted victim, primarily for predatory or defensive reasons. These physiological changes can affect a variety of molecular targets and form the basis of both the detrimental as well as beneficial aspects of these toxic secretions. For this reason, this Editorial and the related Special Issue of *Biomedicines* cover both perspectives in relation to animal poisons, venoms, and toxins.

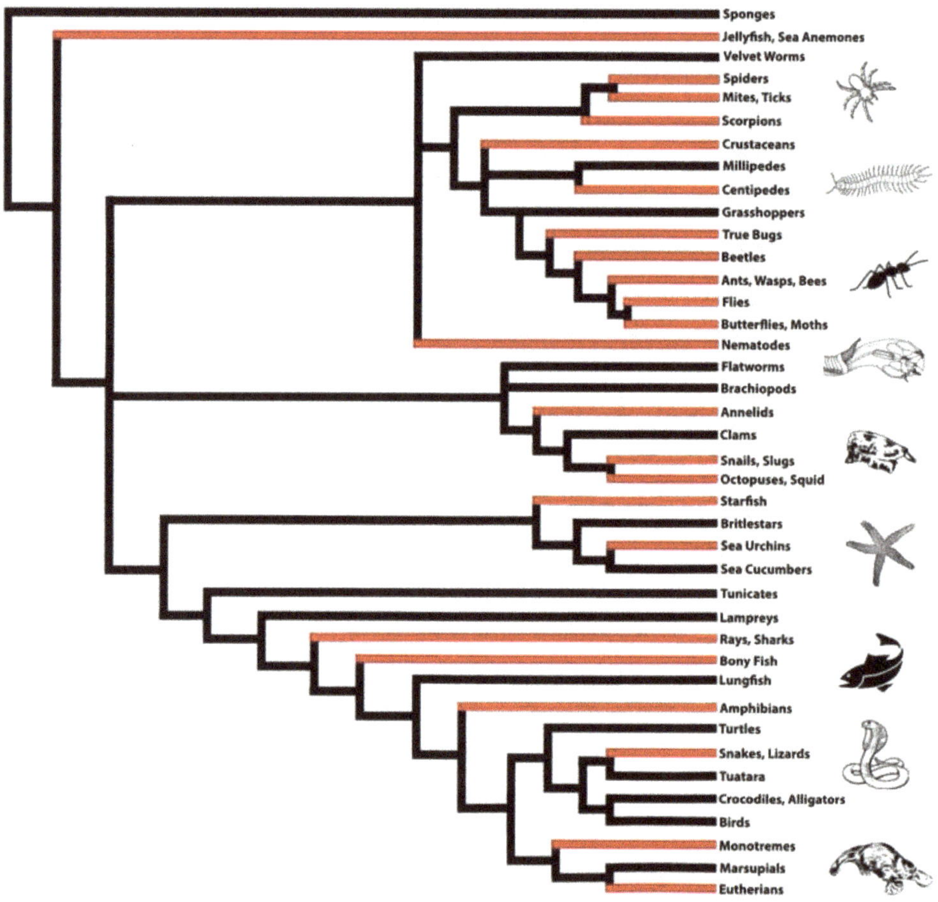

Figure 1. Evolutionary tree of animals (modified from [1]). Lineages with venomous representatives are indicated in red.

2. History of Human Interactions with Venomous Animals

Humans have always been fascinated by venomous and poisonous animals, with their toxic secretions being exploited for traditional medicine for thousands of years. The usage of honeybee venom for a variety of therapeutic applications [11] dates back to at least the second century BC in Eastern Asia [12,13]. Leeches have also been used by many ancient cultures (e.g., Egyptian, Indian, Greek, and Arabian), mainly for bloodletting, but also for the treatment of diseases such as inflammation, skin diseases, rheumatic pain, or reproductive problems [14]. Various Amazonian tribes are known to utilise painful ant stings for their puberty rituals [15]. Another interesting example is poison dart frogs from the family Dendrobatidae, which have been employed by several South American tribes as a source of poison to cover their arrow tips used for hunting [16]. It is a remarkable twist that poison dart frogs do not even produce their toxic alkaloids themselves, but sequester them (in the majority of cases in an unmodified form) from their mostly arthropod diet (e.g., ants and millipedes) [17]. Thus, the human usage of poison dart frog alkaloids can be considered a sequential recycling of toxic compounds originating from arthropods. Furthermore, this example might also blur the separation between venoms and poisons, if venom components are recycled into a poisonous secretion. Some venomous animals such as honeybees have even been domesticated, with records of beekeeping dating back at least 4500 years to Egypt [18] or 3000 years to Israel [19]. In modern agriculture, honeybees are indispensable as production animals for the pollination of a wide variety of crops to ensure the survival of billions of people, with the yield of honey and other bee products merely being an added economic benefit. In the last few decades, a number of other venomous animals have even made the status of human "pets", with a growing global scene of enthusiasts mainly in developed countries keeping venomous snakes, spiders, scorpions, insects, and centipedes in their homes [20].

3. The "Curse": Detrimental Effects of Animal Venoms

In its infancy, venom research was incited by an urgent need for antivenoms to combat human fatalities caused by envenomations from snakes, spiders, and scorpions [21,22]. The most common strategy for developing antivenoms comprises injecting small and then increasing doses of venoms into mammals (e.g., horses, sheep, or rabbits) and then isolating the antibodies produced in their blood as antivenom for treating envenomated humans. The production of heterologous antivenoms was pioneered by Albert Calmette in 1895 to raise cobra antivenom [22] and has since been successfully adapted to a range of other venomous animals. Nowadays, antivenoms are available against a wide range of venomous animals including spiders (*Phoneutria, Loxosceles, Atrax, Latrodectus*), scorpions (only from the family Buthidae, e.g., the genera *Androctonus, Buthus, Centruroides, Leiurus, Parabuthus,* and *Tityus*), ticks (*Ixodes holocyclus* = "paralysis tick"), caterpillars (*Lonomia obliqua*), box jellyfish (*Chironex fleckeri*), stonefish (*Synanceia*), and many species of snake (belonging to the families Elapidae and Viperidae). Modern molecular techniques have also started to tackle a major disadvantage of heterologously produced antivenoms, which is their potential incompatibility with the human immune system. A recent study, for example, showed that oligoclonal mixtures of recombinant human immunoglobulin G can be successfully and cost-efficiently used for neutralising snake venoms [23].

The majority of commercially available antivenoms are already targeted against snakes. Nevertheless, a large deficit still remains in developing effective antivenoms for treating snake envenomations. The reason that snakes have to be considered as the most dangerous venomous animals from a human perspective is not only their large venom amounts but also the fact that most snakes have evolved their venoms to overcome vertebrate prey and therefore many of their toxins also exhibit activity in humans. Another reason is that some snake antivenoms lack cross-reactivity and are therefore only effective to treat envenomations from the particular (or closely related) snake species against which they were raised [24]. Thus, even the use of polyvalent (i.e., raised against several species) antivenoms will be limited to certain geographical areas and cannot simply be applied on a larger or even global scale [24]. Unfortunately, the countries that are most affected by snake envenomations are usually those that are most economically disadvantaged and therefore lack the funding and expertise required for the development of snake antivenoms specific to their region [25]. This became particularly obvious when the commercial production of Fav-Afrique was discontinued in 2014 for economic reasons, which is estimated to have resulted in an additional 10,000 annual deaths in Africa [26]. Due to the global scale of 1.8–5 million annual snake envenomations, the resulting 81,000–138,000 fatalities, and the even larger number of permanent disfigurements and disabilities, snake envenomations have been reclassified as a neglected tropical disease by the World Health Organisation [24–26]. Additionally, due to poor record keeping and many unreported cases in developing countries affected by snake envenomations, these staggering numbers might even be a gross underestimate of the real numbers [24]. While a range of other venomous organisms, including arachnids, hymenopterans, cone snails, and jellyfish, have also been reported to cause human fatalities [27–30], their resulting global fatality numbers are dwarfed by the number of snakebite fatalities. Nevertheless, some of these animals, such as scorpions, can be responsible for a large number of fatalities in those geographical regions where they occur in high population densities [27,31–33].

4. The "Cure": Beneficial Effects of Animal Venoms

In recent decades, the majority of toxinologists have shifted their attention towards potential benefits of toxins from animal venoms for humanity, with various applications, including diagnostics [34], therapeutics [35–42], molecular tools in basic research for studying physiological processes [43–47], and treatments against pests and parasites [48,49]. Most of these applications involve peptide toxins and rely on their exquisite potency and selectivity against their respective molecular targets [50], but also their stability [51] and economical means of production at a large scale [52]. In cases where a molecular target of an animal toxin is also involved in the pathophysiology of a disease, this can then be exploited to develop novel therapeutics [39]. So far, six venom-derived drugs have made it to the market, including an antidiabetic peptide from a lizard, an analgesic peptide and a monomeric insulin from cone snails, a sea anemone peptide for treatment of autoimmune disease, a scorpion peptide for imaging brain tumours during surgery, and a spider peptide bioinsecticide (for further details, see [36]). Moreover, many more animal toxins or toxin-derived drugs are still in the pipeline for a wide variety of potential applications [35,38,40,42]. Importantly, the presence of promising toxin candidates as novel therapeutics or biopesticides is not correlated with their harmful effects on humans. Thus, even venomous species that are completely harmless to humans (which are, by far, the majority of all venomous organisms) might contain potentially interesting toxins in their venoms that could benefit humanity. In addition, the rapid technical advancement of modern -omics techniques has increased not only the speed of venom research but also the depth and quality of generated data and enabled a deeper understanding of various aspects relating to venom evolution and biochemistry. Furthermore, improvements in the sensitivity of modern research equipment have enabled access to venoms from much smaller specimens, such as tiny pseudoscorpions of only a few millimetres in length [53,54]. With the vast majority of venomous animals being less than 1 cm in size, a continuous improvement in the sensitivity of equipment and assays will further increase the quantity and diversity of venomous animals that are accessible to future research. The diversity of venom components is further increased by some animals producing specific venoms for different purposes [55–57] and the potential of microorganisms living inside the venom glands, which also contribute to the chemical complexity of animal venoms [58].

5. Contributions to This Special Issue

This Special Issue of *Biomedicines* comprises 12 research and four review articles about a wide range of venomous or poisonous invertebrates and vertebrates, including sea anemone, cone snails, leeches, spiders, scorpions, ants, caterpillars, frogs, and snakes. The breadth of these contributions covers not only their taxonomic diversity but also both the detrimental and beneficial aspects of animal toxins from a human perspective, which is reflected in the title of this Special Issue: "Animal Venoms—Curse or Cure?". The "curse" aspect of venoms is covered in a number of contributions. For example, the review articles by Ahmadi et al. [59] and Seldeslachts et al. [60] discuss the dangers that venomous scorpions and caterpillars pose to humans, but they also provide insights into current and future treatment options, such as the next-generation recombinant antivenoms [59]. Two contributions from Jeroen Kool's group examine the usefulness of the small-molecule PLA2 inhibitor Varespladib as a potential drug for the treatment of snake bites. In these studies, cutting-edge nanofractionation analytics are employed to determine the effects of Varespladib and other small molecules on the coagulopathic effects of various crotalid and viperid snake venoms [61,62]. The Hodgson lab examined the neutralising abilities of different antivenoms against the effects of venom from the Chinese cobra by using the chick biventer nerve muscle preparation [63]. Another study on Australian snake venoms by Isbister et al. found that phospholipase A2 levels in human snakebite victims could be used as an early indicator of envenomation by Australian elapids (with exception of brown snakes) [64]. The contribution by Nixon et al. reveals that the dimeric ant peptide Mp1a is responsible for a broad range of activities, including the extremely painful symptoms experienced by humans that are stung by jack jumper ants [65]. Potential biosecurity concerns of conotoxins are discussed and largely rejected by Bjorn-Yoshimoto et al. [66], with the benefits of peptides from cone snails by far outweighing their potential negative impacts. Nevertheless, this review article nicely exemplifies how scientifically unsubstantiated political red tape can negatively impact the progress of toxinological research.

Several other contributions to this Special Issue cover the "cure" aspect of animal venoms, which is their potential usage for the benefit of humans. The review by Lemke and Vilcinskas, for example, highlights the resurging interest in leeches, which have been used in traditional medicine for thousands of years [14]. Today's research focusses on a variety of bioactive leech peptides and proteins affecting blood coagulation and inflammation. Spider venom peptides, on the other hand, might be promising candidates for novel analgesics by targeting particular subtypes of voltage-gated sodium (Na_V) channels. Yin et al. [67] not only provide the first characterisation of a toxin from the theraphosid genus *Poecilotheria*. They also demonstrate that, by simply introducing one additional residue, the toxin is converted from a Na_V1.7 activator into an inhibitor, which can be crucial for designing effective analgesic leads. Novel toxins with potential anti-inflammatory activity are further reported from the venom of a sea anemone [68]. In addition to their proposed medical applications, venom components are also useful tools for research. The structural diversity of peptide toxins from venoms, for example, provides an excellent source of novel modulators for studying the pharmacological properties of ion channels and receptors. The article from Wilson et al. [69] describes the new α-conotoxin Pl168 from *Conus planorbis*, belonging to the well-known A superfamily of conus toxins. However, unlike other members of the A superfamily, Pl168 shows no activity on a range of nAChRs or Ca^{2+} and Na^+ channels. Pl168 also comprises a new structural type within the A superfamily, with a presumed novel pharmacological target. Even more potential pharmacological probes could be hidden among the peptides [70] and small molecules [71] found in scorpion venoms. Another study adds to the list of venom compounds with interesting pharmacology by employing a combined transcriptomic and proteomic approach to uncover not only some new bradykinin potentiating peptides but also the first evidence of three-finger toxins from a viperid snake venom [72]. On the other hand, a bradykinin-antagonising peptide was identified from a Chinese frog species and characterised by Zhou et al. [73].

6. Conclusions

I trust that the audience of this Special Issue of *Biomedicines* will enjoy reading the excellent contributions from many of the leading researchers in the field. I further hope that they will inspire the next generation of scientists to turn their attention towards studying the fascinating world of animal venoms and toxins. Despite the horrible and yet too often fatal consequences that venomous animals (in particular, snakes) can have on humans, I believe that their potential benefits for basic research and towards health and food production for billions of people by far outweigh their negative effects. Continuous progress in antivenom development will help in making antivenoms more efficient, cheaper to produce, and more tolerable by reducing unwanted side effects. Thus, continued toxinological research will help in further reducing the negative effects of animal venoms, thereby tipping the scales even more in favour of their beneficial effects for humanity.

Funding: V.H. is funded by a Future Fellowship from the Australian Research Council (FT190100482).

Institutional Review Board Statement: Not applicable.

Informed Consent Statement: Not applicable.

Data Availability Statement: Not applicable.

Acknowledgments: I would like to thank Mande Holford for providing the original version of the figure that I have modified to construct Figure 1.

Conflicts of Interest: The authors declare no conflict of interest.

References

1. Holford, M.; Daly, M.; King, G.F.; Norton, R.S. Venoms to the rescue. *Science* **2018**, *361*, 842–844. [CrossRef]
2. Herzig, V. Arthropod assassins: Crawling biochemists with diverse toxin pharmacopeias. *Toxicon* **2019**, *158*, 33–37. [CrossRef]
3. Senji Laxme, R.R.; Suranse, V.; Sunagar, K. Arthropod venoms: Biochemistry, ecology and evolution. *Toxicon* **2019**, *158*, 84–103. [CrossRef]
4. Walker, A.A.; Robinson, S.D.; Yeates, D.K.; Jin, J.; Baumann, K.; Dobson, J.; Fry, B.G.; King, G.F. Entomo-venomics: The evolution, biology and biochemistry of insect venoms. *Toxicon* **2018**, *154*, 15–27. [CrossRef]
5. Hunter, P. The nature of flight. The molecules and mechanics of flight in animals. *EMBO Rep.* **2007**, *8*, 811–813. [CrossRef] [PubMed]
6. Chu, E.R.; Weinstein, S.A.; White, J.; Warrell, D.A. Venom ophthalmia caused by venoms of spitting elapid and other snakes: Report of ten cases with review of epidemiology, clinical features, pathophysiology and management. *Toxicon* **2010**, *56*, 259–272. [CrossRef]
7. Nisani, Z.; Hayes, W.K. Venom-spraying behavior of the scorpion *Parabuthus transvaalicus* (Arachnida: Buthidae). *Behav. Process.* **2015**, *115*, 46–52. [CrossRef]
8. Szczuka, A.; Godzinska, E.J. The effect of past and present group size on responses to prey in the ant *Formica polyctena* Forst. *Acta Neurobiol. Exp.* **1997**, *57*, 135–150.
9. Safavi-Hemami, H.; Gajewiak, J.; Karanth, S.; Robinson, S.D.; Ueberheide, B.; Douglass, A.D.; Schlegel, A.; Imperial, J.S.; Watkins, M.; Bandyopadhyay, P.K.; et al. Specialized insulin is used for chemical warfare by fish-hunting cone snails. *Proc. Natl. Acad. Sci. USA* **2015**, *112*, 1743–1748. [CrossRef] [PubMed]
10. Xu, X.; Lai, R. The chemistry and biological activities of peptides from amphibian skin secretions. *Chem. Rev.* **2015**, *115*, 1760–1846. [CrossRef] [PubMed]
11. Bogdanov, S. Biological and Therapeutic Properties of Bee Venom. In *The Bee Venom Book;* Bee Product Science: Bern, Switzerland, 2016; pp. 1–23. Available online: https://www.researchgate.net/publication/304011827_Biological_and_therapeutic_properties_of_bee_venom (accessed on 1 April 2021).
12. Lee, J.D.; Park, H.J.; Chae, Y.; Lim, S. An overview of bee venom acupuncture in the treatment of arthritis. *Evid. Based Complement. Alternat. Med.* **2005**, *2*, 79–84. [CrossRef]
13. Yin, C.S.; Koh, H.G. The first documental record on bee venom therapy in Oriental medicine: 2 prescriptions of bee venom in the ancient Mawangdui books of Oriental medicine. *J. Kor. Acup. Mox. Soc.* **1998**, *15*, 143–147.
14. Lemke, S.; Vilcinskas, A. European medicinal leeches-New roles in modern medicine. *Biomedicines* **2020**, *8*, 99. [CrossRef]
15. Balée, W. Part II Indigenous savoir faire: Retention of traditional knowledge. In *Cultural Forests of the Amazon: A Historical Ecology of People and Their Landscapes;* The University of Alabama Press: Tuscaloosa, AL, USA, 2013; pp. 140–148.
16. Albuquerque, U.P.; Melo, J.G.; Medeiros, M.F.; Menezes, I.R.; Moura, G.J.; Asfora El-Deir, A.C.; Alves, R.R.; de Medeiros, P.M.; de Sousa Araujo, T.A.; Alves Ramos, M.; et al. Natural products from ethnodirected studies: Revisiting the ethnobiology of the zombie poison. *Evid. Based Complement. Alternat. Med.* **2012**, *2012*, 202508. [CrossRef]
17. Clark, V.C.; Raxworthy, C.J.; Rakotomalala, V.; Sierwald, P.; Fisher, B.L. Convergent evolution of chemical defense in poison frogs and arthropod prey between Madagascar and the Neotropics. *Proc. Natl. Acad. Sci. USA* **2005**, *102*, 11617–11622. [CrossRef]
18. Kritsky, G. Ancient beekeeping in Egypt: The honey-collection scene from the causeway of Unas of ancient Egypt's fifth dynasty. *Am. Bee J.* **2013**, *153*, 1185–1187.
19. Bloch, G.; Francoy, T.M.; Wachtel, I.; Panitz-Cohen, N.; Fuchs, S.; Mazar, A. Industrial apiculture in the Jordan valley during Biblical times with Anatolian honeybees. *Proc. Natl. Acad. Sci. USA* **2010**, *107*, 11240–11244. [CrossRef] [PubMed]
20. Hauke, T.J.; Herzig, V. Love bites—Do venomous arachnids make safe pets? *Toxicon* **2021**, *190*, 65–72. [CrossRef]
21. Isbister, G.K.; Gray, M.R.; Balit, C.R.; Raven, R.J.; Stokes, B.J.; Porges, K.; Tankel, A.S.; Turner, E.; White, J.; Fisher, M.M. Funnel-web spider bite: A systematic review of recorded clinical cases. *Med. J. Aust.* **2005**, *182*, 407–411. [CrossRef]
22. Hawgood, B.J. Doctor Albert Calmette 1863-1933: Founder of antivenomous serotherapy and of antituberculous BCG vaccination. *Toxicon* **1999**, *37*, 1241–1258. [CrossRef]
23. Laustsen, A.H.; Karatt-Vellatt, A.; Masters, E.W.; Arias, A.S.; Pus, U.; Knudsen, C.; Oscoz, S.; Slavny, P.; Griffiths, D.T.; Luther, A.M.; et al. In vivo neutralization of dendrotoxin-mediated neurotoxicity of black mamba venom by oligoclonal human IgG antibodies. *Nat. Commun.* **2018**, *9*, 3928. [CrossRef] [PubMed]
24. Fry, B.G. Snakebite: When the human touch becomes a bad touch. *Toxins* **2018**, *10*, 170. [CrossRef]

25. Gutierrez, J.M.; Calvete, J.J.; Habib, A.G.; Harrison, R.A.; Williams, D.J.; Warrell, D.A. Snakebite envenoming. *Nat. Rev. Dis. Primers* **2017**, *3*, 17063. [CrossRef]
26. Arnold, C. The snakebite fight. *Nature* **2016**, *537*, 26–28. [CrossRef] [PubMed]
27. Hauke, T.J.; Herzig, V. Dangerous arachnids-Fake news or reality? *Toxicon* **2017**, *138*, 173–183. [CrossRef]
28. Kohn, A.J. Human injuries and fatalities due to venomous marine snails of the family Conidae. *Int. J. Clin. Pharmacol. Ther.* **2016**, *54*, 524–538. [CrossRef] [PubMed]
29. Mariottini, G.L. Hemolytic venoms from marine cnidarian jellyfish—An overview. *J. Venom. Res.* **2014**, *5*, 22–32.
30. Schmidt, J.O. Clinical consequences of toxic envenomations by Hymenoptera. *Toxicon* **2018**, *150*, 96–104. [CrossRef] [PubMed]
31. Chippaux, J.P.; Goyffon, M. Epidemiology of scorpionism: A global appraisal. *Acta Tropica* **2008**, *107*, 71–79. [CrossRef] [PubMed]
32. Dehesa-Davila, M.; Possani, L.D. Scorpionism and serotherapy in Mexico. *Toxicon* **1994**, *32*, 1015–1018. [CrossRef]
33. Furtado, A.A.; Daniele-Silva, A.; Silva-Junior, A.A.D.; Fernandes-Pedrosa, M.F. Biology, venom composition, and scorpionism induced by brazilian scorpion *Tityus stigmurus* (Thorell, 1876) (Scorpiones: Buthidae): A mini-review. *Toxicon* **2020**, *185*, 36–45. [CrossRef]
34. Marsh, N.A. Diagnostic uses of snake venom. *Haemostasis* **2001**, *31*, 211–217. [CrossRef]
35. de Souza, J.M.; Goncalves, B.D.C.; Gomez, M.V.; Vieira, L.B.; Ribeiro, F.M. Animal toxins as therapeutic tools to treat neurodegenerative diseases. *Front. Pharmacol.* **2018**, *9*, 145. [CrossRef]
36. King, G.F. Venoms as a platform for human drugs: Translating toxins into therapeutics. *Expert Opin. Biol. Ther.* **2011**, *11*, 1469–1484. [CrossRef]
37. Norton, R.S. Enhancing the therapeutic potential of peptide toxins. *Expert Opin. Drug Discov.* **2017**, *12*, 611–623. [CrossRef]
38. Ortiz, E.; Gurrola, G.B.; Schwartz, E.F.; Possani, L.D. Scorpion venom components as potential candidates for drug development. *Toxicon* **2015**, *93*, 125–135. [CrossRef] [PubMed]
39. Robinson, S.D.; Undheim, E.A.B.; Ueberheide, B.; King, G.F. Venom peptides as therapeutics: Advances, challenges and the future of venom-peptide discovery. *Expert Rev. Proteom.* **2017**, *14*, 931–939. [CrossRef] [PubMed]
40. Saez, N.J.; Herzig, V. Versatile spider venom peptides and their medical and agricultural applications. *Toxicon* **2019**, *158*, 109–126. [CrossRef] [PubMed]
41. Vetter, I.; Lewis, R.J. Therapeutic potential of cone snail venom peptides (conopeptides). *Curr. Top. Med. Chem.* **2012**, *12*, 1546–1552. [CrossRef] [PubMed]
42. Waheed, H.; Moin, S.F.; Choudhary, M.I. Snake venom: From deadly toxins to life-saving therapeutics. *Curr. Med. Chem.* **2017**, *24*, 1874–1891. [CrossRef]
43. Bohlen, C.J.; Julius, D. Receptor-targeting mechanisms of pain-causing toxins: How ow? *Toxicon* **2012**, *60*, 254–264. [CrossRef]
44. Herzig, V.; Cristofori-Armstrong, B.; Israel, M.R.; Nixon, S.A.; Vetter, I.; King, G.F. Animal toxins—Nature's evolutionary-refined toolkit for basic research and drug discovery. *Biochem. Pharmacol.* **2020**, *181*, 114096. [CrossRef]
45. Kachel, H.S.; Buckingham, S.D.; Sattelle, D.B. Insect toxins—Selective pharmacological tools and drug/chemical leads. *Curr. Opin. Insect Sci.* **2018**, *30*, 93–98. [CrossRef]
46. Osteen, J.D.; Herzig, V.; Gilchrist, J.; Emrick, J.J.; Zhang, C.; Wang, X.; Castro, J.; Garcia-Caraballo, S.; Grundy, L.; Rychkov, G.Y.; et al. Selective spider toxins reveal a role for the Nav1.1 channel in mechanical pain. *Nature* **2016**, *534*, 494–499. [CrossRef]
47. Tsetlin, V.I. Three-finger snake neurotoxins and Ly6 proteins targeting nicotinic acetylcholine receptors: Pharmacological tools and endogenous modulators. *Trends Pharmacol. Sci.* **2015**, *36*, 109–123. [CrossRef] [PubMed]
48. Lovett, B.; Bilgo, E.; Millogo, S.A.; Ouattarra, A.K.; Sare, I.; Gnambani, E.J.; Dabire, R.K.; Diabate, A.; St Leger, R.J. Transgenic *Metarhizium* rapidly kills mosquitoes in a malaria-endemic region of Burkina Faso. *Science* **2019**, *364*, 894–897. [CrossRef] [PubMed]
49. Primon-Barros, M.; Jose Macedo, A. Animal venom peptides: Potential for new antimicrobial agents. *Curr. Top. Med. Chem.* **2017**, *17*, 1119–1156. [CrossRef] [PubMed]
50. Bende, N.S.; Dziemborowicz, S.; Mobli, M.; Herzig, V.; Gilchrist, J.; Wagner, J.; Nicholson, G.M.; King, G.F.; Bosmans, F. A distinct sodium channel voltage-sensor locus determines insect selectivity of the spider toxin Dc1a. *Nat. Commun.* **2014**, *5*, 4350. [CrossRef] [PubMed]
51. Herzig, V.; King, G.F. The cystine knot is responsible for the exceptional stability of the insecticidal spider toxin ω-Hexatoxin-Hv1a. *Toxins* **2015**, *7*, 4366–4380. [CrossRef] [PubMed]
52. Klint, J.K.; Senff, S.; Saez, N.J.; Seshadri, R. Production of recombinant disulfide-rich venom peptides for structural and functional analysis via expression in the periplasm of *E. coli*. *PLoS ONE* **2013**, *8*, e63865. [CrossRef]
53. Kramer, J.; Pohl, H.; Predel, R. Venom collection and analysis in the pseudoscorpion *Chelifer cancroides* (Pseudoscorpiones: Cheliferidae). *Toxicon* **2019**, *162*, 15–23. [CrossRef]
54. Santibanez-Lopez, C.E.; Ontano, A.Z.; Harvey, M.S.; Sharma, P.P. Transcriptomic analysis of pseudoscorpion venom reveals a unique cocktail dominated by enzymes and protease inhibitors. *Toxins* **2018**, *10*, 207. [CrossRef] [PubMed]
55. Dutertre, S.; Jin, A.H.; Vetter, I.; Hamilton, B.; Sunagar, K.; Lavergne, V.; Dutertre, V.; Fry, B.G.; Antunes, A.; Venter, D.J.; et al. Evolution of separate predation- and defence-evoked venoms in carnivorous cone snails. *Nat. Commun.* **2014**, *5*, 3521. [CrossRef]
56. Inceoglu, B.; Lango, J.; Jing, J.; Chen, L.; Doymaz, F.; Pessah, I.N.; Hammock, B.D. One scorpion, two venoms: Prevenom of *Parabuthus transvaalicus* acts as an alternative type of venom with distinct mechanism of action. *Proc. Natl. Acad. Sci. USA* **2003**, *100*, 922–927. [CrossRef] [PubMed]

57. Walker, A.A.; Mayhew, M.L.; Jin, J.; Herzig, V.; Undheim, E.A.B.; Sombke, A.; Fry, B.G.; Meritt, D.J.; King, G.F. The assassin bug *Pristhesancus plagipennis* produces two distinct venoms in separate gland lumens. *Nat. Commun.* **2018**, *9*, 755. [CrossRef] [PubMed]
58. Ul-Hasan, S.; Rodríguez-Román, E.; Reitzel, A.M.; Adams, R.M.M.; Herzig, V.; Nobile, C.J.; Saviola, A.J.; Trim, S.A.; Stiers, E.E.; Moschos, S.A.; et al. The emerging field of venom-microbiomics for exploring venom as a microenvironment, and the corresponding Initiative for Venom Associated Microbes and Parasites (iVAMP). *Toxicon X* **2019**, *4*, 100016. [CrossRef]
59. Ahmadi, S.; Knerr, J.M.; Argemi, L.; Bordon, K.C.F.; Pucca, M.B.; Cerni, F.A.; Arantes, E.C.; Caliskan, F.; Laustsen, A.H. Scorpion venom: Detriments and benefits. *Biomedicines* **2020**, *8*, 118. [CrossRef]
60. Seldeslachts, A.; Peigneur, S.; Tytgat, J. Caterpillar venom: A health hazard of the 21st century. *Biomedicines* **2020**, *8*, 143. [CrossRef] [PubMed]
61. Xie, C.; Albulescu, L.O.; Bittenbinder, M.A.; Somsen, G.W.; Vonk, F.J.; Casewell, N.R.; Kool, J. Neutralizing effects of small molecule inhibitors and metal chelators on coagulopathic Viperinae snake venom toxins. *Biomedicines* **2020**, *8*, 297. [CrossRef]
62. Xie, C.; Albulescu, L.O.; Still, K.B.M.; Slagboom, J.; Zhao, Y.; Jiang, Z.; Somsen, G.W.; Vonk, F.J.; Casewell, N.R.; Kool, J. Varespladib Inhibits the phospholipase A2 and coagulopathic activities of venom components from hemotoxic snakes. *Biomedicines* **2020**, *8*, 165. [CrossRef]
63. Liang, Q.; Huynh, T.M.; Konstantakopoulos, N.; Isbister, G.K.; Hodgson, W.C. An examination of the neutralization of in vitro toxicity of Chinese cobra (*Naja atra*) venom by different antivenoms. *Biomedicines* **2020**, *8*, 377. [CrossRef] [PubMed]
64. Isbister, G.K.; Mirajkar, N.; Fakes, K.; Brown, S.G.A.; Veerati, P.C. Phospholipase A2 (PLA2) as an early indicator of envenomation in Australian elapid snakebites (ASP-27). *Biomedicines* **2020**, *8*, 459. [CrossRef]
65. Nixon, S.A.; Dekan, Z.; Robinson, S.D.; Guo, S.; Vetter, I.; Kotze, A.C.; Alewood, P.F.; King, G.F.; Herzig, V. It takes two: Dimerization is essential for the broad-spectrum predatory and defensive activities of the venom peptide Mp1a from the Jack Jumper Ant *Myrmecia pilosula*. *Biomedicines* **2020**, *8*, 185. [CrossRef]
66. Bjorn-Yoshimoto, W.E.; Ramiro, I.B.L.; Yandell, M.; McIntosh, J.M.; Olivera, B.M.; Ellgaard, L.; Safavi-Hemami, H. Curses or cures: A review of the numerous benefits versus the biosecurity concerns of conotoxin research. *Biomedicines* **2020**, *8*, 235. [CrossRef]
67. Yin, K.; Deuis, J.R.; Dekan, Z.; Jin, A.H.; Alewood, P.F.; King, G.F.; Herzig, V.; Vetter, I. Addition of K22 converts spider venom peptide Pme2a from an activator to an inhibitor of Nav1.7. *Biomedicines* **2020**, *8*, 37. [CrossRef] [PubMed]
68. Gladkikh, I.; Peigneur, S.; Sintsova, O.; Lopes Pinheiro-Junior, E.; Klimovich, A.; Menshov, A.; Kalinovsky, A.; Isaeva, M.; Monastyrnaya, M.; Kozlovskaya, E.; et al. Kunitz-type peptides from the sea anemone *Heteractis crispa* demonstrate potassium channel blocking and anti-inflammatory activities. *Biomedicines* **2020**, *8*, 473. [CrossRef]
69. Wilson, D.T.; Bansal, P.S.; Carter, D.A.; Vetter, I.; Nicke, A.; Dutertre, S.; Daly, N.L. Characterisation of a novel A-superfamily conotoxin. *Biomedicines* **2020**, *8*, 128. [CrossRef] [PubMed]
70. Israel, M.R.; Dash, T.S.; Bothe, S.N.; Robinson, S.D.; Deuis, J.R.; Craik, D.J.; Lampert, A.; Vetter, I.; Durek, T. Characterization of synthetic Tf2 as a Nav1.3 selective pharmacological probe. *Biomedicines* **2020**, *8*, 155. [CrossRef] [PubMed]
71. Evans, E.R.J.; McIntyre, L.; Northfield, T.D.; Daly, N.L.; Wilson, D.T. Small molecules in the venom of the scorpion *Hormurus waigiensis*. *Biomedicines* **2020**, *8*, 259. [CrossRef]
72. Babenko, V.V.; Ziganshin, R.H.; Weise, C.; Dyachenko, I.; Shaykhutdinova, E.; Murashev, A.N.; Zhmak, M.; Starkov, V.; Hoang, A.N.; Tsetlin, V.; et al. Novel bradykinin-potentiating peptides and three-finger toxins from viper venom: Combined NGS venom gland transcriptomics and quantitative venom proteomics of the *Azemiops feae* viper. *Biomedicines* **2020**, *8*, 249. [CrossRef]
73. Zhou, X.; Xu, J.; Zhong, R.; Ma, C.; Zhou, M.; Cao, Z.; Xi, X.; Shaw, C.; Chen, T.; Wang, L.; et al. Pharmacological effects of a novel bradykinin-related peptide (RR-18) from the skin secretion of the Hejiang frog (*Ordorrana hejiangensis*) on smooth muscle. *Biomedicines* **2020**, *8*, 225. [CrossRef] [PubMed]

biomedicines

MDPI

Article

Kunitz-Type Peptides from the Sea Anemone *Heteractis crispa* Demonstrate Potassium Channel Blocking and Anti-Inflammatory Activities

Irina Gladkikh [1,*], Steve Peigneur [2], Oksana Sintsova [1], Ernesto Lopes Pinheiro-Junior [2], Anna Klimovich [1], Alexander Menshov [1], Anatoly Kalinovsky [1], Marina Isaeva [1], Margarita Monastyrnaya [1], Emma Kozlovskaya [1], Jan Tytgat [2] and Elena Leychenko [1,*]

1. G.B. Elyakov Pacific Institute of Bioorganic Chemistry, Far Eastern Branch, Russian Academy of Sciences, 159, Pr. 100 let Vladivostoku, 690022 Vladivostok, Russian; sintsova0@gmail.com (O.S.); annaklim_1991@mail.ru (A.K.); almenshov1990@gmail.com (A.M.); kaaniw@piboc.dvo.ru (A.K.); issaeva@gmail.com (M.I.); rita1950@mail.ru (M.M.); kozempa@mail.ru (E.K.)
2. Toxicology and Pharmacology, University of Leuven (KU Leuven), Campus Gasthuisberg O&N2, Herestraat 49, P.O. Box 922, B-3000 Leuven, Belgium; steve.peigneur@kuleuven.be (S.P.); ernestolopesjr@gmail.com (E.L.P.-J.); jan.tytgat@kuleuven.be (J.T.)

* Correspondence: irinagladkikh@gmail.com (I.G.); leychenko@gmail.com (E.L.)

Received: 17 September 2020; Accepted: 2 November 2020; Published: 4 November 2020

Abstract: The Kunitz/BPTI peptide family includes unique representatives demonstrating various biological activities. Electrophysiological screening of peptides HCRG1 and HCRG2 from the sea anemone *Heteractis crispa* on six Kv1.x channel isoforms and insect *Shaker* IR channel expressed in *Xenopus laevis* oocytes revealed their potassium channels blocking activity. HCRG1 and HCRG2 appear to be the first Kunitz-type peptides from sea anemones blocking Kv1.3 with IC_{50} of 40.7 and 29.7 nM, respectively. In addition, peptides mainly vary in binding affinity to the Kv1.2 channels. It was established that the single substitution, Ser5Leu, in the TRPV1 channel antagonist, HCRG21, induces weak blocking activity of Kv1.1, Kv1.2, and Kv1.3. Apparently, for the affinity and selectivity of Kunitz-fold toxins to Kv1.x isoforms, the number and distribution along their molecules of charged, hydrophobic, and polar uncharged residues, as well as the nature of the channel residue at position 379 (Tyr, Val or His) are important. Testing the compounds in a model of acute local inflammation induced by the introduction of carrageenan administration into mice paws revealed that HCRG1 at doses of 0.1–1 mg/kg reduced the volume of developing edema during 24 h, similar to the effect of the nonsteroidal anti-inflammatory drug, indomethacin, at a dose of 5 mg/kg. ELISA analysis of the animals blood showed that the peptide reduced the synthesis of TNF-α, a pro-inflammatory mediator playing a leading role in the development of edema in this model.

Keywords: sea anemone; Kunitz fold; type 2 potassium channel toxins; electrophysiology; anti-inflammatory activity

1. Introduction

Peptides of the Kunitz/BPTI family contain one of the most evolutionarily ancient and conserved structural motifs, i.e., the Kunitz fold, which is widely distributed among both venomous terrestrial and marine organisms [1]. Historically, the firstly discovered representative of this family, the bovine pancreatic trypsin inhibitor (BPTI) [2], is known as an inhibitor of different serine proteases and capable of carrying out an anti-inflammatory function participating in proliferation and angiogenesis [3–5]. Kunitz-type peptides from snake, spider, scorpion, and sea anemone venoms are encoded by multigene families and form combinatorial libraries of homologous peptides [6–10]. Differing by single amino acid substitutions, some of these peptides not only exhibit protease inhibitory activity, but also can block voltage-gated potassium (Kv) [10–19], calcium (Cav) [20], acid-sensing ion (ASIC) channels [21], and transient receptor potential vanilloid 1 (TRPV1) [22–24]. Furthermore, some of them can interact with integrins [25] and vasopressin receptor 2 [26] as well.

Sea anemone Kv toxins are represented by six unique peptide folds: ShK (type 1), Kunitz-domain (type 2), β-defensin-like (type 3), boundless β-hairpin (type 4), an unknown fold predicted to form an inhibitor cystine knot (type 5), and the PHAB fold (type 6) [27,28]. Type 2 toxins, having the Kunitz fold, include κ1.3-ATTX-As2a-c (AsKC1–AsKC3 or kalicludines 1–3) from *Anemonia sulcata* [16], APEKTx1 from *Anthopleura elegantissima* [17], κ1.3-SHTX-Sha2a (SHTX III) from *Stichodactyla haddoni* [18], and ShPI-1 from *Stichodactyla helianthus* [19]. Kalicludines block Kv1.2 in μM concentrations and strongly inhibit trypsin [16]. APEKTx1, similarly to dendrotoxins (DTX), selectively blocks Kv1.1 channels along with effectively inhibiting trypsin [17]. It was determined that SHTXIII also inhibited trypsin and competed with the binding of α-DTX (alpha-dendrotoxin from mamba snake) in rat synaptosomal membranes at the level of Kv1.1, Kv1.2, and Kv1.6 channels [18]. Since SHTXIII paralyzes crabs, it can block not only mammalian but also crustacean Kv channels [18]. A pseudo wild-type variant of the natural peptide ShPI-1, rShPI-1A, known as an inhibitor of serine, aspartate, and cysteine proteases, was shown to bind to Kv1.1, Kv1.2, and Kv1.6 channels with IC_{50} values in the nM range [19]. Therefore, all known type 2 toxins block Kv channel subtypes widely expressed in neurons of the central nervous system (CNS), in particular Kv1.1, Kv1.2, and Kv1.6 [29].

In contrast to type 2, toxins of types 1, 3, and 5 [30,31] block also the Kv1.3 channelsubtype. Since Kv1.3 channels are expressed in the CNS and immune cells, including microglia, dendritic cells, T (TEM cells), B lymphocytes, and macrophages [32], they mediate autoimmune diseases [33], participate in chronic inflammatory diseases and cancer progression (due to its double role in proliferation and apoptosis regulation) [34]. The most selective toxin ShK from *S. helianthus* with high affinity to Kv1.3 channel (11 pM) [35] has been the subject of intense research, both fundamental and clinical [30,31]. Its designed analog, ShK-186 (Dalazatide), is now undergoing clinical trials on psoriasis [36]. Blocking of Kv1.3 channels decreases the expression levels of pro-inflammatory mediators and may be used in many conditions like neurodegenerative, autoimmune, and chronic diseases accompanied by inflammation. It has been established that the treatment of autoreactive T-lymphocytes by ShK-186 decreases the levels of IL-2, interferon-γ, TNF-α, and IL-4 [37]. Therefore, peptide inhibitors of Kv1.x channels can be assumed as promising compounds for drug design, as well as valuable tools for the investigation of these channels.

Here we report an in vivo anti-inflammatory activity and potassium channel blocking the activity of Kunitz peptides of the sea anemone *Heteractis crispa* by the electrophysiological screening on six isoforms of Kv1.x channels and insect *Shaker* IR channel expressed in *Xenopus laevis* oocytes.

2. Experimental Section

2.1. Purification and Characterization

The native peptides HCRG1 and HCRG2 were isolated as described in [38]. In brief, the peptides were precipitated from a water extract of the sea anemone *Heteractis crispa* (collected by dredging) with 80% acetone; next gel filtration chromatography on an Akrilex P-4 column was carried out, followed by cation-exchange chromatography on a CM-32 cellulose column, with a final purification step using an RP-HPLC Nucleosil C18 column.

The mutant peptide HCRG21 S5L was made using the QuikChange® Site-Directed Mutagenesis Kit (Stratagene, La Jolla, CA, USA), based on the wild type plasmid pET32b-HCRG21 using gene-specific primers (dir 5′-CGTGGTATCTGCTTAGAACCGAAAGTTG-3′; rev 5′-CAACTTTCGGTTCT AAGCAGATACCACG-3′). The resulting mutant plasmid was verified by DNA sequencing, and the target peptide was expressed and purified using the same conditions as was reported for the recombinant peptide HCRG21 [23]. The target peptide was isolated by HPLC on a Jupiter C4 column (10 × 250 mm,

Phenomenex, Torrance, CA, USA), equilibrated by 0.1% TFA, pH 2.2, and eluted in gradient of acetonitrile concentration (Solution B) for 70 min at 3 mL/min.

2.2. MALDI-TOF/MS Analysis

MALDI-TOF/MS spectra of peptides were recorded using an Ultra Flex III MALDI-TOF/TOF mass spectrometer (Bruker, Bremen, Germany) with a nitrogen laser (SmartBeam, 355 nm), reflector and potential LIFT tandem modes of operation. Sinapinic acid was used as a matrix. External calibration was employed using a peptide InhVJ with m/z 6107 [39] and its doubly-charged variant at m/z 3053.

2.3. NMR Spectroscopy

The NMR spectrum was acquired at 30 °C on a Bruker Avance III 700 MHz spectrometer (Bruker Biospin, Billerica, MA, USA) equipped with a triple resonance z-gradient TXO probe. Peptide HCRG21 S5L was dissolved in 90% H_2O/10% D_2O (Deutero GmbH, Kastellaun, Germany) at a concentration of 2 mg/mL. Excitation sculpting with gradients [40] was applied to suppress strong solvent resonance, the chemical shift of their signal was arbitrary chosen as 4.7 ppm. TopSpin 3.6 (Bruker Biospin, Billerica, MA, USA) was used for spectrum acquisition and processing.

2.4. Inhibitory Activity

The trypsin inhibitory activity of HCRG21 S5L was tested through the standard procedure [41] using N-α-benzoyl-D,L-arginine p-nitroanilide hydrochloride (BAPNA). Determination of the peptide trypsin inhibition constant was performed according to the method of Dixon [42] using substrates concentrations of 0.1, 0.16, and 0.256 mM. The concentration of trypsin in the reaction mixture was 50 nM and the tested peptide ranged from 0 up to 512 nM. The inhibitory constants were calculated based on the results of three parallel experiments.

2.5. Expression of Voltage-Gated Ion Channels in Xenopus laevis Oocytes

For the expression of rKv1.1, hKv1.2, hKv1.3, rKv1.4, rKv1.5, rKv1.6, and *Shaker* IR in *Xenopus laevis* oocytes, the linearized plasmids were transcribed using the T7 or SP6 mMESSAGE-mMACHINE transcription kit (Ambion, Austin, TX, USA). The harvesting of stage V–VI oocytes from anaesthetized female *X. laevis* frog was as previously described [43]. Oocytes were injected with 50 nL of cRNA at a concentration of 1 ng/nL using a micro-injector (Drummond Scientific, Broomall, PA, USA). The oocytes were incubated in a solution containing (in mM): NaCl, 96; KCl, 2; $CaCl_2$, 1.8; $MgCl_2$, 2; and HEPES, 5 (pH 7.4), supplemented with 50 mg/L gentamicin sulfate.

2.6. Electrophysiological Studies

The physiological activity in oocytes expressing heterologously the voltage-gated ion channel proteins was determined by the two-electrode voltage-clamp technique, using a Geneclamp 500 amplifier (Molecular Devices, Austin, TX, USA) controlled by the pClamp database system (Axon Instruments, Union City, CA, USA). The measurements were performed at room temperature (18–22 °C). Whole-cell currents were recorded 1–4 days after the mRNA injection. The electrode resistance was 0.7–1.5 MΩ. The signal was amplified, preliminarily filtered by the amplifier embedded four-polar Besselian filter (cutoff frequency 500 Hz) after digitization of the signal at 2000 Hz. Recordings obtained before the activation of the examined currents were used for subtraction of the capacitive and leakage current. The cells were kept at a holding potential of −90 mV. The membrane potential was depolarized to 0 mV for 250 ms with a subsequent pulse to −50 mV for 250 ms in the case of the Kv1.1–Kv1.6 and *Shaker* channels. For statistical analysis, the Student's coefficient ($P < 0.05$) was used. All the results were obtained from at least three independent experiments ($n \geq 3$) and are expressed as mean value ± standard error. The use of the *X. laevis* animals was in accordance with the license number LA1210239 of the Laboratory of Toxicology and Pharmacology, University of Leuven

(Belgium). The use of *X. laevis* was approved by the Ethical Committee for animal experiments of the University of Leuven (P186/2019). All animal care and experimental procedures agreed with the guidelines of the European Convention for the protection of vertebrate animals used for experimental and other scientific purposes (Strasbourg, 18.III.1986).

2.7. Acute Toxicity of HCRG1

The animal studies were performed under the European Convention for the human methods for the animal welfare (Directive 2010/63/EU), the National Standard of the Russian Federation "Good Laboratory Practice" (GOST P 53434-2009, Russia), and was approved by G.B. Elyakov Pacific Institute of Bioorganic Chemistry (Far Eastern Branch, Russian Academy of Sciences) Committee on Ethics of laboratory animal handling 2017/78-A protocol. Adult male ICR line white mice weighing 20–22 g were kept at room temperature with a 12-h light/dark cycle and with ad libitum access to food and water.

HCRG1 was administered once intravenously at doses of 0.1 and 1 mg/kg, control group received saline (0.9% NaCl) (10 mL/kg or 0.250 mL/mouse). Six mice in each group were used. Then, changes in basic physiological parameters, such as motility, behavioral responses, and physical activity, were registered in each group of animals within 24 h.

2.8. Carrageenan-Induced Paw Edema

Tests were performed on male ICR mice, with six individuals in each group. A peptide sample was dissolved in sterile saline and administered intravenously at doses of 0.1 and 1.0 mg/kg. Control animals received an equivalent volume of sterile saline. Indomethacin at a dose of 5 mg/kg was used as a positive control and administered orally to animals. Each mouse received 20 μL of a 1% solution of carrageenan in the hind paw pad after 30 min in the case of saline and tested peptide and after 60 min in the case of indomethacin. Then, the resulting edema was measured at several time points (1, 3, 5, and 24 h) using a plethysmometer (Ugo Basile, Gemonio (VA), Italy).

2.9. Animals Euthanasia Procedure and Blood Sampling

Animals were terminally anaesthetized with sodium pentobarbital (40 mg per mouse *i.p.*, Euthatal, Merial Animal Health, Essex, UK) 24 h after carrageenan injection. Then the thoracic cavity was opened and blood was collected in tubes with the ethylenediaminetetraacetic acid (EDTA) directly from the right atrium of the heart. The whole blood was centrifuged at $2.5 \times 10^3 \times g$ for 10 min to remove cells; the blood serum was then aliquoted and stored at −20 °C. These samples were analyzed for TNF-α in the enzyme-linked immunosorbent assay (ELISA) using a diagnostic kit according to the manufacturer's protocol (CUSABIO BIOTECH Co., Ltd., Houston, TX, USA).

2.10. Molecular Modeling of Kunitz Peptides

The spatial structure models of HCRG1, HCRG2, HCRG21, and HCRG21 S5L were predicted with I-TASSER server [44] and analyzed using UCSF Chimera program (http://www.cgl.ucsf.edu/chimera) [45]. The ShPI-1 (PDB ID 1SHP) from the sea anemone *S. helianthus* was used as a template.

3. Results

3.1. Peptide Purification and Characterization

The peptides HCRG1 and HCRG2 were obtained following the final RP-HPLC step. According to MALDI-TOF/MS data, their molecular weights were 6196 and 6148 Da, respectively, which is consistent with our previously published results [38].

To obtain the mutant peptide HCRG21 S5L, a plasmid-based on pET32b-*hcrg*21 was generated using the site-directed mutagenesis technique. The target peptide was expressed and purified following the same conditions as reported for the recombinant peptide HCRG21 [23]. The retention time of HCRG21 S5L differed from that of HCRG21 and was 36 min (Figure 1). According to the

MALDI-TOF/MS spectra, the molecular weight of the peptide was 6254 Da, which is consistent with the calculated value.

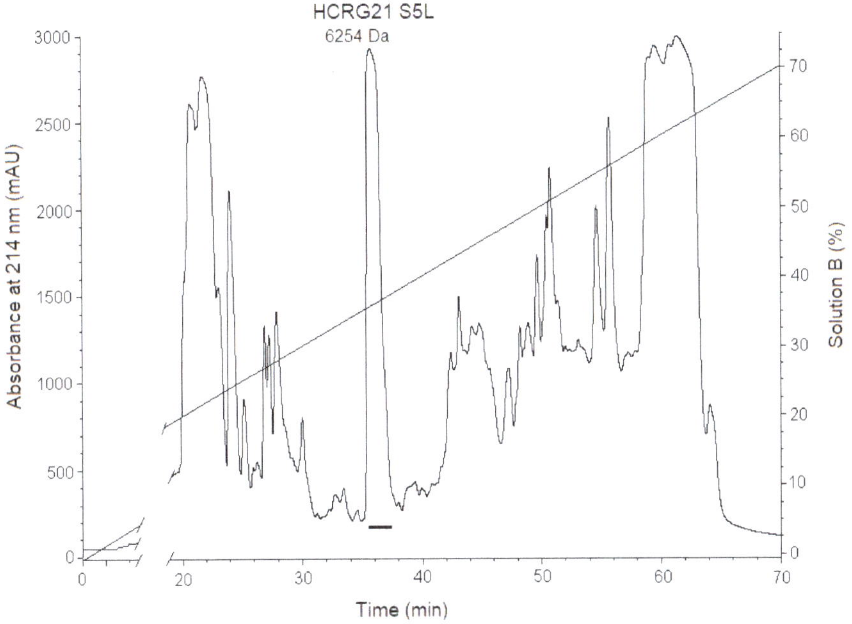

Figure 1. RP-HPLC elution profile of mutant peptide HCRG21 S5L, obtained as the result of hydrolysis of the fusion protein TRX-HCRG21 S5L by BrCN. The fraction containing the mature peptide is underlined. The measured molecular mass of HCRG21 S5L after RP-HPLC is indicated.

To confirm the correct folding of the mutant peptide, the NMR spectroscopy technique was applied. The ^{1}H NMR spectrum (Figure 2) indicates that peptide has a well-defined fold, as evidenced by the presence of resonance signals below 0 ppm and a wide chemical shift dispersion of amide hydrogens (9–6 ppm).

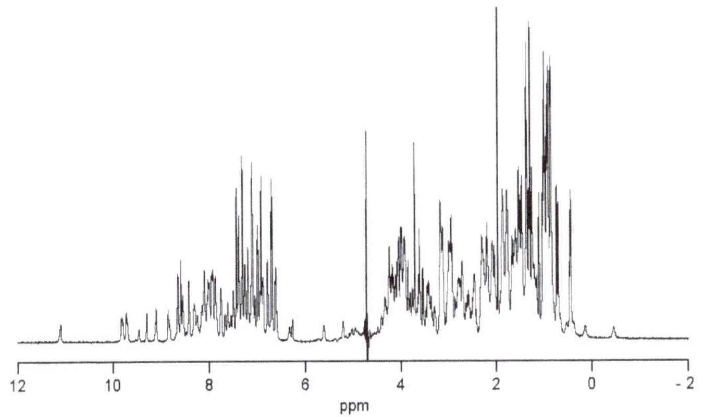

Figure 2. ^{1}H NMR spectrum of HCRG21 S5L.

Peptide HCRG21 S5L was assayed for inhibitory activity against trypsin. The mutant peptide inhibited the trypsin activity with a *Ki* value of 3.4×10^{-7} M (Figure 3) similar to HCRG21

(2×10^{-7} M [23]) and one order higher than for HCRG1 and HCRG2 (2.8×10^{-8} and 5×10^{-8} M, respectively [38]). This is due to the substitution of Thr to Lys in the P1 position which is functionally important for the serine protease inhibition [8,41,46].

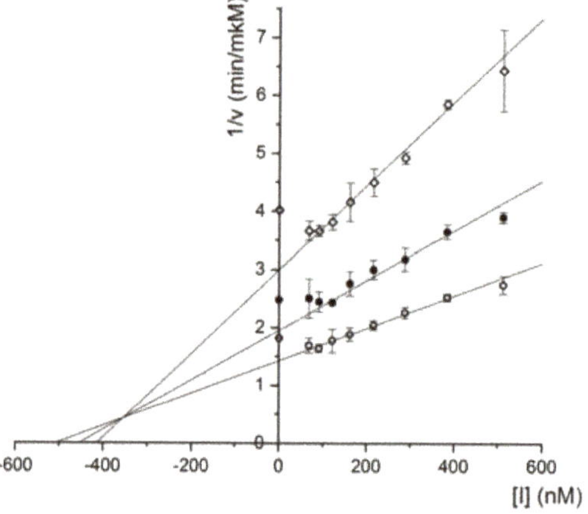

Figure 3. Determination of HCRG21 S5L Ki for trypsin by Dixon method. Substrate concentrations were 0.1 (◊), 0.16 (•), and 0.256 (○) mM. The constants were calculated based on the results of three independent experiments (n ≥ 3).

Comparison of the amino acid sequences of Kv toxins adopting the Kunitz-type fold showed that almost all these peptides contained six Cys residues in a typical pattern (I–VI, II–IV, III–V), except for the scorpion toxin LmKTT-1a and the cone snail toxin Conk-S1, which only had four residues (Figure 4). The sequence identities varied from 44% to 87% for sea anemone toxins and from 33% to 51% for snake, cone snail, spider, and scorpion toxins.

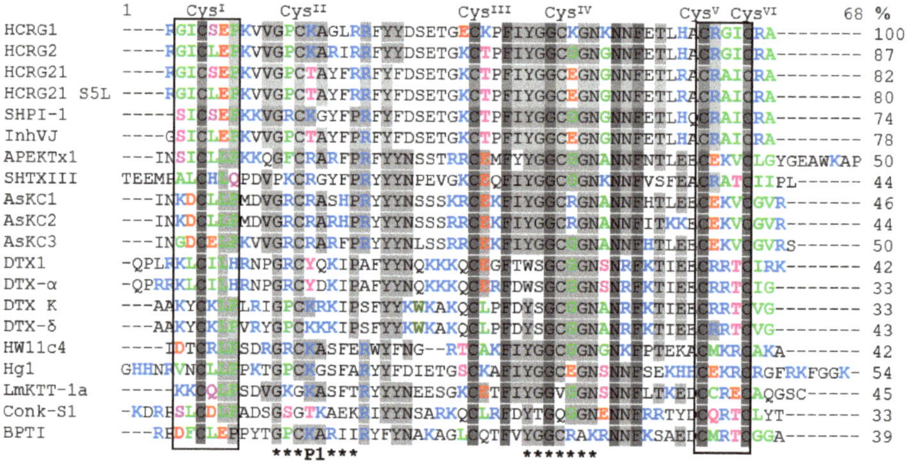

Figure 4. Multiple alignment of Kunitz peptides, blockers of Kv channels and BPTI. APEKTx1 (P61541) from the sea anemone *A. elegantissima*, AsKC1–AsKC3 (Q9TWG0, Q9TWF9, Q9TWF8) from *A. sulcata*, ShPI-1 (P31713) from *S. helianthus*, SHTXIII (B1B5I8) from *S. haddoni*, HCRG1, HCRG2, HCRG21, HCRG21 S5L, and InhVJ from *H. crispa*, HW11c4 (A0A023WBH6) from spider *Ornithoctonus huwena*; LmKTT-1a (P0DJ46) from scorpion *Lychas mucronatus*, Hg1 (P0C8W3) from *Hadrurus gertschi*; DTX1 (P00979), DTX-K (P00981) from snake *Dendroaspis polylepis*, DTX-α (P00980), DTX-δ (P00982) from

Dendroaspis angusticeps; Conk-S1 (P0C1X2) from cone snail *Conus striatus;* BPTI (P00974) from bovine *Bos taurus.* Identical amino acids are shownondark-grey and conservative on light-gray background. Hydrophobic amino acids are indicated by green, positively charged by blue, negatively charged by red, and polar non-charged by pink letters. Frames highlight regions responsible for interaction with Kv channels [19]. Asterisks indicate a reactive site with P1 residue and site of weak interaction with serine proteases.

Garcia-Fernandez R. et al. suggested that functionally important amino acid residues for Kv blocking activity in the Kunitz-type toxin sequences were located in the N- and C-terminal parts of the molecule, in particular around CysI and CysV–CysVI, respectively (Figure 4) [19]. The differences in HCRG1 and HCRG2 were limited only by point substitutions: Ser5Leu, Gly16Arg, Glu28Lys, Lys30Thr, Lys38Gly, and Lys41Gly. Noteworthy, amino acid substitutions of HCRG1 near CysIII and CysIV, Glu28Lys, Lys30Thr, Lys38Gly, and Lys41Gly, were non-conservative replacement in comparison with HCRG2, which might influence the functional activity of these peptides. The main differences between HCRG1, HCRG2, HCRG21, and its mutant were three substitutions: Ser5Leu, Lys14Thr, and Lys/Gly38Glu.

3.2. Electrophysiological Experiments

The native peptides HCRG1 and HCRG2 were screened on a panel of six mammalian voltage-gated potassium (Kv1.1–Kv1.6) and the insect *Shaker* IR channels expressed in *X. laevis* oocytes. Electrophysiological testing revealed that the peptides, at a concentration 1 μM, inhibited approximately 100% of the Kv1.1, Kv1.3, Kv1.6, and *Shaker* IR channel currents. Interestingly, the potassium current through Kv1.2 channels was inhibited by HCRG1 and HCRG2 with 10% and 80% respectively (Figure 5). Notably, HCRG1 and HCRG2 appeared to be the first Kunitz-type peptides from sea anemones blocking Kv1.3. According to the dose–response curves, peptides HCRG1 and HCRG2 mainly differed in binding affinity to the Kv1.2 (Figure 6, Table 1).

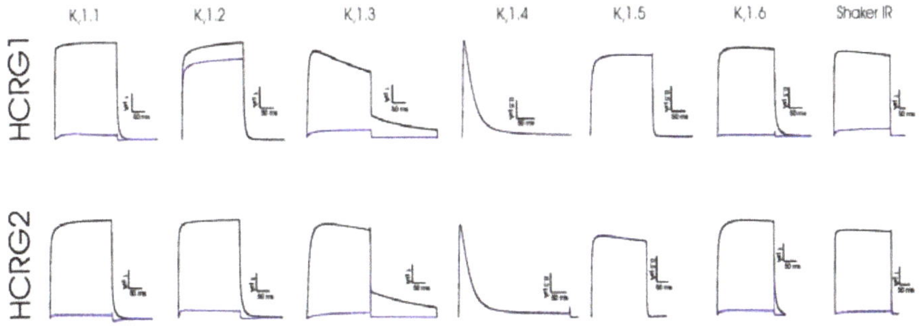

Figure 5. Electrophysiological analysis of HCRG1 and HCRG2 activities on several cloned voltage-gated potassium channel isoforms expressed in *X. laevis* oocytes. Representative whole-cell current traces in control and toxin conditions are shown. The blue line marks steady-state current traces after the application of 1 μM of peptides. Traces shown are representative traces of at least three independent experiments (n ≥ 3).

We tested the mutant peptide HCRG21 S5L on Kv1.1, Kv1.2, and Kv1.3 channels. It was found that, in comparison with HCRG21 which did not exert any activity on the Kv channels, the mutant peptide at a concentration of 10 μM blocked Kv1.1, Kv1.2, and Kv1.3 currents with approximately 33%, 11%, and 14%, respectively (Figure 7). The IC_{50} value on Kv1.1 was much higher than the value obtained for HCRG1 and HCRG2 (Table 1).

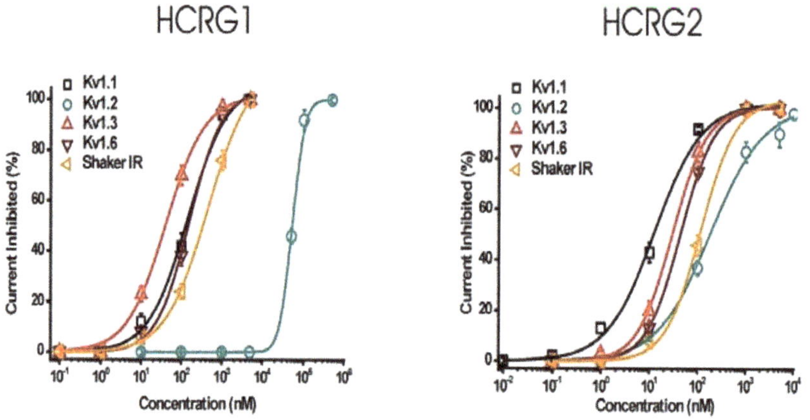

Figure 6. Dose–response curves of HCRG1 and HCRG2 on Kv1.1, Kv1.2, Kv1.3, Kv1.6, and *Shaker* IR channels obtained by plotting the percentage of blocked current as a function of increasing toxin concentrations. Traces shown are representative traces of at least three independent experiments (n ≥ 3).

Table 1. Kunitz-type voltage-gated potassium channel toxins from animal venoms.

Peptide	**IC$_{50}$ (nM)**					**Reference**
	Kv1.1	**Kv1.2**	**Kv1.3**	**Kv1.6**	***Shaker* IR**	
Sea anemones						
HCRG1	142.6 ± 28.1	52,199.0 ± 2751.7	40.7 ± 4.1	154.9 ± 20.4	433.1 ± 43.9	This work
HCRG2	12.6 ± 1.72	181.7 ± 38.5	29.7 ± 1.3	43.9 ± 1.3	114.9 ± 13.9	This work
HCRG21	-	-	-	-	-	[23]
HCRG21 S5L	15,600 ± 0.24	-	-	n.d.	n.d.	This work
ShPI-1	117 ± 15	9 ± 2	-	9 ± 2	-	[19]
APEKTx1	0.9	-	-	-	-	[17]
AsKC1	n.d.	2800	n.d.	n.d.	n.d.	[16]
AsKC2	n.d.	1100	n.d.	n.d.	n.d.	[16]
AsKC3	n.d.	1300	n.d.	n.d.	n.d.	[16]
SHTXIII	270 *	270 *	n.d.	270 *	n.d.	[18]
Snakes						
DTX-α	1.1	0.4	-	9	n.d.	[47]
DTX-I	3.1	0.13	n.d.	+	n.d.	[48]
DTX K	0.03	-	n.d.	-	n.d.	[48]
DTX-δ	0.01	n.d.	n.d.	n.d.	1000	[49]
Cone snail						
Conk-S1	n.d.	n.d.	n.d.	n.d.	1.33	[15]
Scorpions						
LmKTT-1a	>1000	>1000	1580 ± 73	n.d.	n.d.	[50]
Hg1	-	-	6.2	-	-	[10]
Spider						
HW11c4	>10, 000	-	-	n.d.	n.d.	[14]

* ^{125}I α-DTX dendrotoxin binding to synaptosomal membranes, n.d. not determined, - no or weak activity.

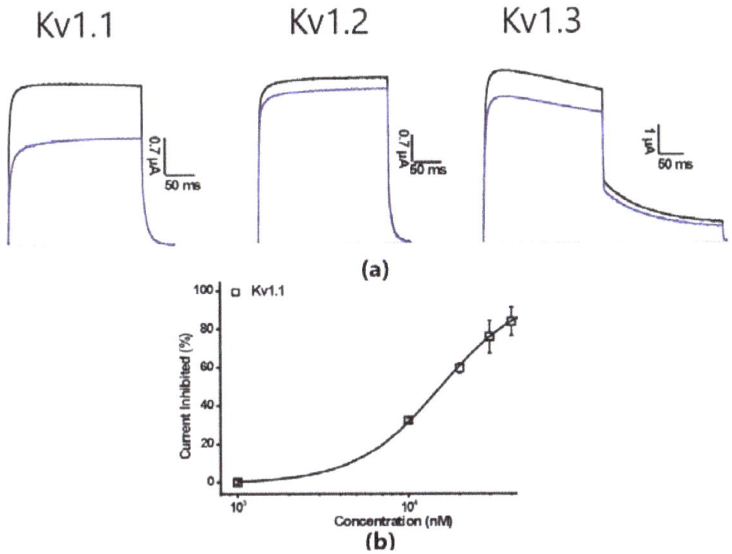

Figure 7. (**a**) Electrophysiological analysis of HCRG21 S5L activity on Kv1.1–Kv1.3 isoforms expressed in *X. laevis* oocytes. Representative whole-cell current traces in control and toxin conditions are shown. The blue line marks steady-state current traces after the application of 10 μM of peptide. (**b**) Dose–response curve for HCRG21 S5L on Kv1.1 channels. Traces shown are representative traces of at least three independent experiments (n ≥ 3).

3.3. Anti-Inflammatory Activity of HCRG1

Carrageenan-induced paw edema is widely used as an in vivo acute inflammatory response model [51]. Since HCRG1 is more specific to Kv1.3, it was tested in a model of acute local inflammation induced by carrageenan administration into mice paws. Before testing, we studied HCRG1 acute intravenous toxicity. After administration of the peptide, the animals exhibited normal behavior and external signs of intoxication (convulsions, asphyxia) or mortality were not detected.

It was found that HCRG1 at doses of 0.1 and 1 mg/kg reduced the volume of developing edema during 24 h. Its effect was close to that of the nonsteroidal anti-inflammatory drug, indomethacin, at a dose of 5 mg/kg (Figure 8A). ELISA analysis of blood taken from animals showed that indomethacin and HCRG1 reduced the synthesis of TNF-α, a proinflammatory mediator that played a leading role in the development of edema and hyperalgesia in that model (Figure 8B) [51].

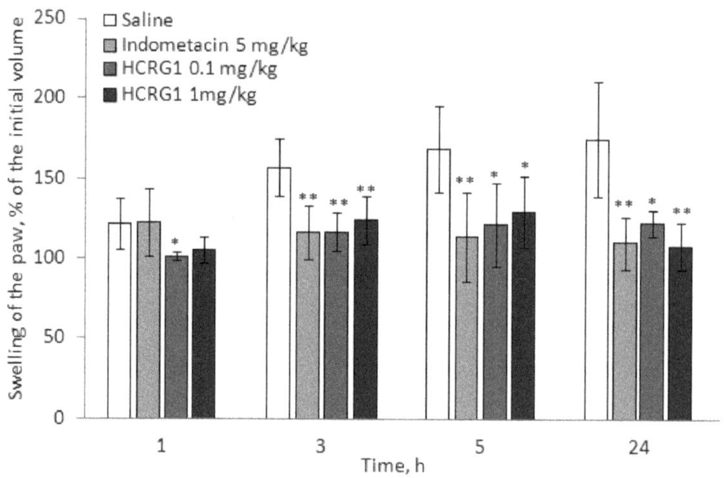

(a)

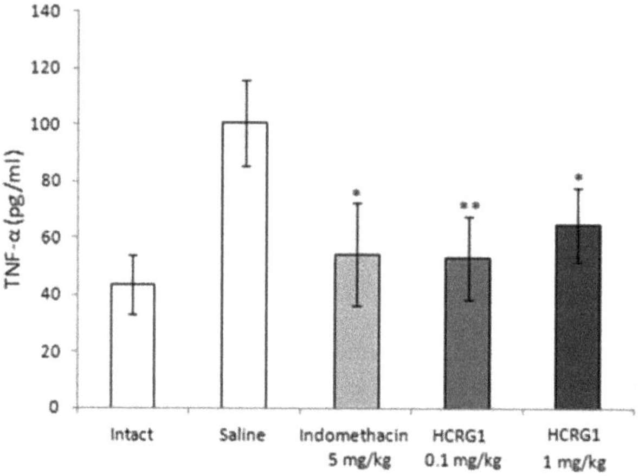

(b)

Figure 8. Effect of peptide HCRG1 on (**a**) paw swelling and (**b**) TNF-α production in mice with acute local inflammation induced by carrageenan administration. Control animals received a similar volume of saline (negative control) or indomethacin solution at a dose of 5 mg/kg (positive control). Intact animals on (**b**) were not subjected to any manipulation. The reliability of differences is calculated by the Student's t-criterion. The value * $p < 0.05$, ** $p < 0.01$ is considered reliable in comparison with the saline group.

4. Discussion

Kunitz-type toxins are members of an ancient family that have been identified in many animal venoms, such as those of snakes, scorpions, spiders, cone snails, and sea anemones. Kunitz-type sea anemone type 2 toxins retained the ability to inhibit serine proteases which might be a venom defense mechanism against the prey's proteases, similar to the toxins found in the venom of scorpions [52]. These peptides are believed to protect their own toxins from self-digestion by proteases. Moreover, they act synergistically with other peptide compounds of the venom and as such, they help to immobilize and kill the prey [1].

Up to now, more than a dozen Kunitz-type peptides produced by sea anemones of *Heteractis* genus (Stichodactylidae) have been described. Moreover, it has been determined that these peptides are encoded by a multigene superfamily composed of distinct GS-, GG-, GN-, and RG-gene families which are produced via a combinatorial library [8]. HCRG1, HCRG2, and HCRG21 are members of HCRG-family which includes 33 mature peptides. HCRG21 shares a high percentage of sequence identity with HCRG1 (82%) and HCRG2 (86%). Moreover, these peptides contain conserved amino acids at the N- and C-termini. Besides trypsin, Kunitz-type peptides from sea anemone *H. crispa* are also able to interact with other serine proteases (chymotrypsin, elastase, kallikrein) [19,39,53], modulate or block TRPV1 channel [22–24], revealing different kind of biological effects such as analgesic [22,54–56], anti-inflammatory [9,41,54,57], antihistamine [41,58], as well as neuroprotective activity [59,60]. However, despite their high degree of homology with the known bifunctional peptides, like kalicludines, SHTXIII, APEKTx1, and ShPI-1 [16,18,19], none of them has shown potassium channels blocking activity.

In this work, we identified a new activity of two previously characterized Kunitz peptides, HCRG1 and HCRG2, from *H. crispa* [38], using electrophysiological screening on six isoforms of Kv1 channels and insect *Shaker* IR channel expressed in *X. laevis* oocytes. Similar to toxin ShPI-1 from *S. helianthus* (Stichodactilidae) [19], HCRG1 and HCRG2 have also been shown to be active against more than one isoform of Kv1.x channels (Figure 5, (Table 1). The main difference compared to all sea anemone type 2 toxins is the ability of HCRG1 and HCRG2 to block Kv1.3 channels. Hence, and to the best of our knowledge, these peptides are the first Kunitz-type sea anemone toxins with activity towards Kv1.3 channels.

Among known Kunitz-type toxins produced by poisonous animals (Table 1), HCRG1 and HCRG2 turned out to be the least selective with respect to Kv1.x isoforms. Kunitz-type toxins from snake and scorpion venoms are more selective and usually modulate Kv1.x isoforms at lower concentrations (Table 1). Notably, HCRG1 inhibits Kv1.3 currents with an IC_{50} value of 40.7 nM, being about 3.5 and 1200 times more powerful blocker for it than for Kv1.1 and Kv1.2, respectively. As for HCRG2, the IC_{50} values differ by 2.5–6 times for all tested channels (Table 1). It is worth noticing that a large amount of a less selective peptide, identical to HCRG2, was found in the mucus of the closely related sea anemone *Heteractis magnifica* during proteomic analysis, which indicates its important place in the venom composition within the genus [9]. For many snake and scorpion toxins, as well as for sea anemone type 1 toxins with the Shk-fold, the amino acid determinants responsible for binding to Kv channels have already been identified. However, for sea anemone type 2 toxins, this question remains unresolved. The importance of a key basic residue (Lys or Arg) associated with a 6.6 ± 1 Å distant key hydrophobic residue (Leu, Tyr or Phe), together with a functional ring of basic amino acids, has been established [17]. Nevertheless, there are known examples of toxins lacking the dyad that still demonstrate blocking activities against Kv channels, suggesting that other epitopes are involved in the high-affinity interaction between the toxin and its target [17,61,62]. It seems that for type 2 toxins with the Kunitz fold, the number and distribution of charged, hydrophobic, and polar uncharged residues are important.

Functionally important amino acid residues in the sequences of sea anemones and other venomous animals Kunitz-type toxins are located in the N- and C-terminal regions of the molecule, in particular around CysI and CysV–CysVI respectively [19]. These amino acid residues form a molecular recognition surface for interaction with Kvs, thanks to the conservative disulfide bond CysI–CysVI which brings together the N- and C-terminal regions of the molecule. Thus, Arg1, Ser5 or Leu5, Arg51, and Arg55 can be responsible for the activity of HCRG1 and HCRG2 (Figure 9). The side chain of Arg1, similar to Arg5 of the peptide Hg1 and Arg4 of the peptides DTX1 and DTX-α, can also make a significant contribution to the binding to Kv. However, HCRG21 and InhVJ which have the same amino acid residues at the indicated positions as HCRG1, HCRG2, and ShPI-1, do not demonstrate activity against Kv channels. Apparently, this is due to the presence in these peptide sequences of the residues Gly1 (for InhVJ), Thr14 and Glu38 (for both) (Figure 4) that impede interaction with the studied Kv channels and, possibly, make them specific to other ion channels [19].

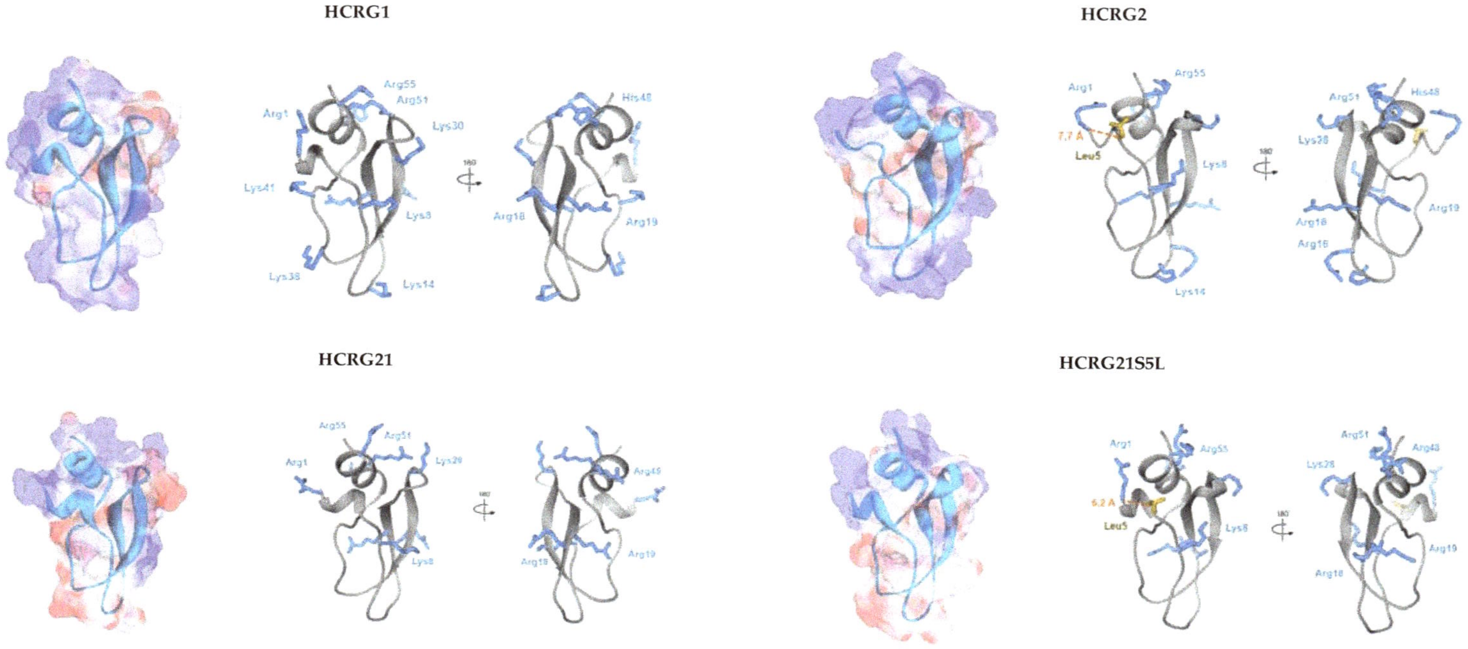

Figure 9. Spatial structures of HCRG1, HCRG2, HCRG21, and HCRG21S5L. 3D-Models of peptides are represented as a ribbon diagram with translucent surfaces accessible to the solvent, painted in accordance with the electrostatic potential: blue indicates the region of positive values, red—negative and gray—neutral. The side chains of positive (Arg and Lys) and hydrophobic (Leu5) amino acid residues are shown as sticks. The distance between the α-carbons of the above amino acid residues is indicated. The ShPI-1 (PDB ID 1SHP) from the sea anemone *S. helianthus* was used as a template. 3D models were made using Discovery Studio and UCSF Chimera.

In the HCRG1 and HCRG2 sequences, unlike those of the Kunitz type peptides AsKC1 and AsKC2 from *A. sulcata*, there is no distinct key residue identifiable for the interaction with Kv channel epitopes, similar to the dyad Lys5/Leu9 typical for dendrotoxins [13,47]. It can be surmised that this role might be partially fulfilled by Arg1/Leu5 residues in HCRG2 (Figure 9), since the affinity of this peptide to Kv1.1 is an order of magnitude higher than for HCRG1. HCRG21 is a full blocker of the TRPV1 channel but completely inactive against Kv1.x channels [23]. Interestingly, a single point mutation, Ser5 to Leu5, introduced for HCRG21 the properties of a weak blocker of Kv1.1, Kv1.2, and Kv1.3 channels (Figure 7). Using site-directed mutagenesis and chemical synthesis, it has been shown that the dyad Lys5 and Leu9 of DTX-α are crucial for channel blockage activity of this toxin [13,47]. We believe that for the peptides HCRG2 and HCRG21 S5L, the Arg1 and Leu5 residues can play the role of such a dyad. According to the results of molecular modeling, these residues are separated by 7.7 Å (HCRG2) and 6.2 Å (HCRG21 S5L) (Figure 9).

Most likely, the higher affinity of HCRG1 for Kv1.3 among the other Kv1 channels is caused by the residues Glu28, Lys30, Lys38, and Lys41, which sets this peptide apart from other sea anemone type 2 toxins (Figure 4). It has been well-established that there is a difference between residues forming the selective channel filter of Kv1.x channels: Asp377-Met378-Tyr379 for Kv1.1, Asp377-Met378-Val379 for Kv1.2, and Asp377-Met378-Hys379 for Kv1.3. The selectivity of different toxins to Kv1.x channel isoforms is dictated by the nature of the residue at position 379 [63]. Structural and functional studies using the site-directed mutagenesis method will further determine the functional significance of the designated amino acids of HCRG1 and HCRG2.

Kv1.3 channels have gained a prominent role for their possibility to control neuroinflammatory and autoimmune diseases [33,64–66]. Inflammation involves several processes including the activation of inflammatory cells, the secretion of pro-inflammatory cytokines and the release of various inflammatory mediators, leading to symptoms of inflammation such as redness, swelling, fever and pain [67]. Previously, we have shown that the peptides HCRG1 and HCRG2 are able to reduce the synthesis of pro-inflammatory mediators, pro-IL-1β, IL-6, and TNF-α, induced by the addition of bacterial lipopolysaccharide to J774A.1 macrophages [36]. These effects can be achieved by inhibiting the proteases linked to inflammatory processes, as well as by blocking of Kv1.3 channels. On one hand, an anti-inflammatory effect was shown for BPTI, known as an inhibitor of different serine proteases, and bikunin, a human Kunitz-type peptide that inhibits the production of thromboxane B2, TNF-α, and IL-8 in macrophages treated with LPS [68]. On the other hand, it has been established that the treatment of autoreactive T-lymphocytes by ShK-186 (analog of ShK from *S. helianthus*) decreased the levels of IL-2, IL-4, interferon-γ, and TNF-α [37]. In this work, we have shown that HCRG1 mice pretreatment (at doses of 0.1 and 1 mg/kg) significantly reduces (~40%) paw edema during 24 h after carrageenan administration. In addition, HCRG1 at a dose of 0.1 mg/kg inhibits the synthesis of TNF-α similar to indomethacin after 24 h (Figure 8B). These data indicate that HCRG1 has an anti-inflammatory effect by inhibiting the secretion of TNF-α, a pro-inflammatory mediator that demonstrates a leading role in the development of edema and hyperalgesia in this model.

In summary, we found out that HCRG1 and HCRG2 from the sea anemone *H. crispa* are new representatives of type 2 toxins demonstrating Kv inhibitory activity similar to other members. Furthermore, they are the first Kunitz-type peptides blocking the activity of prospect pharmacological channel Kv1.3. We first showed the ability of Kunitz-type peptides with dual inhibitory activity, namely towards Kv and serine proteases, to demonstrate anti-inflammatory effects during acute inflammation. We cannot clearly conclude which of the two activities results in the observed effect, but presumably, both can contribute or enhance the peptide action in the organism. Artificial mutant HCRG21 S5L is a curious example of how the substitution of one amino acid residue changes the specificity of sea anemone Kunitz-type toxin from the channel of TRP to Kv family. It shows a fine line between a specific inhibitor of TRPV1 channel and a toxin with a broader function. This manuscript is the starting point for a deeper investigation of the importance of single amino acid residues and the establishment of the evolutionary patterns of Kunitz-type peptides from sea anemones, so similar in their amino acid sequences and so different in the activities.

Author Contributions: Conceptualization, I.G., O.S., E.L., M.M., and J.T.; data curation, S.P.; formal analysis, M.I., A.M., S.P., and E.L.P.-J.; investigation, I.G., O.S., S.P., E.L.P.-J., A.K. (Anna Klimovich), and A.M.; methodology, I.G., O.S., M.I., A.K. (Anatoly Kalinovsky), and S.P.; visualization, A.M. and A.K. (Anatoly Kalinovsky); writing—original draft, I.G. and O.S. writing—review and editing, I.G., O.S., S.P., E.L.P.-J., J.T., M.M., E.K., and E.L. All authors have read and agreed to the published version of the manuscript.

Funding: The studying of native peptides was supported by Grant of the Ministry of Science and Education, Russian Federation 13.1902.21.0012 (Agreement number 075-15-2020-796), the studying of HCRG21 S5L was supported by RSF № 19-74-20088. The MS and NMR spectra were carried out on the equipment of the Collective Facilities Center «The Far Eastern Center for Structural Molecular Research (NMR/MS) PIBOC FEB RAS». J.T. was funded by grants GOC2319 N, GOA4919 N and G0E7120N (F.W.O.-Vlaanderen), and CELSA/17/047 (BOF, KU Leuven). S.P. is supported by KU Leuven funding (PDM/19/164). E.L.P.-J. was funded by scholarships from FAPESP (São Paulo Research Foundation, n. 2016/04761-4) and CAPES (Coordination for the Improvement of Higher Education Personnel, n. 88881.186830/2018-01).

Conflicts of Interest: The authors declare no conflict of interest.

References

1. Mourão, C.B.F.; Schwartz, E.F. Protease inhibitors from marine venomous animals and their counterparts in terrestrial venomous animals. *Mar. Drugs* **2013**, *11*, 2069–2112. [CrossRef]
2. Kunitz, M.; Northrop, J.H. Isolation from beef pancreas of crystalline trypsinogen, trypsin, a trypsin inhibitor, and an inhibitor-trypsin compound. *J. Gen. Physiol.* **1936**, *19*, 991–1007. [PubMed]
3. Ascenzi, P.; Bocedi, A.; Bolognesi, M.; Spallarossa, A.; Coletta, M.; De Cristofaro, R.; Menegatti, E. The bovine basic pancreatic trypsin inhibitor (Kunitz inhibitor): A milestone protein. *Curr. Protein Pept. Sci.* **2003**, *4*, 231–251. [PubMed]
4. Sun, Z.; Lu, W.; Jiang, A.; Chen, J.; Tang, F.; Liu, J.-N. Expression, purification and characterization of aprotinin and a human analogue of aprotinin. *Protein Expr. Purif.* **2009**, *65*, 238–243. [CrossRef]
5. Buczek, O.; Koscielska-Kasprzak, K.; Krowarsch, D.; Dadlez, M.; Otlewski, J. Analysis of serine proteinase-inhibitor interaction by alanine shaving. *Protein Sci.* **2002**, *11*, 806–819. [PubMed]
6. Dai, S.-X.; Zhang, A.-D.; Huang, J.-F. Evolution, expansion and expression of the Kunitz/BPTI gene family associated with long-term blood feeding in Ixodes Scapularis. *BMC Evol. Biol.* **2012**, *12*, 4. [CrossRef]
7. Yuan, C.H.; He, Q.Y.; Peng, K.; Diao, J.B.; Jiang, L.P.; Tang, X.; Liang, S.P. Discovery of a distinct superfamily of kunitz-type toxin (KTT) from Tarantulas. *PLoS ONE* **2008**, *3*. [CrossRef]
8. Isaeva, M.P.; Chausova, V.E.; Zelepuga, E.A.; Guzev, K.V.; Tabakmakher, V.M.; Monastyrnaya, M.M.; Kozlovskaya, E.P. A new multigene superfamily of Kunitz-type protease inhibitors from sea anemone *Heteractis crispa*. *Peptides* **2012**, *34*, 88–97. [CrossRef]
9. Sintsova, O.; Gladkikh, I.; Chausova, V.; Monastyrnaya, M.; Anastyuk, S.; Chernikov, O.; Yurchenko, E.; Aminin, D.; Isaeva, M.; Leychenko, E.; et al. Peptide fingerprinting of the sea anemone *Heteractis magnifica* mucus revealed neurotoxins, Kunitz-type proteinase inhibitors and a new β-defensin α-amylase inhibitor. *J. Proteomics* **2018**, *173*, 12–21. [CrossRef]
10. Chen, Z.Y.; Hu, Y.T.; Yang, W.S.; He, Y.W.; Feng, J.; Wang, B.; Zhao, R.M.; Ding, J.P.; Cao, Z.J.; Li, W.X.; et al. Hg1, novel peptide inhibitor specific for Kv1.3 channels from first scorpion Kunitz-type potassium channel toxin family. *J. Biol. Chem.* **2012**, *287*, 13813–13821. [CrossRef] [PubMed]
11. Harvey, A.L.; Anderson, A.J. Dendrotoxins: Snake toxins that block potassium channels and facilitate neurotransmitter release. *Pharmacol. Ther.* **1985**, *31*, 33–55.
12. Lancelin, J.M.; Foray, M.F.; Poncin, M.; Hollecker, M.; Marion, D. Proteinase inhibitor homologues as potassium channel blockers. *Nat. Struct. Biol.* **1994**, *1*, 246–250. [CrossRef]
13. Owen, D.G.; Hall, A.; Stephens, G.; Stow, J.; Robertson, B. The relative potencies of dendrotoxins as blockers of the cloned expressed in Chinese hamster ovary cells. *Br. J. Pharmacol.* **1997**, *1*, 1029–1034.
14. Jiang, L.; Deng, M.; Duan, Z.; Tang, X.; Liang, S. Molecular cloning, bioinformatics analysis and functional characterization of HWTX-XI toxin superfamily from the spider *Ornithoctonus huwena*. *Peptides* **2014**, *54*, 9–18. [CrossRef]

15. Bayrhuber, M.; Vijayan, V.; Ferber, M.; Graf, R.; Korukottu, J.; Imperial, J.; Garrett, J.E.; Olivera, B.M.; Terlau, H.; Zweckstetter, M.; et al. Conkunitzin-S1 is the first member of a new Kunitz-type neurotoxin family: Structural and functional characterization. *J. Biol. Chem.* **2005**, *280*, 23766–23770. [CrossRef]
16. Schweitz, H.; Bruhn, T.; Guillemare, E.; Moinier, D.; Lancelin, J.-M.M.; Béress, L.; Lazdunski, M.; Beress, L.; Lazdunski, M.; Béress, L.; et al. Kalicludines and Kaliseptine: Two different classes of sea anemone toxins for voltage sensitive K+ cannels. *J. Biol. Chem.* **1995**, *270*, 25121–25126. [CrossRef]
17. Peigneur, S.; Billen, B.; Derua, R.; Waelkens, E.; Debaveye, S.; Béress, L.; Tytgat, J. A bifunctional sea anemone peptide with Kunitz type protease and potassium channel inhibiting properties. *Biochem. Pharmacol.* **2011**, *82*, 81–90. [CrossRef]
18. Honma, T.; Kawahata, S.; Ishida, M.; Nagai, H.; Nagashima, Y.; Shiomi, K. Novel peptide toxins from the sea anemone *Stichodactyla haddoni*. *Peptides* **2008**, *29*, 536–544. [CrossRef] [PubMed]
19. García-Fernández, R.; Peigneur, S.; Pons, T.; Alvarez, C.; González, L.; Chávez, M.A.; Tytgat, J. The kunitz-type protein ShPI-1 inhibits serine proteases and voltage-gated potassium channels. *Toxins (Basel)* **2016**, *8*, 110. [CrossRef]
20. Schweitz, H.; Heurteaux, C.; Bois, P.; Moinier, D.; Romey, G.; Lazdunski, M. Calcicludine, a venom peptide of the Kunitz-type protease inhibitor family, is a potent blocker of high-threshold Ca2+ channels with a high affinity for L-type channels in cerebellar granule neurons. *Proc. Natl. Acad. Sci. USA* **1994**, *91*, 878–882. [CrossRef]
21. Báez, A.; Salceda, E.; Fló, M.; Graña, M.; Fernández, C.; Vega, R.; Soto, E. α-Dendrotoxin inhibits the ASIC current in dorsal root ganglion neurons from rat. *Neurosci. Lett.* **2015**, *606*, 42–47. [CrossRef]
22. Andreev, Y.A.; Kozlov, S.A.; Koshelev, S.G.; Ivanova, E.A.; Monastyrnaya, M.M.; Kozlovskaya, E.P.; Grishin, E.V. Analgesic compound from sea anemone *Heteractis crispa* is the first polypeptide inhibitor of vanilloid receptor 1 (TRPV1). *J. Biol. Chem.* **2008**, *283*, 23914–23921. [CrossRef]
23. Monastyrnaya, M.; Peigneur, S.; Zelepuga, E.; Sintsova, O.; Gladkikh, I.; Leychenko, E.; Isaeva, M.; Tytgat, J.; Kozlovskaya, E. Kunitz-Type Peptide HCRG21 from the Sea Anemone *Heteractis crispa* Is a Full Antagonist of the TRPV1 Receptor. *Mar. Drugs* **2016**, *14*, 229. [CrossRef]
24. Nikolaev, M.V.; Dorofeeva, N.A.; Komarova, M.S.; Korolkova, Y.V.; Andreev, Y.A.; Mosharova, I.V.; Grishin, E.V.; Tikhonov, D.B.; Kozlov, S.A. TRPV1 activation power can switch an action mode for its polypeptide ligands. *PLoS ONE* **2017**, *12*, 1–16. [CrossRef] [PubMed]
25. Papers, J.B.C.; Doi, M.; Mans, B.J.; Louw, A.I.; Neitz, A.W.H. Savignygrin, a Platelet Aggregation Inhibitor from the Soft Tick *Ornithodoros savignyi*, Presents the RGD Integrin Recognition Motif on the Kunitz-BPTI Fold. *J. Biol. Chem.* **2002**, *277*, 21371–21378. [CrossRef]
26. Ciolek, J.; Reinfrank, H.; Sigismeau, S.; Mouillac, B.; Peigneur, S.; Tytgat, J.; Droctov, L.; Mourier, G.; De Pauw, E.; Servent, D.; et al. Green mamba peptide targets type-2 vasopressin receptor against polycystic kidney disease. *Proc. Natl. Acad. Sci. USA* **2017**, *114*, 7154–7159. [CrossRef]
27. Orts, D.J.B.; Moran, Y.; Cologna, C.T.; Peigneur, S.; Madio, B.; Praher, D.; Quinton, L.; De Pauw, E.; Bicudo, J.E.P.W.; Tytgat, J.; et al. BcsTx3 is a founder of a novel sea anemone toxin family of potassium channel blocker. *FEBS J.* **2013**, *280*, 4839–4852. [CrossRef]
28. Madio, B.; Peigneur, S.; Chin, Y.K.Y.; Hamilton, B.R.; Henriques, S.T.; Smith, J.J.; Cristofori, B.; Zoltan, A.; Berin, D.; Paul, A.B.; et al. PHAB toxins: A unique family of predatory sea anemone toxins evolving via intra—Gene concerted evolution defines a new peptide fold. *Cell. Mol. Life Sci.* **2018**, *75*, 4511–4524. [CrossRef]
29. Gutman, G.A.; Chandy, K.G.; Grissmer, S.; Lazdunski, M.; Mckinnon, D.; Pardo, L.A.; Robertson, G.A.; Rudy, B.; Sanguinetti, M.C.; Stu, W.; et al. International Union of Pharmacology. LIII. Nomenclature and Molecular Relationships of Voltage-Gated Potassium Channels. *Pharmacol. Rev.* **2005**, *57*, 473–508. [CrossRef]
30. Norton, R.S.; Chandy, K.G. Venom-derived peptide inhibitors of voltage-gated potassium channels. *Neuropharmacology* **2017**. [CrossRef]
31. Finol-Urdaneta, R.K.; Belovanovic, A.; Micic-Vicovac, M.; Kinsella, G.K.; McArthur, J.R.; Al-Sabi, A. Marine toxins targeting Kv1 channels: Pharmacological tools and therapeutic scaffolds. *Mar. Drugs* **2020**, *18*, 173. [CrossRef]
32. Pérez-Verdaguer, M.; Capera, J.; Serrano-Novillo, C.; Estadella, I.; Sastre, D.; Felipe, A. The voltage-gated potassium channel Kv1.3 is a promising multitherapeutic target against human pathologies. *Expert Opin. Ther. Targets* **2016**, *20*, 577–591. [CrossRef]

33. Rangaraju, S.; Chi, V.; Pennington, M.W.; Chandy, K.G. Kv1.3 Potassium Channels as a Therapeutic Target in Multiple Sclerosis. *Expert Opin. Ther. Targets* **2009**, *13*, 909–924. [CrossRef]
34. Tajti, G.; Wai, D.C.C.; Panyi, G.; Norton, R.S. The voltage-gated potassium channel KV1.3 as a therapeutic target for venom-derived peptides. *Biochem. Pharmacol.* **2020**, 114146. [CrossRef]
35. Castañeda, O.; Sotolongo, V.; Amor, A.M.; Stöcklin, R.; Anderson, A.J.; Harvey, A.L.; Engström, A.; Wernstedt, C.; Karlsson, E. Characterization of a potassium channel toxin from the Caribbean Sea anemone *Stichodactyla helianthus*. *Toxicon* **1995**, *33*, 603–613. [CrossRef]
36. Shen, B.; Cao, Z.; Li, W.; Sabatier, J.-M.M.; Wu, Y. Treating autoimmune disorders with venom-derived peptides. *Expert Opin. Biol. Ther.* **2017**, *17*, 1065–1075. [CrossRef]
37. Chi, V.; Pennington, M.W.; Norton, R.S.; Tarcha, E.J.; Londono, L.M.; Sims-Fahey, B.; Upadhyay, S.K.; Lakey, J.T.; Iadonato, S.; Wulff, H.; et al. Development of a sea anemone toxin as an immunomodulator for therapy of autoimmune diseases. *Toxicon* **2012**, *59*, 529–546. [CrossRef]
38. Gladkikh, I.; Monastyrnaya, M.; Zelepuga, E.; Sintsova, O.; Tabakmakher, V.; Gnedenko, O.; Ivanov, A.; Hua, K.-F.; Kozlovskaya, E. New kunitz-type HCRG polypeptides from the sea anemone *Heteractis crispa*. *Mar. Drugs* **2015**, *13*, 6038–6063. [CrossRef]
39. Gladkikh, I.; Monastyrnaya, M.; Leychenko, E.; Zelepuga, E.; Chausova, V.; Isaeva, M.; Anastyuk, S.; Andreev, Y.; Peigneur, S.; Tytgat, J.; et al. Atypical reactive center Kunitz-type inhibitor from the sea anemone *Heteractis crispa*. *Mar. Drugs* **2012**, *10*, 1545–1565. [CrossRef] [PubMed]
40. Hwang, T.L.; Shaka, A.J. Water Suppression That Works. Excitation Sculpting Using Arbitrary Wave-Forms and Pulsed-Field Gradients. *J. Magn. Reson. Ser. A* **1995**, *112*, 275–279. [CrossRef]
41. Sintsova, O.V.; Monastyrnaya, M.M.; Pislyagin, E.A.; Menchinskaya, E.S.; Leychenko, E.V.; Aminin, D.L.; Kozlovskaya, E.P. Anti-inflammatory activity of a polypeptide from the *Heteractis crispa* sea anemone. *Russ. J. Bioorg. Chem.* **2015**, *41*, 590–596. [CrossRef]
42. Dixon, M. The determination of enzyme inhibitor constants. *Biochem. J.* **1953**, *55*, 170–171. [CrossRef]
43. Liman, E.R.; Tytgat, J.; Hess, P. Subunit stoichiometry of a mammalian K+ channel determined by construction of multimeric cDNAs. *Neuron* **1992**, *9*, 861–871. [CrossRef]
44. Yang, J.; Zhang, Y. I-TASSER server: New development for protein structure and function predictions. *Nucleic Acids Res.* **2015**, *43*, W174–W181. [CrossRef]
45. Pettersen, E.F.; Goddard, T.D.; Huang, C.C.; Couch, G.S.; Greenblatt, D.M.; Meng, E.C.; Ferrin, T.E. UCSF Chimera—A visualization system for exploratory research and analysis. *J. Comput. Chem.* **2004**, *25*, 1605–1612. [CrossRef]
46. Helland, R.; Otlewski, J.; Sundheim, O.; Dadlez, M.; Smalås, A.O. The crystal structures of the complexes between bovine beta-trypsin and ten P1 variants of BPTI. *J. Mol. Biol.* **1999**, *287*, 923–942. [CrossRef] [PubMed]
47. Harvey, A.L. Twenty years of dendrotoxins. *Toxicon* **2001**, *39*, 15–26. [CrossRef]
48. Robertson, B.; Owen, D.; Stow, J.; Butler, C.; Newland, C. Novel effects of dendrotoxin homologues on subtypes of mammalian Kv1 potassium channels expressed in Xenopus oocytes. *FEBS Lett.* **1996**, *383*, 26–30. [CrossRef]
49. Imredy, J.P.; MacKinnon, R. Energetic and structural interactions between δ-dendrotoxin and a voltage-gated potassium channel. *J. Mol. Biol.* **2000**, *296*, 1283–1294. [CrossRef]
50. Chen, Z.; Luo, F.; Feng, J.; Yang, W.; Zeng, D.; Zhao, R.; Cao, Z.; Liu, M.; Li, W.; Jiang, L.; et al. Genomic and Structural Characterization of Kunitz-Type Peptide LmKTT-1a Highlights Diversity and Evolution of Scorpion Potassium Channel Toxins. *PLoS ONE* **2013**, *8*, 1–10. [CrossRef] [PubMed]
51. Rocha, A.C.C.; Fernandes, E.S.; Quintão, N.L.M.; Campos, M.M.; Calixto, J.B. Relevance of tumour necrosis factor-α for the inflammatory and nociceptive responses evoked by carrageenan in the mouse paw. *Br. J. Pharmacol.* **2006**, *148*, 688–695. [CrossRef]
52. Ma, H.; Xiao-Peng, T.; Yang, S.-L.; Lu, Q.-M.; Lai, R. Protease inhibitor in scorpion (*Mesobuthus eupeus*) venom prolongs the biological activities of the crude venom. *Chin. J. Nat. Med.* **2016**, *14*, 607–614. [CrossRef]
53. Kvetkina, A.N.; Kaluzhskiy, L.A.; Leychenko, E.V.; Isaeva, M.P. New Targets of Kunitz-Type Peptide from Sea Anemone *Heteractis magnifica*. *Dokl. Biochem. Biophys.* **2019**, *487*, 1–4. [CrossRef] [PubMed]
54. Andreev, Y.A.; Kozlov, S.A.; Korolkova, Y.V.; Dyachenko, I.A.; Bondarenko, D.A.; Skobtsov, D.I.; Murashev, A.N.; Kotova, P.D.; Rogachevskaja, O.A.; Kabanova, N.V.; et al. Polypeptide modulators of TRPV1 produce analgesia without hyperthermia. *Mar. Drugs* **2013**, *11*, 5100–5115. [CrossRef]

55. Tabakmakher, V.M.; Sintsova, O.V.; Krivoshapko, O.N.; Zelepuga, E.A.; Monastyrnaya, M.M.; Kozlovskaya, E.P. Analgesic effect of novel Kunitz-type polypeptides of the sea anemone *Heteractis crispa*. *Dokl. Biochem. Biophys.* **2015**, *461*, 232–235. [CrossRef]
56. Sintsova, O.V.; Palikov, V.A.; Palikova, Y.A.; Klimovich, A.A.; Gladkikh, I.N.; Andreev, Y.A.; Monastyrnaya, M.M.; Kozlovskaya, E.P.; Dyachenko, I.A.; Kozlov, S.A.; et al. Peptide Blocker of Ion Channel TRPV1 Exhibits a Long Analgesic Effect in the Heat Stimulation Model. *Dokl. Biochem. Biophys.* **2020**, *493*, 215–217. [CrossRef]
57. Sokotun, I.N.; Gnedenko, O.V.; Leychenko, A.V.; Monastyrnaya, M.M.; Kozlovskaya, E.P.; Molnar, A.A.; Ivanov, A.S.; Gnedenko, O.V.; Leychenko, E.V.; Monastyrnaya, M.M.; et al. Study of the interaction of trypsin inhibitor from the sea anemone *Radianthus macrodactylus* with proteases. *Biochem. Suppl. Ser. B Biomed. Chem.* **2007**, *1*, 139–142. [CrossRef]
58. Sintsova, O.V.; Pislyagin, E.A.; Gladkikh, I.N.; Monastyrnaya, M.M.; Menchinskaya, E.S. Kunitz-Type Peptides of the Sea Anemone Heteractis crispa: Potential Anti-Inflammatory Compounds. *Russ. J. Bioorg. Chem.* **2017**, *43*, 91–97. [CrossRef]
59. Kvetkina, A.N.; Leychenko, E.V.; Yurchenko, E.A.; Pislyagin, E.A.; Peigneur, S.; Tytgat, J.; Isaeva, M.; Aminin, D.; Kozlovskaya, E.P. A New Iq-Peptide of the Kunitz Type from the *Heteractis magnifica* Sea Anemone Exhibits Neuroprotective Activity in a Model of Alzheimer's Disease. *Russ. J. Bioorg. Chem.* **2018**, *44*, 416–423. [CrossRef]
60. Kvetkina, A.; Leychenko, E.; Chausova, V.; Zelepuga, E.; Chernysheva, N.; Guzev, K.; Pislyagin, E.; Yurchenko, E.; Menchinskaya, E.; Aminin, D.; et al. A new multigene HCIQ subfamily from the sea anemone *Heteractis crispa* encodes Kunitz-peptides exhibiting neuroprotective activity against 6-hydroxydopamine. *Sci. Rep.* **2020**, *10*, 4205. [CrossRef]
61. Shon, K.J.; Stocker, M.; Terlau, H.; Stühmer, W.; Jacobsen, R.; Walker, C.; Grilley, M.; Watkins, M.; Hillyard, D.R.; Gray, W.R.; et al. κ-Conotoxin PVIIA is a peptide inhibiting the Shaker K+ channel. *J. Biol. Chem.* **1998**, *273*, 33–38. [CrossRef]
62. Huys, I.; Xu, C.Q.; Wang, C.Z.; Vacher, H.; Martin-Eauclaire, M.F.; Chi, C.W.; Tytgat, J. BmTx3, a scorpion toxin with two putative functional faces separately active on A-type K+ and HERG currents. *Biochem. J.* **2004**, *378*, 745–752. [CrossRef] [PubMed]
63. Gilquin, B.; Braud, S.; Eriksson, M.A.L.; Roux, B.; Bailey, T.D.; Priest, B.T.; Garcia, M.L.; Ménez, A.; Gasparini, S. A variable residue in the pore of Kv1 channels is critical for the high affinity of blockers from sea anemones and scorpions. *J. Biol. Chem.* **2005**, *280*, 27093–27102. [CrossRef] [PubMed]
64. Wang, X.; Li, G.; Guo, J.; Zhang, Z.; Zhang, S.; Zhu, Y.; Cheng, J.; Yu, L.; Ji, Y.; Tao, J. Kv1.3 Channel as a Key Therapeutic Target for Neuroinflammatory Diseases: State of the Art and Beyond. *Front. Neurosci.* **2020**, *13*. [CrossRef]
65. Sarkar, S.; Nguyen, H.M.; Malovic, E.; Luo, J.; Langley, M.; Palanisamy, B.N.; Singh, N.; Manne, S.; Neal, M.; Gabrielle, M.; et al. Kv1.3 modulates neuroinflammation and neurodegeneration in Parkinson's disease. *J. Clin. Investig.* **2020**, *130*, 4195–4212. [CrossRef]
66. Rangaraju, S.; Raza, S.A.; Pennati, A.; Deng, Q.; Dammer, E.B.; Duong, D.; Pennington, M.W.; Tansey, M.G.; Lah, J.J.; Betarbet, R.; et al. A systems pharmacology-based approach to identify novel Kv1.3 channel-dependent mechanisms in microglial activation. *J. Neuroinflamm.* **2017**, *14*, 128. [CrossRef] [PubMed]
67. Mansouri, M.T.; Hemmati, A.A.; Naghizadeh, B.; Mard, S.A.; Rezaie, A.; Ghorbanzadeh, B. A study of the mechanisms underlying the anti-inflammatory effect of ellagic acid in carrageenan-induced paw edema in rats. *Indian J. Pharmacol.* **2015**, *47*, 292–298. [CrossRef] [PubMed]
68. Shigetomi, H.; Onogi, A.; Kajiwara, H.; Yoshida, S.; Furukawa, N.; Haruta, S.; Tanase, Y.; Kanayama, S.; Noguchi, T.; Yamada, Y.; et al. Anti-inflammatory actions of serine protease inhibitors containing the Kunitz domain. *Inflamm. Res.* **2010**, *59*, 679–687. [CrossRef]

Publisher's Note: MDPI stays neutral with regard to jurisdictional claims in published maps and institutional affiliations.

biomedicines

MDPI

Review

European Medicinal Leeches—New Roles in Modern Medicine

Sarah Lemke [1] **and Andreas Vilcinskas** [1,2,*]

1 Institute for Insect Biotechnology, Justus-Liebig-University Giessen, Heinrich-Buff-Ring 26-32, D-35392 Giessen, Germany; Sarah.Lemke@agrar.uni-giessen.de
2 Fraunhofer Institute for Molecular Biology and Applied Ecology IME, Department of Bioresources, Ohlebergsweg 12, D-35392 Giessen, Germany
* Correspondence: Andreas.Vilcinskas@agrar.uni-giessen.de

Received: 30 March 2020; Accepted: 24 April 2020; Published: 27 April 2020

Abstract: Before the advent of modern medicine, natural resources were widely used by indigenous populations for the prevention and treatment of diseases. The associated knowledge, collectively described as folk medicine or traditional medicine, was largely based on trial-and-error testing of plant extracts (herbal remedies) and the use of invertebrates, particularly medicinal maggots of the blowfly *Lucilia sericata* and blood-sucking leeches. The widespread use of traditional medicine in the West declined as scientific advances allowed reproducible testing under controlled conditions and gave rise to the modern fields of biomedical research and pharmacology. However, many drugs are still derived from natural resources, and interest in traditional medicine has been renewed by the ability of researchers to investigate the medical potential of diverse species by high-throughput screening. Likewise, researchers are starting to look again at the benefits of maggot and leech therapy, based on the hypothesis that the use of such animals in traditional medicine is likely to reflect the presence of specific bioactive molecules that can be developed as drug leads. In this review, we consider the modern medical benefits of European medicinal leeches based on the systematic screening of their salivary proteins.

Keywords: medicinal leeches; drug discovery; *Hirudo* spec.; antistasins; hirudin; eglins; saratins

---

1. The Biology of Medicinal Leeches

European medicinal leeches of the genus *Hirudo* are blood-feeding annelids. The most relevant species are *H. orientalis* (Asian leech), *H. medicinalis* (European leech) and *H. verbana* (Hungarian leech). All three species are ectoparasites that live in freshwater ponds and slowly flowing streams, where they locate their vertebrate hosts by sensing heat, chemicals or movement [1,2]. Leeches attach to the host body surface and cut the skin using hundreds of calcified teeth [3]. They can then draw blood for up to one hour while secreting saliva into the wound. The secreted salivary proteins and peptides reach the vascular system of the host via thousands of tiny salivary gland cell ducts [4]. After ingestion by the leech, the host blood is compressed in the crop by the excretion of water and salts [5,6]. The remaining highly viscous blood comprises plasma proteins and blood cells and can be stored in the crop for up to one year [7]. It is thought that the morphology of the concentrated erythrocytes remains stable during storage [8], which means that proteolysis induced by host proteases released from leukocytes is inhibited [5]. Furthermore, leeches inevitably make contact with (and thus ingest) some bacteria on the surface of the host's skin during feeding, but the stored blood does not become overrun with pathogens. Indeed, foremost symbiotic core bacteria such as *Aeromonas veronii*, *A. hydrophila* and *Rikinella*-like species survive in the alimentary tract of the leech [9–11]. It is supposed that symbionts like *A. veronii* support the digestion of host blood by facilitating hemolysis [10,12,13] and may also help to suppress the growth of other bacteria in the crop of the leech [9]. In most parasitic leeches the host blood is stored in the crop, while food digestion and the absorption of nutrients occur predominantly in the intestine. It can be assumed that medicinal leech enzymes (e.g., endopeptidases, aminopeptidases, phosphatases) promote digestion processes [14].

2. The Pharmacological Potential of Medicinal Leeches

Medicinal leeches were used by Egyptian, Indian, Greek and Arab physicians thousands of years ago. The main application was bloodletting, but leeches were also recommended for the treatment of systemic ailments such as inflammation, skin diseases, rheumatic pain or problems with the reproductive system [15]. As an advocate of leech therapy, the Greek physician Galen of Pergamon (130–201 AD) described leeches as an effective treatment for numerous diseases. Later, in the Middle Ages, leech therapy was popular because it was less painful than conventional treatments and was recommended even for diseases of the nervous system and eyes. The use of leeches declined in the age of modern medicine, but medical interest was rekindled when one of the strongest natural anticoagulants—hirudin—was discovered in leech saliva by John Berry Haycraft in 1884, further characterized by Fritz Markwardt in the 1950s [15].

In the 1960s, physicians rediscovered the pharmacological potential of leech saliva. For example, medicinal leeches were used to prevent vascular disorders after reconstructive surgery [16], to re-establish disrupted blood vessel networks and as an alternative to anti-inflammatory drugs. Most reports concerning medicinal leech therapy focus on cosmetic and reconstructive surgery. However, leech therapy has been tested for many conditions over the past two decades, including migraine [17,18], knee osteoarthritis [19–25], cardiovascular disease [26–28], skin disorders [29], diabetic foot ulcers [30–32], priapism [33], macroglossia [34,35], cancer [36,37] and skin wounds [38,39]. For most of these conditions only individual case studies were published [39], but migraine and knee osteoarthritis are exceptions. Migraine is a primary neurological disorder and, for most patients, a lifelong illness associated with headaches, vomiting, nausea, photophobia and phonophobia. In a case series of seven patients who were unresponsive to conventional drugs, post-auricular leech therapy was shown to significantly reduce the frequency of migraine headaches, which the authors attributed to the presence of potent anesthetic, anti-inflammatory and vasodilator substances in the leech saliva [17]. Osteoarthritis is a disorder of the joints that is prevalent in older people (>65 years) and causes pain after activity and stiffness after rest [40]. A meta-analysis of seven articles published between 2000 and 2017 showed that leech therapy could improve the symptoms of knee osteoarthritis and reduce pain [39]. Importantly, leeches placed on the knee often achieved comparable or even better pain relief than conventional drugs, and patients reported that mobility was restored and the benefits of leech therapy were sometimes still evident after six months [41]. Although the benefits of leech therapy were evident from these studies, the salivary compounds responsible for these effects and the underlying molecular mechanisms were not characterized in detail.

3. Salivary Proteins: Natural Drugs from Medicinal Leeches

Antagonistic interactions between parasites and their hosts have led to an evolutionary "arms race", during which ectoparasites adapted to feed on host body fluids [42,43]. To ingest and digest host blood, medicinal leeches synthesize more than 100 salivary proteins and peptides [44–47]. The molecules are secreted during feeding and target physiological pathways involved in host defense, working as analgesics (kininases), anticoagulants (hirudin, calin, saratin and apyrase), anti-inflammatories (eglins, bdellins and tryptase inhibitor), cell matrix-degrading proteins (hyaluronidase) or antimicrobials [7,45,47–58]. Salivary transcriptome data from *Macrobdella decora* [59] and *Hirudo nipponia* [60], as well as expressed sequence tag libraries constructed from the salivary glands of *H. verbana*, *M. decora* and *Aliolimnatis fenestrata* [61], provided insight into the spectrum proteins found in leech saliva. For European medicinal leeches, the combined transcriptomic analysis of salivary gland cells and proteomic analysis of saliva in *H. medicinalis*, *H. orientalis* and *H. verbana* revealed a much wider repertoire of components than previously known [44], indicating that only ~15% of the salivary proteins in these species were identified and characterized (Table 1).

Analysis of the salivary transcriptomes of *H. medicinalis*, *H. orientalis* and *H. verbana* revealed the presence of transcripts representing 189, 86 and 344 salivary proteins, respectively [44]. The three closely related species were found to share 39 orthologous clusters, whereas 50 orthologous clusters were shared by any two of the three species [44]. Many of these newly discovered leech salivary proteins are either associated with blood feeding or related to proteins found in animal venoms [44]. The salivary proteins predicted from transcriptomic and proteomic data can be assigned to various functional groups based on their structural similarities, including metalloproteases representing the M12, M13 and M28 families, hyaluronidases, apyrases, adenosine deaminases, antistasins, cysteine-rich secretory proteins (CRISPs), eglins, cystatins, PAN/apple domain proteins, α2-macroglobulins, low-density lipoprotein receptors, R-type lectins, and salivary proteins containing a von Willebrand factor type A (vWA) domain. These proteins are likely to be involved in the regulation of blood coagulation, the temporary adjustment of blood pressure, the regulation of inflammation, the suppression of microbial growth or the digestion of blood in the crop [44]. Interestingly, differential gene expression analysis indicated that genes encoding salivary proteins, such as hirudin, eglins, saratins and destabilases, were also expressed in other leech tissues, showing that at least some leech "salivary proteins" are not restricted to the saliva and may have additional physiological functions [44]. Some leech-specific anticoagulants were also found in leeches that do not feed on blood, such as *Whitmania pigra* [62]. Interestingly, these anticoagulants were upregulated after feeding [62] just as they are in blood-feeding leeches [63].

The identified metalloprotease families in leech salivary encompass astacins (M12), neprilysins (M13) and aminopeptidase S (M28). Members of these metalloprotease families were also determined in the salivary secretion of medicinal maggots of *Lucilia sericata* [64]. Astacin-like metalloproteases are endopeptidases, which were originally identified in the crayfish *Astacus astacus*, which contribute to digestion. A homologues were found in the venom of the brown spiders *Loxosceles*, with the recombinant form able to induce morphological changes, such as loss of adhesion of muscular aorta cells in vitro and hydrolyzed purified fibrinogen and fibronectin [65]. Mammalian neprilysin is involved in reproduction and the modulation of neuronal activity and blood pressure [66]. Interestingly, the transcriptomic analysis of the salivary glands from medicinal maggots *L. sericata* elucidated a diversification of proteolytic enzymes [64], whereas the most diverse groups of molecules in the saliva of leeches represented protease inhibitors.

Many leech salivary proteins, including antistasin-like inhibitors, hirudins, hirudin-like factors and Kunitz-type proteinase inhibitors, show remarkable diversity [44,78], possibly reflecting target-oriented evolution [83] promoted by gene duplication events [84]. Gene duplication events are likely to have promoted the acquisition of two major salivary protein families—salivary blood coagulation inhibitors and platelet aggregation inhibitors—in blood-feeding ticks [85]. Gene recruitment also supports the diversification of salivary protein isoforms, based on the hypothesis that regulatory evolution is fundamental for adaptive evolution [86]. Accordingly, at least some venom and salivary proteins were recruited from other tissues, where they fulfilled distinct biological functions. The recruitment of alternative splice variants and 5′ exon evolution might explain the adaptation of vampire bats to hematophagy and may be a more common source of genomic complexity in sanguivorous animals than the evolution of new genes [86]. This led to the identification of novel and convergently recruited venom proteins in blood-feeding leeches and vampire bats [86].

Table 1. Leech salivary proteins from *H. medicinalis, H. verbana* or *H. orientalis*. Isoforms of individual proteins are not shown.

Salivary Protein	Mechanism of Action	Biological Significance	Reference
Hirustasin (Mass: 5.866 kDa)	Tissue kallikrein inhibitor and inhibitor of trypsin, chymotrypsin and neutrophil cathepsin G	Anti-inflammatory	[55]
Apyrase (Mass: 45 kDa)	Cleavage of adenosine 5′-diphosphate	Inhibitor of platelet aggregation	[67]
Bdellin B-3 (Mass: 6.141 kDa)	Inhibitor of plasmin, trypsin and sperm acrosin	Anti-inflammatory	[68]
Calin (Mass: 65 kDa)	Prevents the binding of von Willebrand factor to collagen	Inhibitor of platelet aggregation	[50,69]
Collagenase (Mass: 50 kDa)	Cleavage of collagen	Collagen digestion	[70]
Destabilase (Mass: 12.6–12.9 kDa)	Cleavage of fibrin clots, cleavage of peptidoglycans in bacterial walls	Anticoagulant/antimicrobial	[71–73]
Eglin C (Mass: 8.1 kDa)	Neutrophil elastase inhibitor, cathepsin G inhibitor	Anti-inflammatory	[74,75]
Hirudin (Mass: 7.1 kDa)	Thrombin inhibitor	Anticoagulant	[48,76]
Hirudin-like factors (Mass: 4.27–6.67; isoforms HLF1-HLF3)	Unknown for the three European species		[77,78]
Hyaluronidase (Mass: 27.5 kDa)	Cleavage of hyaluronic acid	Extracellular matrix digestion	[79]
Leech-derived tryptase inhibitor (Mass: 4.7 kDa)	Mast cell tryptase inhibitor	Anti-inflammatory	[56,57]
Leech carboxypeptidase inhibitor (Mass: 7.2 kDa)	Carboxypeptidase B inhibitor	Unclear	[80]
Saratin (Mass: 12 kDa)	Inhibits the binding of von Willebrand factor to collagen	Inhibitor of platelet aggregation	[51,81]
Yagin (Mass: 15.4 kDa)	Factor Xa inhibitor	Anticoagulant	[82]

Evolutionary models explaining the adaptation of leech salivary proteins to specific hosts are still a matter of debate. Current challenges include the lack of well-characterized proteins in terms of mode of action and target. The isoproteins in leech saliva may have more than one target in the host, or their activity may be dependent on pH, temperature, the season or the developmental phase. Both the redundancy of salivary proteins (multiple proteins directed against the same target) and the potential cooperative interactions among multiple salivary proteins should be considered. The interplay of several salivary proteins can be seen in the bloodsucking arthropod *Rhodnius prolixus*, which produces four isoforms of salivary nitrophorin. All of them are vasodilators (working in cooperation) and histamine suppressors, but one is a strong inhibitor of factor IXa, another is a weaker anticoagulant and the remaining two isoforms appear to have lost their anticoagulant activity [87].

4. Antistasins as a Representative Leech Salivary Protein Family

Several antistasins were identified in leech species, including (1) the prototype antistasin, isolated from the salivary glands of the Mexican leech, *Haementeria officials*; (2) hirustasin and bdellastasin, identified in *H. medicinalis*; (3) ghilanten, identified in *Haementeria ghilianii*; (4) piguamerin, identified in *H. nipponia*; and (5) guamerin I (*H. nipponia*) and guamerin II, isolated from *Whitmania edentula* [88–93]. All of these cysteine-rich proteins contain several repeated motifs, each consisting of six conserved cysteine and two conserved glycine residues [94], but differ widely in terms of structure and function [89].

The prototype antistasin is a polypeptide of 119 amino acids that includes 10 disulfide bridges and a twofold internal repeat, suggesting that it arose following a gene duplication event [54,95]. This protein is a potent competitive inhibitor of coagulation factor Xa, a serine protease which cleaves antistasin at position Arg^{34} to yield a 10-kDa fragment [91]. The presence of antistasin therefore maintains host blood in a liquid state [54]. The medical applications of antistasin are not restricted to its role as an anticoagulant because its ability to inhibit serine proteases was also shown to prevent the spread of tumors, probably by reducing the likelihood of metastasis [96].

Additional antistasin-type proteins known to inhibit factor Xa include ghilanten [93] and yagin [82]. In contrast, guamerin I [97] and guamerin II [88] are specific inhibitors of neutrophil and pancreas elastases, whereas hirustasin is a potent inhibitor of trypsin, chymotrypsin, cathepsin G and tissue kallikrein [55]. In contrast to hirustasin, piguamerin does not inhibit tissue kallikrein, but does inhibit plasma kallikrein and trypsin [89]. The P1 residue of the reactive site determines the specificity of serine protease inhibitors [98]. If it is lysine or arginine, the inhibitor targets trypsin and trypsin-like enzymes. However, if it is tyrosine, phenylalanine, leucine or methionine, then chymotrypsin or chymotrypsin-like enzymes are more likely targets [99]. If it is alanine or serine, the inhibitor will tend to target elastase-like enzymes [98,99]. This was confirmed for a serine protease inhibitor containing antistasin and whey acidic protein (WAP) domains (StmAW-SPI) isolated from the tropical sea cucumber *Stichopus monotuberculatus* [98].

5. Leech Salivary Proteins as Drug Leads

Natural products from plants and animals provide an astonishingly diverse source of active compounds for drug development and clinical trials [100] and can be used as tools for pharmacological or biotechnological applications [101]. Medicinal leeches are promising for the treatment of diseases associated with pain, inflammation or blood disorders. However, the use of living animals poses a risk of infection. Leeches carry bacteria in their digestive tract [10,11] and on their skin, and these bacteria could infect patients undergoing treatment. The use of antibiotic prophylaxis to minimize post-operative leech-borne infections only partially addresses this issue and encourages the emergence of multidrug-resistant pathogens in a clinical setting [102]. One strategy to avoid contact with leeches altogether is the extraction and purification of individual salivary components and their production as recombinant proteins to be administered using sterile equipment. Linked sets of proteomic and transcriptomic data are needed to explore bioactive proteins and peptides derived from natural animal sources such as leech saliva [101]. Such combined analysis (e.g., RNA-Seq + MALDI-TOF-MS or

NanoLC-ESI-MS) allows researchers to compare salivary gland transcripts containing signal peptides with salivary proteins secreted into the host wound. Because European medical leeches have thousands of single salivary glands cells and their saliva secretion mechanisms are still unknown, it is necessary to prepare salivary gland cell tissues for proteomics. Comparative proteomic analysis of unfed leeches and fed leeches enabled researchers to separate proteins and to distinguish between secretory and nonsecretory proteins [63]. The combination of proteomics and transcriptomics followed by a conserved domain search made it possible to predict the functional domains of salivary proteins that may be responsible for the observed therapeutic effects of leeches, leading to the identification of new anti-inflammatory, analgesic or pro-coagulant leads (Figure 1). The pharmacological potential of a protein can only be established if its target is known, and this is best achieved by expressing the drug lead as a recombinant protein so that ample amounts are available for testing in vitro, in cells, in tissue-based assays and in animal models. Multiple assays are available for the detection of targets related to blood coagulation, pain pathways, antimicrobial activity, cytotoxicity and inflammation. Recombinant leech proteins can be expressed in bacteria [77,103], yeast [104–106], insect cells [107] or a cell-free expression system, or leech peptides can be prepared by chemical synthesis. Correct folding is important but difficult to control, because leech salivary proteins often contain numerous cysteine residues that form disulfide bonds and these structures must be replicated to ensure that synthetic and recombinant proteins remain stable and functional. Eglins are an identified leech salivary protein family without cysteine residues [74,75], while other described salivary proteins possess six cysteine residues (hirudin, hirudin-like factors, leech-derived tryptase inhibitor, bdellin-B3; saratin; [48,51,56,57,68,76,77,81]), eight cysteine residues (leech carboxypeptidase inhibitor; [80]), 10 cysteine residues (hirustasin; [55]) or 14 cysteine residues (destabilase; [71–73]). The formation of disulfide bonds is one of the most important post-translational modifications, ensuring the bioactivity of the protein and underpinnig the assignment of the protein to a given class or family [101]. Correct folding can be confirmed by X-ray crystallography or nuclear magnetic resonance (NMR) spectroscopy, but large quantities of protein are required. In contrast, preliminary structural analysis with limited sample quantities is possible using approaches such as electron capture dissociation (ECD) or electron transfer dissociation (ETD) coupled with liquid chromatography mass spectrometry (LC-MS) using a triple quadrupole ion trap mass spectrometer [108].

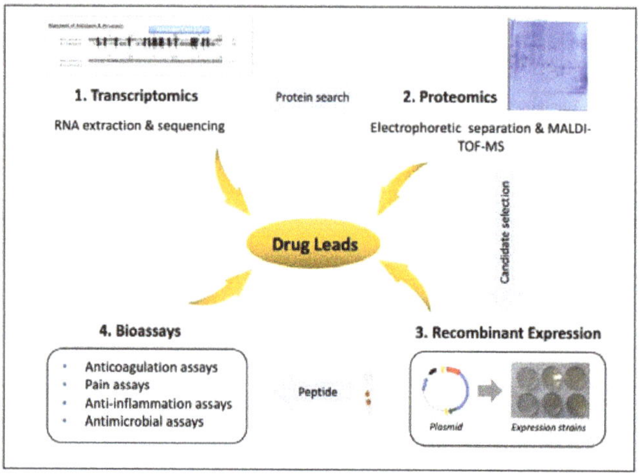

Figure 1. Workflow for the analysis of leech salivary proteins as drug leads. To analyze individual leech salivary proteins, a combination of transcriptomics and proteomics provides the protein sequences. Recombinant proteins are expressed to test their activities in cells, tissues and animal models, for example, to determine whether they possess anticoagulation, analgesic, anti-inflammatory or antimicrobial effects.

Author Contributions: All authors have read and agreed to the published version of the manuscript.

Funding: The authors acknowledge the generous funding by the Hessen State Ministry of Higher Education, Research and the Arts (HMWK) for the project "Animal Venomics" via the LOEWE Center "Translational Biodiversity Genomics".

Acknowledgments: The authors thank Richard M. Twyman for editing the manuscript.

Conflicts of Interest: The authors declare no conflict of interest.

References

1. Dickinson, M.H.; Lent, C.M. Feeding behavior of the medicinal leech, *Hirudo medicinalis* L. *J. Comp. Physiol. A* **1984**, *154*, 449–455. [CrossRef]
2. Elliott, J.M.; Tullett, P.A. The effects of temperature, atmospheric pressure and season on the swimming activity of the medicinal leech, *Hirudo medicinalis* (Hirudinea; Hirudinidae), in a Lake District tarn. *Freshwater Biol.* **1986**, *16*, 405–415. [CrossRef]
3. Hammersen, F. The muscle structure in the pharyngeal wall of *Hirudo medicinalis* and *Haemopsis sanguisuga*. *Z. Zellforsch. Mikrosk. Anat.* **1963**, *60*, 797–814. [CrossRef] [PubMed]
4. Marshall, C.G.; Lent, C.M. Excitability and secretory activity in the salivary gland cells of jawed leeches (Hirudinea: Gnathobdellida). *J. Exp. Biol.* **1988**, *137*, 89–105. [PubMed]
5. Lent, C.M.; Fliegner, K.H.; Freedman, E.; Dickinson, M.H. Ingestive behaviour and physiology of the medicinal leech. *J. Exp. Biol.* **1988**, *137*, 513–527. [PubMed]
6. Zerbst-Boroffka, I. Ion transport mechanism in basal and diuretic nephridia of the leech, *Hirudo medicinalis* L. *Comp. Biochem. Physiol.* **1973**, *86*, 151–154. [CrossRef]
7. Roters, F.J.; Zebe, E. Protease inhibitors in the alimentary tract of the medicinal leech *Hirudo medicinalis*: In vivo and in vitro studies. *J. Comp. Physiol. B* **1992**, *162*, 85–92. [CrossRef]
8. Roters, F.J. Untersuchungen über Die Verdauungsphysiologie des Blutegels *Hirudo medicinalis*. Ph.D. Thesis, University of Münster, Münster, Germany, 1985.
9. Indergand, S.; Graf, J. Ingested blood contributes to the specificity of the symbiosis of *Aeromonas veronii* biovar sobria and *Hirudo medicinalis*, the medicinal leech. *Appl. Environ. Microbiol.* **2000**, *66*, 4735–4741. [CrossRef]
10. Maltz, M.A.; Bomar, L.; Lapierre, P.; Morrison, H.G.; McClure, E.A.; Sogin, M.L.; Graf, J. Metagenomic analysis of the medicinal leech gut microbiota. *Front. Microbiol.* **2014**, *5*, 151. [CrossRef]
11. Siddall, M.E.; Min, G.S.; Fontanella, F.M.; Phillips, A.J.; Watson, S.C. Bacterial symbiont and salivary peptide evolution in the context of leech phylogeny. *Parasitology* **2011**, *138*, 1815–1827. [CrossRef]
12. Bomar, L.; Maltz, M.; Colston, S.; Graf, J. Directed culturing of microorganisms using metatranscriptomics. *Mbio* **2011**, *2*, e00012-11. [CrossRef] [PubMed]
13. Maltz, M.A.; Graf, J. The Type II Secretion System Is Essential for Erythrocyte Lysis and Gut Colonization by the Leech Digestive Tract Symbiont *Aeromonas veronii*. *Appl. Environ. Microbiol.* **2011**, *77*, 597–603. [CrossRef] [PubMed]
14. Dziekońska-Rynko, J.; Bielecki, A.; Palińska, K. Activity of selected hydrolytic enzymes from leeches (Clitellata: Hirudinida) with different feeding strategies. *Biologia* **2009**, *64*, 370–376. [CrossRef]
15. Abdualkader, A.M.; Ghawi, A.M.; Alaama, M.; Awang, M.; Merzouk, A. Leech therapeutic applications. *Indian J. Pharm. Sci.* **2013**, *75*, 127–137. [PubMed]
16. Deganc, M.; Zdravic, F. Venous congestion of flaps treated by application of leeches. *Br. J. Plast. Surg.* **1960**, *13*, 187–192. [CrossRef]
17. Ansari, S.; Fasihuzzaman, N.; Jabeen, A.; Sultana, A.; Khan, A.Q. Post-auricular leech therapy reduced headache & migraine days in chronic migraine. *J. Drug Deliv. Ther.* **2019**, *9*, 75–80.
18. Bakhshi, M.; Jalalian, B.; Valian, M.; Shariati, S.; Saeidi, T.; Ranjbar, H. Can leech therapy be used as an alternative treatment for controlling migraine headache? A Pilot Study. *Acta Fac. Med. Naissensis* **2015**, *32*, 189–197. [CrossRef]
19. Andereya, S.; Stanzel, S.; Maus, U.; Mueller-Rath, R.; Mumme, T.; Siebert, C.H.; Stock, F.; Schneider, U. Assessment of leech therapy for knee osteoarthritis: A randomized study. *Acta Orthop.* **2008**, *79*, 235–243. [CrossRef]

20. Michalsen, A.; Moebus, S.; Spahn, G.; Esch, T.; Langhorst, J.; Dobos, G.J. Leech therapy for symptomatic treatment of knee osteoarthritis: Results and implications of a pilot study. *Leech* **2002**, *84*, 88.
21. Michalsen, A.; Klotz, S.; Lüdtke, R.; Moebus, S.; Spahn, G.; Dobos, G.J. Effectiveness of leech therapy in osteoarthritis of the knee: A randomized, controlled trial. *Ann. Intern. Med.* **2003**, *139*, 724–730. [CrossRef]
22. Rai, P.K.; Singh, A.K.; Singh, O.P.; Rai, N.P.; Dwivedi, A.K. Efficacy of leech therapy in the management of osteoarthritis (Sandhivata). *Ayu* **2011**, *32*, 213–217. [CrossRef] [PubMed]
23. Shiffa, M.; Siddiquib, M.A.; Sultana, A.; Zaman, F.; Fahamiya, N.; Akhtarc, M.U. Comparative clinical evaluation of leech therapy in the treatment of knee osteoarthritis. *Eur. J. Integr.* **2013**, *5*, 261–269. [CrossRef]
24. Stange, R.; Moser, C.; Hopfenmueller, W.; Mansmann, U.; Buehring, M.; Uehleke, B. Randomised controlled trial with medical leeches for osteoarthritis of the knee. *Complement. Ther. Med.* **2012**, *20*, 1–7. [CrossRef] [PubMed]
25. Zaidi, S.M.; Abbas Jamil, S.S.; Sultana, A.; Zaman, F.; Fuzail, M. Safety and efficacy of leeching therapy for symptomatic knee osteoarthritis using Indian medicinal leech. *Indian J. Tradit. Knowl.* **2009**, *8*, 437–442.
26. Hanif, H.; Nouri, M.; Amirjamshidi, A. Medicinal leech therapy in neurosurgical practice. *J. Inj. Violence Res.* **2012**, *4*, 72.
27. Kusnetsova, L.P.; Lusov, V.A.; Volov, N.A.; Smirnova, N.A.; Bogdanova, L.S. Hirudotherapy in complex treatment of chronic heart failure. *Russ. J. Cardiol.* **2008**, *2*, 28–30.
28. Nargiza, E.; Mirdjuraev, E.; Ergasheva, N. Leech therapy to prevent ischemic stroke: p1231. *Eur. J. Neurol.* **2010**, *17*, 170.
29. Shankar, K.P.; Rao, S.D.; Umar, S.N.; Gopalakrishnaiah, V. A clinical trial for evaluation of leech application in the management of Vicarcikā (Eczema). *Anc. Sci. Life* **2014**, *33*, 236–241. [CrossRef]
30. Amarprakash, P.D. Case study of leech application in diabetic foot ulcer. *Int. J. Res. Ayurveda Pharm.* **2012**, *3*, 748–751.
31. Na, H.J. The Effects of live leech (*Hirudo Medicinalis*) therapy on diabetic foot: A clinical case report. *Korean J. Orient. Med.* **2003**, *24*, 136–138.
32. Zaidi, S.A. Unani treatment and leech therapy saved the diabetic foot of a patient from amputation. *Int. Wound J.* **2016**, *13*, 263–264. [CrossRef] [PubMed]
33. Asgari, S.A.; Rostami, S.; Teimoori, M. Leech therapy for treating priapism: Case report. *Iran. J. Public Health* **2017**, *46*, 985–988. [PubMed]
34. Bumpous, J.M.; Byrne, P.J.; Bernstein, P.E. The use of medicinal leeches to treat macroglossia secondary to blunt trauma. *Otolaryngol. Head Neck Surg.* **2001**, *125*, 649–650. [CrossRef] [PubMed]
35. Ramzan, M.; Droog, W.; Sleeswijk Visser, S.; van Roessel, E.W.; Meynaar, I.A. Leech got your tongue? Haematoma of the tongue treated with medicinal leeches: A case report. *Neth. J. Crit. Care* **2010**, *14*, 268–270.
36. Kalender, M.E.; Comez, G.; Sevinc, A.; Dirier, A.; Camci, C. Leech therapy for symptomatic relief of cancer pain. *Pain Med.* **2010**, *11*, 443–445. [CrossRef] [PubMed]
37. Philip, J.; Armitage, D.W.; Phillips, K.R.; Parr, N.J. Leech therapy for penoscrotal oedema in patients with hormone-refractory prostate carcinoma. *BJU Int.* **2003**, *91*, 579–580. [CrossRef]
38. Darestani, K.D.; Mirghazanfari, S.M.; Moghaddam, K.G.; Hejazi, S. Leech therapy for linear incisional skin-wound healing in rats. *J. Acupunct. Meridian Stud.* **2014**, *7*, 194–201. [CrossRef]
39. Ghods, R.; Abdi, M.; Pourrahimi, M.; Dabaghian, F.H. Leech therapy indications: A scoping review. *Tradit. Med. Res.* **2019**, *4*, 118–130.
40. Gunawan, F.; Wibowo, Y.R.; Bunawan, N.C.; Turner, J.H. Controversy: Hirudotherapy (leech therapy) as an alternative treatment for osteoarthritis. *Acta Med. Indones.* **2015**, *47*, 176–180.
41. Pilcher, H. Medicinal leeches: Stuck on you. *Nature* **2004**, *432*, 10–11. [CrossRef]
42. Talbot, B.; Balvín, O.; Vonhof, M.J.; Broders, H.G.; Fenton, B.; Keyghobadi, N. Host association and selection on salivary protein genes in bed bugs and related blood-feeding ectoparasites. *R. Soc. Open Sci.* **2017**, *4*, 170446. [CrossRef] [PubMed]
43. Van Valen, L. A new evolutionary law. In *Evolutionary Theory*; Band 1; University of Chicago Press: Chicago, IL, USA, 1973; pp. 1–30.
44. Babenko, V.V.; Podgorny, O.V.; Manuvera, V.A.; Kasianov, A.S.; Manolov, A.I.; Grafskaia, E.N.; Shirokov, D.A.; Kurdyumov, A.S.; Vinogradov, D.V.; Nikitina, A.S.; et al. Draft genome sequences of *Hirudo medicinalis* and salivary transcriptome of three closely related medicinal leeches. *BioRxiv* 2018. [CrossRef]

45. Baskova, I.P.; Zavalova, L.L. Proteinase inhibitors from the medicinal leech *Hirudo medicinalis*. *Biochemistry* **2001**, *66*, 703–714. [PubMed]
46. Baskova, I.P.; Zavalova, L.L.; Basanova, A.V.; Moshkovskii, S.A.; Zgoda, V.G. Protein profiling of the medicinal leech salivary gland secretion by proteomic analytical methods. *Biochemistry* **2004**, *69*, 770–775. [CrossRef]
47. Hildebrandt, J.-P.; Lemke, S. Small bite, large impact—Saliva and salivary molecules in the medical leech, *Hirudo medicinalis*. *Naturwissenschaften* **2011**, *98*, 995–1008. [CrossRef]
48. Ascenzi, P.; Amiconi, G.; Bode, W.; Bolognesi, M.; Coletta, M.; Menegatti, E. Proteinase inhibitors from the European medicinal leech *Hirudo medicinalis*: Structural, functional and biomedical aspects. *Mol. Asp. Med.* **1995**, *16*, 215–313. [CrossRef]
49. Baskova, I.P.; Khalil, S.; Nartikova, V.F.; Paskhina, T.S. Inhibition of plasma kallikrein. Kininase and kinin-like activities of preparations from the medicinal leeches. *Thromb. Res.* **1992**, *67*, 721–730. [CrossRef]
50. Deckmyn, H.; Stassen, J.M.; Vreys, I.; Van Houtte, E.; Sawyer, R.T.; Vermylen, J. Calin from *Hirudo medicinalis*, an inhibitor of platelet adhesion to collagen, prevents platelet-rich thrombosis in hamsters. *Blood* **1995**, *85*, 712–719. [CrossRef]
51. Gronwald, W.; Bomke, J.; Maurer, T.; Domogalla, B.; Huber, F.; Schumann, F.; Kremer, W.; Fink, F.; Rysiok, T.; Frech, M.; et al. Structure of the leech protein saratin and characterization of its binding to collagen. *J. Mol. Biol.* **2008**, *381*, 913–927. [CrossRef]
52. Haycraft, J.B. On the action of a secretion obtained from the medicinal leech on the coagulation of the blood. *Proc. R. Soc. Lond. B* **1884**, *36*, 478–487.
53. Linker, A.; Meyer, K.; Hoffman, P. The production of hyaluronate oligosaccharides by leech hyaluronidase and alkali. *J. Biol. Chem.* **1960**, *235*, 924–927. [PubMed]
54. Mittl, P.R.; Di Marco, S.; Fendrich, G.; Pohlig, G.; Heim, J.; Sommerhoff, C.; Fritz, H.; Priestle, J.P.; Grütter, M.G. A new structural class of serine protease inhibitors revealed by the structure of the hirustasin-kallikrein complex. *Structure* **1997**, *5*, 253–264. [CrossRef]
55. Söllner, C.; Mentele, R.; Eckerskorn, C.; Fritz, H.; Sommerhoff, C.P. Isolation and characterization of hirustasin, an antistasin-type serine-proteinase inhibitor from the medical leech *Hirudo medicinalis*. *Eur. J. Biochem.* **1994**, *219*, 937–943. [CrossRef] [PubMed]
56. Sommerhoff, C.P.; Söllner, C.; Mentele, R.; Piechottka, G.P.; Auerswald, E.A.; Fritz, H. A Kazal-type inhibitor of human mast cell tryptase: Isolation from the medical leech *Hirudo medicinalis*, characterization, and sequence analysis. *Biol. Chem. Hoppe Seyler* **1994**, *375*, 685–694. [CrossRef]
57. Stubbs, M.T.; Morenweiser, R.; Stürzebecher, J.; Bauer, M.; Bode, W.; Huber, R.; Piechottka, G.P.; Matschiner, G.; Sommerhoff, C.P.; Fritz, H.; et al. The three-dimensional structure of recombinant leech-derived tryptase inhibitor in complex with trypsin. Implications for the structure of human mast cell tryptase and its inhibition. *J. Biol. Chem.* **1997**, *272*, 19931–19937. [CrossRef]
58. Vilahur, G.; Duran, X.; Juan-Babot, O.; Casani, L.; Badimon, L. Antithrombotic effects of saratin on human atherosclerotic plaques. *Thromb. Haemost.* **2004**, *92*, 191–226. [CrossRef]
59. Min, G.-S.; Sarkar, I.N.; Siddall, M.E. Salivary Transcriptome of the North American Medicinal Leech, *Macrobdella decora*. *J. Parasitol.* **2010**, *96*, 1211–1221. [CrossRef]
60. Lu, Z.; Shi, P.; You, H.; Liu, Y.; Chen, S. Transcriptomic analysis of the salivary gland of medicinal leech *Hirudo nipponia*. *PLoS ONE* **2018**, *13*, e0205875. [CrossRef]
61. Kvist, S.; Min, G.-S.; Siddall, M.E. Diversity and selective pressures of anticoagulants in three medicinal leeches (Hirudinida: Hirudinidae, Macrobdellidae). *Ecol. Evol.* **2013**, *3*, 918–933. [CrossRef]
62. Khan, M.S.; Guan, D.-L.; Kvist, S.; Ma, L.B.; Xie, J.X.; Xu, S.Q. Transcriptomics and differential gene expression in *Whitmania pigra* (Annelida: Clitellata: Hirudinida: Hirudinidae): Contrasting feeding and fasting modes. *Ecol. Evol.* **2019**, *9*, 4706–4719. [CrossRef]
63. Lemke, S.; Müller, C.; Hildebrandt, J.-P. Be ready at any time: Postprandial synthesis of salivary proteins in salivary gland cells of the haematophagous leech *Hirudo verbana*. *J. Exp. Biol.* **2016**, *219*, 1139–1145. [CrossRef]
64. Franta, Z.; Vogel, H.; Lehmann, R.; Rupp, O.; Goesmann, A.; Vilcinskas, A. Next generation sequencing identifies five major classes of potentially therapeutic enzymes secreted by *Lucilia sericata* medical maggots. *BioMed Res. Int.* **2016**, *2016*, 8285428. [CrossRef] [PubMed]

65. Chaves-Moreira, D.; Matsubara, F.; Schemczssen-Graeff, Z.; De Bona, E.; Heidemann, V.; Guerra-Duarte, C.; Gremski, L.; Chávez-Olórtegui, C.; Senff-Ribeiro, A.; Chaim, O.; et al. Brown Spider (Loxosceles) venom toxins as potential biotools for the development of novel therapeutics. *Toxins* **2019**, *11*, 355. [CrossRef] [PubMed]
66. Feygina, E.; Katrukha, G.; Semenov, G. Neutral Endopeptidase (Neprilysin) in Therapy and Diagnostics: Yin and Yang. *Biochemistry* **2019**, *84*, 1346–1358. [CrossRef] [PubMed]
67. Rigbi, M.; Orevi, M.; Eldor, A. Platelet aggregation and coagulation inhibitors in leech saliva and their roles in leech therapy. In *Seminars in Thrombosis and Hemostasis*; Thieme Medical Publishers, Inc.: New York, NY, USA, 1996; Volume 22, pp. 273–278.
68. Fink, E.; Rehm, H.; Gippner, C.; Bode, W.; Eulitz, M.; Machleidt, W.; Fritz, H. The primary structure of bdellin B-3 from the leech Hirudo medicinalis. Bdellin B-3 is a compact proteinase inhibitor of a "non-classical" Kazal type. It is present in the leech in a high molecular mass form. *Biol. Chem. Hoppe Seyler* **1986**, *367*, 1235–1242. [CrossRef] [PubMed]
69. Munro, R.; Jones, C.P.; Sawyer, R.T. Calin—A platelet adhesion inhibitor from the saliva of the medicinal leech. *Blood Coagul. Fibrinolysis* **1991**, *2*, 179–184. [CrossRef]
70. Rigbi, M.; Levy, H.; Iraqi, F.; Teitelbaum, M.; Orevi, M.; Alajoutsijarvi, A.; Horovitz, A.; Galun, R. The saliva of the medicinal leech *Hirudo medicinalis*—I. Biochemical characterization of the high molecular weight fraction. *Comp. Biochem. Physiol. B* **1987**, *87*, 567–573. [CrossRef]
71. Baskova, I.P.; Zavalova, L.L. Polyfunctionality of lysozyme destabilase from the medicinal leech. *Russ. J. Bioorg. Chem.* **2008**, *34*, 304–309. [CrossRef]
72. Zavalova, L.L.; Baskova, I.P.; Lukyanov, S.A.; Sass, A.V.; Snezhkov, E.V.; Akopov, S.B.; Artamonova, I.I.; Archipova, V.S.; Nesmeyanov, V.A.; Kozlov, D.G.; et al. Destabilase from the medicinal leech is a representative of a novel family of lysozymes. *Biochim. Biophys. Acta (BBA) Protein Struct. Mol. Enzymol.* **2000**, *1478*, 69–77. [CrossRef]
73. Zavalova, L.L.; Yudina, T.G.; Artamonova, I.I.; Baskova, I.P. Antibacterial non-glycosidase activity of invertebrate destabilase-lysozyme and of its helical amphipathic peptides. *Chemotherapy* **2006**, *52*, 158–160. [CrossRef]
74. Braun, N.J.; Bodmer, J.L.; Virca, G.D.; Metz-Virca, G.; Maschler, R.; Bieth, J.G.; Schnebli, H.P. Kinetic studies on the interaction of eglin c with human leukocyte elastase and cathepsin G. *Biol. Chem. Hoppe Seyler* **1987**, *368*, 299–308. [CrossRef] [PubMed]
75. Junger, W.G.; Hallstrom, S.; Redl, H.; Schlag, G. Inhibition of human, ovine, and baboon neutrophil elastase with eglin c and secretory leukocyte proteinase inhibitor. *Biol. Chem. Hoppe Seyler* **1992**, *373*, 119–122. [CrossRef] [PubMed]
76. Markwardt, F. Untersuchungen über hirudin. *Naturwiss* **1955**, *42*, 537–538. [CrossRef]
77. Müller, C.; Mescke, K.; Liebig, S.; Mahfoud, H.; Lemke, S.; Hildebrandt, J.-P. More than just one: Multiplicity of Hirudins and Hirudin-like Factors in the Medicinal Leech, *Hirudo medicinalis*. *Mol. Genet. Genom.* **2016**, *291*, 227–240. [CrossRef] [PubMed]
78. Müller, C.; Haase, M.; Lemke, S.; Hildebrandt, J.-P. Hirudins and hirudin-like factors in *Hirudinidae*: Implications for function and phylogenetic relationships. *Parasitol. Res.* **2017**, *116*, 313–325. [CrossRef]
79. Hovingh, P.; Linker, A. Hyaluronidase activity in leeches (Hirudinea). *Comp. Biochem. Physiol. B Biochem. Mol. Biol.* **1999**, *124*, 319–326. [CrossRef]
80. Reverter, D.; Vendrell, J.; Canals, F.; Horstmann, J.; Aviles, F.X.; Fritz, H.; Sommerhoff, C.P. A carboxypeptidase inhibitor from the medical leech Hirudo medicinalis. Isolation, sequence analysis, cDNA cloning, recombinant expression, and characterization. *J. Biol. Chem.* **1998**, *273*, 32927–32933. [CrossRef]
81. Domogalla, B. NMR-Lösungsstruktur des Proteins Saratin, Strukturelle Charakterisierung der Saratin-Kollagen-Interaktion und des Carausius Morosus-hyperthrehalosämischen Hormons (Cam-HrTH-I). Ph.D. Thesis, University of Regensburg, Regensburg, Germany, 2005.
82. Kornowski, R.; Eldor, A.; Werber, M.M.; Ezov, N.; Zwang, E.; Nimrod, A.; Chernine, A.; Finkelstein, A.; Panet, A.; Laniado, S.; et al. Enhancement of recombinant tissue-type plasminogen activator thrombolysis with a selective factor Xa inhibitor derived from the leech *Hirudo medicinalis*: Comparison with heparin and hirudin in a rabbit thrombosis model. *Coron. Artery Dis.* **1996**, *7*, 903–909. [CrossRef]

83. Schwarz, A.; Cabezas-Cruz, A.; Kopecký, J.; Valdés, J.J. Understanding the evolutionary structural variability and target specificity of tick salivary Kunitz peptides using next generation transcriptome data. *BMC Evol. Biol.* **2014**, *14*, 4. [CrossRef]
84. Andersen, J.F. Structure and mechanism in salivary proteins from blood-feeding arthropods. *Toxicon* **2010**, *56*, 1120–1129. [CrossRef]
85. Mans, B.J.; Neitz, A.W.H. Adaptation of ticks to a blood-feeding environment: Evolution from a functional perspective. *Insect Biochem. Mol. Biol.* **2004**, *34*, 1–17. [CrossRef] [PubMed]
86. Phillips, C.D.; Baker, R.J. Secretory gene recruitments in vampire bat salivary adaptation and potential convergences with sanguivorous leeches. *Front. Ecol. Evol.* **2015**. [CrossRef]
87. Champagne, D.E. Antihemostatic molecules from saliva of blood-feeding arthropods. *Pathophysiol. Haemost. Thromb.* **2005**, *34*, 221–227. [CrossRef] [PubMed]
88. Kim, D.R.; Hong, S.J.; Ha, K.S.; Joe, C.O.; Kang, K.W. A cysteine-rich serine protease inhibitor (Guamerin II) from the non-blood sucking leech *Whitmania edentula*: Biochemical characterization and amino acid sequence analysis. *J. Enzym. Inhib.* **1996**, *10*, 81–91. [CrossRef]
89. Kim, D.R.; Kang, K.W. Amino acid sequence of piguamerin, an antistasin-type protease inhibitor from the blood sucking leech *Hirudo nipponia. Eur. J. Biochem.* **1998**, *254*, 692–697. [CrossRef]
90. Kim, H.; Chu, T.T.; Kim, D.Y.; Kim, D.R.; Nguyen, C.M.; Choi, J.; Lee, J.R.; Hahn, M.J.; Kim, K.K. The crystal structure of guamerin in complex with chymotrypsin and the development of an elastase-specific inhibitor. *J. Mol. Biol.* **2008**, *376*, 184–192. [CrossRef]
91. Nutt, E.M.; Jain, D.; Lenny, A.B.; Schaffer, L.; Siegl, P.K.; Dunwiddie, C.T. Purification and characterization of recombinant antistasin: A leech-derived inhibitor of coagulation factor Xa. *Arch. Biochem. Biophys.* **1991**, *285*, 37–44. [CrossRef]
92. Rester, U.; Bode, W.; Moser, M.; Parry, M.A.; Huber, R.; Auerswald, E. Structure of the complex of the antistasin-type inhibitor bdellastasin with trypsin and modelling of the bdellastasin-microplasmin system. *J. Mol. Biol.* **1999**, *293*, 93–106. [CrossRef]
93. Rester, U.; Bode, W.; Sampaio, C.A.M.; Auerswald, E.; Lopes, A.P.Y. Cloning, purification, crystallization and preliminary X-ray diffraction analysis of the antistasin-type inhibitor ghilanten (domain I) from *Haementeria ghilianii* in complex with porcine beta-trypsin. *Acta Crystallogr. D Biol. Crystallogr.* **2001**, *57*, 1038–1041. [CrossRef]
94. Joo, S.S.; Won, T.J.; Kim, J.S.; Yoo, Y.M.; Tak, E.S.; Park, S.Y.; Park, H.Y.; Hwang, K.W.; Park, S.C.; Lee, D.I. Inhibition of Coagulation Activation and Inflammation by a Novel Factor Xa Inhibitor Synthesized from the Earthworm *Eisenia andrei. Biol. Pharm. Bull.* **2009**, *32*, 253–258. [CrossRef]
95. Holstein, T.W.; Mala, C.; Kurz, E.; Bauer, K.; Greber, M.; David, C.N. The primitive metazoan Hydra expresses antistasin, a serine protease inhibitor of vertebrate blood coagulation: cDNA cloning, cellular localization and developmental regulation. *FEBS Lett.* **1992**, *309*, 288–292. [CrossRef]
96. Han, J.H.; Law, S.W.; Keller, P.M.; Kniskern, P.J.; Silberklang, M.; Tung, J.-S.; Gasic, T.B.; Gasic, G.J.; Friedman, P.A.; Ellis, R.W. Cloning and expression of cDNA encoding antistasin, a leech-derived protein having anti-coagulant and anti-metastatic properties. *Proc. Natl. Acad. Sci. USA* **1989**, *83*, 1084–1088. [CrossRef]
97. Jung, H.I.; Kim, S.I.; Ha, K.S.; Joe, C.O.; Kang, K.W. Isolation and characterization of guamerin, a new human leukocyte elastase inhibitor from *Hirudo nipponia. J. Biol. Chem.* **1995**, *270*, 13879–13884. [CrossRef] [PubMed]
98. Yan, A.; Ren, C.; Chen, T.; Jiang, X.; Sun, H.; Hu, C. Identification and functional characterization of a novel antistasin/WAP-like serine protease inhibitor from the tropical sea cucumber, *Stichopus monotuberculatus. Fish Shellfish Immunol.* **2016**, *59*, 203–212. [CrossRef] [PubMed]
99. Laskowski, M., Jr.; Kato, I. Protein inhibitors of proteinases. *Annu. Rev. Biochem.* **1980**, *49*, 593–626. [CrossRef]
100. Harvey, A.L.; Edrada-Ebel, R.; Quinn, R.J. The re-emergence of natural products for drug discovery in the genomics era. *Nat. Rev. Drug Discov.* **2015**, *14*, 111–129. [CrossRef]
101. Kaas, Q.; Craik, D.J. Bioinformatics-Aided Venomics. *Toxins* **2015**, *7*, 2159–2187. [CrossRef]
102. Verriere, B.; Sabatier, B.; Carbonnelle, E.; Mainardi, J.L.; Prognon, P.; Whitaker, I.; Lantieri, L.; Hivelin, M. Medicinal leech therapy and Aeromonas spp. infection. *Eur. J. Clin. Microbiol. Infect. Dis.* **2016**, *35*, 1001–1006. [CrossRef]
103. Strube, K.H.; Kröger, B.; Bialojan, S.; Otte, M.; Dodt, J. Isolation, sequence analysis, and cloning of haemadin. An anticoagulant peptide from the Indian leech. *J. Biol. Chem.* **1993**, *268*, 8590–8595.

104. Marco, S.D.; Fendrich, G.; Knecht, R.; Strauss, A.; Pohlig, G.; Heim, J.; Priestle, J.-P.; Sommerhoff, C.P.; Grütter, M.G. Recombinant hirustasin: Production in yeast, crystallization, and interaction with serine proteases. *Protein Sci.* **1997**, *6*, 109–118. [CrossRef]
105. Pohlig, G.; Fendrich, G.; Knecht, R.; Eder, B.; Piechottka, G.; Sommerhoff, C.P.; Heim, J. Purification, characterization and biological evaluation of recombinant leech-derived tryptase inhibitor (rLDTI) expressed at high level in the yeast *Saccharomyces cerevisiae*. *Eur. J. Biochem.* **1996**, *241*, 619–626. [CrossRef] [PubMed]
106. Rosenfeld, S.A.; Nadeau, D.; Tirado, J.; Hollis, G.F.; Knabb, R.M.; Jia, S. Production and purification of recombinant hirudin expressed in the methylotrophic yeast *Pichia pastoris*. *Protein Expr. Purif.* **1996**, *8*, 476–482. [CrossRef] [PubMed]
107. Kollewe, C.; Vilcinskas, A. Production of recombinant proteins in insect cells. *Am. J. Bioch. Biotech.* **2013**, *9*, 255–271. [CrossRef]
108. Wu, S.-L.; Jiang, H.; Lu, Q.; Dai, S.; Hancock, W.S.; Karger, B.L. Mass Spectrometric Determination of Disulfide Linkages in Recombinant Therapeutic Proteins Using On-line LC-MS with Electron Transfer Dissociation (ETD). *Anal. Chem.* **2009**, *81*, 112–122. [CrossRef] [PubMed]

biomedicines

MDPI

Review

Curses or Cures: A Review of the Numerous Benefits Versus the Biosecurity Concerns of Conotoxin Research

Walden E. Bjørn-Yoshimoto [1], Iris Bea L. Ramiro [1], Mark Yandell [2,3], J. Michael McIntosh [4,5,6], Baldomero M. Olivera [4], Lars Ellgaard [7] and Helena Safavi-Hemami [1,4,8,*]

1 Department of Biomedical Sciences, University of Copenhagen, 2200 Copenhagen N, Denmark; walden@sund.ku.dk (W.E.B.-Y.); iris.ramiro@sund.ku.dk (I.B.L.R.)
2 Eccles Institute of Human Genetics, University of Utah, Salt Lake City, UT 84112, USA; myandell@genetics.utah.edu
3 Utah Center for Genetic Discovery, University of Utah, Salt Lake City, UT 84112, USA
4 School of Biological Sciences, University of Utah, Salt Lake City, UT 84112, USA; mcintosh.mike@gmail.com (J.M.M.); olivera@biology.utah.edu (B.M.O.)
5 George E. Whalen Veterans Affairs Medical Center, Salt Lake City, UT 84148, USA
6 Department of Psychiatry, University of Utah, Salt Lake City, UT 84108, USA
7 Department of Biology, Linderstrøm-Lang Centre for Protein Science, University of Copenhagen, 2200 Copenhagen N, Denmark; lellgaard@bio.ku.dk
8 Department of Biochemistry, University of Utah, Salt Lake City, UT 84112, USA
* Correspondence: safavihelena@sund.ku.dk

Received: 30 June 2020; Accepted: 19 July 2020; Published: 22 July 2020

Abstract: Conotoxins form a diverse group of peptide toxins found in the venom of predatory marine cone snails. Decades of conotoxin research have provided numerous measurable scientific and societal benefits. These include their use as a drug, diagnostic agent, drug leads, and research tools in neuroscience, pharmacology, biochemistry, structural biology, and molecular evolution. Human envenomations by cone snails are rare but can be fatal. Death by envenomation is likely caused by a small set of toxins that induce muscle paralysis of the diaphragm, resulting in respiratory arrest. The potency of these toxins led to concerns regarding the potential development and use of conotoxins as biological weapons. To address this, various regulatory measures have been introduced that limit the use and access of conotoxins within the research community. Some of these regulations apply to all of the ≈200,000 conotoxins predicted to exist in nature of which less than 0.05% are estimated to have any significant toxicity in humans. In this review we provide an overview of the many benefits of conotoxin research, and contrast these to the perceived biosecurity concerns of conotoxins and research thereof.

Keywords: conotoxin; conopeptide; cone snail; venom; envenomations; fatalities; drugs; biosecurity; biomedicine

1. Introduction

This article is divided into four sections. In the introductory section we provide an overview of the definition and classification of conotoxins, their chemical and pharmacological diversity, and a brief history of the methodologies used for conotoxin discovery. In the second section we highlight measurable scientific and societal benefits of conotoxin research with a view toward the future. The third section addresses biosecurity concerns and past and current regulations of conotoxins. In this section we discuss fatalities resulting from cone snail envenomations, toxicity data of selected conotoxins, the potential misuse of conotoxins as biological weapons, and their fictional use as murder weapons in the literature and popular media. In the concluding remarks, we assess the effectiveness and justification of regulations and suggest revisions of some current regulatory measures.

1.1. Conotoxin Definition, Classification, and Discovery

Venomous cone snails comprise a large and diverse lineage of marine gastropods within the family of Conidae (superfamily Conoidea) [1–4]. Based on molecular phylogenetic data, cone snails can be grouped into ≈57 distinct clades (or subgenera) [5], all of which use venom for prey capture (examples shown in Figure 1).

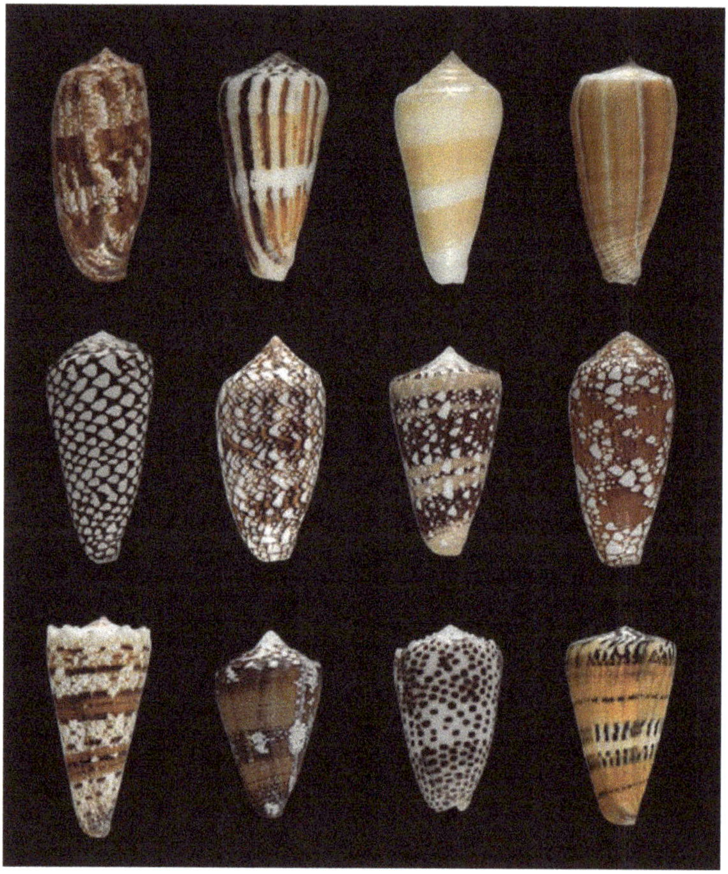

Figure 1. Shells of selected cone snail species from nine subgenera (for subgenus classification see [5]). Top row: fish-hunting cone snails (from left to right: *Conus geographus* (*Gastridium*), *Conus magus* and *Conus consors* (*Pionoconus*), *Conus purpurascens* (*Chelyconus*)), middle row: snail-hunting cone snails (*Conus marmoreus* (*Conus*), *Conus textile* and *Conus ammiralis (Cylinder)*, *Conus omaria* (*Darioconus*)), bottom row: worm-hunting species (*Conus imperialis* and *Conus regius* (*Stephanoconus*), *Conus pulicarius* (*Puncticulis*), *Conus mustelinus* (*Rhizoconus*)). Shells not to scale.

In the most basic sense, a conotoxin is a toxin identified from any of the ≈1000 living cone snails. The majority of conotoxins are gene-derived peptides that are synthesized at the ribosome and further processed in the endoplasmic reticulum (ER) and Golgi apparatus of the secretory cells of the venom gland. Small molecules of non-peptidic nature have also been isolated from cone snail venom. These have traditionally not been defined as "conotoxins", but instead named according to their characteristic chemical structures (for example [6,7]). Cone snail small molecules have not been subject to regulation and will therefore not be further discussed in this review.

The majority of conotoxins identified to date contain disulfide bonds that are formed between cysteine residues to confer structural stability and resistance against proteolytic degradation [8]. However, not all conotoxins contain cysteines and it has been suggested that conotoxins should be classified into those that are cysteine-rich (i.e., containing more than one disulfide bond) and those that are cysteine-poor (i.e., containing only one or no disulfide bonds). The term "conopeptide" was suggested to describe the latter group. However, this distinction has not received traction in the field and both terms conotoxin and conopeptide are now being used interchangeably [9].

Three biochemical and pharmacological features have been used to broadly classify conotoxins into distinct groups: their pharmacological target and activity (typically designated by a Greek letter), their cysteine framework (designated by Roman numerals) and their gene superfamily (designated by Latin letters). For example, conotoxins **αA-GI** and **αM-MIIIJ** both target the nicotinic acetylcholine receptor (nAChR) as represented by the Greek letter **α** but their genes and cysteine frameworks do not share any homology; one belongs to the **A** gene superfamily and has a type **I** cysteine framework while the other belongs to the **M** gene superfamily and has a type **III** cysteine framework. To date, more than 10 distinct pharmacological classes, 50 gene superfamilies, and 28 cysteine frameworks have been described [10], and more are likely to be discovered in the future.

The five best studied pharmacological classes of conotoxins all target ion channels expressed in the nervous and locomotor systems: **α** (inhibitors of nAChR), **ω** (inhibitors of voltage-gated calcium channels, VGCC), **κ** (inhibitors of voltage-gated potassium channels, VGKC), **μ** (inhibitors of voltage-gated sodium channels, VGSC), and **δ** (delayers of activation of voltage-gated sodium channels, VGSC) (Table 1). Not all pharmacological classes of conotoxins have a Greek letter designation. Instead, some have been named according to their sequence homology or similarity to other peptides (e.g., conopressins share sequence homology to vasopressin-oxytocin and coninsulins to insulin) or according to their phenotypic effect in mice (e.g., Conantokins, toxins that induce a sleep-like state in mice, were named after the Filipino word for sleep, "antok") (Table 1).

Table 1. Pharmacological families of conotoxins (in alphabetical order, modified from [10]).

Pharmacological Family	Molecular Target	Molecular Mechanism	Reference Conotoxin	Reference
α (alpha)	Nicotinic acetylcholine receptors (nAChR)	Receptor antagonists	GI	[11]
γ (gamma)	Neuronal pacemaker cation channels	Channel activator, potentially indirect effect	PnVIIA	[12]
δ (delta)	Voltage-gated Na channel	Delay channel inactivation	PVIA	[13]
ι (iota)	Voltage-gated Na channels	Channel activators	RXIA	[14]
κ (kappa)	Voltage-gated K channels	Channel blockers	PVIIA	[15]
μ (mu)	Voltage-gated Na channels	Channel blockers	GIIIA	[16]
ϱ (rho)	α1 adrenoreceptors	Allosteric inhibitor	TIA	[17]
σ (sigma)	5-hydroxytryptamine 3 receptor (HTR3A)	Receptor antagonist	GVIIIA	[18]
τ (tao)	Somatostatin receptor (SSTR)	Receptor antagonist	CnVA	[19]
χ (chi)	Norepinephrine Transporter	Inhibitor	MrIA	[17]
ω (omega)	Voltage-gated Ca channels	Channel blockers	GVIA	[20]
Φ (phi)	Promotes cell proliferation	Not determined	MiXXVIIA	[21]
Examples of pharmacological families without Greek letter designation				
Conantokins	N-methyl-D-aspartate receptor (NMDAR)	Receptor antagonists	Conantokin-G	[22]
Coninsulins	Insulin receptor	Receptor agonists	Con-Insulin G1	[23]
Conopressins	Vasopressin receptor	Receptor agonists and antagonists	Lys-Conopressin-G	[24]

1.2. Conotoxin Discovery

In the early days of conotoxin discovery, dating back to the 1960s, conotoxins were directly isolated from dissected venom, usually by bioassay-directed fractionation and sequencing (for example [11, 25–27]). Thus, discovery was focused on the biological activity of a newly identified toxin, and as such, the toxin's pharmacological activity and classification was usually determined. A common assay used to identify new toxins was by intracranial (IC; into the brain) or intraperitoneal (IP; into the abdominal cavity) injection of fractionated venom compounds into mice followed by observational recording [11,22,25–30]. Sequencing of active components required several rounds of purification from the complex venom mixture. As the conotoxins that elicited the most severe phenotypes when injected in mice could be more easily traced during purification, most conotoxins identified early on were those that were potently active in vertebrates and elicited severe effects such as seizures, shaking, paralysis, respiratory distress, or death [11,22,25–30]. Conotoxins that did not elicit a strong physiological response were not pursued or not reported (for example, see [31]). This may have resulted in the perception that most conotoxins have severe toxicity in vertebrates. Additionally, early studies predominantly focused on the venom of fish-hunting (piscovorous) cone snails. However, fish hunters constitute fewer than 20% of the total species diversity of cone snails [32]. The vast majority of cone snails prey on worms (vermivorous), and a small fraction of species prey on other mollusks (molluscivorous). Conotoxins isolated from piscovorous species are more likely to show toxicity in vertebrates than those isolated from vermivorous and molluscivorous species. Indeed, as conotoxin research expanded to the venoms of worm- and snail-hunting species and to more diverse sets of toxins from fish-hunters (e.g., α-conotoxins that target neuronal nAChRs, coninsulins, conopressins), the number of conotoxins with no or very low phenotypic activity in vertebrates steadily increased [10,33]. The vast majority of conotoxins isolated from venom to date have little to no toxicity in vertebrates.

The advent of genome sequencing in the 2000s dramatically changed how conotoxins could be identified; toxin sequences could now be readily deduced from genomic DNA or mRNA without the need to physically isolate toxins from venom. This led to a dramatic increase in the rate of conotoxin discovery; today more than 20,000 conotoxin sequences have been identified with thousands more anticipated to be sequenced in the coming years. The vast majority of these conotoxins have never been directly isolated from venom and their pharmacological activity remains unknown. For toxin sequences that share significant homology with toxins of known pharmacologies, activity can sometimes be predicted, but potencies and subtype selectivity profiles are difficult to predict. Activities of conotoxin sequences that do not share significant homology with known toxins are impossible to predict and, one may argue, these should not even be called conotoxins until a biological activity or presence in venom has been verified. To address this issue we previously proposed the usage of "conotoxin candidate" or "putative conotoxin" until future evidence can verify that a newly identified sequence indeed encodes a biologically active toxin (and is not merely predicted to do so) [34]. However, currently, there is no consensus in the field about how to best define newly identified conotoxin sequences.

While the difficulty of defining and classifying toxin sequences from large datasets has not been perceived as a limitation in the field of conotoxin research, the lack of a clear definition combined with the complexity of biological activities and toxicities has complicated the generation of well-reasoned regulations for research on, and access to, conotoxins (see Section 3.4).

2. Conotoxin "Cures"—Scientific and Societal Benefits of Conotoxin Research

2.1. The Conotoxin Drug Ziconotide (Tradename Prialt®)

ω-Conotoxin MVIIA (or ziconotide) is arguably the most famous conotoxin discovered to date. First isolated from the venom of the magician cone, *Conus magus*, at the University of Utah in 1982 [26], it was developed as a drug for the treatment of intractable pain by the biotech company Neurex Corp, approved by the United States Food and Drug Administration (FDA) in 2004, and marketed as Prialt® (the primary alternative to morphine) (Table 2). The history of the discovery of ω-conotoxin MVIIA has recently been reviewed in more detail elsewhere [35]. Here, we focus on the initial scientific goals that led to the discovery of ω-MVIIA and the societal benefits of this conotoxin today.

Table 2. Overview of conotoxin drug leads.

Conotoxin	Molecular Target	Clinical Indication	Stage in Development	Company
MVIIA (ziconotide, Prialt®)	$Ca_v2.2$ channel	Refractory chronic and cancer pain	Approved	TerSera Therapeutics, Riemser Pharma GmbH, Eisai Co., Ltd.
α-RgIA4 (KCP-400)	nAChR (subtype α9α10)	Neuropathic Pain	Pre-clinical (ongoing)	Kineta, Inc.
Mini-Ins (conotoxin insulin analog)	Insulin receptor	Type 1 diabetes	Pre-clinical (ongoing)	Monolog LLC
Contulakin-G (CGX-1160)	Neurotensin receptor	Neuropathic Pain	Phase I (on hold, demise of company)	Cognetix, Inc.
α-Vc1.1 (ACV1)	nAChR (subtype α9α10)	Neuropathic Pain	Phase I (discontinued, lack of efficacy)	Metabolic Pharmaceuticals
ω-CVID	$Ca_v2.2$ channel	Chronic Pain	Phase II (discontinued)	Amrad, Inc.
χ-MrIA (Xen2174)	Norepinephrine transporter	Postoperative pai	Phase II (discontinued)	Xenome, Inc.
Conantokin-G (CGX-1007)	NMDA receptor (subtype NR2B)	Intractable Epilepsy	Pre-clinical (discontinued, demise of company)	Cognetix, Inc.
κ-PVIIA (CGX-1051)	K_v1 subfamily	Cardioprotection	Pre-clinical (discontinued, demise of company)	Cognetix, Inc.

ω-MVIIA was discovered as part of an initiative into understanding why the venom of fish-hunting cone snails could be paralytic. In fish, ω-MVIIA was found to block neuromuscular transmission at the presynaptic terminus by inhibiting a specific voltage-gated calcium channel [36,37]. However, in the early 1980s, calcium channels had not been defined at a molecular level and it was uncertain how many different voltage-gated calcium channels were present in the vertebrate nervous system. The isolation of ω-MVIIA and a related peptide from *Conus geographus*, ω-GVIA, provided key pharmacological tools to define different types of voltage-gated calcium channels. Both peptides were selective for a calcium channel subtype that had not previously been recognized (initially known as the N-type calcium channel, and later as $Ca_v2.2$). While exploring the potential biomedical applications of ω-MVIIA, experiments conducted by Neurex Corp with a radiolabeled analog revealed specific binding to layers of the spinal cord dorsal horn previously established to be important for the perception of pain [38]. This finding paved the way for the subsequent development of ω-MVIIA as an analgesic [39].

The commercial drug Prialt® is an exact synthetic copy of ω-MVIIA. When approved by the FDA in 2004, Prialt was a welcome addition to the repertoire of anesthesiologists as an agent with a non-opioid mechanism. Unlike opioids, Prialt does not cause addiction or respiratory depression, but at high doses can lead to other severe, albeit not fatal, side effects, including psychomotor effects ranging from mild ataxia and auditory hallucinations (typically completely reversible with a small dose reduction) to more debilitating ataxia and psychosis. Furthermore, because Prialt acts by targeting $Ca_v2.2$ channels expressed in the central nervous system, it must be administered intrathecally using an implanted pump. This is an invasive and relatively costly procedure that has been a barrier to more widespread use. Thus, clinically, Prialt was often used a last resort. However, due to the lack of availability of effective, non-opioid therapeutics, recent guidelines now encourage the use of Prialt as a first-line agent in various pain conditions including neuropathic and nociceptive pain [40].

Furthermore, Prialt has been increasingly used in combination with an intrathecal opioid, exploiting the potentially synergistic effect of Prialt and opioids in the treatment of refractory chronic and cancer pain [41].

2.2. Conotoxin Drug Leads

In addition to the clinical development of ω-MVIIA several other conotoxins have been at various stages of development as drug leads for pain, epilepsy, heart disease, and diabetes (for recent reviews on these toxins see [35,42–44]). Table 2 provides an overview of these drug leads. Despite their promising therapeutic applications, none of these conotoxins has (yet) reached clinical approval. It is difficult to assess the underlying reasons for this because information on commercial developments of drug leads is typically not made accessible to the public when the development of a compound is discontinued (e.g., information on lack of efficacy in clinical trials, safety concerns, change in a company's development program, demise of a company, intellectual property disputes, etc.). Where known, we list the current development status of conotoxin drug leads and the reason for why past development efforts were halted (Table 2).

Regardless of their drug development status, many of these toxins have become valuable pharmacological and biomedical tools for the study of signaling pathways important in health and disease.

2.3. Diagnostic Tool

One hallmark feature of conotoxins is their target specificity for closely related subtypes of receptors and ion channels. The selectivity profile of ω-conotoxin GVIA from the venom of *Conus geographus*, a homolog of the approved drug Prialt, led to its development as a diagnostic tool for Lambert–Eaton myasthenic syndrome (LEMS). LEMS is an autoimmune disorder, which results in muscle weakness, and is associated with lung cancer. LEMS is caused by the production of antibodies against presynaptic voltage-gated calcium channels (VGCCs), which results in the inhibition of acetylcholine release at the neuromuscular junction [45–47]. While it has historically been difficult to differentiate LEMS from symptomatically related disorders, in 1989 Sher and coworkers showed that antibodies against VGCCs produced in LEMS could immunoprecipitate ^{125}I-ω-conotoxin GVIA-bound N-type VGCCs ($Ca_v2.2$), which are elevated in about half of LEMS patients [45,48]. This laid the basis for a diagnostic radio immunoprecipitation assay to differentiate LEMS from similar disorders, such as myasthenia gravis. By labeling solubilized cell membrane expressing $Ca_v2.2$ with ^{125}I-labeled ω-conotoxin GVIA, and exposing this to LEMS patient serum, antibodies against $Ca_v2.2$ can bind the receptor-conotoxin complex. These are then precipitated, and the radioactivity can then be detected, indicating that the patient serum contains $Ca_v2.2$ antibodies. This diagnosis was later improved by the use of a different conotoxin that binds P/Q-type VGCCs ($Ca_v2.1$), ω-conotoxin MVIIC. Antibodies against $Ca_v2.1$ are elevated in about 85 % of LEMS patients [49,50]. Differentiating these disorders is critical for guiding clinical care [51]. The emergence of medically relevant diagnostic tools provides an important example for the societal benefits of conotoxin research.

2.4. Cosmetics

Similarly to botulinium toxin (Botox®), conotoxins that have myorelaxant properties can be developed as anti-wrinkle creams or injectable formulations. One such conotoxin is μ-CIIIC, originally isolated from the fish-hunting cone snail *Conus consors* as part of the European Commission-funded CONCO project ("CONCO: the cone snail genome project for health"). μ-CIIIC preferentially blocks the skeletal muscle sodium channel, $Na_v1.4$, and the neuronal sodium channel $Na_v1.2$ [52]. Due to the blocking of $Na_v1.4$, it can act as a myorelaxant. μ-CIIIC was initially investigated as a drug for the treatment of pain and as a local anesthetic but is now sold as the active ingredient in a non-prescription cosmetic anti-wrinkle product under the name "XEP™-018".

2.5. Research Tools

Conotoxins that target mammalian receptors are often selective for certain receptor subtypes, or subunit compositions. This feature renders conotoxins excellent tools for a plethora of studies in the areas of pharmacology, neuroscience, biochemistry, and structural biology. Table 3 lists a small number of these conotoxins, and examples of their use in basic biology and biomedical research. There is of course overlap with clinically developed conotoxins (Table 2), which are also often used as research tools. For instance, ω-conotoxin MVIIA (the drug Prialt), has been used as a tool compound in thousands of studies.

Another conotoxin that has been extensively used as a research tool in the scientific literature (> 3000 publications) is ω-conotoxin GVIA, a potent and selective blocker of the presynaptic N-type calcium channels, $Ca_V2.2$. The $Ca_V2.2$ channels play a crucial role in neurotransmitter release in response to action potentials in the kidneys, where they regulate the dilation of arteries, and in the heart, where they regulate cardiac excitability [53–55]. Hence, ω-conotoxin GVIA has been used extensively in numerous studies of various topics, including neurotransmission, pain, cardiology, epilepsy, renal function, and nuclear signaling (selected references in Table 3).

Another example is the α-conotoxin, ImI, from the vermivorous *Conus imperialis* (as well as the subsequently discovered α-conotoxin, ImII [56]). ImI and ImII are inhibitors of the neuronal α7 subtype of the nAChRs [57]. These toxins, like most other subtype- or subunit-selective conotoxins, have been used to elucidate the importance of receptor subunits in numerous biological- and pathophysiological studies [58–60]. However, they have also seen other more specialized uses. For instance, in a 2014 study Heghinian and co-workers used several different α-conotoxins to perform structurally guided mutations in the *D. melanogaster* α7 nAChR, allowing this receptor to display similar selectivity for various conotoxins as the mammalian counterpart. This, in turn, resulted in *D. melanogaster* cholinergic synapses that mimic the synaptic behavior of vertebrate synapses, improving the suitability of these mutant flies as a tool for in vivo drug discovery [61].

In a 2015 study, Lin and co-workers utilized the specificity of α-ImI for cellular targeting of the chemotherapy drug, paclitaxel [62]. The authors showed that linking paclitaxel-containing micelles to α-ImI significantly decreased the mass of tumors in mice when compared to either unlinked paclitaxel-filled micelles or free paclitaxel. In addition, they observed a lower systemic toxicity of the α-ImI-linked micelles.

In addition, several conotoxins have served as tools in structural biology to elucidate specific receptor binding sites or mechanisms of receptor activation. For instance, the X-ray crystal structure of the conotoxin con-ikot-ikot from *Conus striatus* [63] in complex with the GluR2 AMPA receptor subunit revealed the molecular mechanism underlying receptor activation [64]. Another example is the conotoxin Con-Insulin G1 from *Conus geographus* that revealed a minimum binding motif of insulin at the human insulin receptor [65].

Conotoxins undergo post-translational processing (folding and modification) in the ER and Golgi prior to packaging and secretion into the lumen of the venom gland. Due to their small size, chemical diversity, and high degree of post-translational modifications, conotoxins are ideal candidates to study general principles of peptide folding, modification, and secretion. Several conotoxins have been repeatedly used as model substrates for studies into enzyme-assisted peptide biosynthesis and folding, such as α-GI [66,67], μ-SmIIIA [68,69], and conantokin-G [70,71].

Lastly, conotoxins are among the most rapidly evolving gene products known in nature and have served as tools in a diverse range of studies on the effects of feeding ecology, prey taxa, dietary breadth, age and geographical heterogeneity on the evolution of venom genes [72–76], and studies on the role of gene duplication and positive selection on venom gene expression and diversification [77–79].

Table 3. Examples of conotoxins used as research tools.

Conotoxin	Target	Feature	Useful in Field(s) of Research
α-GI, μ-SmIIIA, Conantokin-G	Various targets	Substrates for enzymes involved in peptide biosynthesis	Elucidating peptide biosynthesis and folding [68–70]
α-ImI	α7 nAChR	Subtype selectivity [56]	Targeted drug delivery in cancer [62], engineering *D. melanogaster* as better human disease model [61], chromaffin cell signaling [57]
α-MII	nAChR	Subtype selective [80]	Inflammation [81], reward and addiction [82,83]
α-Vc1.1 and α-Rg1A	α9α10 nAChR	Subtype selective [84,85]	Neuropathic pain and inflammation [86–88], immunology [89–91]
Con-ikot-ikot	AMPA receptor	Disrupts desensitization, stabilizes open conformation [63,64]	Receptor crystallization [64]
Con-Insulin G1	Insulin receptor	Minimized binding motif at the insulin receptor [65]	Receptor binding and drug design [92]
κ-PVIIA	Voltage-gated K^+ channels	Voltage-sensitive binding/blocking of voltage-gated K-channels [15]	Cancer [93], cardioprotection in ischemia [94]
κM-RIIIJ	Voltage-gated K^+ channels	Subtype selectivity [95,96]	Neuronal profiling [5,6,97,98], channel subtype expression profiling [96,99]
ω-GVIA	Voltage-gated Ca^{2+} channels	Subtype selective [37,99]	Neurotransmission [100–102], pain [103], cardiology [55], epilepsy [104], renal function [105], nuclear signaling [106]
ω-MVIIC	Voltage-gated Ca^{2+} channels	Inhibits various subtypes broadly [107,108]	Epilepsy [109], long-term depression [110], pain [111,112]

2.6. Conotoxin Research—A View toward the Future

Recent advances in throughput and sensitivity of next-generation DNA and peptide sequencing have resulted in a massive increase in the rate of conotoxin discovery (for example [34,113]). This is unlikely to decrease any time soon given that the cost of sequencing continues to fall. In combination with the generation of easier, less computationally heavy bioinformatic tools for data analysis, conotoxin discovery can now be done without the need of expensive or highly specialized equipment. The increasing rate of conotoxin discovery is being met with advances in methodologies for conotoxin production (for example [114–116]), high-content target screening and identification (for example [117–119]), and with a newly sparked interest in peptide-based drug development by the pharma industry [120]. We anticipate that this combination will lead to the development and design of many more conotoxin-based biomedical tools and pharmacological agents in the future.

3. Conotoxin "Curses"—Biosecurity Concerns

3.1. Cone Snail Envenomations and Human Fatalities

From the very first report of a human fatality from a cone snail sting ≈350 years ago, through to 2017, 141 cases of human envenomations have been recorded, of which 36 were fatal [121]. No human fatalities have been reported for the past 20 years. Most, if not all, of the 36 human fatalities caused by cone snail stings have been attributed to a single species, *Conus geographus* [121]. All of these were accidental, and there have been no reports of the use of cone snail venom as a weapon for murder.

In humans, symptoms from cone snail envenomations vary depending on several factors, including cone snail species. Often, pain or numbness is reported, but symptoms can include edema, vision impairment, fatigue and faintness, dyspnea, loss of reflexes, and nausea. Some victims have noticed a burning sensation at the site of the sting, while others have reported that the sting itself initially went unnoticed. Subsequently, reports of faintness, palpebral ptosis, dysphagia, as well as vision and speech impairment are common in more severe cases, though in some cases no obvious symptoms have been reported prior to the onset of muscle paralysis, which in the worst case can lead to death due to respiratory or cardiac arrest within a few hours [122–124]. No effective antivenom exists against cone snail venom.

While the venom of a small subset of the ≈800 species of cone snails is toxic to humans, the number of human envenomations by these animals pales in comparison to those reported for other venomous animals. Snake bites undoubtedly comprise the largest contribution of serious human envenomations by any group of animals. While exact data can be difficult to obtain, the World Health Organization estimates that ≈2.7 million people are envenomated by snakes every year, resulting in 81,000–138,000 deaths per year, and 400,000 permanent disabilities, including amputations [125]. The large number of deaths from snake bites result, in part, from a much larger rate of human–snake encounters. Nevertheless, it is clear that snake envenomations present a significantly larger concern to human health and life, compared to cone snails.

Another large contributor to human envenomations are scorpions, with an estimated 1.2 million global envenomations, and more than 3250 deaths each year [126]. One of the most venomous stings, the eastern red scorpion *Hottentotta tamulus*, has an estimated fatality rate of ≈30% when untreated. Similarly to cone snails, no effective antivenom exists for *H. tamulus* venom, though treatment with the anti-hypertension drug prazosin can lower this fatality rate to 2–4% [127,128].

As with cone snails, other venomous animals have also been an important source of biological, and biomedical research, research tools, as well as drugs and drug leads. Snake venom has provided several clinically important drugs, including blood pressure medication, coagulants, and anticoagulants [129–131]. Numerous scorpion venom components are likewise being investigated for biomedical uses, including novel peptide antimicrobial drugs [132].

3.2. Fictional Use of Conotoxins as Bioweapons

As envenomation by some species can be deadly, cone snails and their toxins have gained notoriety, both in national biodefense considerations (see Section 3.4), as well as in fiction. Some of these have recently been reviewed elsewhere [121,133].

For instance, in the Michael Crichton novel "The Lost World" (the sequel to "Jurassic Park"), as well as in the movie and video game adaptations of the novel, the "Lindstradt air gun", a gun shooting a dart containing "enhanced venom" from the cone snail *Conus purpurascens* is used to kill or paralyze dinosaurs. In the movie, *Conus purpurascens* venom is described as the most powerful neurotoxin in the world that acts within 1/2000th of a second, which is stated to be faster than the velocity of nerve conduction.

In a 1972 episode of the television show Hawaii five-0 (season 4, episode 20: "Cloth of Gold"), a *Conus textile*, also called the "cloth of gold", is intended to be used as a murder weapon. Instead it ends up being used as a tool for suicide by the main antagonist who presses it against his throat and is stung.

The Danish/Swedish television show, "Broen" ("The Bridge", season 4, episode 5), featured the venom of *Conus geographus* (although an image of *Conus textile* was shown) as a weapon for murder. The toxin used was allegedly manufactured in a conotoxin production facility in Hamburg, Germany.

Another example is an episode of the animated British children's show "Octonauts" (season 3, episode 3) that featured a cone snail shooting poison-loaded harpoons at crew members after being lost inside an underwater vessel.

Conotoxins have also appeared in several written murder mysteries, such as in James Patterson's 2018 thriller "Murder in Paradise" or the novel "Murder on the Mataniko Bridge" by Ann Kengalu.

3.3. *Conotoxin Toxicity*

Contrary to their appearance as powerful murder weapons in fiction, no real-life incident for the nefarious use of a cone snail, its venom or toxin components has ever been reported. In this section, we report on the toxicity of some conotoxins in mammals that inspired both their use as weapons in fiction, and the introduction of regulatory measures for scientists working with conotoxins.

Due to the way conotoxins were traditionally identified (i.e., by behavioral bioassays in mice, see Section 1.2), the toxins that are the most potent in mammals were typically among the first to be identified [11,26,27]. As discussed above, these include a toxin from *C. geographus*, α-conotoxin GI, a potent inhibitor of nicotinic acetylcholine receptors of the neuromuscular junction [134–136] (Table 4). α-conotoxin GI significantly contributes to the comparably high fatality rate of *C. geographus* envenomations where it is believed to induce muscle paralysis and, ultimately, respiratory arrest due to paralysis of the diaphragm [137]. This toxin was described more than 40 years ago, and yet, to our knowledge, no incidents have ever been reported of its misuse. On the contrary, α-conotoxin GI been a valuable research tool in neurosciences and biochemistry (Table 3). As with all cone snail species, the venom of *C. geographus* contains more than 100 different toxins, the majority of which are not considered harmful to humans. As with α-conotoxin GI, numerous other *C. geographus* toxins have been valuable as drug leads and biomedical tools as well as one diagnostic agent (see Sections 2.2, 2.3 and 2.5).

Since conotoxins comprise a large and diverse class of compounds with many different biomolecular targets in various species, the mammalian toxicity of different conotoxins likewise covers a range of orders of magnitude. The median lethal dose (LD_{50}) of α-conotoxin GI is 12 μg/kg when injected intraperitoneally (IP) in mice [11]. Indeed, several conotoxins in the α-conotoxin family that target muscle-type nicotinic acetylcholine receptors of the neuromuscular junction, are quite potent toxins in mammals. However, this group forms a very small subset of α-conotoxins (most target neuronal nAChR subtypes and have very little to no toxicity in mammals) and a minuscule percentage of all conotoxins. For the vast majority of other conotoxins, the toxicity in mammals is so low that no LD_{50} has ever been determined. This not only includes many toxins from worm- or snail hunting species that have little to no effect in vertebrates, but also numerous toxins from fish hunters. For instance, the venom of *C. geographus* contains a vasopressin-like toxin (conopressin-G) that elicits a grooming behavior in mice when injected intracerebrally [24], and insulin-like toxins (coninsulins), that are used by the snail to induce low blood sugar in fish prey but activate the mammalian insulin receptor at much lower potency than human insulin [138]. As stated above, even within the family of α-conotoxins, most toxins have very low to no toxicity in mammals. For instance, α-conotoxin GIC, also from *C. geographus*, targets neuronal nAChRs, does not block human neuromuscular nAChR subunit compositions in electrophysiological assays, nor do mice display any motor deficits or paralysis when injected with up to 5 nmol IP (corresponding to >250 μg/kg) [139].

While certain conotoxins are indeed toxic to humans, these toxins are significantly less potent than certain toxins produced in other animals (see Table 4). For instance, even the most lethal conotoxin is more than one order of magnitude less potent than both textilotoxin, a protein toxin from the eastern brown snake, *Pseudonaja textilis*, as well as ciguatoxins and maitotoxins, which are produced by various dinoflagellate species.

Furthermore, conotoxins appear to only be toxic when injected. While not every route of administration has been described, attempts have been made to improve the oral activity of conotoxin drug leads. An example is the α-conotoxin Vc1.1, where numerous modifications were tested in order to increase its oral bioactivity. The analog obtained with the highest oral bioactivity was still ≈1000 fold less potent when administered orally, than when injected [86,140].

Table 4. Comparison of the median lethal dose (LD_{50}) of different toxins and toxic substances.

Toxin	LD50 in Mice (μg/kg)	Route of Administration	Type of Toxin	Source	Known Antivenom/ Antidote	Reference
α-conotoxin GI	12	IP	Peptide	*Conus geographus*	No	[11]
ω-conotoxin GVIA	≈60	IP	Peptide	*Conus geographus*	No	[141]
Textilotoxin	1	IP	Protein	*Pseudonaja textilis*	Depends *	[142]
Volkensin	1.38–1.73	IP	Protein	*Adenia volkensii*	No	[143]
Ciguatoxin-1	0.25	IP and oral	Polycyclic poylethers	Various dinoflagellates	No	[144]
Maitotoxin	0.13	IP	Polycyclic poylethers	Various dinoflagellates	No †	[145]
Palytoxin	0.15	IV	Polycyclic poylethers	*Palythoa* corals and dinoflagellates (or bacteria living on these)	No	[146]
Batrachotoxin	2	SC	Alkaloid	Various beetles, birds, and frogs	No	[147]
Saxitoxin	10	IP	Alkaloid	Various marine dinoflagellates	In guinea pigs #	[148]
Tetrodotoxin	8	IV	Alkaloid	Various marine bacteria (e.g., *Pseudoalteromonas tetraodonis*) symbiotically living with numerous marine animals, e.g., *Tetraodontidae* fish, *Hapalochlaena* octopodes, and *Naticidae* snails	No †	[149]

† Supportive treatment provided [150]. * After initial binding phase completed, antivenom seems to have no effect [151,152]. # 4-Aminopyridine (marketed as Ampyra in the US, and used to manage symptoms of multiple sclerosis) has been shown to reverse the effect of saxitoxin poisoning in guinea pigs [153].

3.4. Past and Current Regulations of Research on Conotoxins

Worldwide, various governing bodies are responsible for maintaining lists of regulated substances that are deemed biosecurity concerns. Items on these regulatory lists are subject to certain restrictions in their export and use, including in research. These lists contain various pathogens (e.g., Ebola virus, sheeppox virus) but also include toxins of biological origin. Most of these toxins have a well-defined chemical identity and biological activity, e.g., tetrodotoxin, botulinum toxin, or T2-mycotoxin. However, for conotoxins, this is not the case, and the term "conotoxin" or "conotoxins" is used without additional classification. For example, at the time of writing, the European Union (EU) includes "conotoxin" as a controlled substance [154] and Australian regulations cover "conotoxins" [155], both of which are virtually identical to how the United States regulated conotoxins prior to a 2012 revision. Thus, these two lists not only include conotoxins that have toxicity in vertebrates, but also those that elicit little or no physiological response in vertebrates and those with unknown biological activity. Given the chemical, structural, and biological diversity of conotoxins (see Section 1.1) regulating conotoxins as a single entity is clearly problematic. It is worth noting that to the best of our knowledge, no regulatory agency has ever had "snake toxins" or "scorpion toxins" as a regulated substance in the same manner as "conotoxins". Neither does any country, to the best of our knowledge, regulate any of the specific components of any animal venoms, even ones that are more potent toxins in mammals than any conotoxin (see Table 4 for examples). Without a clear definition of the term "conotoxin", as currently the case in many countries, interpretation is often left to the individual evaluating a given case, who is typically not an expert in the field.

To address this, some countries have more narrowly defined their classification of regulated conotoxins. For example, until 2012, the select agent list in the United States included "conotoxins". This has since been revised to only include the paralytic α-conotoxins containing a very distinct sequence pattern, which corresponds to the sequence motifs found in the conotoxins that block muscle-type nicotinic acetylcholine receptors ([156]; "*Short, paralytic alpha conotoxins containing the following amino acid sequence* $X_1CCX_2PACGX_3X_4X_5X_6CX_7$ *where C = Cysteine residues with the 1st and 3rd Cysteine, and the 2nd and 4th Cysteine forming specific disulfide bridges;* X_1 *= any amino acid(s) or Des-X;* X_2 *= Asparagine or Histidine; P = Proline; A = Alanine; G = Glycine;* X_3 *= Arginine or Lysine;* X_4 *= Asparagine, Histidine, Lysine, Arginine, Tyrosine, Phenylalanine or Tryptophan;* X_5 *= Tyrosine, Phenylalanine, or Tryptophan;* X_6 *= Serine, Threonine, Glutamate, Aspartate, Glutamine, or Asparagine;* X_7 *= Any amino acid(s); "Des X" = "an amino acid does not have to be present at this position."*). This narrower definition was also recently adopted by the Danish Center of Biosecurity and Biopreparedness (CBB) [157].

In 1985, the "Australia Group" was formed as an informal arrangement aimed at allowing members to harmonizing export, while minimizing the risk of this export aiding in chemical and biological weapon proliferation [158]. At the time of writing, the Australia Group has 44 members, including Australia, New Zealand, the United States, Argentina, Mexico, Japan, the Republic of Korea, the United Kingdom, Switzerland, and members of the European Union. Conotoxins are listed as biological agents, thus requiring members to control their international trade with the exception of medical or clinical formulations of conotoxins designated for human use.

The exact implementation of the regulations, in regard to research activities utilizing conotoxins, varies in different countries, but typically researchers are allowed to work with threshold amounts (often 100 mg is used), while being subject to lower regulatory requirements for handling, training, and/or reporting to authorities, whereas higher amounts of conotoxin are typically subject to more stringent restrictions and requirements. Where regulatory agencies have differentiated various conotoxins, this typically applies to a very select group of paralytic and potent toxins in mammals, such as the paralytic α-conotoxins. If differences between conotoxins are not specified, these limitations are typically interpreted to mean that even small amounts of any conotoxin are regulated in this manner, regardless of the toxicity of the specific conotoxin in question.

It is interesting to note that the crude cone snail venom, even from the most venomous species, has never been regulated. Only "conotoxin" components of the venom are regulated, even in cases where the term "conotoxins" is used to encompass every single component of the venom. This is despite the fact that the venom components elicit a synergistic effect, in fact being more potent as crude venom than as the individual components that are regulated [15,159].

3.5. Potential Use of Conotoxins as Bioweapons

Although, to our knowledge, there has not been a single incident on the use of cone snail venom or conotoxins outside of legitimate research and drug development programs, the regulatory measures described in the previous Section 3.4 reflect concerns about the potential misuse of conotoxins in bioterrorism.

One such concern is that conotoxins could potentially be aerosolized and thus more easily spread and inhaled by potential victims. The bioavailibilities upon pulmonary inhalation greatly varies between different compounds [160–163] making it difficult to predict whether any conotoxin would retain toxicity in an aerosolized form. If indeed they did, this would provide an alternate route of administration. However, the toxin would still need to be formulated for aerosolization purposes, and formulating peptides for aerosol delivery is not trivial. Producing the appropriate particle sizes, as well as the being able to retain peptide integrity during the process remains challenging [164].

Another potential concern is that some conotoxins could be injected thereby acting as a murder weapon. However, this also applies to many other biological and non-biological compounds that are lethal when directly injected into the human body, many of which have never been regulated.

The small amount needed for some conotoxins could potentially render them difficult to detect, complicating the determination of the cause of death. The pharmacokinetics of conotoxins in humans are not well described. It has been reported that for α-conotoxin GI, no breakdown was detected after a 3-h incubation in human plasma [165], and for α-conotoxin MII, more than 60% remained after 24 h of incubation in human plasma [166], though the in vivo clearance of these and other conotoxins could be much faster due to metabolism outside of systemic circulation [167]. While modern forensic testing methods are able to detect peptide concentration in plasma of ≈0.1 parts-per-billion [168], it is possible that a conotoxin could metabolize beyond this limit before an autopsy would be performed. A further and likely more pressing concern could be that no antivenom exists. This means that even if a victim could receive care in time, life-saving medical interventions are limited to supportive care (for example, for α-conotoxin GI mouth to mouth or mechanical ventilation can be performed until the paralysis wears off). This, however, is also true for numerous compounds that are not regulated, several of them being more potent than any conotoxin (see Table 4).

Another avenue for potentially using conotoxins as bioweapons could be their incorporation into the genomes of pathogenic viruses and bacteria genomes in order to enhance their deadliness. According to an interview with a former scientist in the United States senate a program of such nature was allegedly carried out in the Soviet Union. This program allegedly led to the generation of a smallpox virus that carried conotoxin sequences before it was ultimately terminated [169]. As stated in the interview these conotoxins contained two specific cystine bridges and, thus, were likely α-conotoxins. While this report could have led to the strict regulations regarding conotoxin research, it should be noted that many other toxins could be used in such a manner and research on dangerous pathogens, including the smallpox virus, is already strictly regulated.

In 2017, El-Aziz and co-workers published a method for in vivo neutralization of toxic peptides using DNA oligonucleotides [170]. As a proof of concept, they used α-conotoxin PrXA from *Conus parius*, a fast acting and potent toxin targeting the nAChRs of the skeletal muscles. They showed that the oligonucleotides ("adaptamers") could efficiently counteract the binding to receptors, inhibition of diaphragm contraction, and death induced by this conotoxin in mice. While not yet available for clinical use, the World Health Organization has classified envenomations as category A (the highest priority concern available), mostly due to snake bites. Since this approach could also be useful for toxins from other animals, including snakes, these promising efforts could lead to the generation of effective medical treatment options in the future.

4. Concluding Remarks

4.1. Concluding Remarks on Conotoxin "Cures"

Since the dawn of conotoxin research ≈60 years ago [6,171,172], the number of new conotoxins being identified has exploded. Through the decades, their increasing chemical and pharmacological diversity became apparent and, to date, >5000 research articles have been published in this field of research. Furthermore, conotoxins have been used as tools in thousands of additional research studies, many of which could only be conducted due to the unique properties of certain conotoxins. From a basic understanding of receptor subunit compositions, receptor structures, and peptide folding and expression, to more physiological studies on such diverse topics as epilepsy, inflammation, cancer, pain, cardiology, renal function, and addiction (see Table 3), and even clinical studies and an FDA approved drug (see Table 2), these peptides have already provided immense benefits to basic and applied research and society. With the advances in genomics sequencing, the number of available conotoxin sequences is rapidly increasing. Every new sequence is a new opportunity for furthering research into novel biology, as well as clinical treatments. As long as researchers can use these valuable tools in their research, novel discoveries will continue for many more decades to come.

4.2. Concluding Remarks on Conotoxin "Curses"

A few select conotoxins are indeed toxic to humans, but the vast majority are not. It seems self-evident that the harmless conotoxins should not be subject to regulations. However, here we argue that even for the more potent toxins, regulations on researchers are unlikely to prevent their use in bioterrorism, but instead will impede research that, as outlined above, provides many impactful benefits. As we have explained, even the most potent conotoxins appear to be poor candidates for the development of biological weapons (see Section 3.5). Moreover, knowledge of toxin sequences and their synthesis has been publicly available for decades, and the reagents and equipment needed are, to the best of our knowledge, not regulated. In fact, some of these toxins can be readily purchased from commercial providers. However, as discussed, the actual formulation of conotoxins for an aerosol delivery is likely to prove challenging, and it is unclear whether conotoxins would even be bioavailable in such a formulation. With cheap, easy alternatives readily available and proven effective (e.g., phosgene gas), there would seem to be little incentive to pursue this. Consider too, that if successful, recent efforts in developing oligonucleotide-based blockers of peptide toxins may provide broadly applicable treatments. This would further lower the potential of conotoxins as bioweapons. Likewise, concerns about using conotoxins as injectable weapons, while possible, seem largely irrelevant outside of fiction, considering the plethora of other toxins or toxic substances that could easily replace conotoxins in such a scenario.

4.3. Suggestions

First, the lack of a clear definition of "conotoxin" or "conotoxins" in legislative work is highly problematic. At the very least, a clear distinction should be made between different conotoxins. If, after a careful consideration of the available literature, any regulatory authority still sees a reason to keep certain conotoxins on the list of potential bioweapon threats, it is essential that these are clearly differentiated from other conotoxins.

Second, it is our opinion that listing even the most potent toxins will have little effect in regard to their potential use in bioterrorism. As discussed, toxin sequences and information on synthesis and recombinant production are publicly available and have been for decades. Limiting the use of these toxins in research is unlikely to reduce a potential bioterror threat. Instead, it is a barrier to research in this important field.

Funding: B.M.O. and M.Y. acknowledges funding from the US National Institutes of Health (GM122869), and JMM from GM136430, GM103801 and US Department of Defense W81XWH170413 (to BMO and JMM). L.E. acknowledges funding from the Independent Research Fund Denmark | Technology and Production Sciences (7017-00288), and H.S.-H. acknowledges funding from the Velux Foundation (Villum grant 19063).

Conflicts of Interest: J.M.M., B.M.O. and H.S.-H. hold patents on some of the conotoxins listed in this review.

References

1. Abdelkrim, J.; Aznar-Cormano, L.; Fedosov, A.E.; Kantor, Y.I.; Lozouet, P.; Phuong, M.A.; Zaharias, P.; Puillandre, N. Exon-Capture-Based Phylogeny and Diversification of the Venomous Gastropods (Neogastropoda, Conoidea). *Mol. Biol. Evol.* **2018**, *35*, 2355–2374. [CrossRef] [PubMed]
2. Puillandre, N.; Bouchet, P.; Duda, T.F., Jr.; Kauferstein, S.; Kohn, A.J.; Olivera, B.M.; Watkins, M.; Meyer, C. Molecular phylogeny and evolution of the cone snails (Gastropoda, Conoidea). *Mol. Phylogenetics Evol.* **2014**, *78*, 290–303. [CrossRef] [PubMed]
3. Fleming, C.J. 1822, taxID: 14107. MolluscaBase. Available online: http://molluscabase.org/ (accessed on 14 July 2020).
4. World Register of Marine Species (WoRMS), tax ID 14107. Available online: https://www.marinespecies.org (accessed on 14 July 2020).
5. Puillandre, N.; Duda, T.F.; Meyer, C.; Olivera, B.M.; Bouchet, P. One, four or 100 genera? A new classification of the cone snails. *J. Molluscan Stud.* **2014**, *80*. [CrossRef] [PubMed]
6. Kohn, A.J.; Saunders, P.R.; Wiener, S. Preliminary studies on the venom of the marine snail. *Conus. Ann. N. Y. Acad. Sci.* **1960**, *90*, 706–725. [CrossRef]
7. Neves, J.L.; Lin, Z.; Imperial, J.S.; Antunes, A.; Vasconcelos, V.; Olivera, B.M.; Schmidt, E.W. Small Molecules in the Cone Snail Arsenal. *Org. Lett.* **2015**, *17*, 4933–4935. [CrossRef]
8. Safavi-Hemami, H.; Foged, M.M.; Ellgaard, L. Evolutionary Adaptations to Cysteine-Rich Peptide Folding. In *Oxidative Folding of Peptides and Proteins*; Feige, M.J., Ed.; Royal Society of Chemistry: London, UK, 2018.

9. Puillandre, N.; Koua, D.; Favreau, P.; Olivera, B.M.; Stocklin, R. Molecular phylogeny, classification and evolution of conopeptides. *J. Mol. Evol.* **2012**, *74*, 297–309. [CrossRef]
10. Olivera, B.M.; Safavi-Hemami, H.; Horvarth, M.P.; Teichert, R.W. Conopeptides, Marine Natural Products from Venoms: Biomedical Applications and Future Research Applications. In *Marine Biomedicine: From Beach to Bedside*; Baker, B.J., Ed.; CRC Press: Boca Raton, FL, USA, 2015; ISBN 9780367575304.
11. Cruz, L.J.; Gray, W.R.; Olivera, B.M. Purification and properties of a myotoxin from *Conus geographus* venom. *Arch. Biochem. Biophys.* **1978**, *190*, 539–548. [CrossRef]
12. Fainzilber, M.; Nakamura, T.; Lodder, J.C.; Zlotkin, E.; Kits, K.S.; Burlingame, A.L. Gamma-Conotoxin-PnVIIA, a gamma-carboxyglutamate-containing peptide agonist of neuronal pacemaker cation currents. *Biochemistry* **1998**, *37*, 1470–1477. [CrossRef]
13. Shon, K.J.; Grilley, M.M.; Marsh, M.; Yoshikami, D.; Hall, A.R.; Kurz, B.; Gray, W.R.; Imperial, J.S.; Hillyard, D.R.; Olivera, B.M. Purification, Characterization, Synthesis, and Cloning of the Lockjaw Peptide from *Conus purpurascens* Venom. *Biochemistry* **1995**, *34*, 4913–4918. [CrossRef]
14. Jimenez, E.C.; Shetty, R.P.; Lirazan, M.; Rivier, J.; Walker, C.; Abogadie, F.C.; Yoshikami, D.; Cruz, L.J.; Olivera, B.M. Novel excitatory *Conus* peptides define a new conotoxin superfamily. *J. Neurochem.* **2003**, *85*, 610–621. [CrossRef]
15. Terlau, H.; Shon, K.J.; Grilley, M.; Stocker, M.; Stuhmer, W.; Olivera, B.M. Strategy for rapid immobilization of prey by a fish-hunting marine snail. *Nature* **1996**, *381*, 148–151. [CrossRef] [PubMed]
16. Cruz, L.J.; Gray, W.R.; Olivera, B.M.; Zeikus, R.D.; Kerr, L.; Yoshikami, D.; Moczydlowski, E. *Conus geographus* toxins that discriminate between neuronal and muscle sodium channels. *J. Biol. Chem.* **1985**, *260*, 9280–9288.
17. Sharpe, I.A.; Gehrmann, J.; Loughnan, M.L.; Thomas, L.; Adams, D.A.; Atkins, A.; Palant, E.; Craik, D.J.; Adams, D.J.; Alewood, P.F.; et al. Two new classes of conopeptides inhibit the alpha 1-adrenoceptor and noradrenaline transporter. *Nat. Neurosci.* **2001**, *4*, 902–907. [CrossRef] [PubMed]
18. England, L.J.; Gulyas, J. Inactivation of a serotonin-gated ion channel by a polypeptide toxin from marine snails (vol 281, pg 575, 1998). *Science* **1998**, *282*, 417.
19. Petrel, C.; Hocking, H.G.; Reynaud, M.; Upert, G.; Favreau, P.; Biass, D.; Paolini-Bertrand, M.; Peigneur, S.; Tytgat, J.; Gilles, N.; et al. Identification, structural and pharmacological characterization of τ-CnVA, a conopeptide that selectively interacts with somatostatin sst3 receptor. *Biochem. Pharmacol.* **2013**, *85*, 1663–1671. [CrossRef]
20. Olivera, B.M.; McIntosh, J.M.; Cruz, L.J.; Luque, F.A.; Gray, W.R. Purification and sequence of a presynaptic peptide toxin from *Conus geographus* venom. *Biochemistry* **1984**, *23*, 5087–5090. [CrossRef] [PubMed]
21. Jin, A.H.; Dekan, Z.; Smout, M.J.; Wilson, D.; Dutertre, S.; Vetter, I.; Lewis, R.J.; Loukas, A.; Daly, N.L.; Alewood, P.F. Conotoxin Φ-MiXXVIIA from the Superfamily G2 Employs a Novel Cysteine Framework that Mimics Granulin and Displays Anti-Apoptotic Activity. *Angew. Chem.* **2017**, *56*, 14973–14976. [CrossRef]
22. Olivera, B.M.; McIntosh, J.M.; Clark, C.; Middlemas, D.; Gray, W.R.; Cruz, L.J. A sleep-inducing peptide from *Conus geographus* venom. *Toxicon* **1985**, *23*, 277–282. [CrossRef]
23. Safavi-Hemami, H.; Gajewiak, J.; Karanth, S.; Robinson, S.D.; Ueberheide, B.; Douglass, A.D.; Schlegel, A.; Imperial, J.S.; Watkins, M.; Bandyopadhyay, P.K.; et al. Specialized insulin is used for chemical warfare by fish-hunting cone snails. *Proc. Natl. Acad. Sci. USA* **2015**, *112*, 1743–1748. [CrossRef]
24. Cruz, L.J.; de Santos, V.; Zafaralla, G.C.; Ramilo, C.A.; Zeikus, R.; Gray, W.R.; Olivera, B.M. Invertebrate vasopressin/oxytocin homologs. Characterization of peptides from *Conus geographus* and *Conus striatus* venoms. *J. Biol. Chem.* **1987**, *262*, 15821–15824.
25. Clark, C.; Olivera, B.M.; Cruz, L.J. A toxin from the venom of the marine snail *Conus geographus* which acts on the vertebrate central nervous system. *Toxicon* **1981**, *19*, 691–699. [CrossRef]
26. McIntosh, M.; Cruz, L.J.; Hunkapiller, M.W.; Gray, W.R.; Olivera, B.M. Isolation and structure of a peptide toxin from the marine snail *Conus magus*. *Arch. Biochem. Biophys.* **1982**, *218*, 329–334. [CrossRef]
27. Gray, W.R.; Luque, A.; Olivera, B.M.; Barrett, J.; Cruz, L.J. Peptide toxins from *Conus geographus* venom. *J. Biochem.* **1981**, *256*, 4734–4740.
28. Feldman, D.H.; Olivera, B.M.; Yoshikami, D. Omega *Conus geographus* toxin—A peptide that blocks calcium channels. *FEBS Lett.* **1987**, *214*, 295–300. [CrossRef]
29. Craig, A.G.; Zafaralla, G.; Cruz, L.J.; Santos, A.D.; Hillyard, D.R.; Dykert, J.; Rivier, J.E.; Gray, W.R.; Imperial, J.; DelaCruz, R.G.; et al. An O-glycosylated neuroexcitatory *Conus* peptide. *Biochemistry* **1989**, *37*, 16019–16025. [CrossRef]

30. Cruz, L.J.; Krupryszewski, G.; LeCheminant, G.W.; Gray, W.R.; Olivera, B.M.; Rivier, J. Mu-conotoxin GIIIA, a peptide ligand for muscle sodium channels: Chemical synthesis, radiolabeling, and receptor characterization. *Biochemistry* **1989**, *28*, 3437–3442. [CrossRef]
31. Rybin, M.J.; O'Brien, H.; Ramiro, I.B.L.; Azam, L.; McIntosh, J.M.; Olivera, B.M.; Safavi-Hemami, H.; Yoshikami, D. αM-Conotoxin MIIIJ Blocks Nicotinic Acetylcholine Receptors at Neuromuscular Junctions of Frog and Fish. *Toxins* **2020**, *12*, 197. [CrossRef]
32. Olivera, B.M.; Seger, J.; Horvath, M.P.; Fedosov, A.E. Prey-Capture Strategies of Fish-Hunting Cone Snails: Behavior, Neurobiology and Evolution. *Brain Behav. Evol.* **2015**, *86*, 58–74. [CrossRef]
33. Robinson, S.D.; Norton, R.S. Conotoxin gene superfamilies. *Mar. Drugs* **2014**, *12*, 6058–6101. [CrossRef]
34. Li, Q.; Watkins, M.; Robinson, S.D.; Safavi-Hemami, H.; Yandell, M. Discovery of Novel Conotoxin Candidates Using Machine Learning. *Toxins* **2018**, *10*, 503. [CrossRef]
35. Safavi-Hemami, H.; Brogan, S.E.; Olivera, B.M. Pain therapeutics from cone snail venoms: From Ziconotide to novel non-opioid pathways. *J. Proteom.* **2019**, *190*, 12–20. [CrossRef] [PubMed]
36. Kerr, L.M.; Yoshikami, D. A venom peptide with a novel presynaptic blocking action. *Nature* **1984**, *308*, 282–284. [CrossRef] [PubMed]
37. McCleskey, E.W.; Fox, A.P.; Feldman, D.H.; Cruz, L.J.; Olivera, B.M.; Tsien, R.W.; Yoshikami, D. Omega-conotoxin: Direct and persistent blockade of specific types of calcium channels in neurons but not muscle. *Proc. Natl. Acad. Sci. USA* **1987**, *84*, 4327–4331. [CrossRef]
38. Todd, A.J. Neuronal circuitry for pain processing in the dorsal horn. *Nat. Rev. Neurosci.* **2010**, *11*, 823–836. [CrossRef] [PubMed]
39. Miljanich, G.P. Ziconotide: Neuronal calcium channel blocker for treating severe chronic pain. *Curr. Med. Chem.* **2004**, *11*, 3029–3040. [CrossRef] [PubMed]
40. Deer, T.R.; Pope, J.E.; Hayek, S.M.; Bux, A.; Buchser, E.; Eldabe, S.; De Andrés, J.A.; Erdek, M.; Patin, D.; Grider, J.S.; et al. The Polyanalgesic Consensus Conference (PACC): Recommendations on Intrathecal Drug Infusion Systems Best Practices and Guidelines. *Neuromodulation J. Int. Neuromodulation Soc.* **2017**, *20*, 96–132. [CrossRef]
41. Webster, L.R. The Relationship Between the Mechanisms of Action and Safety Profiles of Intrathecal Morphine and Ziconotide: A Review of the Literature. *Pain Med.* **2015**, *16*, 1265–1277. [CrossRef]
42. Pennington, M.W.; Czerwinski, A.; Norton, R.S. Peptide therapeutics from venom: Current status and potential. *Bioorg. Med. Chem.* **2018**, *26*, 2738–2758. [CrossRef]
43. King, G.F. Venoms as a platform for human drugs: Translating toxins into therapeutics. *Expert Opin. Biol. Ther.* **2011**, *11*, 1469–1484. [CrossRef]
44. Robinson, S.D.; Safavi-Hemami, H. Venom peptides as pharmacological tools and therapeutics for diabetes. *Neuropharmacology* **2017**. [CrossRef]
45. Sher, E.; Gotti, C.; Canal, N.; Scoppetta, C.; Piccolo, G.; Evoli, A.; Clementi, F. Specificity of calcium channel autoantibodies in Lambert-Eaton myasthenic syndrome. *Lancet* **1989**, *2*, 640–643. [CrossRef]
46. Lennon, V.A.; Kryzer, T.J.; Griesmann, G.E.; O'Suilleabhain, P.E.; Windebank, A.J.; Woppmann, A.; Miljanich, G.P.; Lambert, E.H. Calcium-channel antibodies in the Lambert-Eaton syndrome and other paraneoplastic syndromes. *N. Engl. J. Med.* **1995**, *332*, 1467–1474. [CrossRef]
47. Mareska, M.; Gutmann, L. Lambert-Eaton myasthenic syndrome. *Semin. Neurol.* **2004**, *24*, 149–153. [CrossRef] [PubMed]
48. Leys, K.; Lang, B.; Johnston, I.; Newsom-Davis, J. Calcium channel autoantibodies in the Lambert-Eaton myasthenic syndrome. *Ann. Neurol.* **1991**, *29*, 307–314. [CrossRef] [PubMed]
49. Motomura, M.; Johnston, I.; Lang, B.; Vincent, A.; Newsom-Davis, J. An improved diagnostic assay for Lambert-Eaton myasthenic syndrome. *J. Neurol. Neurosurg. Psychiatry* **1995**, *58*, 85–87. [CrossRef]
50. Lang, B.; Waterman, S.; Pinto, A.; Jones, D.; Moss, F.; Boot, J.; Brust, P.; Williams, M.; Stauderman, K.; Harpold, M.; et al. The role of autoantibodies in Lambert-Eaton myasthenic syndrome. *Ann. N. Y. Acad. Sci.* **1998**, *841*, 596–605. [CrossRef]
51. Skeie, G.O.; Apostolski, S.; Evoli, A.; Gilhus, N.E.; Illa, I.; Harms, L.; Hilton-Jones, D.; Melms, A.; Verschuuren, J.; Horge, H.W. Guidelines for treatment of autoimmune neuromuscular transmission disorders. *Eur. J. Neurol.* **2010**, *17*, 893–902. [CrossRef]

52. Favreau, P.; Benoit, E.; Hocking, H.G.; Carlier, L.; D' hoedt, D.; Leipold, E.; Markgraf, R.; Schlumberger, S.; Córdova, M.A.; Gaertner, H.; et al. A novel μ-conopeptide, CnIIIC, exerts potent and preferential inhibition of NaV1.2/1.4 channels and blocks neuronal nicotinic acetylcholine receptors. *Br. J. Pharmacol.* **2012**, *166*, 1654–1668. [CrossRef]
53. Westenbroek, R.E.; Hell, J.W.; Warner, C.; Dubel, S.J.; Snutch, T.P.; Catterall, W.A. Biochemical properties and subcellular distribution of an N-type calcium channel alpha 1 subunit. *Neuron* **1992**, *9*, 1099–1115. [CrossRef]
54. Hayashi, K.; Wakino, S.; Sugano, N.; Ozawa, Y.; Homma, K.; Saruta, T. Ca2+ channel subtypes and pharmacology in the kidney. *Circ. Res.* **2007**, *100*, 342–353. [CrossRef]
55. Li, D.; Paterson, D.J. Pre-synaptic sympathetic calcium channels, cyclic nucleotide-coupled phosphodiesterases and cardiac excitability. *Semin. Cell Dev. Biol.* **2019**, *94*, 20–27. [CrossRef] [PubMed]
56. Ellison, M.; McIntosh, J.M.; Olivera, B.M. Alpha-conotoxins ImI and ImII. Similar alpha 7 nicotinic receptor antagonists act at different sites. *J. Biol. Chem.* **2003**, *278*, 757–764. [CrossRef] [PubMed]
57. Broxton, N.M.; Down, J.G.; Gehrmann, J.; Alewood, P.F.; Satchell, D.G.; Livett, B.G. Alpha-conotoxin ImI inhibits the alpha-bungarotoxin-resistant nicotinic response in bovine adrenal chromaffin cells. *J. Neurochem.* **1999**, *72*, 1656–1662. [CrossRef] [PubMed]
58. Terlau, H.; Olivera, B.M. *Conus* Venoms: A Rich Source of Novel Ion Channel-Targeted Peptides. *Physiol. Rev.* **2004**, *84*, 41–68. [CrossRef]
59. Azam, L.; McIntosh, J.M. Alpha-conotoxins as pharmacological probes of nicotinic acetylcholine receptors. *Acta Pharmacol. Sin.* **2009**, *30*, 771–783. [CrossRef]
60. Giribaldi, J.; Dutertre, S. α-Conotoxins to explore the molecular, physiological and pathophysiological functions of neuronal nicotinic acetylcholine receptors. *Neurosci. Lett.* **2018**, *679*, 24–34. [CrossRef]
61. Heghinian, M.D.; Mejia, M.; Adams, D.J.; Godenschwege, T.A.; Marí, F. Inhibition of cholinergic pathways in Drosophila melanogaster by α-conotoxins. *FASEB J. Off. Publ. Fed. Am. Soc. Exp. Biol.* **2015**, *29*, 1011–1018. [CrossRef]
62. Mei, D.; Lin, Z.; Fu, J.; He, B.; Gao, W.; Ma, L.; Dai, W.; Zhang, H.; Wang, X.; Wang, J.; et al. The use of α-conotoxin ImI to actualize the targeted delivery of paclitaxel micelles to α7 nAChR-overexpressing breast cancer. *Biomaterials* **2015**, *42*, 52–65. [CrossRef]
63. Walker, C.S.; Jensen, S.; Ellison, M.; Matta, J.A.; Lee, W.Y.; Imperial, J.S.; Duclos, N.; Brockie, P.J.; Madsen, D.M.; Isaac, J.T.R.; et al. A Novel *Conus* Snail Polypeptide Causes Excitotoxicity by Blocking Desensitization of AMPA Receptors. *Curr. Biol.* **2009**, *19*, 900–908. [CrossRef]
64. Chen, L.; Durr, K.L.; Gouaux, E. X-ray structures of AMPA receptor-cone snail toxin complexes illuminate activation mechanism. *Science* **2014**, *345*, 1021–1026. [CrossRef]
65. Menting, J.G.; Gajewiak, J.; MacRaild, C.A.; Chou, D.H.; Disotuar, M.M.; Smith, N.A.; Miller, C.; Erchegyi, J.; Rivier, J.E.; Olivera, B.M.; et al. A minimized human insulin-receptor-binding motif revealed in a *Conus geographus* venom insulin. *Nat. Struct. Mol. Biol.* **2016**, *23*, 916–920. [CrossRef] [PubMed]
66. Buczek, O.; Olivera, B.M.; Bulaj, G. Propeptide Does Not Act as an Intramolecular Chaperone but Facilitates Protein Disulfide Isomerase-Assisted Folding of a Conotoxin Precursor. *Biochemistry* **2004**, *43*, 1093–1101. [CrossRef] [PubMed]
67. Safavi-Hemami, H.; Bulaj, G.; Olivera, B.M.; Williamson, N.A.; Purcell, A.W. Identification of *Conus* peptidylprolyl cis-trans isomerases (PPIases) and assessment of their role in the oxidative folding of conotoxins. *J. Biol. Chem.* **2010**, *285*, 12735–12746. [CrossRef] [PubMed]
68. Safavi-Hemami, H.; Li, Q.; Jackson, R.L.; Song, A.S.; Boomsma, W.; Bandyopadhyay, P.K.; Gruber, C.W.; Purcell, A.W.; Yandell, M.; Olivera, B.M.; et al. Rapid expansion of the protein disulfide isomerase gene family facilitates the folding of venom peptides. *Proc. Natl. Acad. Sci. USA* **2016**, *113*, 3227–3232. [CrossRef] [PubMed]
69. Fuller, E.; Green, B.R.; Catlin, P.; Buczek, O.; Nielsen, J.S.; Olivera, B.M.; Bulaj, G. Oxidative folding of conotoxins sharing an identical disulfide bridging framework. *FEBS J.* **2005**, *272*, 1727–1738. [CrossRef] [PubMed]
70. Bandyopadhyay, P.K.; Colledge, C.J.; Walker, C.S.; Zhou, L.-M.; Hillyard, D.R.; Olivera, B.M. Conantokin-G Precursor and Its Role in g-Carboxylation by a Vitamin K-dependent Carboxylase from a *Conus* Snail. *J. Biol. Chem.* **1998**, *273*, 5447–5450. [CrossRef]

71. Bulaj, G.; Buczek, O.; Goodsell, I.; Jimenez, E.C.; Kranski, J.; Nielsen, J.S.; Garrett, J.E.; Olivera, B.M. Efficient oxidative folding of conotoxins and the radiation of venomous cone snails. *Proc. Natl. Acad. Sci. USA* **2003**, *100*, 14562–14568. [CrossRef]
72. Safavi-Hemami, H.; Lu, A.; Li, Q.; Fedosov, A.E.; Biggs, J.; Showers Corneli, P.; Seger, J.; Yandell, M.; Olivera, B.M. Venom Insulins of Cone Snails Diversify Rapidly and Track Prey Taxa. *Mol. Biol. Evol.* **2016**, *33*, 2924–2934. [CrossRef]
73. Chang, D.; Duda, T.F., Jr. Age-related association of venom gene expression and diet of predatory gastropods. *BMC Evol. Biol.* **2016**, *16*, 27. [CrossRef]
74. Duda, T.F.; Palumbi, S.R. Gene expression and feeding ecology: Evolution of piscivory in the venomous gastropod genus *Conus*. *Proc. R. Soc. Lond. Ser. B-Biol. Sci.* **2004**, *271*, 1165–1174. [CrossRef]
75. Phuong, M.A.; Mahardika, G.N. Targeted sequencing of venom genes from cone snail genomes reveals coupling between dietary breadth and conotoxin diversity. *bioRxiv* **2017**. [CrossRef]
76. Phuong, M.A.; Mahardika, G.N.; Alfaro, M.E. Dietary breadth is positively correlated with venom complexity in cone snails. *BMC Genom.* **2016**, *17*, 401. [CrossRef] [PubMed]
77. Chang, D.; Duda, T.F.J. Extensive and continuous duplication facilitates rapid evolution and diversification of gene families. *Mol. Biol. Evol.* **2012**, *29*, 2019–2029. [CrossRef] [PubMed]
78. Duda, T.F.; Palumbi, S.R. Molecular genetics of ecological diversification: Duplication and rapid evolution of toxin genes of the venomous gastropod *Conus*. *Proc. Natl. Acad. Sci. USA* **1999**, *96*, 6820–6823. [CrossRef] [PubMed]
79. Puillandre, N.; Watkins, M.; Olivera, B.M. Evolution of *Conus* peptide genes: Duplication and positive selection in the A-superfamily. *J. Mol. Evol.* **2010**, *70*, 190–202. [CrossRef]
80. Cartier, G.E.; Yoshikami, D.; Gray, W.R.; Luo, S.; Olivera, B.M.; McIntosh, J.M. A New a-Conotoxin Which Targets α3β2 Nicotinic Acetylcholine Receptors. *J. Biol. Chem.* **1996**, *271*, 7522–7528. [CrossRef]
81. Safronova, V.G.; Vulfius, C.A.; Shelukhina, I.V.; Mal'tseva, V.N.; Berezhnov, A.V.; Fedotova, E.I.; Miftahova, R.G.; Kryukova, E.V.; Grinevich, A.A.; Tsetlin, V.I. Nicotinic receptor involvement in regulation of functions of mouse neutrophils from inflammatory site. *Immunobiology* **2016**, *221*, 761–772. [CrossRef]
82. Sanjakdar, S.S.; Maldoon, P.P.; Marks, M.J.; Brunzell, D.H.; Maskos, U.; McIntosh, J.M.; Bowers, M.S.; Damaj, M.I. Differential roles of α6β2* and α4β2* neuronal nicotinic receptors in nicotine- and cocaine-conditioned reward in mice. *Neuropsychopharmacol. Off. Publ. Am. Coll. Neuropsychopharmacol.* **2015**, *40*, 350–360. [CrossRef]
83. Zhao-Shea, R.; Liu, L.; Soll, L.G.; Improgo, M.R.; Meyers, E.E.; McIntosh, J.M.; Grady, S.R.; Marks, M.J.; Gardner, P.D.; Tapper, A.R. Nicotine-mediated activation of dopaminergic neurons in distinct regions of the ventral tegmental area. *Neuropsychopharmacol. Off. Publ. Am. Coll. Neuropsychopharmacol.* **2011**, *36*, 1021–1032. [CrossRef]
84. Ellison, M.; Haberlandt, C.; Gomez-Casati, M.E.; Watkins, M.; Elgoyhen, A.B.; McIntosh, J.M.; Olivera, B.M. Alpha-RgIA: A novel conotoxin that specifically and potently blocks the alpha9alpha10 nAChR. *Biochemistry* **2006**, *45*, 1511–1517. [CrossRef]
85. Vincler, M.; Wittenauer, S.; Parker, R.; Ellison, M.; Olivera, B.M.; McIntosh, J.M. Molecular mechanism for analgesia involving specific antagonism of alpha9alpha10 nicotinic acetylcholine receptors. *Proc. Natl. Acad. Sci. USA* **2006**, *103*, 17880–17884. [CrossRef] [PubMed]
86. Satkunanathan, N.; Livett, B.G.; Gayler, K.; Sandall, D.; Down, J.G.; Khalil, Z. Alpha-conotoxin Vc1.1 alleviates neuropathic pain and accelerates functional recovery of injured neurones. *Brain Res.* **2005**, *1059*, 149–158. [CrossRef]
87. McIntosh, J.M.; Absalom, N.; Chebib, M.; Elgoyhen, A.B.; Vincler, M. Alpha9 nicotinic acetylcholine receptors and the treatment of pain. *Biochem. Pharmacol.* **2009**, *78*, 693–702. [CrossRef] [PubMed]
88. Di Cesare Mannelli, L.; Cinci, L.; Micheli, L.; Zanardelli, M.; Pacini, A.; McIntosh, J.M.; Ghelardini, C. Alpha-conotoxin RgIA protects against the development of nerve injury-induced chronic pain and prevents both neuronal and glial derangement. *Pain* **2014**, *155*, 1986–1995. [CrossRef] [PubMed]
89. Richter, K.; Sagawe, S.; Hecker, A.; Küllmar, M.; Askevold, I.; Damm, J.; Heldmann, S.; Pöhlmann, M.; Ruhrmann, S.; Sander, M.; et al. C-Reactive Protein Stimulates Nicotinic Acetylcholine Receptors to Control ATP-Mediated Monocytic Inflammasome Activation. *Front. Immunol.* **2018**, *9*, 1604. [CrossRef]

90. Richter, K.; Koch, C.; Perniss, A.; Wolf, P.M.; Schweda, E.K.H.; Wichmann, S.; Wilker, S.; Magel, I.; Sander, M.; McIntosh, J.M.; et al. Phosphocholine-Modified Lipooligosaccharides of Haemophilus influenzae Inhibit ATP-Induced IL-1β Release by Pulmonary Epithelial Cells. *Molecules* **2018**, *23*, 1979. [CrossRef]
91. Grau, V.; Richter, K.; Hone, A.J.; McIntosh, J.M. Conopeptides [V11L;V16D] ArIB and RgIA4: Powerful Tools for the Identification of Novel Nicotinic Acetylcholine Receptors in Monocytes. *Front. Pharmacol.* **2018**, *9*, 1499. [CrossRef]
92. Xiong, X.; Menting, J.; Disotuar, M.; Smith, N.; Delanie, C.; Ghabash, G.; Agrawal, R.; Wang, X.; He, X.; Fisher, S.; et al. A structurally minimized insulin based on cone-snail venom insulin principles. *Nat. Struct. Mol. Biol.* **2020**, *27*, 615–624. [CrossRef]
93. Dave, K.; Lahiry, A. Conotoxins: Review and docking studies to determine potentials of conotoxin as an anticancer drug molecule. *Curr. Top. Med. Chem.* **2012**, *12*, 845–851. [CrossRef]
94. Lubbers, N.L.; Campbell, T.J.; Polakowski, J.S.; Bulaj, G.; Layer, R.T.; Moore, J.; Gross, G.J.; Cox, B.F. Postischemic administration of CGX-1051, a peptide from cone snail venom, reduces infarct size in both rat and dog models of myocardial ischemia and reperfusion. *J. Cardiovasc. Pharmacol.* **2005**, *46*, 141–146. [CrossRef]
95. Chen, P.; Dendorfer, A.; Finol-Urdaneta, R.K.; Terlau, H.; Olivera, B.M. Biochemical characterization of kappaM-RIIIJ, a Kv1.2 channel blocker: Evaluation of cardioprotective effects of kappaM-conotoxins. *J. Biol. Chem.* **2010**, *285*, 14882–14889. [CrossRef] [PubMed]
96. Cordeiro, S.; Finol-Urdaneta, R.K.; Köpfer, D.; Markushina, A.; Song, J.; French, R.J.; Kopec, W.; de Groot, B.L.; Giacobassi, M.J.; Leavitt, L.S.; et al. Conotoxin κM-RIIIJ, a tool targeting asymmetric heteromeric K(v)1 channels. *Proc. Natl. Acad. Sci. USA* **2019**, *116*, 1059–1064. [CrossRef] [PubMed]
97. Teichert, R.W.; Raghuraman, S.; Memon, T.; Cox, J.L.; Foulkes, T.; Rivier, J.E.; Olivera, B.M. Characterization of two neuronal subclasses through constellation pharmacology. *Proc. Natl. Acad. Sci. USA* **2012**, *109*, 12758–12763. [CrossRef]
98. Teichert, R.W.; Smith, N.J.; Raghuraman, S.; Yoshikami, D.; Light, A.R.; Olivera, B.M. Functional profiling of neurons through cellular neuropharmacology. *Proc. Natl. Acad. Sci. USA* **2012**, *109*, 1388–1395. [CrossRef] [PubMed]
99. Coleman, S.K.; Newcombe, J.; Pryke, J.; Dolly, J.O. Subunit composition of Kv1 channels in human CNS. *J. Neurochem.* **1999**, *73*, 849–858. [CrossRef]
100. Huang, R.; Wang, Y.; Li, J.; Jiang, X.; Li, Y.; Liu, B.; Wu, X.; Du, X.; Hang, Y.; Jin, M.; et al. Ca(2+)-independent but voltage-dependent quantal catecholamine secretion (CiVDS) in the mammalian sympathetic nervous system. *Proc. Natl. Acad. Sci. USA* **2019**, *116*, 20201–20209. [CrossRef]
101. Dooley, D.J.; Lupp, A.; Hertting, G.; Osswald, H. Omega-conotoxin GVIA and pharmacological modulation of hippocampal noradrenaline release. *Eur. J. Pharmacol.* **1988**, *148*, 261–267. [CrossRef]
102. Hansen, T.; Tarasova, O.S.; Khammy, M.M.; Ferreira, A.; Kennard, J.A.; Andresen, J.; Staehr, C.; Brain, K.L.; Nilsson, H.; Aalkjaer, C. [Ca(2+)] changes in sympathetic varicosities and Schwann cells in rat mesenteric arteries-Relation to noradrenaline release and contraction. *Acta Physiol.* **2019**, *226*, e13279. [CrossRef]
103. Scott, D.A.; Wright, C.E.; Angus, J.A. Actions of intrathecal omega-conotoxins CVID, GVIA, MVIIA, and morphine in acute and neuropathic pain in the rat. *Eur. J. Pharmacol.* **2002**, *451*, 279–286. [CrossRef]
104. Nigam, A.; Hargus, N.J.; Barker, B.S.; Ottolini, M.; Hounshell, J.A.; Bertram, E.H., III; Perez-Reyes, E.; Patel, M.K. Inhibition of T-Type calcium channels in mEC layer II stellate neurons reduces neuronal hyperexcitability associated with epilepsy. *Epilepsy Res.* **2019**, *154*, 132–138. [CrossRef]
105. Tarif, N.; Bakris, G.L. Preservation of renal function: The spectrum of effects by calcium-channel blockers. *Nephrol. Dial. Transplant.* **1997**, *12*, 2244–2250. [CrossRef] [PubMed]
106. Dolmetsch, R.E.; Pajvani, U.; Fife, K.; Spotts, J.M.; Greenberg, M.E. Signaling to the nucleus by an L-type calcium channel-calmodulin complex through the MAP kinase pathway. *Science* **2001**, *294*, 333–339. [CrossRef] [PubMed]
107. Hillyard, D.R.; Monje, V.D.; Mintz, I.M.; Bean, B.P.; Nadasdi, L.; Ramachandran, J.; Miljanich, G.; Azimi-Zoonooz, A.; McIntosh, J.M.; Cruz, L.J.; et al. A new *Conus* peptide ligand for mammalian presynaptic Ca2+ channels. *Neuron* **1992**, *9*, 69–77. [CrossRef]
108. McDonough, S.I.; Swartz, K.J.; Mintz, I.M.; Boland, L.M.; Bean, B.P. Inhibition of calcium channels in rat central and peripheral neurons by omega-conotoxin MVIIC. *J. Neurosci. Off. J. Soc. Neurosci.* **1996**, *16*, 2612–2623. [CrossRef]

109. Tian, G.F.; Azmi, H.; Takano, T.; Xu, Q.; Peng, W.; Lin, J.; Oberheim, N.; Lou, N.; Wang, X.; Zielke, H.R.; et al. An astrocytic basis of epilepsy. *Nat. Med.* **2005**, *11*, 973–981. [CrossRef]
110. Carter, B.C.; Jahr, C.E. Postsynaptic, not presynaptic NMDA receptors are required for spike-timing-dependent LTD induction. *Nat. Neurosci.* **2016**, *19*, 1218–1224. [CrossRef] [PubMed]
111. Zhang, Y.; Qin, W.; Qian, Z.; Liu, X.; Wang, H.; Gong, S.; Sun, Y.G.; Snutch, T.P.; Jiang, X.; Tao, J. Peripheral pain is enhanced by insulin-like growth factor 1 through a G protein-mediated stimulation of T-type calcium channels. *Sci. Signal.* **2014**, *7*, ra94. [CrossRef]
112. Wang, H.; Wei, Y.; Pu, Y.; Jiang, D.; Jiang, X.; Zhang, Y.; Tao, J. Brain-derived neurotrophic factor stimulation of T-type Ca(2+) channels in sensory neurons contributes to increased peripheral pain sensitivity. *Sci. Signal.* **2019**, *12*. [CrossRef]
113. Phuong, M.A.; Mahardika, G.N. Targeted Sequencing of Venom Genes from Cone Snail Genomes Improves Understanding of Conotoxin Molecular Evolution. *Mol. Biol. Evol.* **2018**, *35*, 1210–1224. [CrossRef]
114. Turchetto, J.; Sequeira, A.F.; Ramond, L.; Peysson, F.; Bras, J.L.; Saez, N.J.; Duhoo, Y.; Blemont, M.; Guerreiro, C.I.; Quinton, L.; et al. High-throughput expression of animal venom toxins in Escherichia coli to generate a large library of oxidized disulphide-reticulated peptides for drug discovery. *Microb. Cell Factories* **2017**, *16*, 6. [CrossRef]
115. Sequeira, A.F.; Turchetto, J.; Saez, N.J.; Peysson, F.; Ramond, L.; Duhoo, Y.; Blémont, M.; Fernandes, V.O.; Gama, L.T.; Ferreira, L.M.; et al. Gene design, fusion technology and TEV cleavage conditions influence the purification of oxidized disulphide-rich venom peptides in Escherichia coli. *Microb. Cell Factories* **2017**, *16*, 4. [CrossRef] [PubMed]
116. Nielsen, L.D.; Foged, M.M.; Albert, A.; Bertelsen, A.B.; Soltoft, C.L.; Robinson, S.D.; Petersen, S.V.; Purcell, A.W.; Olivera, B.M.; Norton, R.S.; et al. The three-dimensional structure of an H-superfamily conotoxin reveals a granulin fold arising from a common ICK cysteine framework. *J. Biol. Chem.* **2019**, *294*, 8745–8759. [CrossRef] [PubMed]
117. Teichert, R.W.; Memon, T.; Aman, J.W.; Olivera, B.M. Using constellation pharmacology to define comprehensively a somatosensory neuronal subclass. *Proc. Natl. Acad. Sci. USA* **2014**, *111*, 2319–2324. [CrossRef] [PubMed]
118. MacRae, C.A.; Peterson, R.T. Zebrafish as tools for drug discovery. *Nat. Rev. Drug Discov.* **2015**, *14*, 721–731. [CrossRef]
119. Tay, B.; Stewart, T.A.; Davis, F.M.; Deuis, J.R.; Vetter, I. Development of a high-throughput fluorescent no-wash sodium influx assay. *PLoS ONE* **2019**, *14*, e0213751. [CrossRef]
120. Fosgerau, K.; Hoffmann, T. Peptide therapeutics: Current status and future directions. *Drug Discov. Today* **2015**, *20*, 122–128. [CrossRef]
121. Kohn, A.J. *Conus* Envenomation of Humans: In Fact and Fiction. *Toxins* **2018**, *11*, 10. [CrossRef]
122. Kizer, K.W. Marine envenomations. *J. Toxicol. Clin. Toxicol.* **1983**, *21*, 527–555. [CrossRef]
123. McIntosh, J.M.; Jones, R.M. Cone venom–from accidental stings to deliberate injection. *Toxicon* **2001**, *39*, 1447–1451. [CrossRef]
124. Halford, Z.A.; Yu, P.Y.; Likeman, R.K.; Hawley-Molloy, J.S.; Thomas, C.; Bingham, J.P. Cone shell envenomation: Epidemiology, pharmacology and medical care. *Diving Hyperb. Med.* **2015**, *45*, 200–207.
125. World Health Organization Snakebite Report. Available online: https://www.who.int/snakebites/disease/en/ (accessed on 14 July 2020).
126. Chippaux, J.P.; Goyffon, M. Epidemiology of scorpionism: A global appraisal. *Acta Trop.* **2008**, *107*, 71–79. [CrossRef] [PubMed]
127. Kularatne, S.A.; Dinamithra, N.P.; Sivansuthan, S.; Weerakoon, K.G.; Thillaimpalam, B.; Kalyanasundram, V.; Ranawana, K.B. Clinico-epidemiology of stings and envenoming of Hottentotta tamulus (Scorpiones: Buthidae), the Indian red scorpion from Jaffna Peninsula in northern Sri Lanka. *Toxicon* **2015**, *93*, 85–89. [CrossRef] [PubMed]
128. Rodrigo, C.; Gnanathasan, A. Management of scorpion envenoming: A systematic review and meta-analysis of controlled clinical trials. *Syst. Rev.* **2017**, *6*, 74. [CrossRef] [PubMed]
129. Slagboom, J.; Kool, J.; Harrison, R.A.; Casewell, N.R. Haemotoxic snake venoms: Their functional activity, impact on snakebite victims and pharmaceutical promise. *Br. J. Haematol.* **2017**, *177*, 947–959. [CrossRef] [PubMed]

130. Saab, F.; Ionescu, C.; Schweiger, M.J. Bleeding risk and safety profile related to the use of eptifibatide: A current review. *Expert Opin. Drug Saf.* **2012**, *11*, 315–324. [CrossRef] [PubMed]
131. Serrano, S.M. The long road of research on snake venom serine proteinases. *Toxicon* **2013**, *62*, 19–26. [CrossRef]
132. Ortiz, E.; Gurrola, G.B.; Schwartz, E.F.; Possani, L.D. Scorpion venom components as potential candidates for drug development. *Toxicon* **2015**, *93*, 125–135. [CrossRef]
133. Tenorio, M.J. Conotoxins: Weapons of Mass Destruction? *Cone Collect.* **2013**, *22*, 6–7.
134. McManus, O.B.; Musick, J.R.; Gonzalez, C. Peptides isolated from the venom of *Conus geographus* block neuromuscular transmission. *Neurosci. Lett.* **1981**, *25*, 57–62. [CrossRef]
135. McManus, O.B.; Musick, J.R. Postsynaptic block of frog neuromuscular transmission by conotoxin GI. *J. Neurosci. Off. J. Soc. Neurosci.* **1985**, *5*, 110–116. [CrossRef]
136. Groebe, D.R.; Gray, W.R.; Abramson, S.N. Determinants involved in the affinity of alpha-conotoxins GI and SI for the muscle subtype of nicotinic acetylcholine receptors. *Biochemistry* **1997**, *36*, 6469–6474. [CrossRef]
137. Almquist, R.G.; Kadambi, S.R.; Yasuda, D.M.; Weitl, F.L.; Polgar, W.E.; Toll, L.R. Paralytic activity of (des-Glu1)conotoxin GI analogs in the mouse diaphragm. *Int. J. Pept. Protein Res.* **1989**, *34*, 455–462. [CrossRef] [PubMed]
138. Ahorukomeye, P.; Disotuar, M.M.; Gajewiak, G.; Karanth, S.; Watkins, M.; Robinson, S.D.; Flórez Salcedo, P.; Smith, N.A.; Smith, B.J.; Schlegel, A.; et al. Fish-hunting cone snail venoms are a rich source of minimized ligands of the vertebrate insulin receptor. *eLife* **2019**, *8*, e41574. [CrossRef] [PubMed]
139. McIntosh, J.M.; Dowell, C.; Watkins, M.; Garrett, J.E.; Yoshikami, D.; Olivera, B.M. A-Conotoxin GIC from *Conus geographus*, a Novel Peptide Antagonist of Nicotinic Acetylcholine Receptors. *J. Biol. Chem.* **2002**, *277*, 33610–33615. [CrossRef] [PubMed]
140. Clark, R.J.; Jensen, J.E.; Nevin, S.T.; Callaghan, B.P.; Adams, D.J.; Craik, D.J. The engineering of an orally active conotoxin for the treatment of neuropathic pain. *Angew. Chem.* **2010**, *49*, 6545–6548. [CrossRef] [PubMed]
141. Suszkiw, J.B.; Murawsky, M.M.; Shi, M. Further characterization of phasic calcium influx in rat cerebrocortical synaptosomes: Inferences regarding calcium channel type(s) in nerve endings. *J. Neurochem.* **1989**, *52*, 1260–1269. [CrossRef]
142. Xiao, H.; Pan, H.; Liao, K.; Yang, M.; Huang, C. Snake Venom PLA(2), a Promising Target for Broad-Spectrum Antivenom Drug Development. *BioMed Res. Int.* **2017**, *2017*, 6592820. [CrossRef] [PubMed]
143. Stirpe, F.; Barbieri, L.; Abbondanza, A.; Falasca, A.I.; Brown, A.N.; Sandvig, K.; Olsnes, S.; Pihl, A. Properties of volkensin, a toxic lectin from Adenia volkensii. *J. Biol. Chem.* **1985**, *260*, 14589–14595.
144. Lewis, R.J.; Sellin, M.; Poli, M.A.; Norton, R.S.; MacLeod, J.K.; Sheil, M.M. Purification and characterization of ciguatoxins from moray eel (Lycodontis javanicus, Muraenidae). *Toxicon* **1991**, *29*, 1115–1127. [CrossRef]
145. Yokoyama, A.; Murata, M.; Oshima, Y.; Iwashita, T.; Yasumoto, T. Some chemical properties of maitotoxin, a putative calcium channel agonist isolated from a marine dinoflagellate. *J. Biochem.* **1988**, *104*, 184–187. [CrossRef]
146. Moore, R.E.; Scheuer, P.J. Palytoxin: A new marine toxin from a coelenterate. *Science* **1971**, *172*, 495–498. [CrossRef] [PubMed]
147. Tokuyama, T.; Daly, J.; Witkop, B.; Karle, I.L.; Karle, J. The structure of batrachotoxinin A, a nol vesteroidal alkaloid from the Colombian arrow poison frog, Phyllobates aurotaenia. *J. Am. Chem. Soc.* **1968**, *90*, 1917–1918. [CrossRef] [PubMed]
148. Halstead, B.W.; Schantz, E.J.; World Health Organization. *Paralytic Shellfish Poisoning*; World Health Organization: Geneva, Switzerland, 1984; Volume 79, ISBN 9241700793.
149. Stonik, V.A.; Stonik, I.V. Studies on marine toxins: Chemical and biological aspects. *Stud. Mar. Toxins Chem. Biol. Asp.* **2010**, *79*, 5. [CrossRef]
150. Cohen, J.A.; Guardia III, C.F.; Mowchun, J.J.; Stommel, E.W. Demyelinating Diseases of the Peripheral Nerves. In *Nerves and Nerve Injuries*; Academic Press: Cambridge, MA, USA, 2015; pp. 895–934. [CrossRef]
151. Jones, R.G.; Lee, L.; Landon, J. The effects of specific antibody fragments on the 'irreversible' neurotoxicity induced by Brown snake (Pseudonaja) venom. *Br. J. Pharmacol.* **1999**, *126*, 581–584. [CrossRef] [PubMed]
152. Tyler, M.I.; Barnett, D.; Nicholson, P.; Spence, I.; Howden, M.E. Studies on the subunit structure of textilotoxin, a potent neurotoxin from the venom of the Australian common brown snake (*Pseudonaja textilis*). *Biochim. Biophys. Acta* **1987**, *915*, 210–216. [CrossRef]

153. Benton, B.J.; Keller, S.A.; Spriggs, D.L.; Capacio, B.R.; Chang, F.C. Recovery from the lethal effects of saxitoxin: A therapeutic window for 4-aminopyridine (4-AP). *Toxicon* **1998**, *36*, 571–588. [CrossRef]
154. Europa Council Reculation (EC) No 428/2009. Available online: http://data.europa.eu/eli/reg/2009/428/2012-06-15 (accessed on 14 July 2020).
155. Australian Government Federal Register of Legislation Defence and Strategic Goods List 2019. Available online: https://www.legislation.gov.au/Details/F2019L00424/Html/Text (accessed on 14 July 2020).
156. US Centers for Disease Control and Prevention Select Agents and Toxins List. Available online: https://www.selectagents.gov/SelectAgentsandToxinsList.html (accessed on 14 July 2020).
157. Center for Biosikring og Bioberedskab Liste over Kontrolbelagte Biologiske Stoffer. Available online: https://www.biosikring.dk/681/#c4878 (accessed on 14 July 2020).
158. The Australia Group. Available online: https://www.dfat.gov.au/publications/minisite/theaustraliagroupnet/site/en/index.html (accessed on 14 July 2020).
159. Olivera, B.M.; Gray, W.R.; Zeikus, R.; McIntosh, J.M.; Varga, J.; Rivier, J.; Desantos, V.; Cruz, L.J. Peptide neurotoxins from fish-hunting cone snails. *Science.* **1985**, *230*, 1338–1343. [CrossRef]
160. Patton, J.S.; Trinchero, P.; Platz, R.M. Bioavailability of pulmonary delivered peptides and proteins: α-interferon, calcitonins and parathyroid hormones. In Proceedings of the Sixth International Symposium on Recent Advances in Drug Delivery Systems, Salt Lake City, UT, USA, 21–24 February 1993; pp. 79–85.
161. Adjei, A.; Garren, J. Pulmonary delivery of peptide drugs: Effect of particle size on bioavailability of leuprolide acetate in healthy male volunteers. *Pharm. Res.* **1990**, *7*, 565–569. [CrossRef]
162. Agu, R.U.; Ugwoke, M.I.; Armand, M.; Kinget, R.; Verbeke, N. The lung as a route for systemic delivery of therapeutic proteins and peptides. *Respir. Res.* **2001**, *2*, 198–209. [CrossRef]
163. Hickey, A.J.; da Rocha, S.R. *Pharmaceutical Inhalation Aerosol Technology*, 3rd ed.; CRC Press: Boca Raton, FL, USA, 2019; Volume 3, p. 746.
164. Johnson, K.A. Preparation of peptide and protein powders for inhalation. *Adv. Drug Deliv. Rev.* **1997**, *26*, 3–15. [CrossRef]
165. Yu, S.; Yang, B.; Yan, L.; Dai, Q. Sensitive Detection of α-Conotoxin GI in Human Plasma Using a Solid-Phase Extraction Column and LC-MS/MS. *Toxins* **2017**, *9*, 235. [CrossRef] [PubMed]
166. Clark, R.J.; Fischer, H.; Dempster, L.; Daly, N.L.; Rosengren, K.J.; Nevin, S.T.; Meunier, F.A.; Adams, D.J.; Craik, D.J. Engineering stable peptide toxins by means of backbone cyclization: Stabilization of the alpha-conotoxin MII. *Proc. Natl. Acad. Sci. USA* **2005**, *102*, 13767–13772. [CrossRef] [PubMed]
167. Di, L. Strategic approaches to optimizing peptide ADME properties. *AAPS J.* **2015**, *17*, 134–143. [CrossRef]
168. Smith, M.L.; Vorce, S.P.; Holler, J.M.; Shimomura, E.; Magluilo, J.; Jacobs, A.J.; Huestis, M.A. Modern instrumental methods in forensic toxicology. *J. Anal. Toxicol.* **2007**, *31*, 237–253. [CrossRef]
169. Infectious Diseases Society of America. Available online: https://www.idsociety.org (accessed on 6 October 2004).
170. El-Aziz, T.M.A.; Ravelet, C.; Molgo, J.; Fiore, E.; Pale, S.; Amar, M.; Al-Khoury, S.; Dejeu, J.; Fadl, M.; Ronjat, M.; et al. Efficient functional neutralization of lethal peptide toxins in vivo by oligonucleotides. *Sci. Rep.* **2017**, *7*, 7202. [CrossRef]
171. Endean, R.; Rudkin, C. Studies of the venoms of some *Conidae*. *Toxicon* **1963**, *1*, 49–64. [CrossRef]
172. Kohn, A.J. Piscivorous Gastropods of the Genus *Conus*. *Proc. Natl. Acad. Sci. USA* **1956**, *42*, 168–171. [CrossRef]

biomedicines

MDPI

Article

Characterisation of a Novel A-Superfamily Conotoxin

David T. Wilson [1], Paramjit S. Bansal [1], David A. Carter [2], Irina Vetter [2,3], Annette Nicke [4], Sébastien Dutertre [5] and Norelle L. Daly [1,*]

1 Centre for Molecular Therapeutics, Australian Institute of Tropical Health and Medicine, James Cook University, Smithfield, QLD 4878, Australia; david.wilson4@jcu.edu.au (D.T.W.); paramjit.bansal@jcu.edu.au (P.S.B.)
2 Centre for Pain Research, Institute for Molecular Bioscience, The University of Queensland, St Lucia, QLD 4072, Australia; d.carter@imb.uq.edu.au (D.A.C.); i.vetter@imb.uq.edu.au (I.V.)
3 School of Pharmacy, The University of Queensland, Woolloongabba, QLD 4102, Australia
4 Walther Straub Institute of Pharmacology and Toxicology, Faculty of Medicine, LMU Munich, Nußbaumstraße 26, 80336 Munich, Germany; annette.nicke@lrz.uni-muenchen.de
5 Institut des Biomolécules Max Mousseron, UMR 5247, Université de Montpellier, CNRS, 34095 Montpellier, France; sebastien.dutertre@umontpellier.fr
* Correspondence: norelle.daly@jcu.edu.au; Tel.: +61-7-4232-1815

Received: 3 May 2020; Accepted: 18 May 2020; Published: 20 May 2020

Abstract: Conopeptides belonging to the A-superfamily from the venomous molluscs, *Conus*, are typically α-conotoxins. The α-conotoxins are of interest as therapeutic leads and pharmacological tools due to their selectivity and potency at nicotinic acetylcholine receptor (nAChR) subtypes. Structurally, the α-conotoxins have a consensus fold containing two conserved disulfide bonds that define the two-loop framework and brace a helical region. Here we report on a novel α-conotoxin Pl168, identified from the transcriptome of *Conus planorbis*, which has an unusual 4/8 loop framework. Unexpectedly, NMR determination of its three-dimensional structure reveals a new structural type of A-superfamily conotoxins with a different disulfide-stabilized fold, despite containing the conserved cysteine framework and disulfide connectivity of classical α-conotoxins. The peptide did not demonstrate activity on a range of nAChRs, or Ca^{2+} and Na^{+} channels suggesting that it might represent a new pharmacological class of conotoxins.

Keywords: conopeptide; NMR spectroscopy; disulfide framework

1. Introduction

Cone snail venoms comprise mainly small peptides, termed conotoxins, and represent one of the most extensive libraries of bioactive compounds from marine creatures. Conotoxins generally have selectivity and potency for a range of ion channels and G-protein coupled receptors and consequently have been useful as pharmacological tools and therapeutic leads [1]. Several conotoxins have been tested in clinical trials, with an N-type calcium channel blocker from *Conus magus* (ω-MVIIA) approved by the Federal Drug Administration (FDA) as Prialt® for the treatment of chronic pain [2–4]. While the majority of studies aimed at developing conotoxins as drug leads focussed on treatment of pain (e.g., ω-CVID and χ-MrIA [5]) other studies have expanded the potential applications of conotoxins. Conantokin G, a *N*-methyl-D-aspartate (NMDA) antagonist from *Conus geographus*, has been of interest for development as an anticonvulsant [6], while more recent studies have shown antimycobacterial activity (O1_cal29b from *Californiconus californicus*) [7] and inhibitory effects against the growth of lung cancer cells (TxID from *Conus textile*) [8]. The venom of a single species can contain hundreds of different peptides and with at least 750 different species of cone snails [9,10], it is estimated that more than 1 million unique peptides exist [10]. However, despite extensive study in the field, we have currently sampled less than 1% of this diversity [10].

Conotoxins have been classified into various gene superfamilies based on signal sequence conservation, in addition to classification into families based on cysteine framework and receptor targets [11]. The number of disulfide bonds is typically 2-4, but the connectivity can vary even amongst conotoxins containing the same number of cysteine residues, as can the bioactivity. The known cone snail venom peptide sequences and their known functions have been collated in the database Conoserver [12,13]. Twenty-nine superfamilies and thirty different cysteine frameworks have been identified in Conoserver to date, highlighting the diversity in the sequences of conotoxins. The A-superfamily is one of the most well characterised, with the majority containing cysteine framework I (CC-C-C). This framework is primarily associated with the α-conotoxin family, members of which specifically antagonise the nicotinic acetylcholine receptors (nAChRs) [14,15]. nAChRs are ligand-gated ion channels involved in a range of physiological and pathophysiological processes, including muscle contraction, pain sensation and nicotine addiction. They are classified as muscle-type and neuronal, and have been implicated in neurological disorders such as Parkinson's and Alzheimer's diseases [16] making them potential drug targets. nAChRs exist as homopentamers or heteropentamers comprising a range of different subunits [17]. α-Conotoxins are one of the most medically relevant families of conotoxins, highlighted by a cyclic version of Vc1.1 displaying oral activity in an animal model of neuropathic pain [3,18]. Additional engineering studies have further highlighted the potential of this peptide in drug design [19,20].

α-Conotoxins are generally less than 20 residues in length, have a CysI-CysIII, CysII-CysIV disulfide connectivity and the majority have a 4/7 loop spacing, which represents 4 residues in the first inter-cysteine loop and 7 in the second loop (Figure 1a). A well-studied example containing this loop spacing is Vc1.1 [21]. Several other loop spacings have been identified in the α-conotoxin family, and the size of the loops correlates to some extent with specificity for different nAChR subtypes. For example, 3/4 α-conotoxins target homomeric neuronal nAChRs, 3/5 α-conotoxins target muscle-type nAChRs and 4/4, 4/6 and 4/7 α-conotoxins target different heteromeric and/or homomeric neuronal nAChRs [14].

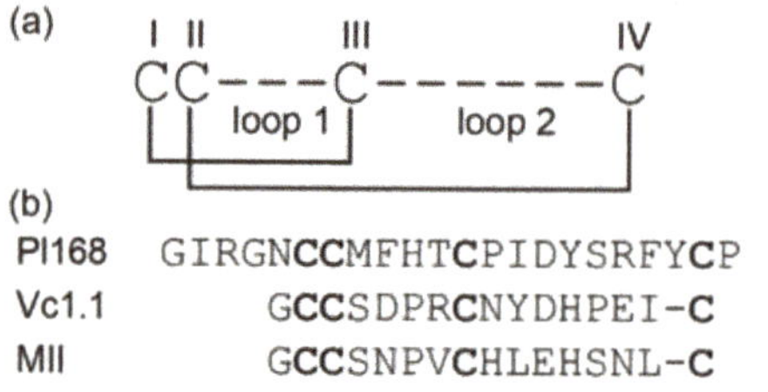

Figure 1. Framework and sequences of α-conotoxins. (**a**) Framework I is represented highlighting the two inter-cysteine loops; the number of residues within each of these loops is used to define the α-conotoxin class. In addition, the globular disulfide bond connectivity present in α-conotoxins is also shown. (**b**) The sequence of Pl168 from *Conus planorbis*, which contains a 4/8 framework. The sequences of related 4/7 α-conotoxins, Vc1.1 and MII are also shown. Cysteine residues are highlighted in bold.

The structures of several α-conotoxins have been determined using nuclear magnetic resonance (NMR) spectroscopy. This technique is well suited to the determination of the structures of α-conotoxins because of their small size, high aqueous solubility and relatively well-defined structures [22]. In addition, some studies used X-ray crystallography to study α-conotoxins either in isolation or in complex with binding partners. Despite the variation in inter-cysteine loop sizes across the family, the majority of α-conotoxins are characterised by a small helical structure, which is braced by the CysI-CysIII disulfide bond. The additional disulfide bond connecting CysII-CysIV generally tethers the C-terminal region to the N-terminus.

Here we show that a minor change in the inter-cysteine loop spacing in framework I can have a significant impact on the structure and bioactivity. Pl168, a 22-residue framework I peptide that contains an unusual 4/8 spacing, was identified in the transcriptome of *Conus planorbis* as a new α-conotoxin [23]. The sequence of Pl168, along with the sequences of two well characterised α-conotoxins, Vc1.1 and

MII, are given in Figure 1b. The three-dimensional structure of Pl168 differs significantly from the characteristic α-conotoxin fold and the peptide does not block a range of nAChRs or Ca^{2+} and Na^{+} channels, indicating that it might represent a new pharmacological class of A-superfamily toxin.

2. Experimental Section

2.1. Peptide Synthesis, Purification and Characterisation

Synthetic Pl168 was manually synthesised using standard solid-phase peptide synthesis fluorenylmethyloxycarbonyl (Fmoc) methods and 2-chlorotrityl-chloride resin. The Fmoc protected amino acids (Auspep, Australia) were activated using *O*-(1*H*-6-Chlorobenzotriazole-1-yl)-1,1,3,3-tetramethyluronium hexafluorophosphate (HCTU) (Iris, Germany) and coupled on resin with *N*,*N*-diisopropylethylamine (DIPEA) (Auspep, Australia)/dimethylformamide (DMF) (Auspep, Australia) by stepwise solid-phase peptide synthesis chemistry. Cleavage of the peptide chain from the solid support was achieved with a mixture of trifluoroacetic acid (TFA) (Auspep, Australia):triisopropylsilane (TIPS) (Auspep, Australia):H_2O (95%:2.5%:2.5% *v*/*v*) followed by purging with nitrogen to evaporate TFA. The peptide was then precipitated in ice-cold diethyl ether (Auspep, Australia) and dissolved in 50% acetonitrile (Sigma, Australia):50% H_2O:0.1% TFA (*v*/*v*) and subsequently lyophilised to dryness. Crude peptide was purified by reversed-phase high performance liquid chromatography (RP-HPLC) on a Phenomenex Jupiter C_{18} preparative column (300 Å, 10 μm, 250 × 21.2 mm) (Phenomenex, Torrance, CA, USA), using a gradient of 0-60% solvent B (Solvent A: 99.95% H_2O:0.05% TFA; Solvent B: 90% acetonitrile:10% H_2O:0.045%TFA) over 60 min. Collected fractions were analysed using a SCIEX 5800 matrix-assisted laser desorption ionisation (MALDI) time-of-flight (TOF)/TOF mass spectrometer (SCIEX, Foster City, CA, USA) and then lyophilised. Formation of the disulfide bonds was carried out in ammonium bicarbonate pH 8.0 (Sigma, Australia) at room temperature and the major isomer from the oxidation reaction purified using RP-HPLC and the mass confirmed using MALDI-TOF mass spectrometry (SCIEX, Foster City, CA, USA).

2.2. NMR Spectroscopy

Lyophilised peptide was dissolved in 90% H_2O:10% D_2O at a concentration of approximately 0.2 mM. All NMR spectra were acquired on a Bruker 600 MHz AVANCE III NMR spectrometer (Bruker, Karlsruhe, Germany) equipped with a cryogenically cooled probe. Two-dimensional ^1H-^1H TOCSY, ^1H-^1H NOESY, ^1H-^1H DQF-COSY, and collected at 290 K were used for sequence-specific assignments and structure calculations. Thus, ^1H-^{15}N HSQC, and ^1H-^{13}C HSQC spectra were acquired for carbon and nitrogen chemical shifts, respectively. All spectra were recorded with a 1 s interscan delay using standard Bruker pulse sequences with an excitation sculpting scheme for solvent suppression. Two-dimensional spectra were collected over 4096 data points in the f2 dimension and 512 increments in the f1 dimension over a spectral width of 12 ppm. Homonuclear NOESY and TOCSY spectra were acquired with a mixing time of 200 and 250 ms, and a spin lock time of 80 ms, respectively. All spectra were processed using Bruker TopSpin (Version 3.5pl7) and assigned using CCPNMR analysis [24] based on the approach described in Wüthrich et al. [25]. The αH secondary shifts were determined by subtracting random coil ^1H NMR chemical shifts from the experimental αH chemical shifts [26].

2.3. Structure Calculations

Structures were calculated with the CYANA program using an automated NOE assignment protocol [27]. Torsion-angle restraints were predicted using TALOS-N [28] and hydrogen bonds predicted based on preliminary structures calculated without disulfide bond restraints. Calculations were also performed with the three possible disulfide bond connectivities to determine the most likely connectivity. A set of 100 final structures was calculated with the globular disulfide connectivity and 20 structures with the lowest target function chosen to present the final ensemble. Structures were visualized and the root-mean-square deviation (RMSD) values were assessed using MOLMOL [29].

2.4. Electrophysiological Measurements

Rat nAChR cDNAs were provided by J. Patrick, Baylor College of Medicine, Houston, TX, and subcloned into the oocyte expression vector pNKS2. The cRNA was synthesized with the SP6 mMessage mMachine kit (Ambion, Austin, TX, USA), and *Xenopus laevis* (Nasco International) oocytes were kindly provided by Prof. Luis Pardo, Göttingen). Oocytes were injected with 50 nL aliquots of cRNA (0.05 mg/mL). The nAChR subunits of heteromeric receptors were mixed at the ratio of 1:1 (α3:β2) or 5:1 (α4:β2).

Recordings were performed as described [30] in ND96 (96 mM NaCl, 2 mM KCl, 1 mM $CaCl_2$, 1 mM $MgCl_2$, and 5 mM 4-(2-hydroxyethyl)-1-piperazineethanesulfonic acid (HEPES) at pH 7.4). Briefly, current responses to 100 μM acetylcholine (ACh) or 100 μM nicotine (in the case of α7) were recorded at −70 mV using a Turbo Tec 05X Amplifier (NPI Electronic, Tamm, Germany) and Cell Works software. A fast and reproducible solution exchange (<300 ms) was achieved with a 50 μL funnel-shaped oocyte chamber combined with a fast solution flow (~150 μL s^{-1}) fed through a custom-made manifold mounted immediately above the oocyte. Agonist pulses were applied for 2 s at 4 min intervals. Peptide up to 100 μM was applied for 3 min in a static bath.

2.5. FLIPR^{Tetra} Ion Channel Assays

The effect of Pl168 on human ion channels was assessed using a high-throughput Ca^{2+} imaging assay as previously described [31–34]. In brief, SH-SY5Y human neuroblastoma cells (ATCC) were cultured in Roswell Park Memorial Institute (RPMI) medium supplemented with L-glutamine (1 mM) and 15% foetal bovine serum and maintained at 37 °C/5% CO_2. Cells were plated on black-walled 384-well imaging plates (Corning, NY, USA) 48 h prior to loading with Calcium 4 No-wash dye (Molecular Devices, Sunnyvale, CA) in physiological salt solution (PSS, composition in mM: 140 NaCl, 11.5 glucose, 5.9 KCl, 1.4 $MgCl_2$, 1.2 NaH_2PO_4, 5 $NaHCO_3$, 1.8 $CaCl_2$, 10 HEPES, pH 7.4). Fluorescence responses (excitation 470–495 nm; emission 515–575 nm) were measured at 1 s intervals using a FLIPR^{Tetra} fluorescence imaging plate reader (Molecular Devices, Sunnyvale, CA), with peptide (30 μM) added 300 s prior to stimulation of ion channel specific responses, followed by a further 300 reads. $Ca_V2.2$ responses were elicited by addition of KCl (90 mM)/$CaCl_2$ (5 mM) in the presence of nifedipine (10 μM); α7 nAchR responses by choline (30 μM) in the presence of PNU-120596 (10 μM); α3-containing nAChR responses by nicotine (30 μM); Ca_V1 responses by KCl (90 mM)/$CaCl_2$ (5 mM) in the presence of ω-conotoxin CVIF (10 μM); and Na_V responses by veratridine (50 μM). Data was analysed using ScreenWorks 3.2.0.14 (Molecular Devices, Sunnyvale, CA, USA) and expressed as response over baseline, with baseline defined as 10 reads prior to agonist addition.

3. Results

3.1. Peptide Synthesis and Characterisation

To allow structural and functional characterisation of Pl168, the peptide was synthesised using Fmoc chemistry and oxidation of the cysteine residues to form disulfide bonds was carried out in ammonium bicarbonate pH 8.0 at room temperature. A major isomer was present in the oxidation reaction and was purified using RP-HPLC and the mass analysed using MALDI-TOF mass spectrometry. The sample was lyophilised and stored at 4 °C until subsequent analyses were carried out.

3.2. Structural Characterisation

The three-dimensional structure of Pl168 was determined using NMR spectroscopy. The spectra display sharp peaks, and only one conformation is evident based on the number of amide proton peaks. This qualitative analysis suggests that the two proline residues in the sequence are not in cis/trans isomerisation, a phenomenon which is relatively common in small peptides. Backbone and side-chain assignments were determined using established procedures [25] and dihedral angle restraints were predicted based on the chemical shift assignments using TALOS [28]. Slowly exchanging amide protons were analysed by dissolving lyophilized peptide in 100% D_2O and recording one-dimensional and TOCSY spectra over time. More than eight amide protons were evident in the spectra following 10 min of dissolution in D_2O, with three (Thr11, Tyr20 and Cys21) still present after three hours. The protection of amide protons from the solvent indicates they are involved in hydrogen bonds. Preliminary structures were calculated using CYANA, based on the predicted dihedral angle restraints and incorporating a protocol for automated assignment of the NOESY inter-residue cross-peaks to derive distance restraints. Analysis of the preliminary structures and slowly exchanging amide protons allowed the incorporation of hydrogen bond restraints into the calculations.

Initial structures were calculated without disulfide bond restraints. Analysis of these structures indicated that Cys6 forms a disulfide bond with Cys12, based on 11 out of 15 structures having sulfur-sulfur distances for these two cysteine residues in close proximity. The sulfur atoms of Cys7 and Cys21 were not in close proximity to other cysteine residues. The presence of the Cys6-Cys12 disulfide bond implies that the peptide contains the globular disulfide connectivity (CysI-CysIII, CysII-CysIV) present in α-conotoxins. To confirm this is the likely connectivity, structures were calculated with the three different disulfide connectivities (Table 1). Consistent with the structures calculated without disulfide bond restraints, the globular disulfide bond connectivity had the lowest target function of all three connectivities. An overlay of the 20 lowest energy structures incorporating the globular connectivity, and the secondary structure present in Pl168 is given in Figure 2. The main elements of secondary structure are α-helices from Cys6 to Phe9, and Ile14 to Tyr20. The N-terminal region, prior to the first cysteine residue, is disordered in the structures, consistent with the lack of NOEs in this region. By contrast, residues 6–21 are well defined. The structural statistics for the final ensemble of structures are given in Table 2.

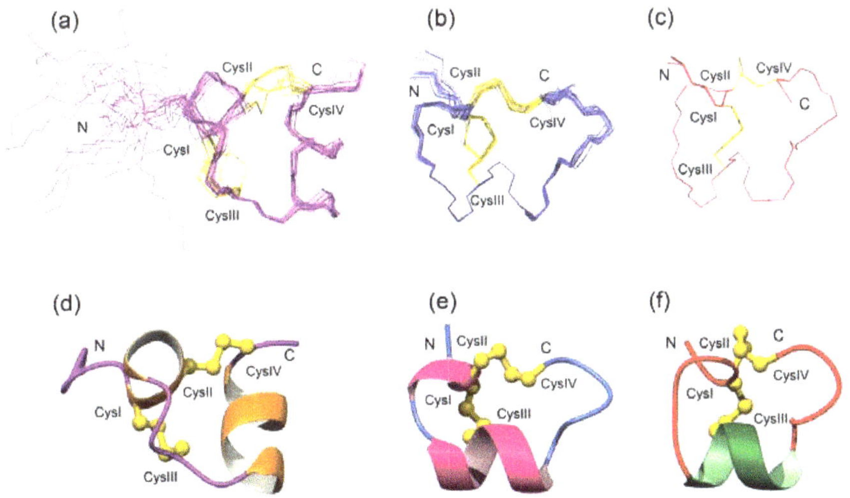

Figure 2. Three-dimensional structures of Pl168 (**a**,**d**), Vc1.1 (**b**,**e**; PDB code 2h8s) and MII (**c**,**f**; PDB code 1mii). Superposition of the lowest energy structures are shown at the top of the diagram and the ribbon representation showing the secondary structure shown at the bottom. The disulfide bonds are shown as yellow lines on the top of the figure, and in ball-and-stick format on the bottom.

Table 1. Analysis of Pl168 structures calculated with the three possible disulfide bond connectivities.

Connectivity	Fold	Target Function [1]
Cys6-Cys12, Cys7-Cys21	Globular	0.046 ± 0.037
Cys6-Cys21, Cys7-Cys12	Ribbon	1.23 ± 0.099
Cys6-Cys7, Cys12-Cys21	Beads	3.3 ± 0.090

[1] Average target function from 15 structures calculated using CYANA.

Table 2. Structural statistics for pl168 with a globular disulfide connectivity.

Experimental Restraints	
Interproton distance restraints	
Intraresidue	57
Sequential	50
Medium range (i–j < 5)	17
Long range (i–j ≥ 5)	8
Total	132
Dihedral-angle restraints	30
Hydrogen bonds (2 per bond)	12
R.m.s. deviations from mean coordinate structure (Å) (in residues 6–21)	
Backbone atoms	0.44 +/− 0.14
All heavy atoms	1.51 +/− 0.25
Ramachandran Statistics *	
% in most favoured region	77.8
% in additionally allowed region	22.2

* Based on the PROCHECK analysis https://servicesn.mbi.ucla.edu/PROCHECK/.

3.3. *Electrophysiology*

The influence of Pl168 on a range of cloned nAChR subtypes expressed in *Xenopus laevis* oocytes was assessed by two-electrode voltage clamp measurements as previously described [30]. No effect was observed on the $\alpha 7$, $\alpha 4\beta 2$, $\alpha 3\beta 2$ or muscle-type nAChRs at peptide concentrations up to 100 μM.

3.4. *FLIPR^{Tetra} Ion Channel Assays*

The effect of Pl168 (30 μM) on ion channel responses (response over baseline; mean ± S.E.M, $n = 4$) was assessed using fluorescent Ca^{2+} imaging in the human neuroblastoma cell line SH-SY5Y endogenously expressing nAchR, Ca_V and Na_V channels. Pl168 (30 μM) had no effect on $\alpha 7$ nAChR responses (control, 2.6 ± 0.14; Pl168, 2.5 ± 0.06), no effect on nicotine-induced $\alpha 3$ nAChR responses (control, 0.69 ± 0.05; Pl168, 0.54 ± 0.09), no effect on L-type (Ca_V1) voltage-gated Ca^{2+} channel responses (control, 1.8 ± 0.23; Pl168, 1.9 ± 0.14) or voltage-gated Na^+ channel responses (control, 0.65 ± 0.07; Pl168, 0.74 ± 0.07), and only a small (18%) inhibition of N-type ($Ca_V2.2$) voltage-gated Ca^{2+} channel responses (control, 0.17 ± 0.008; Pl168, 0.14 ± 0.01) (Figure 3). Addition of the peptide also caused no increase in Ca^{2+}, suggesting it does not act as an agonist at endogenously expressed ion channels or receptors linked to Ca^{2+} signalling.

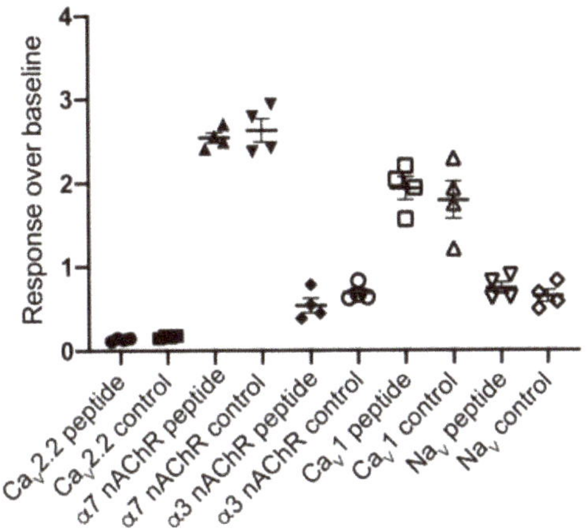

Figure 3. The effect of Pl168 (30 μM) on ion channel responses assessed using fluorescent Ca^{2+} imaging in the human neuroblastoma cell line SH-SY5Y endogenously expressing nAChR, Ca_V and Na_V channels. No effect was observed with the exception of a small (18%) inhibition of N-type ($Ca_V2.2$) voltage-gated Ca^{2+} channel responses. (•) Pl168 (30 μM) on $Ca_V2.2$ channels; (■) Control KCl (90 mM)/$CaCl_2$ (5 mM) in the presence of nifedipine (10 μM) on $Ca_V2.2$ channels; (▲) Pl168 (30 μM) on α7 nAchRs; (▼) Control α7 nAchR response by choline (30 μM) in the presence of PNU-120596 (10 μM); (◆) Pl168 (30 μM) on α3 nAchRs; (O) Control α3-containing nAChR response by nicotine (30 μM); (□) Pl168 (30 μM) on Ca_V1 channels; (△) Control Ca_V1 response by KCl (90 mM)/$CaCl_2$ (5 mM) in the presence of ω-conotoxin CVIF (10 μM); (▽) Pl168 (30 μM) on Na_V channels; (◇) Control Na_V channel response by veratridine (50 μM).

4. Discussion

We have determined the three-dimensional structure of an A-superfamily conotoxin containing an unusual 4/8 spacing and shown that it represents a new structural sub-family. α-Conotoxins, the major family of A-superfamily peptides, have been well studied with more than 70 structures submitted to the Protein Data Bank. In general, the fold is very similar across the family, but we show here that an additional residue in loop 2 appears to have a significant effect on the structural fold.

Pl168 was synthesized without selective protection of the cysteine residues, but nonetheless a major isomer was produced, which was purified and structurally analysed using NMR spectroscopy. Structural analysis indicated that the globular disulfide bond connectivity was present in the synthetic version of Pl168. The Pl168 sequence was identified from transcriptomic data and therefore a co-elution with the native material was not possible. Although unlikely, it is conceivable that the native peptide present in the venom displays a different connectivity given that the folding conditions can have a significant influence on the isomers present. For instance, a recent study showed that recombinant expression of the α-conotoxin TxIA resulted in the ribbon isomer in contrast to synthetic studies which allowed production of the globular isomer [35]. In the absence of a direct comparison of the synthetic peptide with native material we cannot say definitively that this connectivity is present in the venom, but the well-defined structure displayed by the synthetic version of Pl168 and the propensity of A-superfamily framework I toxins to contain the globular connectivity is consistent with the synthetic peptide being equivalent to the native peptide.

The structures of Pl168 comprise two helical regions connected by a loop region. Comparison of Pl168 with the 4/7 conotoxin Vc1.1 indicates that the folds are similar in that both are characterised by α-helices braced by two disulfide bonds as shown in Figure 2. It should be noted, however, that not all the Vc1.1 structures in the ensemble [36] contain the N-terminal helix, and many α-conotoxins only contain the one helical region centered around CysIII as shown for α-conotoxin MII [37] (Figure 2).

However, the structural differences between α-conotoxins such as Vc1.1 and MII, and Pl168 relate to the bracing of the disulfide bonds. Whereas CysIII in Vc1.1 and MII is located within the α-helix, Cys III in Pl168 is present in the loop region and this distinction prevents an effective superposition of these structures. These structural differences, and the presence of a related peptide in *Conus planorbis* with only one residue different to Pl168 (Y20N mutation; GenBank: ADJ67509.1), suggests that Pl168 could represent a new structural class and possibly a new sub-family of conotoxins.

Extensive mutational studies have been done on a range of α-conotoxins, which have identified residues important for bioactivity, including a recent study on MilIA, the first conotoxin isolated from *Conus milneedwardsi* [38]. Interestingly, mutations in MilIA allowed elucidation of residues important in switching between muscle and neuronal nAChRs preference. However, the α-conotoxin family is large with diverse inter-cysteine loop sequences and there does not appear to be a common pharmacophore. The lack of activity of Pl168 against a range of nAChRs suggests that the overall three-dimensional structural and side-chain orientations are not optimal for interaction with the mammalian nAChRs tested in this study. However, given the range of different nAChRs subunits, it is still possible that it inhibits a subtype not tested or a prey-specific nAChR (*C. planorbis* feeds on polychete worms). Although Pl168 contains a conserved signal sequence with other α-conotoxins, it might target another receptor or ion channel as peptides from the A-superfamily are very diverse in their sequence and bioactivity [11]. However, the lack or minimal activity against Ca^+ and Na^+ channels suggests that a wide screen is required to determine the bioactivity of this peptide.

Author Contributions: Conceptualization, S.D., N.L.D. and D.T.W.; methodology, S.D., N.L.D., D.T.W., P.S.B., D.A.C., A.N., I.V.; formal analysis, S.D., N.L.D. and D.T.W; investigation, N.L.D., P.S.B., D.A.C., A.N.; resources, N.L.D., S.D., I.V., A.N.; data curation, S.D., N.L.D.; writing, N.L.D., D.T.W., writing, review and editing, all authors.; visualization, N.L.D., D.T.W.; funding acquisition, N.L.D., S.D., I.V., A.N. All authors have read and agreed to the published version of the manuscript.

Funding: The James Cook University NMR facility was partially funded by the Australian Research Council (LE160100218). This work was partially supported by an Australian Research Council Future Fellowship (FF110100226) awarded to N.L.D.

Acknowledgments: We thank Anna Durner and Anna Puttko for assistance.

Conflicts of Interest: The authors declare no conflict of interest.

References

1. Mir, R.; Karim, S.; Kamal, M.A.; Wilson, C.; Mirza, Z. Conotoxins: Structure, Therapeutic Potential and Pharmacological Applications. *Curr. Pharm. Des.* **2016**, *22*, 582–589. [CrossRef] [PubMed]
2. Schmidtko, A.; Lotsch, J.; Freynhagen, R.; Geisslinger, G. Ziconotide for treatment of severe chronic pain. *Lancet* **2010**, *375*, 1569–1577. [CrossRef]
3. Durek, T.; Craik, D.J. Therapeutic conotoxins: A US patent literature survey. *Expert Opin. Ther. Pat.* **2015**, *25*, 1159–1173. [CrossRef] [PubMed]
4. Safavi-Hemami, H.; Brogan, S.E.; Olivera, B.M. Pain therapeutics from cone snail venoms: From Ziconotide to novel non-opioid pathways. *J. Proteomics* **2019**, *190*, 12–20. [CrossRef] [PubMed]
5. Lewis, R.J. Discovery and development of the chi-conopeptide class of analgesic peptides. *Toxicon* **2012**, *59*, 524–528. [CrossRef] [PubMed]
6. Barton, M.E.; White, H.S.; Wilcox, K.S. The effect of CGX-1007 and CI-1041, novel NMDA receptor antagonists, on NMDA receptor-mediated EPSCs. *Epilepsy Res.* **2004**, *59*, 13–24. [CrossRef] [PubMed]
7. Bernaldez-Sarabia, J.; Figueroa-Montiel, A.; Duenas, S.; Cervantes-Luevano, K.; Beltran, J.A.; Ortiz, E.; Jimenez, S.; Possani, L.D.; Paniagua-Solis, J.F.; Gonzalez-Canudas, J.; et al. The Diversified O-Superfamily in Californiconus californicus Presents a Conotoxin with Antimycobacterial Activity. *Toxins* **2019**, *11*, 128. [CrossRef]
8. Qian, J.; Liu, Y.Q.; Sun, Z.H.; Zhangsun, D.T.; Luo, S.L. Identification of nicotinic acetylcholine receptor subunits in different lung cancer cell lines and the inhibitory effect of alpha-conotoxin TxID on lung cancer cell growth. *Eur. J. Pharm.* **2019**, *865*, 172674. [CrossRef]

9. Himaya, S.W.A.; Lewis, R.J. Venomics-accelerated cone snail venom peptide discovery. *Int. J. Mol. Sci.* **2018**, *19*, 788. [CrossRef]
10. Jin, A.H.; Muttenthaler, M.; Dutertre, S.; Himaya, S.W.A.; Kaas, Q.; Craik, D.J.; Lewis, R.J.; Alewood, P.F. Conotoxins: Chemistry and biology. *Chem. Rev.* **2019**, *119*, 11510–11549. [CrossRef]
11. Robinson, S.D.; Norton, R.S. Conotoxin gene superfamilies. *Mar. Drugs* **2014**, *12*, 6058–6101. [CrossRef]
12. Kaas, Q.; Westermann, J.C.; Halai, R.; Wang, C.K.; Craik, D.J. ConoServer, a database for conopeptide sequences and structures. *Bioinformatics* **2008**, *24*, 445–446. [CrossRef] [PubMed]
13. Kaas, Q.; Yu, R.; Jin, A.H.; Dutertre, S.; Craik, D.J. ConoServer: Updated content, knowledge, and discovery tools in the conopeptide database. *Nucleic Acids Res.* **2012**, *40*, 325–330. [CrossRef] [PubMed]
14. Giribaldi, J.; Dutertre, S. Alpha-conotoxins to explore the molecular, physiological and pathophysiological functions of neuronal nicotinic acetylcholine receptors. *Neurosci. Lett.* **2018**, *679*, 24–34. [CrossRef] [PubMed]
15. Azam, L.; McIntosh, J.M. Alpha-conotoxins as pharmacological probes of nicotinic acetylcholine receptors. *Acta Pharm. Sin.* **2009**, *30*, 771–783. [CrossRef] [PubMed]
16. Shimohama, S.; Kawamata, J. Roles of nicotinic acetylcholine receptors in the pathology and treatment of Alzheimer's and Parkinson's diseases. In *Nicotinic Acetylcholine Receptor Signaling in Neuroprotection*; Akaike, A., Shimohama, S., Misu, Y., Eds.; Springer: Singapore, 2018; pp. 137–158. [CrossRef]
17. Hurst, R.; Rollema, H.; Bertrand, D. Nicotinic acetylcholine receptors: From basic science to therapeutics. *Pharm. Ther.* **2013**, *137*, 22–54. [CrossRef]
18. Clark, R.J.; Jensen, J.; Nevin, S.T.; Callaghan, B.P.; Adams, D.J.; Craik, D.J. The engineering of an orally active conotoxin for the treatment of neuropathic pain. *Angew. Chem. Int. Ed. Engl.* **2010**, *49*, 6545–6548. [CrossRef]
19. Castro, J.; Grundy, L.; Deiteren, A.; Harrington, A.M.; O'Donnell, T.; Maddern, J.; Moore, J.; Garcia-Caraballo, S.; Rychkov, G.Y.; Yu, R.; et al. Cyclic analogues of alpha-conotoxin Vc1.1 inhibit colonic nociceptors and provide analgesia in a mouse model of chronic abdominal pain. *Br. J. Pharm.* **2018**, *175*, 2384–2398. [CrossRef]
20. Yu, R.; Seymour, V.A.; Berecki, G.; Jia, X.; Akcan, M.; Adams, D.J.; Kaas, Q.; Craik, D.J. Less is More: Design of a Highly Stable Disulfide-Deleted Mutant of Analgesic Cyclic alpha-Conotoxin Vc1.1. *Sci. Rep.* **2015**, *5*, 13264. [CrossRef]
21. Sadeghi, M.; Carstens, B.B.; Callaghan, B.P.; Daniel, J.T.; Tae, H.S.; O'Donnell, T.; Castro, J.; Brierley, S.M.; Adams, D.J.; Craik, D.J.; et al. Structure-activity studies reveal the molecular basis for GABAB-Receptor mediated inhibition of high voltage-activated calcium channels by alpha-conotoxin Vc1.1. *ACS Chem. Biol.* **2018**, *13*, 1577–1587. [CrossRef]
22. Marx, U.C.; Daly, N.L.; Craik, D.J. NMR of conotoxins: Structural features and an analysis of chemical shifts of post-translationally modified amino acids. *Magn. Reson. Chem.* **2006**, *44*, 41–50. [CrossRef] [PubMed]
23. Jin, A.H.; Vetter, I.; Himaya, S.W.; Alewood, P.F.; Lewis, R.J.; Dutertre, S. Transcriptome and proteome of *Conus planorbis* identify the nicotinic receptors as primary target for the defensive venom. *Proteomics* **2015**, *15*, 4030–4040. [CrossRef] [PubMed]
24. Skinner, S.P.; Fogh, R.H.; Boucher, W.; Ragan, T.J.; Mureddu, L.G.; Vuister, G.W. CcpNmr AnalysisAssign: A flexible platform for integrated NMR analysis. *J. Biomol. NMR* **2016**, *66*, 111–124. [CrossRef] [PubMed]
25. Wüthrich, K. *NMR of Proteins and Nucleic Acids*; Wiley-Interscience: New York, NY, USA, 1986.
26. Wishart, D.S.; Bigam, C.G.; Holm, A.; Hodges, R.S.; Sykes, B.D. 1H, 13C and 15N random coil NMR chemical shifts of the common amino acids. I. Investigations of nearest-neighbor effects. *J. Biomol. NMR* **1995**, *5*, 67–81. [CrossRef] [PubMed]
27. Wurz, J.M.; Kazemi, S.; Schmidt, E.; Bagaria, A.; Guntert, P. NMR-based automated protein structure determination. *Arch. Biochem. Biophys.* **2017**, *628*, 24–32. [CrossRef]
28. Shen, Y.; Bax, A. Protein backbone and sidechain torsion angles predicted from NMR chemical shifts using artificial neural networks. *J. Biomol. NMR* **2013**, *56*, 227–241. [CrossRef]
29. Koradi, R.; Billeter, M.; Wuthrich, K. MOLMOL: A program for display and analysis of macromolecular structures. *J. Mol. Graph.* **1996**, *14*. [CrossRef]
30. Beissner, M.; Dutertre, S.; Schemm, R.; Danker, T.; Sporning, A.; Grubmuller, H.; Nicke, A. Efficient binding of 4/7 alpha-conotoxins to nicotinic alpha4beta2 receptors is prevented by Arg185 and Pro195 in the alpha4 subunit. *Mol. Pharm.* **2012**, *82*, 711–718. [CrossRef] [PubMed]

31. Mueller, A.; Starobova, H.; Inserra, M.C.; Jin, A.H.; Deuis, J.R.; Dutertre, S.; Lewis, R.J.; Alewood, P.F.; Daly, N.L.; Vetter, I. alpha-Conotoxin MrIC is a biased agonist at alpha7 nicotinic acetylcholine receptors. *Biochem. Pharm.* **2015**, *94*, 155–163. [CrossRef] [PubMed]
32. Sousa, S.R.; McArthur, J.R.; Brust, A.; Bhola, R.F.; Rosengren, K.J.; Ragnarsson, L.; Dutertre, S.; Alewood, P.F.; Christie, M.J.; Adams, D.J.; et al. Novel analgesic omega-conotoxins from the vermivorous cone snail Conus moncuri provide new insights into the evolution of conopeptides. *Sci. Rep.* **2018**, *8*, 13397. [CrossRef]
33. Vetter, I.; Mozar, C.A.; Durek, T.; Wingerd, J.S.; Alewood, P.F.; Christie, M.J.; Lewis, R.J. Characterisation of Na(v) types endogenously expressed in human SH-SY5Y neuroblastoma cells. *Biochem. Pharm.* **2012**, *83*, 1562–1571. [CrossRef]
34. Vetter, I.; Lewis, R.J. Characterization of endogenous calcium responses in neuronal cell lines. *Biochem. Pharm.* **2010**, *79*, 908–920. [CrossRef] [PubMed]
35. El Hamdaoui, Y.; Wu, X.; Clark, R.J.; Giribaldi, J.; Anangi, R.; Craik, D.J.; King, G.F.; Dutertre, S.; Kaas, Q.; Herzig, V.; et al. Periplasmic expression of 4/7 alpha-Conotoxin TxIA analogs in E. coli favors ribbon isomer formation—Suggestion of a binding bode at the alpha7 nAChR. *Front. Pharm.* **2019**, *10*, 577. [CrossRef] [PubMed]
36. Clark, R.J.; Fischer, H.; Nevin, S.T.; Adams, D.J.; Craik, D.J. The synthesis, structural characterization, and receptor specificity of the alpha-conotoxin Vc1.1. *J. Biol. Chem.* **2006**, *281*, 23254–23263. [CrossRef] [PubMed]
37. Hill, J.M.; Oomen, C.J.; Miranda, L.P.; Bingham, J.P.; Alewood, P.F.; Craik, D.J. Three-dimensional solution structure of alpha-conotoxin MII by NMR spectroscopy: Effects of solution environment on helicity. *Biochemistry* **1998**, *37*, 15621–15630. [CrossRef] [PubMed]
38. Peigneur, S.; Devi, P.; Seldeslachts, A.; Ravichandran, S.; Quinton, L.; Tytgat, J. Structure-function elucidation of a new alpha-conotoxin, MilIA, from *Conus milneedwardsi*. *Mar. Drugs* **2019**, *17*, 535. [CrossRef]

biomedicines

MDPI

Review

Scorpion Venom: Detriments and Benefits

Shirin Ahmadi [1,2,*], Julius M. Knerr [1], Lídia Argemi [1], Karla C. F. Bordon [3], Manuela B. Pucca [1,4], Felipe A. Cerni [1,3], Eliane C. Arantes [3], Figen Çalışkan [2,5] and Andreas H. Laustsen [1,*]

1 Department of Biotechnology and Biomedicine, Technical University of Denmark, DK-2800 Kongens Lyngby, Denmark; juliusknerr@aol.com (J.M.K.); lidia.argemimuntadas@gmail.com (L.A.); manu.pucca@ufrr.br (M.B.P.); felipe_cerni@hotmail.com (F.A.C.)
2 Department of Biotechnology and Biosafety, Graduate School of Natural and Applied Sciences, Eşkisehir Osmangazi University, TR-26040 Eşkisehir, Turkey; fcalis@ogu.edu.tr
3 Department of BioMolecular Sciences, School of Pharmaceutical Sciences of Ribeirão Preto, University of São Paulo, Ribeirão Preto—São Paulo 14040-903, Brazil; karla@fcfrp.usp.br (K.C.F.B.); ecabraga@fcfrp.usp.br (E.C.A.)
4 Medical School, Federal University of Roraima, Boa Vista, Roraima 69310-000, Brazil
5 Department of Biology, Faculty of Science and Letters, Eskisehir Osmangazi University, TR-26040 Eskisehir, Turkey
* Correspondence: shiahm@dtu.dk (S.A.); ahola@bio.dtu.dk (A.H.L.); Tel.: +45-7164-6042 (S.A.); +45-2988-1134 (A.H.L.)

Received: 2 April 2020; Accepted: 7 May 2020; Published: 12 May 2020

Abstract: Scorpion venom may cause severe medical complications and untimely death if injected into the human body. Neurotoxins are the main components of scorpion venom that are known to be responsible for the pathological manifestations of envenoming. Besides neurotoxins, a wide range of other bioactive molecules can be found in scorpion venoms. Advances in separation, characterization, and biotechnological approaches have enabled not only the development of more effective treatments against scorpion envenomings, but have also led to the discovery of several scorpion venom peptides with interesting therapeutic properties. Thus, scorpion venom may not only be a medical threat to human health, but could prove to be a valuable source of bioactive molecules that may serve as leads for the development of new therapies against current and emerging diseases. This review presents both the detrimental and beneficial properties of scorpion venom toxins and discusses the newest advances within the development of novel therapies against scorpion envenoming and the therapeutic perspectives for scorpion toxins in drug discovery.

Keywords: scorpion venom; potassium channel toxins; calcins; scorpionism; fungicide; parasiticide; bradykinin potentiating peptide; analgesics; antivenom

1. Introduction

According to national public health data, about 1.5 million scorpion envenomings, resulting in 2000–3000 deaths, are recorded annually worldwide [1,2]. While large regions in the Northern Hemisphere, such as the United States, Canada, Europe, and Russia, as well as Australia in the Southern Hemisphere are not associated with severe scorpionism [3], more than two billion people living in northern Saharan Africa, African Sahel, South Africa, Near and Middle East, southern India, eastern Andes, Mexico, and South America are at risk of being stung by scorpions [1]. Climate change together with urban expansion and poor city sanitation management in many of these areas have increased the likelihood of encountering scorpions. For instance, in Brazil alone, malign incidences with scorpions have nearly doubled from 64,000 to 124,000 annual envenoming cases since 2012 [4].

To date, over 2000 scorpion species have been described. The vast majority of the scorpion species that are dangerous to humans belong to the Buthidae family [5], but some species in the families of

Scorpionidae and Hemiscorpiidae have also been classified as harmful [6,7]. Geographical distributions of most of these medically significant species correlate with the local prevalence of scorpionism. Hence, the density of dangerous species is especially high in northern Africa, Iran, Saudi Arabia, Brazil, Mexico, and Venezuela [3,8,9]. Local pain is often the first symptom of scorpion envenoming, which may set in only minutes after a sting has occurred. Depending on the scorpion species, the symptoms can progress to severe complications over the course of a few hours. Inducing a massive release of neurotransmitters, scorpion venom neurotoxins usually cause sweating, nausea, vomiting, hypersalivation, restlessness, and, in more severe cases, arrhythmia, unconsciousness, and heart failure, which may lead to death [10]. However, in spite of the hazardous and life-threatening effects of scorpion envenoming, therapeutic properties of scorpion body parts and venoms in ancient medicine have been utilized by humans for thousands of years [10]. Nowadays, the potential therapeutic value of different scorpion venom compounds is being increasingly investigated, as these compounds may represent promising leads for the development of new pharmaceuticals.

In this review, we survey the field of scorpion venom research from different angles focusing both on the detrimental and beneficial properties of scorpion venom toxins. First, scorpion venom compounds together with clinical manifestations and symptoms of different levels of scorpionism are introduced. Then, currently available treatments and research into new alternatives, i.e., next-generation antivenoms, are discussed. Finally, the latest reported results from the scientific literature focusing on the widespread potential applications of scorpion venom compounds are presented.

2. Scorpion Venom Compounds

Scorpions use their venom to defend against predators and to capture prey. The composition of scorpion venom is highly complex and heterogeneous. Up until now, small scorpion venom peptides are the most studied compounds, mainly due to their diversity and broad pharmacological properties. Accordingly to their structure, these small peptides are classified into three large superfamilies: peptides containing cysteine-stabilized (CS) α/β motifs, calcins, and non-disulfide bridged peptides (NDBPs) [11]. However, enzymes (larger proteins), mixtures of inorganic salts, free amino acids, nucleotides, amines, and lipids are also found in scorpion venom [12].

2.1. *Peptides Containing CS α/β Motifs*

These peptides consist of an α-helix joined to a double or triple-stranded β-sheet via a disulfide bridge (Figure 1) [12]. These molecules present two completely conserved disulfide bonds in the C_i–C_j and C_{i+4}–C_{j+2} positions; although some of them also exhibit an extra link connecting the two endings of the peptide chain [11]. All scorpion peptides containing CS α/β motifs act in a similar way. Their interaction with ion channels result in blocking or modulation of the normal mode of action of these channels [12]. Members of this superfamily can be subdivided into long or short scorpion toxin families, corresponding to their respective structures.

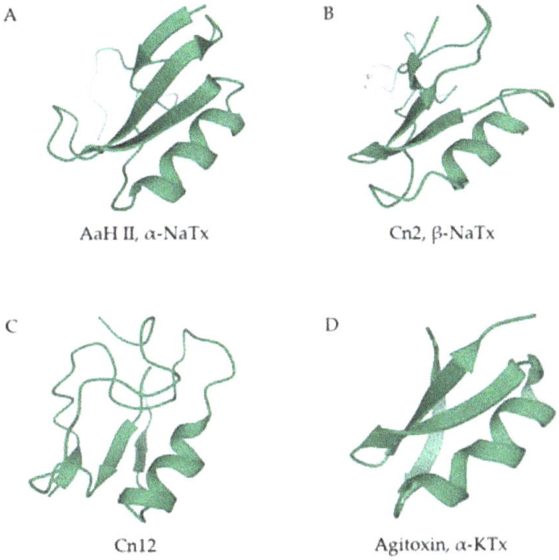

Figure 1. Ribbon diagrams of the 3D structure of selected scorpion venom peptides containing the cysteine-stabilized (CS) α/β motif. (**A**) AaHII from *Androctonus australis* is a classical α-NaTx. (**B**) Cn2 from *Centruroides noxius* venom is a classical β-NaTx. (**C**) Cn12, also from *C. noxius* venom, shows structural resemblance to β-NaTxs, but exhibits an α-NaTx function. (**D**) Agitoxin 1 from *Leiurus hebraeus* (previously *L. quinquestriatus hebraeus*) is an α-KTx toxin. The Protein Database accession numbers are 1PTX for AhHII; 1CN2 for Cn2, 1PE4 for Cn12, and 1AGT for agitoxin 1. KTx: potassium channel toxins, NaTx: sodium channel toxins.

2.1.1. Long Scorpion Toxins

Peptides from the long scorpion toxin superfamily are 55–76 residue-long molecules with generally four disulfide bridges [13]. Due to their mode of action, they can also be called sodium channel toxins (NaTxs), as their main targets are sodium ion channels [12]. This family can be further divided into two groups, α and β-NaTxs, depending on their specific interaction with the voltage-gated Na^+ channels (Figure 1A,B). α-NaTxs block site 3 of sodium ion channels, and therefore inhibit the inactivation of the channels and prolong their action potential. In contrast, β-NaTxs interact with site 4 of Na^+ channels and shift the activation voltage of the channels to a more negative potential, which results in channel inactivation (opposite to the effects of site 3 toxins) [14]. It is noteworthy that not all NaTxs can be assigned to these two groups. For example, Cn12, from *Centruroides noxius*, and Ts2, from *Tityus serrulatus* venom, structurally resemble a β-NaTx but exhibit an α-NaTx effect (Figure 1C) [15,16]. In addition, AaH IT4, a toxin from *Androctonus australis hector*, displays both α and β-NaTx effects [11].

2.1.2. Short Scorpion Toxins

The short scorpion toxin family is composed of peptides of 23–64 residues in length with three or four disulfide bridges. These peptides, also known as potassium channel toxins (KTxs), mainly act as potassium ion channel blockers (Figure 1D) [17]. Considering their sequences and cysteine pairs, KTxs can be divided into α, β, γ, κ, δ, λ, and ε-KTx groups [18,19]. The α-KTx group, which is considered to be the largest subgroup of the short scorpion toxin family, contains 23–42 residue-long peptides with three or four disulfide bridges [20]. The β-KTx group comprises longer chain peptides of 50–57 residues in length [21]. The γ-KTx group can be found in the genera *Centruroides*, *Mesobuthus*, and *Buthus*, and it mainly blocks the human *Ether-à-go-go*-Related Gene (hERG) channels [22]. Instead of having a CS α/β structure, similar to the α, β, and γ-KTx subfamilies, toxins of the κ-KTx group are composed of two parallel short α-helices connected by a β-turn that is stabilized by two disulfide bridges, yet their interaction with potassium ion channels is similar to that of the α-KTx group [23].

Although the δ, λ, and ε-KTx groups do not contain a CS α/β motif, they are mentioned in the continuation of other KTxs. The δ-KTx group contains a Kunitz-type structural fold with a double-stranded antiparallel β-sheet flanked by an α-helix in both the C-terminal and N-terminal segments. Since the Kunitz-type structural folds are the active domains of proteins that inhibit the function of serine proteases, δ-KTxs exert both protease and potassium channel-inhibiting properties [24]. The λ-KTx group, similar to calcins, contain an inhibitor cystine knot (ICK) motif (see Section 2.2) that contains a triple-stranded antiparallel β-sheet stabilized by three cystine linkages [25,26]. The ε-KTx group has recently been defined and, so far, it has just two members, Ts11 and Ts12 from *T. serrulatus* venom. Ts11 shows less than 50% identity with KTxs from other subfamilies. Ts11, similar to λ -KTxs, contains an ICK motif. However, λ-KTxs possess only three disulfide bridges, while Ts11 has four disulfide bridges assembled in a unique pattern [19].

2.2. Calcins

This small, but growing, family of scorpion toxins consists of calcium channel-modulating peptides, such as imperacalcin (imperatoxin), maurocalcin, hemicalcin, hadrucalcin, opicalcin, urocalcin, and vejocalcin [27]. Sharing high sequence similarity (>78% identity), calcins include an ICK motif stabilized by three disulfide bridges [28]. Calcins mainly act as agonists of ryanodine receptors (RyRs), which are intracellular ligand-activated calcium channels that are found in endoplasmic/sarcoplasmic reticulum membranes. RyRs play an essential role during excitation–contraction coupling in cardiac and skeletal muscles by releasing Ca^{2+} from intracellular reservoirs [29]. In general, calcins induce long-lasting subconductance states on the RyR channels, which lead to an increase in the intracellular Ca^{2+} level and subsequently contractile paralysis [30].

Calcins also present the ability to pass through cell membranes without causing their lysis [31]. It has been hypothesized that the clustering of positively charged, basic residues on one side of the calcins gives them a dipole moment that possibly interacts with negatively charged membrane lipid rafts, such as gangliosides. Once these toxins interact with the outer membrane, interaction between the hydrophobic regions of the toxin and the inner membrane is favored, and the toxin is transiently translocated. Further electrostatic interactions with negatively charged molecules from the cytoplasm trigger the entrance of calcins into the cell without disrupting its membrane [32]. This feature makes the calcins excellent candidates for intracellular drug delivery, since they can enter cells without disrupting them, even when large membrane-impermeable molecules are conjugated to them [33].

A calcium channel modulator, distinct from the toxins that act on RyRs was recently identified through transcriptome analysis of *T. serrulatus* and designated as a cell-penetrating peptide (CPP)-Ts. The synthetic CPP-Ts is the first described scorpion toxin that activates Ca^{2+} signaling through the nuclear inositol 1,4,5-trisphosphate receptors. This toxin, together with the calcium channel toxin-like BmCa1 from *Mesobuthus martensii*, forms a new subfamily of calcium toxins and shows promising anticancer effects (see Section 4.8) [34].

It is noteworthy that calcins are not the only cell-penetrating scorpion toxins. The transient receptor potential cation channel subfamily V, member 1 (TRPV1) is a chemosensory ion channel, which is also known as the wasabi receptor. Generally, TRPV1 is activated through a unique mechanism involving the covalent modification of specific cysteine residues located within the channel's cytoplasmic N-terminus. Recently, it has been reported that Wasabi Receptor Toxin (WaTx), from *Urodacus manicatus* venom, is capable of activating this receptor. This means that WaTx can cross the plasma membrane and bind to the same allosteric nexus that is covalently modified by other agonists [35].

2.3. Non-Disulfide Bridged Peptides (NDBPs)

NDBPs are small, 13–56 amino acid-long peptides with a very heterogeneous composition. Compared to scorpion peptides with disulfide bridges, NDBPs do not present a conserved or predictable structure-function relationship [36]. Most of these peptides are cationic molecules that display notable structural flexibility. In aqueous solutions, these peptides exhibit a random coil conformation. However, under membrane-mimicking environments, such as 50%–60% of aqueous trifluoroethanol, they readily adopt an amphipathic α-helical structure [37]. This characteristic enables them to interact with a broad spectrum of biological targets; however, they do not have any known specific molecular targets [38,39].

2.4. Enzymes

Few enzymes have been found in scorpion venoms, in part because up until recently, interest has been focused on small proteins and peptides. However, during the past years, hyaluronidases, phospholipases, and metalloproteases, among other enzymes, have been detected in venoms of different scorpion species.

Different hyaluronidases have been identified in different families of scorpions, including Buthidae, Bothriuridae, and Urodacidae [40]. It is known that these enzymes potentiate the toxicity of venom by disrupting the integrity of the extracellular matrix and connective tissues surrounding blood vessels at sting point, and they thereby ease the systemic diffusion of other relevant scorpion toxins [41]. It has recently been demonstrated that hyaluronidases also play an essential role in venom distribution from the bloodstream to the target organs [42]. The same study also indicated that the neutralization of hyaluronidases could be considered as a first-aid strategy in scorpion envenoming treatment.

Phospholipases are known to be potent hemolytic agents, as they disrupt cell membranes by hydrolyzing phospholipids. They can also cause tissue necrosis and hemorrhages. Phospholipase activity has been detected in several scorpion species, including *Opisthacanthus cayaporum* [43] and *Heterometrus laoticus* [44].

Generally, venoms from *Tityus* species exhibit significant proteolytic activity, and the first scorpion metalloprotease was discovered in the venom of *T. serrulatus* [45]. Metalloproteases and serine proteases have also been detected in *T. discrepans* venom [46] and, apart from *Tityus* species, in the venom of *Hemiscorpius lepturus* [47]. It is believed that proteases play a key role in activating toxin precursors through post-translational modifications [48]. In addition, these enzymes inhibit platelet aggregation, modulate cytokine production, and activate the complement system [49,50]. Altogether, these effects facilitate the diffusion of scorpion venom toxins via the degradation of matrix proteins.

2.5. Other Venom Compounds

Only a very limited number of studies on non-peptidic scorpion venom compounds have been reported. However, it has been shown that the venoms of some scorpions, including *M. tamulus*, contain serotonin, which is a monoamine that may cause vomiting and considerable local pain in scorpion envenomings [51]. The metal and salt composition of some scorpion species have also been evaluated by Al-Asmari et al. [52]. In their study, they found copper, zinc, calcium, magnesium, iron, lead, manganese, arsenic, and nickel ions in the venom of *A. bicolor*, *A. crassicauda*, and *Leiurus quinquestriatus*. They suggested that these components are associated with enzyme activity, as they probably act as enzyme cofactors. In addition, two 1,4-benzoquinone compounds, with antimicrobial activity, have recently been isolated from the venom of *Diplocentrus melici*, a scorpion species endemic to Mexico [53] (see Table 1). Moreover, it has been reported that one of the low-molecular-weight compounds with anticoagulant activity isolated from the *Heterometrus laoticus* venom is adenosine, which is a well-known inhibitor of platelet aggregation [54,55].

3. Detriments of Scorpion Venom: Scorpion Envenoming

Scorpion envenomings can cause severe pathological effects and even death in humans. The intensity of an envenoming usually depends on the victim's sensitivity and body mass, the anatomical location of the sting, the amount of injected venom, and the scorpion species. Commonly, based on the severity of symptoms, scorpion envenomings are classified into three levels: mild, moderate, and severe (Figure 2) [56,57]. Mild envenomings result in local inflammatory reactions, whereas moderate and severe envenomings may provoke lethal systemic responses.

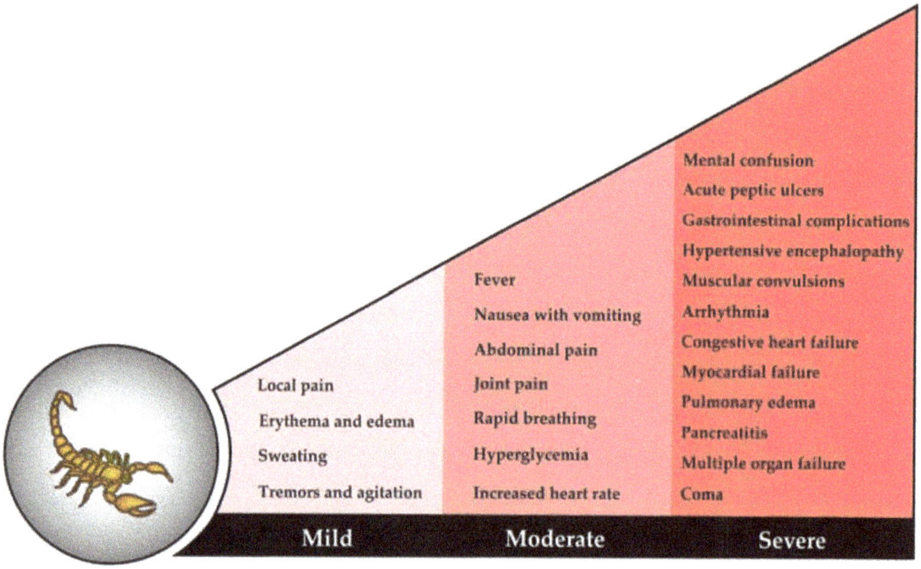

Figure 2. Clinical manifestations and symptoms of mild, moderate, and severe scorpion envenomings. Typical symptoms of mild stings last for minutes to hours and include great local pain, a reddened and swollen site of sting (erythema and edema), numbness, sweating, body tremors, and agitation. More intense stings from scorpions with venom containing cytolytic toxins may result in blood blisters, hemorrhages, and necrosis of the surrounding tissue. In moderate envenoming cases, the body additionally reacts with fever, abdominal and joint pain, hyperglycemia, abnormally rapid breathing, increased heart rate, and nausea with vomiting. These symptoms can reside for days and are mostly caused by neurotoxins: Na^+, K^+, and Ca^{2+} ion channel modulators. Neurotoxins can also cause severe envenomings, which can lead to cardiovascular, neurological, pulmonary, and/or gastrointestinal complications, such as pulmonary edema, myocardial failure, arrhythmia, congestive heart failure, extreme muscular convulsion, hypertensive encephalopathy, acute peptic ulcers, pancreatitis and lethal multiple organ failure, mental confusion, and coma. After several days, most victims of lethal scorpion stings die from cardiac or respiratory failure.

3.1. Scorpion Envenoming Treatment

Generally, the first treatment strategies that are undertaken after an envenoming event focus on pain relief and possibly intravenous hydration to decrease the negative effects of strong salivation and sweating. In order to relieve acute pain after a scorpion sting, either cooling by ice or intravenous injection of paracetamol or nonsteroidal anti-inflammatory drugs, such as diclofenac and indomethacin, or topical administration of lidocaine cream at the site of the sting can be used [58]. However, it is not surprising that the analgesic effect of lidocaine might be superior to the former treatments [59]. Further substances that are considered for application in envenoming cases are prazosin (which counteracts catecholamine-induced hypertension) [60], antihistamines and steroids (which reduce inflammatory responses) [61], sodium phenobarbital (which prevents convulsions and lung edema) [8,62], and calcium gluconate (which eases muscle spasms) [63]. While partially being used in practice, there does not seem to be a general consensus on the efficacy and possible adverse effects of these treatment options. Yet, in the case of prazosin, it has been shown that the mortality and the mean residence time in the hospital could be significantly reduced by the administration of two doses of the drug, one immediate and one three hours after the envenoming incident [64]. Additionally, small molecules, such as heparin, ethylenediaminetetraacetic acid EDTA, and aristolochic acid have been shown to neutralize scorpion venom enzymes, such as hyaluronidases, phospholipases A_2, and metalloproteases. Thus, these molecules might be considered as a starting point for the development of future treatments [5]. In more severe envenoming cases, antivenoms are employed to neutralize the venom and diminish the morbidity and mortality of scorpion stings (Figure 3).

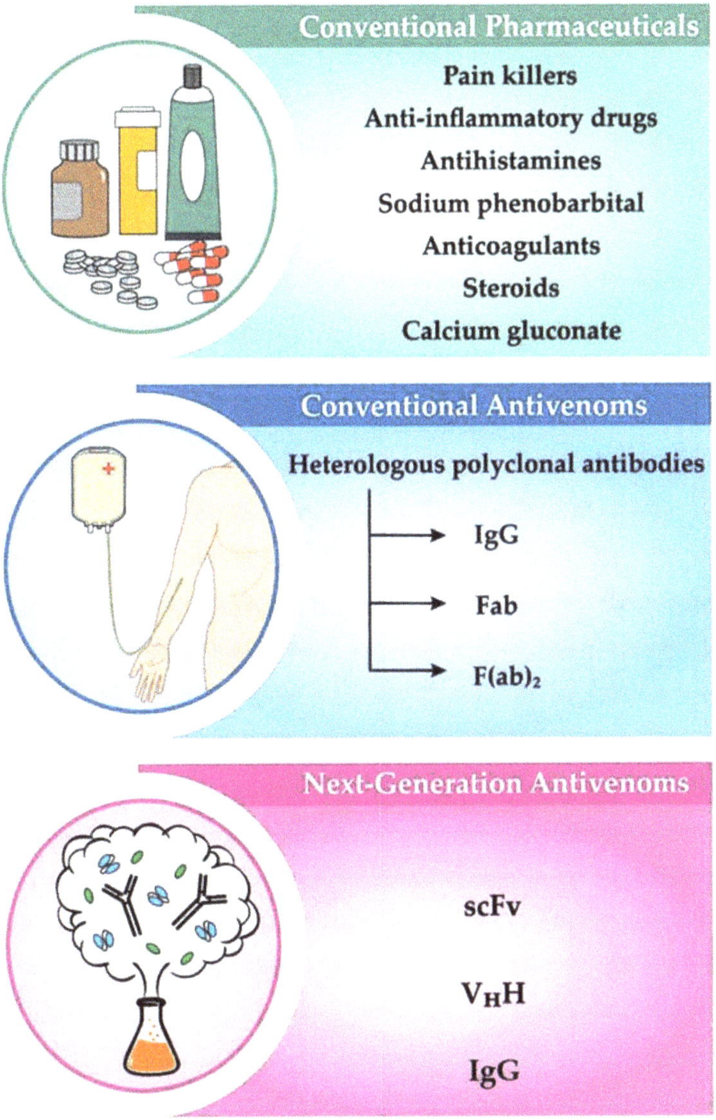

Figure 3. Scorpion envenoming treatments. Conventional pharmaceuticals are used for mild envenomings, while antivenom therapy is applied in moderate and severe cases. Recombinant antivenoms are suggested to have higher therapeutic value over the conventional antivenoms and may become the future mainstay of treatment.

3.1.1. Conventional Plasma-Derived Antivenoms

Conventional plasma-derived antivenoms are produced by the purification (and digestion) of polyclonal immunoglobulin G (IgG) molecules harvested from the plasma of hyperimmunized animals, such as horses or sheep. These polyclonal antivenoms can cause severe adverse reactions due to their heterologous origin [65] and are known from the field of snakebite envenoming to generally possess low percentages of venom-neutralizing antibodies [66,67]. Moreover, conventional antivenoms may have limited efficacy against the medically most important toxins, such as small neurotoxins, as these toxins are often weakly immunogenic and therefore fail to raise a strong antibody response in the production animal [68]. Nonetheless, the administration of these types of antivenoms is effective for clinical use and has been life-saving since the 1900s. Thus, plasma-derived antivenoms are still the standard of treatment for systemic scorpion envenomings [69].

Recently, in pursuit of finding alternatives to equine IgGs for scorpion envenoming treatment, strategies involving avian egg-yolk-derived immunoglobulin Ys (IgYs) have been developed [70]. In contrast to equine IgGs, avian IgY antibodies are obtained noninvasively from egg yolks from laying hens that have been immunized with scorpion venom. These IgY molecules have been argued to activate the mammalian complement system much less than animal-derived IgGs and not interact with rheumatoid factors. They are produced in amounts comparable to those found in the plasma of large mammals and have been argued to be more affordable. Previous studies on IgY-based antivenoms against snake and scorpion venoms have demonstrated that neutralizing antibodies can be raised by this method, albeit with lower neutralizing capacity than antibodies present in plasma-derived antivenoms [71]. Nevertheless, there has been a slightly increased interest in the use of egg-yolk-derived IgY antibodies for antivenom manufacture [72–75]. As an example, in a recent study, it was demonstrated using a rescue assay involving mice that the lethality of *A. australis hector* (*Aah*) venom could be neutralized with IgY antibodies. However, in addition to having the same drawbacks as equine IgGs in terms of polyclonality and batch-to-batch variation, avian-derived IgYs are phylogenetically even more distantly related to mammals [76] and still require the use of production animals for their manufacture. Therefore, it seems likely that the development of next-generation antivenoms based on recombinant monoclonal antibodies and antibody fragments may be a more promising research avenue for developing effective, safe, and cost-competitive antivenoms with defined therapeutic composition for future envenoming therapy.

3.1.2. Recombinant Antivenoms

In the field of next-generation antivenoms, the development of phage display technology and recent advances in toxicovenomics have enabled researchers to pursue new therapeutic strategies with the purpose of creating better envenoming therapies [77]. These technology-driven approaches have made it possible to identify the most toxic, and thus medically relevant, components in a given venom, and to efficiently and systematically discover human monoclonal antibodies against these components. In turn, this has paved the way for developing recombinant antivenoms with anticipated improved safety profiles compared to conventional antivenoms. As an example, using phage display technology, the discovery of a human monoclonal single-chain variable fragment (scFv) antibody against *T. serrulatus* toxins, serrumab, was reported in 2012 [78]. This monoclonal antibody was demonstrated to have a high neutralizing capacity against β-toxins from *T. serrulatus*, while it was also capable of cross-neutralizing toxins from *C. suffusus suffusus* and *L. quinquestriatus*. More recently, in 2019, the field of recombinant scorpion antivenoms took another step forward when the discovery of a broadly-neutralizing monoclonal scFv antibody (scFv 10FG2) capable of neutralizing an estimated 13 different neurotoxins from different scorpion species belonging to the *Centruroides* genus was reported [79]. Using a rescue assay, this study demonstrated that scFv 10FG2 was capable of neutralizing 3 LD_{50}s of freshly obtained whole venoms from five different scorpion species, belonging to the *Centruroides* genus, in 1:10 and 1:20 molar ratios of venom to antibody. The implementation of broadly-neutralizing antibodies in the formulation of recombinant antivenoms is a significant simplification in their pharmaceutical composition, since the inclusion of only a few broadly-neutralizing antibodies may be sufficient to neutralize the entire venoms of several different species. Reducing the product complexity of recombinant antivenoms is an important challenge to solve to enable cost-competitive manufacture of such medicines [80,81].

Next to scFvs, single-domain V_HH antibodies, also known as nanobodies (Nb), are being intensively explored for their utility in relation to recombinant antivenoms. Nbs are native to the immune system of camelids and sharks and constitute the smallest natural antibody fragments known to date [82]. The low molecular mass of Nbs allows for their distribution into deep tissues throughout the body [83,84]. This property, in addition to their high ex vivo stability and low immunogenicity, makes them an interesting format for the development of next-generation scorpion antivenoms [5,85]. As an example of their utility, a preclinical study on a bispecific Nb, targeting AahI and AahII toxins from *A. australis* venom, demonstrated that this Nb was able to provide in vivo protection against 100 LD_{50}s of intracerebroventricularly administered AahI (toxin to Nb molar ratio of 1:2) and 5 LD_{50}s of subcutaneously administered whole venom. These results were significantly better than controls, in which equimolar amounts of traditional equine antibody fragments were unable to neutralize 2 LD_{50}s of subcutaneously administered whole venom [86]. Finally, using a murine model, it was demonstrated that low molecular mass toxin–Nb complexes seemed to be quickly cleared through glomerular filtration, while uptake in the liver remained low [87]. Thus, these studies demonstrated that Nbs may possess promising pharmacokinetic and pharmacodynamic characteristics. Similar studies on *H. lepturus* and *Hottentotta saulcyi* with comparable results also support the notion that Nbs may find their utility for developing novel treatments for scorpion envenomings [83,88].

Finally, monoclonal IgGs are another recombinant antibody format that has been investigated for its ability to neutralize animal toxins. As an example, in vivo lethality studies assessing the neutralization capacity of several murine monoclonal IgGs have shown positive results for the neutralization of *A. australis* and *C. noxius* toxins [66]. In the future, however, it is likely that research in this area will focus more on human monoclonal IgGs, rather than non-human IgGs, as human IgGs have a range of benefits over heterologous IgGs. An overview of the benefits and drawbacks of different antibody formats can be found elsewhere [66].

4. Benefits of Scorpion Venom: Ongoing Research on Scorpion Toxins with Potential Therapeutic Applications

It is widely reported in the literature that scorpion venom is a rich source of bioactive compounds, and as such, their toxins are of interest to the pharmaceutical and biotech industries [89]. However, despite the fact that substantial research efforts are ongoing and the prospects for scorpion-derived therapeutic peptides are very promising, chlorotoxin is the only toxin from scorpion venom that has been taken into clinical trials [90]. Moreover, no scorpion toxin-based drug is currently found in the market [91]. In this section, potential applications of scorpion venom compounds, which have been the subject of therapeutic research, are presented (Figure 4), with a focus on results recently reported in the scientific literature. A comprehensive overview of such compounds, including older research reports, can be found elsewhere [12].

4.1. Antibacterial Effects

In the past century, antimicrobial drugs revolutionized the control of diseases caused by microorganisms, such as bacteria, fungi, viruses, and parasites. However, due to the global problem of antimicrobial resistance (AMR) development, new antimicrobial agents are crucially needed for the 21st century. These agents must be discovered at a rate that is sufficiently fast to combat the evolving rate of multidrug resistance (MDR) in microorganisms [92]. Natural product research holds promise for providing new molecules as a basis for novel antimicrobial drug development. In 1991, it was reported that the folding pattern of charybdotoxin, a KTx isolated from *L. quinquestriatus hebraeus* venom, was strikingly similar to that of the insect antibacterial component, defensin [93]. This discovery set the stage for studies on scorpion-derived antimicrobial peptides (AMPs), which have led to a large number of discoveries that may be of relevance for therapeutic applications. Comprehensive reviews on the different classes of AMPs found in the venom of several scorpion species can be found elsewhere [94,95]. Here, the focus will be directed only on more recent discoveries, with an overview of AMPs with bactericidal activity that have been reported in the last five years, which is summarized in Table 1.

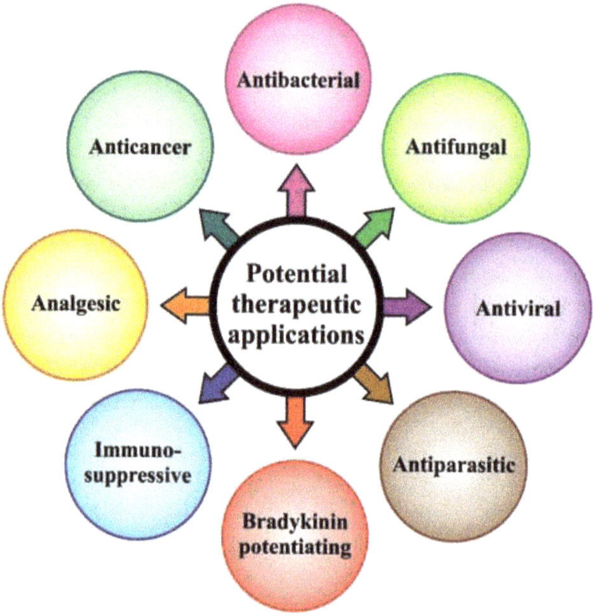

Figure 4. The potential therapeutic applications of scorpion venom compounds discussed in this article.

Table 1. Scorpion-derived compounds with antibacterial activities. MDR: multidrug resistance.

Year	Scorpion Species	Antibacterial Agent	MW (S–S Bridge)	Target	Reference
2015	*A. aeneas*	AaeAP1 AaeAP2	2016.18 Da (0) 1986.15 Da (0)	*S. aureus*	[96]
2015	*C. margaritatus*	Cm38	2149 Da (2)	*Klebsiella pneumonia*	[97]
2015	*T. stigmurus*	Stigmurin	1795.22 Da (0)	Gram-positive bacteria including *S. aureus* and Methicillin-resistant *S. aureus* (MRSA)	[98]
2016	*M. gibbosus*	Low molecular mass chitosan *	3220 Da (0)	Bacterial species in general, including *Listeria monocytogenes*, *Bacillus subtilis*, *Salmonella enteritidis*, and the yeast *Candida albicans*	[99]
2016	*Scorpio maurus palmatus* (synthetic)	Smp-24 Smp-43	2578 Da (0) 4654.3 Da (0)	Highest activity against Gram-positive bacteria, limited activity against *C. albicans*	[100]
2017	*Isometrus maculatus*	Im-4 Im-5 Im-6	1714 Da (0) 2803.7 Da (0) 1707 Da (0)	Gram-positive bacteria Gram-positive and Gram-negative bacteria Gram-positive bacteria	[101]
2018	*T. obscurus*	ToAP2	9486 Da (0)	*Mycobacterium massiliense*	[102]
2018	*M. eupeus*	Meucin-49 Meucin-18	5574.93 Da (?) 2107.13 Da (0)	Gram-positive bacteria Gram-negative bacteria	[103]

Table 1. *Cont.*

Year	Scorpion Species	Antibacterial Agent	MW (S–S Bridge)	Target	Reference
2018	*M. martensii* *M. gibbosus* *M. eupeus*	Marcin-18 Megicin-18 Meucin-18	2135.63 Da (0?) 2068.04 Da (?) 2107.13 Da (0)	Gram-positive bacteria, including some clinical antibiotic-resistant strains	[104]
2018	*Liocheles australasiae*	LaIT2 N-LaIT2	6628.2 Da (3) 3326 Da (?)	Gram-negative bacteria	[105]
2018	*T. stigmurus*	StigA6 StigA16	1908 Da (0?) 1949 Da (0?)	Gram-positive and Gram-negative bacteria	[106]
2019	*D. melici*	Red 1,4-benzoquinone: 3,5-dimethoxy-2-(methylthio) cyclohexa-2,5-diene-1,4-dione * Blue 1,4-benzoquinone: 5-methoxy-2,3-bis(methylthio)cyclohexa-2,5-diene-1,4-dione *	168.15 Da	*S. aureus* *M. tuberculosis*, including an MDR strain	[53]
2017	*U. yaschenkoi*	UyCT1 UyCT3 UyCT5 Uy17 Uy192 Uy234	1603.9 Da (0) 1433.7 Da (0) 1442.7 Da (0) 1369.43 Da (0) 1459.98 Da (0) 1986.19 Da (0)	Gram-positive and Gram-negative bacteria	[107]
2019	*U. yaschenkoi*	Uy234 Uy17 Uy192	1986.19 Da (0) 1369.43 Da (0) 1459.98 Da (0)	MDR bacteria, including β-hemolytic *Streptococcus* strains	[108]
2017	*U. manicatus*	Um2 Um3 Um4 Um5	2034.56 Da (?) 1577.23 Da (?) 1428.58 Da (?) 1508.82 Da (?)	Gram-positive and Gram-negative bacteria	[107]
2019	*T. serrulatus* (hemolymph)	Serrulin	3564 Da (?)	Gram-positive and Gram-negative bacteria	[109]
2019	*A. australis hector*	G-TI	7390 Da (4, predicted)	*B. cereus*	[110]

The compounds mentioned in Table 1 are from the scorpion venom, unless otherwise specified. Whenever data on the number of disulfide bridges were not available for a compound, a question mark (?) is used. Non-peptidic compounds are marked with a star (*).

Recently, the spotlight has been put on the general and intrinsic multifunctionality of scorpion venom components, including AMPs [103]. For instance, native scorpion AMPs, UyCT3, and UyCT5 from *U. yaschenkoi* and an enhanced UyCT peptide (designated as D3) were demonstrated to be potential bioinsecticides and promising candidates for the engineering of aphid-resistant crops. When pea aphids (*Acyrthosiphon pisum*) that are known as severe agricultural pests were fed with these AMPs, the AMPs displayed activity against aphid bacterial symbionts and reduced the number of symbionts, leading to a reduction in pest survival and delay in pest reproduction [111]. Meucin-49 from *M. eupeus* also showed insecticidal activity in addition to having broad-spectrum activity against Gram-positive and Gram-negative bacteria [103]. The red and blue benzoquinones from *D. melici* are multifunctional components that, besides showing antibacterial activity, also exert cytotoxic effects on neoplastic cell lines. In mouse models of MDR tuberculosis infection, blue benzoquinone showed comparable activity to commercially available antibiotics, while it did not cause adverse side effects in healthy mice [53]. Similarly, the low molecular mass chitosan obtained from *M. gibbosus* had a strong inhibitory effect against the bacterium *L. monocytogenes* and the yeast *C. albicans*. In addition, its antibacterial activity against *B. subtilis* and *S. enteritidis* was higher than the antibiotic, gentamicin [99].

Despite the multifunctionality and desirable potent action against microbes, natural scorpion AMPs generally have cytotoxic effects on eukaryotic cells, which is an obstacle that must be overcome. To this end, protein engineering techniques have been used to improve the potency and spectra of antimicrobial activity of the natural scorpion AMPs [107,112,113]. Employing these techniques, it has been demonstrated that scorpion AMPs can be effectively used as scaffolds to design more specific and less harmful antibiotics [114,115]. In addition, combining low concentrations of fast-killing scorpion AMPs with classical antibiotics is another approach that can be pursued in order to circumvent their cytotoxic effects against eukaryotic cells [116]. All in all, using natural scorpion AMPs as scaffolds for the rational design of novel antimicrobial agents and mixed formulations of antibiotics opens a new window of research to be pursued in the future.

4.2. Antifungal Effects

The most important opportunistic fungal pathogens that are responsible for high mortality, especially in hospitalized and immunocompromised/critically ill patients, belong to the *Candida*, *Aspergillus*, *Cryptococcus*, and *Pneumocystis* genera [117]. It has been reported that the prevalence of invasive fungal infections has increased from 6.3% in 1999 to 20% in 2013 [118]. Among the aforementioned genera, *Candida* is the most common cause of fungal infections worldwide, and invasive candidiasis occurs in more than 100,000 patients every year [119]. Antifungal drug resistance among *Candida* species is increasingly reported, and the emergence of MDR *C. glabrata*, which can acquire resistance following exposure to antifungal agents, presents significant challenges in many medical centers [120]. Moreover, only three drug classes are licensed for monotherapy against *Candida* infections including azoles, polyenes, and echinocandins [120]. Therefore, new antifungal drug candidates from additional drug classes are sought after. A summary of the scorpion-derived antifungal agents reported in the last five years is found in Table 2.

Table 2. Reported work on scorpion derived antifungal agents.

Year	Scorpion Species	Antifungal Agent	MW (S–S Bridge)	Target	Reference
2015	*T. stigmurus*	Stigmurin	1795.22 Da (0)	*C. albicans*, *C. krusei*, and *C. glabrata*	[98]
2015	*A. aeneas*	AaeAP1 AaeAP2	2016.18 Da (0) 1986.15 Da (0)	*C. albicans*	[96]
2016	*T. stigmurus*	Hypotensin TistH	2700 Da (0)	*C. albicans*, *C. tropicalis* and *Aspergillus flavus*	[121]
2016	*T. obscurus*	ToAcP, ToAP1, ToAP2, ToAP3, ToAP4	? (0)	*Cryptococcus neoforman* and *Candida species*	[122]
2017	*T. serrulatus*	Ts1	8300 Da (3)	*A. nidulans*	[123]
2018	*T. stigmurus*	StigA6 StigA16	1908 Da (0?) 1949 Da (0?)	*C. albicans*, *C. krusei*, and *C. glabrata*	[106]
2019	*T. serrulatus* (hemolymph)	Serrulin	3564 Da (0)	*A. niger* and *C. albicans*	[109]

The compounds mentioned in Table 1 are from the scorpion venom, unless otherwise specified. Whenever data on the molecular weight and/or the number of disulfide bridges were not available for a compound, a question mark (?) is used.

Stigmurin, selected and synthesized based on a transcriptomic analysis of the *T. stigmurus* venom gland, exhibits both antibacterial and antifungal activity. It is effective against the Gram-positive bacterial species, *S. aureus*, including methicillin-resistant strains. Stigmurin has also been demonstrated to be effective against the fungi *C. albicans*, *C. krusei*, and *C. glabrata*, with low toxicity against healthy human erythrocytes [98]. These data suggested that stigmurin could be considered for the treatment of candidiasis. More recently, two analog peptides, StigA6 and StigA16, were designed from the original peptide that demonstrated improved antimicrobial and antifungal activity. These peptides could inhibit the growth of both Gram-positive and Gram-negative bacteria, as well as *C. albicans*,

C. krusei, and *C. glabrata*, at lower minimal inhibitory doses compared to stigmurin [106]. StigA6 and StigA16 also showed high antiparasitic activity against *Trypanosoma cruzi* (see Section 4.4). This study demonstrated that rational design using scorpion toxins as scaffolds may be useful for obtaining leads with improved therapeutic features against a wide range of pathogens, including fungi.

4.3. Antiviral Effects

Few antiviral vaccines and drugs are commercially available against the more than 200 viruses known to infect humans [124], which is a situation that has been highlighted by the current SARS-CoV-2 pandemic and puts an emphasis on the importance of discovery and development of new antiviral agents. To this end, venomous animals are considered by many researchers as promising sources for such discoveries [124,125]. While some scorpion toxins show specific antiviral effects against just one type of virus, other toxins are active against several different viruses. Mucroporin-M1, a derivative of mucroporin from the *Lychas mucronatus* venom, presents antiviral activities against three RNA viruses (measles (MeV), severe acute respiratory syndrome-related coronavirus (SARS-CoV), and influenza H5N1). Binding assays demonstrated that there is a significant and specific interaction between immobilized mucroporin-M1 on CM5 biosensor chips and MeV. Following the mixing of 1×10^3 plaque-forming units per milliliter (PFU/mL) of MeV with different concentrations of mucroporin-M1 and incubating the mixture for 1 h at 37 °C, two probable mechanisms of action were assessed. These assessments included measurements of the direct effects of mucroporin-M1 on the virus through the inhibition of MeV plaque formation and evaluation of the compound's ability to compromise the infectivity of the virus through the suppression of MeV replication. The results showed that MeV infectivity could be inhibited almost completely by 10 μg/mL of mucroporin-M1 within 40 min. In a similar way, mucroporin-M1 showed inhibitory effects against both SARS-CoV and H5N1 pseudoviruses [126]. Later, it was demonstrated that mucroporin-M1 can inhibit the replication of the Hepatitis B virus through the activation of the mitogen-activated protein kinase (MAPK) pathway and downregulation of HNF4α in vitro and in vivo [127]. Given the dual inhibitory activities against viruses and bacteria, mucroporin-M1 may be considered as a lead compound for treating viral and bacterial co-infections. Mucroporin-M1 also serves as an example demonstrating the potential of peptides from scorpion venoms to be used as scaffolds for designing multifunctional antiviral agents.

Another example is the recombinant peptide, rEv37, from the scorpion *Euscorpiops validus*, which was been demonstrated to possess inhibitory effects against dengue virus type 2 (DENV-2), hepatitis C virus (HCV), Zika virus (ZIKV), and herpes simplex virus type 1 infections at non-cytotoxic concentrations. The inhibitory effects of rEv37 against DENV-2, HCV, and ZIKV infections were determined in the hepatoma cell line Huh7 via real-time fluorescent quantitative PCR for mRNA in the infected cells. rEv37 was able to reduce the level of DENV-2, HCV, and ZIKV infection at the mRNA level at a concentration of 10 μM by 91%, 97%, and 87%, respectively. Since the cellular entry processes of these four viruses are similar, it has been suggested that a specific molecular mechanism, in which the rEv37 peptide alkalizes acidic organelles to prevent low pH-dependent fusion of the viral membrane to the endosomal membrane, blocks the release of the viral genome from the endosome to the cytoplasm and thus restricts viral late entry [128]. The propensity to cause adverse reactions, lack of or low efficacy, and high price of the very few vaccines and therapeutics that are available against the aforementioned viruses [129,130] emphasize that rEv37 may be a relevant lead that possibly could be developed into an antiviral drug.

Smp76, a scorpine-like peptide from the venom of *S. maurus palmatus*, is another recent example of a scorpion-derived agent that is effective against different viruses. The recombinantly expressed peptide (rSmp76) can inhibit RNA replication and protein synthesis of DENV-2 and ZIKV in primary mouse macrophages, the human lung adenocarcinoma cell line (A549), the Huh7 cell line, and the human monocytic cell line (THP-1) in a dose-dependent manner. At a concentration of 10 mM, the inhibitory effects of rSmp76 were 75.7% against infections caused by DENV-2 (*TSV01*) and its more virulent strain (NGC), while for ZIKV infection, inhibition was evaluated to be 73.8%. Although the detailed molecular mechanisms of the rSmp76-induced inhibitory effects need to be elucidated, it seems that the mechanism of inhibition did not include direct inactivation of the viral particles. It has been suggested that rSmp76 suppresses an established viral infection by upregulating interferon-β expression through the phosphorylation of the interferon regulatory factor 3, which enhances type-I IFN responses and thus inhibits viral infection [131]. Since the achievement of viral clearance is very difficult, antiviral agents, such as rSmp76, that can suppress established viral infections are considered to be more efficient than traditional antiviral therapeutics, which exert their antiviral effects through the direct inactivation of viral particles or the inhibition of viral cell entry [131]. Enhancing the protective effects of host innate immunity, such as interferon (IFN) activation, by antiviral agents, such as rSmp76, may potentially circumvent the development of drug resistance and the effects of genetic variability in the viral genome [132]. These examples, selected from dozens of ongoing studies, demonstrate the potential of scorpion-derived peptides to be developed as antiviral therapeutics.

4.4. Antiparasitic Effects

Parasitic diseases are considered a health problem, particularly in developing countries, where people are frequently infected by parasites belonging to the genera, *Plasmodium*, *Trypanosoma*, and *Leishmania*, among others [133,134]. Since antiparasitic therapeutic agents available for clinical use are often toxic [135], there is an urgent need for the discovery and development of novel therapeutics [136].

Scorpion toxins have been demonstrated to possess inhibitory effects against a number of parasites. Scorpine, purified from *Pandinus imperator* venom, was the first isolated scorpion toxin that demonstrated antiprotozoan effects against *Plasmodium berghei* [137]. Later on, recombinantly expressed scorpine produced 98% mortality in the sexual stage of *P. berghei* and 100% reduction in *P. falciparum* parasitemia [138]. Similarly, meucin-24 and meucin-25, two linear NDBPs synthesized from a cDNA library of the *M. eupeus* venom gland, demonstrated antimalarial activity. Both peptides inhibited the development of *P. berghei* and killed intra-erythrocytic *P. falciparum* parasites at micromolar concentrations without harming mammalian cells [139], making them potential candidates for antimalarial therapies.

Scorpion-derived agents can be effective against other parasites as well. *Taenia solium* (pork tapeworm) is a parasite responsible for taeniasis (intestinal infection) and cysticercosis (tissue infection) in humans [140]. In 2010, *T. solium* cysticercosis was added to the list of major Neglected Tropical Diseases of the World Health Organization (WHO) [141]. *T. crassiceps* is another species of the Taeniidae family of tapeworms that, due to extensive antigen similarity with *T. solium*, functions as an experimental model to test and screen promising antigens before testing them in pigs [142]. It has been demonstrated using in vitro assays that Hge36, a naturally occurring truncated form of a scorpine-like peptide from the *Hoffmannihadrurus gertschi* venom, can reduce the viability of *T. crassiceps* larval cysts at submicromolar concentrations while having a minimal effect on human lymphocytes [143]. This study demonstrated that scorpion-derived agents may hold potential as therapeutic agents for human cysticercosis disease.

Human African trypanosomiasis (sleeping sickness) and American trypanosomiasis (Chagas disease) are induced upon infection with the protozoan parasites, *T. brucei* and *T. cruzi*, respectively. Being considered endemic in Latin America, Chagas disease is a potentially life-threatening illness that affects 6–7 million lives according to the WHO [144]. In an in vitro assay, it was recently demonstrated that stigmurin and its analogs, StigA6, StigA16, StigA25, and StigA31, show high antiparasitic activity against epimastigote forms of *T. cruzi* that is a form naturally found in the gut of infected insect vectors [106,113]. StigA6 and StigA16 have also been shown to have activity against trypomastigote forms of *T. cruzi*, which are mainly found in the blood of patients in the acute phase of Chagas disease. In addition, these peptides demonstrate higher antiparasitic activity at a lower concentration compared to benznidazole, which together with nifurtimox are currently available as Chagas disease medicines [106]. Therefore, StigA6 and StigA16 may be utilized in the development of therapeutics against Chagas disease.

It has been demonstrated that Leishmania parasites are sensitive to peptides with antimicrobial and ion channel inhibitory activity. Since scorpion venoms are rich sources of such peptides, Borges et al. demonstrated that *T. discrepans* crude venom and its main fractions (TdI, II, and III) could inhibit the growth of promastigote forms (the motile, long-elongated flagellated infective form of the Leishmania parasite that develops in the midgut of the sandfly) of *L. mexicana*, *L. braziliensis*, and *L. chagasi* that eventually led to parasite death in vitro [145]. Unfortunately, to the best of our knowledge, leishmanicidal activity of compounds from the venoms of other scorpion species/families has not been reported, and it should be investigated whether the leshmanicidal effects are restricted to the genus *Tityus*.

4.5. Bradykinin-Potentiating Effects

Bradykinin is a potent endothelium-dependent vasodilator peptide with hypotensive properties that belongs to the kinin group of proteins. The angiotensin-converting enzyme (ACE) inactivates bradykinin by degrading it [146,147]. The inhibition of ACE via bradykinin-potentiating peptides (BPPs), such as captopril, which is derived from a peptide found in the venom of the lancehead viper (*Bothrops jararaca*), has been established as a clinically approved strategy for preventing hypertension [148].

The multifunctionality of scorpion toxins is in the limelight once again regarding the bradykinin-potentiating effects of scorpion venoms. It has been demonstrated that the C-terminal fragment of BmKbpp, an AMP from *M. martensii* venom with antibacterial and antifungal activities, shows significant sequence similarity with the peptide K12, which is a known ACE inhibitor from *B. occitanus* venom. In an in vitro assay using guinea pig ileum segments of nearly 3 cm in length, both BmKbpp whole peptide and its C-terminal fragment (BmKbpp-C) demonstrated bradykinin-potentiating activity at a concentration of 50 nM. However, BmKbpp whole peptide and BmKbpp-C were less potent than peptide K12, with BmKbpp-C being more active than the whole peptide [149]. The sequence similarity between a fragment of a toxin and BPPs is also observed for *T. serrulatus* venom peptides. The N-terminal of Ts3, an α-toxin acting on voltage-gated sodium channels, demonstrated a striking sequence similarity with Ts10 (former Peptide T) that is a known BPP [150]. Ts10 was originally reported as an ACE inhibitor, since it could inhibit the ACE-catalyzed hydrolysis of bradykinin [151]. Later, using male Wistar rats and their aortic rings, in vitro and in vivo assays demonstrated that the N-terminal of Ts3 ($Ts3_{1\text{-}14[C12S]}$) and Ts10 were not able to directly inhibit ACE activity; instead, they induced a strong vasodilatory effect that could be reversed in the presence of the nitric oxide (NO) synthase inhibitor, N(ω)-nitro-L-arginine methyl ester (L-NAME). This suggests that Ts10 and $Ts3_{1\text{-}14[C12S]}$ play their role by activating molecular targets in the vascular endothelium, which leads to NO production and eventually vasodilation [150]. In addition, it has been reported that *T. serrulatus* hypotensins (TsHpt-I, II, III, and IV) and TistH from *T. stigmurus* also potentiate bradykinin through improvement of the endothelial function and NO release in rats [152,153]. These cases show that scorpion peptides can potentiate bradykinin through mechanisms other than ACE inhibition.

Besides vasodilation and hypotension, scorpion-derived BPPs play important roles in other physiological processes. It is estimated that a considerable number of cancer patients receive radiation therapy during their course of illness [154]. However, radiation therapy might lead to side effects, including radiation-induced heart disease (RIHD) in patients having lymphoma, breast, lung, and esophageal cancer [155,156]. It has been demonstrated that BPPs obtained from *L. quinquestriatus* improved cardiomyopathy induced by γ-radiation in rats, probably by acting as a scavenger of free radicals to protect the heart from negative effects derived from radiation exposure [157].

4.6. Immunosuppressive Effects

Several scorpion toxins can modulate the immune system [158]. Indeed, the contribution of released inflammatory mediators (e.g., cytokines, eicosanoids, and reactive oxygen species) and activation of the complement system is well explored in the envenoming pathophysiology following scorpion stings [57,158,159]. For instance, an increase in the regulatory cytokines, interleukin (IL)-10 and IL-4, has been observed in experimental envenomings by *A. australis hector* and *C. noxius*, as well as in real human envenomings by *T. serrulatus* [160–163]. Although most of the studied scorpion toxins exhibit pro-inflammatory effects and activate the immune system [20,58,160,164,165], a few of them demonstrate potential therapeutic applications by controlling the immune responses and acting as immunosuppressive agents.

The most studied class of immunosuppressive scorpion toxins is the blockers of voltage-gated potassium channel type 1.3 ($K_V1.3$). Although many cells express $K_V1.3$, most of the studies have focused on effector memory T cells (T_{EM}) due to the high expression profiles of $K_V1.3$. The T_{EM} cells are a subpopulation of T cells regarded as an attractive pharmacological target because of their role in the development of autoimmune diseases [166]. A recent review covering the structure and function of these channels, as well as the therapeutic implications of blocking $K_V1.3$ using toxins derived from scorpion venom, has summarized the studies of more than 60 scorpion toxins from the *Androctonus*, *Buthus*, *Mesobuthus*, *Lychas*, *Parabuthus*, *Leiurus*, *Centruroides*, and *Tityus* genera [167].

Beside $K_V1.3$ channels, other ion channels, such as $K_V3.1$ and $K_V2.1$, have also been demonstrated to be important for T-cell activation and function [168,169]. Pucca et al. described Ts6 and Ts15, from *T. serrulatus*, which block $K_V2.1$ and inhibit the proliferation and function of different T-cell subpopulations in vitro. The study also showed that Ts15 was capable of inhibiting delayed-type hypersensitivity (DTH) response in vivo, indicating the potential of the peptide to be developed into a treatment for autoimmune diseases [169]. Another study performed by Xiao et al. described the immunosuppressive and anti-inflammatory properties of St20, a disulfide-bridged α-KTx found in the venom of *Scorpiops tibetanus*. In vitro functional studies showed that this peptide was able to inhibit the expression of the cell surface marker CD69, as well as the secretion of IL-2, tumor necrosis factor (TNF)-α, and IFN-γ in activated human T cells. In vivo experiments using a rat autoimmune disease model showed that DTH was ameliorated in the presence of St20 [170]. Thus, new immunosuppressive therapeutic drugs may be derived from scorpion venom toxins, which can be optimized in regard to structure and function, possibly facilitating the future use of such agents in clinical settings.

4.7. Analgesic Effects

Generally, scorpion stings are reported as very painful events. Most known scorpion toxins are known to modulate voltage-gated ion channels (mainly sodium and potassium channels) [20]. Voltage-gated sodium (Na_V) channels play a key role in nociception (pain) [171]. The Na_V channels comprise a family of nine homologous α-subunits ($Na_V1.1$–$Na_V1.9$), which together with β-units (β1–β4) generate the ion-conducting pore [172]. However, only four Na_V channel subtypes are involved in pain: $Na_V1.1$, $Na_V1.6$, $Na_V1.7$, and $Na_V1.9$ [173–176]. Throughout the last decades, scorpion toxins capable of inducing pain mediated by these channels have been widely explored [20,177–180]. Most recently, two peptides, Hj1a and Hj2a, have been isolated from the *Hottentotta jayakari* venom that are potent agonists of $Na_V1.1$. Demonstrating dual α/β activity by modifying both the activation and inactivation properties of the channel, Hj1a and Hj2a may be used as alternative tools for developing selective $Na_V1.1$ modulators for the treatment of epileptic diseases, such as Dravet syndrome [181]. In addition, scorpion toxins that induce pain, mediated by different ion channels, such as voltage-gated potassium channel 4.2 ($K_V4.2$) [182] and TRPV1 [35,183], have also been encountered.

Moreover, scorpion toxins capable of controlling pain (i.e., analgesics) have been reported in the literature. Many of these analgesic toxins are not toxic to mammals, as they belong to a group of insect-specific neurotoxic α or β-toxins that interact with Na_V, K_V, and/or Ca_V pathways [114,184–188]. During the last two decades, over 20 scorpion venom-derived peptides and proteins have been reported to exert anti-nociceptive effects in vitro and in vivo. Due to the absence of toxicity in mammals and comparable effects to standard of care medications, such as carbamazepine, most of the scorpion-derived proteins are intriguing agents that could be used for future development of analgesics. The scorpion *M. martensii* (previously known as *B. martensii* Karsch) has been thoroughly studied as the source of more than 15 analgesic peptides [189,190]. Analgesic properties have also been reported in *A. mauretanicus mauretanicus* (AmmVIII, α-anatoxin), *L. quinquestriatus quinquestriatus* (LqqIT2, β-toxin), *H. laoticus* (Hetlaxin, α-toxin), *B. occitanus tunetanus* (BotAF, β-toxin), and *T. serrulatus* (TsNTxP) (Table 3). However, there is still much unexplored venom territory for future discovery in the field of analgesic venom components.

In 2019, Rigo et al. reported the presence of anti-nociceptive effects of a non-toxic protein from *T. serrulatus*, TsNTxP [191]. This protein is described to be structurally similar to Na_V-modulating neurotoxins, such as Ts7. However, TsNTxP is non-toxic to animals. Effects of TsNTxP were studied in 184 adult male and female Swiss mice in regard to acute and neuropathic pain. The results demonstrated that TsNTxP has potent anti-nociceptive properties in both models, which is potentially due to a substantial reduction of glutamate release. These results, combined with the lack of acute adverse effects, suggest that TsNTxP may possibly be utilized in future pain treatment.

Table 3. Summary of known anti-nociceptive scorpion toxins.

Toxin Name	Scorpion Species	MW (S–S Bridge)	Target	Reference
BmK AS	*M. martensii*	7701 Da (4)	TTX-R (Na_V1.8, 1.9), TTX-S (Na_V1.3); reduction of neural excitability; skeletal muscle RyR	[192–195]
BmK IT2	*M. martensii*	6650 Da (4)	TTX-R and TTX-S Na_V	[192,196]
BmK IT-AP	*M. martensii*	8157 Da (4)	N/A	[197]
BmK dITAP3	*M. martensii*	6740 Da (4)	N/A	[187]
BmK AEP/BmK ANEP	*M. martensii*	6738 Da (4)	Na_V1.1, Na_V1.3, Na_V1.6, Na_V1.7	[198–200]
BmK AS1	*M. martensii*	7712 Da (4)	TTX-R and TTX-S Na_V, skeletal-muscle RyR-1	[201]
BmK AGAP	*M. martensii*	7281 Da (4)	Prevention of peripheral and spinal MAPKs expression; Decrease of spinal c-Fos expression; Na_V1.7, Na_V1.8, Na_V1.4, Na_V1.5; Ca_V	[185,202–205]
BmK Ang P1	*M. martensii*	8141 Da (4)	N/A	[206]
BmK Ang M1	*M. martensii*	7040 Da (4)	Na_V, K_V	[114,207]
BmK(M)9	*M. martensii*	7106 Da (4)	Na_V1.4, Na_V1.5, Na_V1.7	[208,209]
BmK AGP-SYPU1	*M. martensii*	7227 Da (4)	N/A	[210]
BmK AGP-SYPU2	*M. martensii*	7457 Da (4)	Na_V	[211,212]
BmK AGAP-SYPU2	*M. martensii*	7253 Da (4)	Na_V (suspected)	[213]
BmK-YA	*M. martensii*	871 Da (0)	μ, κ, δ-opioid receptor	[188]
BmKBTx	*M. martensii*	6800 Da (3)	Na_V1.7	[214]
BmNaL-3SS2	*M. martensii*	7338.26 Da (3)	Na_V1.7	[214]
AmmVIII	*A. mauretanicus mauretanicus*	7383 Da (4)	Na_V1.2, endogenous opioid system, no data on other Na_Vs yet	[186]
LqqIT2	*L. quinquestriatus quinquestriatus*	6845 Da (4)	Endogenous opioid system, no data on other Na_Vs yet	[186]
TsNTxP	*T. serrulatus*	6702 (4)	N/A (possibly glutamate release)	[191]
BotAF	*B. occitanus tunetanus*	7446 Da (4)	Peripheral or spinal mechanisms	[198]
Hetlaxin	*H. laoticus*	3665 Da (4)	K_V1.3, K_V1.1	[184,215]

4.8. Anticancer Effects

The discovery of specific and selective anticancer drugs that can directly act on tumors, display a synergistic effect with existing chemotherapeutics, or function as cargoes for drugs with low bioavailability is significantly on the rise [216]. Chlorotoxin (CTx) from *L. quinquestriatus* venom is a molecule that interacts with chloride channels. CTx was the first scorpion-derived agent that demonstrated inhibitory effects on glioma cell migration and invasion. It also exhibited the advantage of being able to penetrate deep into tumor tissue [217,218]. Since the discovery of CTx, the list of scorpion crude venoms and isolated toxins with anticancer activity has been growing rapidly, hence a comprehensive review of all reported compounds exceeds the scope of this review, but can be found elsewhere [216–219]. Here, we present a few cherry-picked recent studies with the most significant findings.

T. serrulatus crude venom was tested in 2019 for possible anticancer effects against the SiHa and HeLa cervical cancer cell lines, and the venom was shown to induce apoptosis in HeLa cells [220]. Wang et al. had previously obtained similar results with the crude venoms of *H. liangi* and *M. martensii*. The two venoms were tested for potential anticancer effects toward HeLa cells, and both venoms showed dose-dependent anti-proliferative and apoptosis-inducing effects through upregulation of the CDK-inhibitor, p21. However, neither of the venoms showed significant effects on non-cancer HUVEC-21 cells, suggesting specificity toward cancer cells [221]. Additionally, the venoms of *A. crassicauda* and *L. quinquestriatus* have been examined using breast (MDA-MB-231) and colorectal (HCT-8) cancer cell lines [222]. This examination revealed that the venoms exhibited significant time and dose-dependent cytotoxicity, and that they caused an increase in the number of apoptotic cells and reactive oxygen species for both cancer cell lines when the cell lines were subjected to the venoms. The observed arrests in the cell cycle could be an indication of tumor suppressor p21 upregulation and could, hence, suggest selectivity toward cancer cells. Anticancer properties have been recently associated to the crude venom of *Rhopalurus junceus* and a mix of five peptides from the same venom [223,224]. Despite generating promising results, further investigations on the aforementioned scorpion crude venoms are needed to characterize the effective anticancer constituents among other venom components.

In 2018, Li et al. constructed a scorpion venom library of *A. australis* and *A. mauretanicus* that led to the discovery of a highly potent novel anticancer peptide from *A. mauretanicus* named Gonearrestide. This peptide was subsequently tested against several colorectal cancer cell lines (DLD-1, Hke3, Dks8, and HCT116) and the glioma cell line, U-251. Extensive in vitro, in vivo, and ex vivo studies on HCT116 cells demonstrated that this peptide possessed high specificity toward cancer cells, could significantly arrest the cell cycle in the G1 phase, and could thus strongly inhibit tumor growth. Additionally, proliferation and cytotoxicity studies with the non-cancer human epithelial cell lines FHC (colon), MCF-10A (breast), and human erythrocytes only identified negligible off-target effects of Gonearrestide [225]. Another study by BenAissa et al. investigated the activity of the negatively charged fractions of *A. australis* venom against DU145 prostate cancer cells and successfully identified strong anti-proliferative effects mediated by the $Na_V1.6$-directed peptide AaHIV [226]. However, regardless of its potent anti-proliferative effects, this peptide was not able to inhibit cell migration. Another study on AGAP and AGAP-SYPU2 from *M. martensii* venom (see Section 4.7 for their analgesic effects) demonstrated that these two peptides possessed in vivo antitumor properties in mouse Ehrlich ascites tumor models and mouse S-180 fibrosarcoma models [213,227]. Furthermore, AGAP showed strong anticancer effects, including the inhibition of stemness, epithelial–mesenchymal transition, migration, and invasion toward MCF-7 and MDA-MB-231 breast cancer cells [228]. It also inhibited the voltage-gated proton channel Hv1 [229], which has been investigated as a possible target for cancer therapy and has been extensively reviewed elsewhere [230]. Two studies on a third *M. martensii* peptide, BmKn2, indicated that this peptide could selectively induce apoptosis in cancerous human oral cells, while normal cells were affected to a much lesser extent [231,232]. Another interesting study highlights a newly discovered short (14 residues) peptide from *B. occitanus tunetanus*, RK1, with potent anticancer effects toward glioblastoma (U87) and melanoma (IGR39) cancers [233]. While showing no apparent in vivo neurotoxicity toward intracerebroventricularly injected mice, RK1 was demonstrated to possess cytotoxicity against U87 and IGR139 cells in vitro, and it was able to inhibit cell proliferation and migration of these two cancer cell lines. RK1 also inhibited angiogenesis in a chicken chorioallantoic membrane model. A cell-penetrating peptide (CPP) from *T. serrulatus* venom, named CPP-Ts, is the final promising member of the long list of scorpion-derived agents with anticancer effects discussed here. Using a CPP-Ts-derived peptide (subpeptide$^{14-39}$), a study demonstrated that this peptide has selective internalization properties in specific cancer cell lines, such as SK-MEL-188, HEP G2, Caco-2, MDA-MB-231, A549, and DU 145, which make it a potential intranuclear delivery tool for cancer cell targeting [34]. These handful of studies from the growing body of recently published papers indicate the potential of utilizing scorpion venoms as a source for discovering new cancer therapeutics.

5. Conclusions

The large diversity of scorpion venom components has fueled a wide range of studies on these molecules, from toxicology to antivenom development and therapeutic applications. In particular, therapeutic applications of scorpion venom compounds have attracted a lot of attention due to the urgent need for either finding or improving treatments against a broad spectrum of diseases. The emergence and spread of superbugs (AMR microorganisms) represent an increasingly serious threat to global public health, which is projected to get much worse in the years ahead. Therefore, the exploration of the utility of novel bioactive molecules, scaffolds, and mechanisms of action represents a potentially powerful approach to develop new antimicrobial therapeutics and diagnostic tools for current and future diseases. Dozens of scorpion-derived bioactive molecules have been shown to possess promising pharmacological properties, of which around 100 have been mentioned in this review. These pharmacological properties of scorpion-derived bioactive molecules include antimicrobial, immunosuppressive, bradykinin-potentiating, analgesic, and anticancer effects among others. In addition to chlorotoxin, which has already entered clinical trials, the CPP-Ts peptide (which is a potential intranuclear delivery tool for targeting cancer cells) is likely to be a molecule receiving significant scientific interest in the future. However, before venom-derived biotherapeutics can be introduced to the market, a number of technological issues must be overcome, including obtaining access to material (venoms and toxins), characterizing isolated venom components, establishing manufacturing approaches for novel compounds, and reducing the potential propensity to cause adverse effects, especially for long-term therapy. Nevertheless, the scientific literature reviewed here shows several examples of promising scorpion venom-derived proteins and peptides that may be used as leads for the development of new biotherapeutics. Thus, if the data observed in vitro and in preclinical models translates well to the clinical setting, there may indeed be great promise in exploiting the benefits of scorpion toxins.

Author Contributions: Writing—original draft preparation, S.A., M.B.P., K.C.F.B., J.M.K., L.A.; writing—review and editing, S.A., A.H.L., F.Ç., E.C.A.; visualization, F.A.C.; supervision, S.A., A.H.L. All authors have read and agreed to the published version of the manuscript.

Funding: We thank the Villum Foundation (grant 00025302) for financial support.

Conflicts of Interest: The authors declare no conflicts of interest.

References

1. Chippaux, J.-P.; Goyffon, M. Epidemiology of scorpionism: A global appraisal. *Acta Trop.* **2008**, *107*, 71–79. [CrossRef] [PubMed]
2. WHO. *Report of the Eleventh Meeting of the WHO Strategic and Technical Advisory Group for Neglected Tropical Diseases*; World Health Organization: Geneva, Switzerland, 2018; pp. 1–28. [CrossRef]
3. Chippaux, J.-P. Emerging options for the management of scorpion stings. *Drug Des. Dev. Ther.* **2012**, *6*, 165–173. [CrossRef] [PubMed]
4. Reckziegel, G.C.; Pinto, V.L.; Reckziegel, G.C.; Pinto, V.L. Scorpionism in Brazil in the years 2000 to 2012. *J. Venom. Anim. Toxins Incl. Trop. Dis.* **2014**, *20*, 46. [CrossRef] [PubMed]
5. Laustsen, A.H.; Solà, M.; Jappe, E.C.; Oscoz, S.; Lauridsen, L.P.; Engmark, M. Biotechnological Trends in Spider and Scorpion Antivenom Development. *Toxins* **2016**, *8*, 226. [CrossRef] [PubMed]
6. Lourenço, W.R. The evolution and distribution of noxious species of scorpions (Arachnida: Scorpiones). *J. Venom. Anim. Toxins Incl. Trop. Dis.* **2018**, 24. [CrossRef]
7. Hauke, T.J.; Herzig, V. Dangerous arachnids—Fake news or reality? *Toxicon* **2017**, *138*, 173–183. [CrossRef]
8. Mullen, G.; Durden, L. Medical and Veterinary Entomology. *Ann. Trop. Med. Parasitol.* **2019**, 3. [CrossRef]

9. Ward, M.J.; Ellsworth, S.A.; Nystrom, G.S. A global accounting of medically significant scorpions: Epidemiology, major toxins, and comparative resources in harmless counterparts. *Toxicon* **2018**, *151*, 137–155. [CrossRef]
10. Petricevich, V.L. Scorpion Venom and the Inflammatory Response. Available online: https://www.hindawi.com/journals/mi/2010/903295/ (accessed on 12 January 2020).
11. De la Vega, R.C.R.; Vidal, N.; Possani, L.D. Chapter 59—Scorpion Peptides. In *Handbook of Biologically Active Peptides*, 2nd ed.; Kastin, A.J., Ed.; Academic Press: Boston, MA, USA, 2013; pp. 423–429, ISBN 978-0-12-385095-9.
12. Ortiz, E.; Gurrola, G.B.; Schwartz, E.F.; Possani, L.D. Scorpion venom components as potential candidates for drug development. *Toxicon* **2015**, *93*, 125–135. [CrossRef]
13. Valdivia, H.H.; Martin, B.M.; Ramírez, A.N.; Fletcher, P.L.; Possani, L.D. Isolation and pharmacological characterization of four novel Na+ channel-blocking toxins from the scorpion *Centruroides noxius* Hoffmann. *J. Biochem.* **1994**, *116*, 1383–1391. [CrossRef]
14. Goyffon, M.; Tournier, J.-N. Scorpions: A Presentation. *Toxins* **2014**, *6*, 2137–2148. [CrossRef] [PubMed]
15. Caliskan, F. Scorpion Venom Research Around the World: Turkish Scorpions. In *Toxinology: Scorpion Venoms*; Gopalakrishnakone, P., Ed.; Springer: Dordrecht, The Netherlands, 2013; pp. 1–19, ISBN 978-94-007-6647-1.
16. Del Río-Portilla, F.; Hernández-Marín, E.; Pimienta, G.; Coronas, F.V.; Zamudio, F.Z.; Rodríguez de la Vega, R.C.; Wanke, E.; Possani, L.D. NMR solution structure of Cn12, a novel peptide from the Mexican scorpion *Centruroides noxius* with a typical beta-toxin sequence but with alpha-like physiological activity. *Eur. J. Biochem.* **2004**, *271*, 2504–2516. [CrossRef] [PubMed]
17. Rodríguez de la Vega, R.C.; Possani, L.D. Current views on scorpion toxins specific for K+-channels. *Toxicon* **2004**, *43*, 865–875. [CrossRef] [PubMed]
18. Tytgat, J.; Chandy, K.G.; Garcia, M.L.; Gutman, G.A.; Martin-Eauclaire, M.F.; van der Walt, J.J.; Possani, L.D. A unified nomenclature for short-chain peptides isolated from scorpion venoms: Alpha-KTx molecular subfamilies. *Trends Pharm. Sci.* **1999**, *20*, 444–447. [CrossRef]
19. Cremonez, C.M.; Maiti, M.; Peigneur, S.; Cassoli, J.S.; Dutra, A.A.A.; Waelkens, E.; Lescrinier, E.; Herdewijn, P.; de Lima, M.E.; Pimenta, A.M.C.; et al. Structural and Functional Elucidation of Peptide Ts11 Shows Evidence of a Novel Subfamily of Scorpion Venom Toxins. *Toxins* **2016**, *8*, 288. [CrossRef]
20. Pucca, M.B.; Peigneur, S.; Cologna, C.T.; Cerni, F.A.; Zoccal, K.F.; Bordon, K.d.C.F.; Faccioli, L.H.; Tytgat, J.; Arantes, E.C. Electrophysiological characterization of the first *Tityus serrulatus* alpha-like toxin, Ts5: Evidence of a pro-inflammatory toxin on macrophages. *Biochimie* **2015**, *115*, 8–16. [CrossRef]
21. Cerni, F.A.; Pucca, M.B.; Amorim, F.G.; de Castro Figueiredo Bordon, K.; Echterbille, J.; Quinton, L.; De Pauw, E.; Peigneur, S.; Tytgat, J.; Arantes, E.C. Isolation and characterization of Ts19 Fragment II, a new long-chain potassium channel toxin from *Tityus serrulatus* venom. *Peptides* **2016**, *80*, 9–17. [CrossRef]
22. Jiménez-Vargas, J.M.; Restano-Cassulini, R.; Possani, L.D. Toxin modulators and blockers of hERG K(+) channels. *Toxicon* **2012**, *60*, 492–501. [CrossRef]
23. Srinivasan, K.N.; Sivaraja, V.; Huys, I.; Sasaki, T.; Cheng, B.; Kumar, T.K.S.; Sato, K.; Tytgat, J.; Yu, C.; San, B.C.C.; et al. kappa-Hefutoxin1, a novel toxin from the scorpion *Heterometrus fulvipes* with unique structure and function. Importance of the functional diad in potassium channel selectivity. *J. Biol. Chem.* **2002**, *277*, 30040–30047. [CrossRef]
24. Chen, Z.; Luo, F.; Feng, J.; Yang, W.; Zeng, D.; Zhao, R.; Cao, Z.; Liu, M.; Li, W.; Jiang, L.; et al. Genomic and Structural Characterization of Kunitz-Type Peptide LmKTT-1a Highlights Diversity and Evolution of Scorpion Potassium Channel Toxins. *PLoS ONE* **2013**, *8*, e60201. [CrossRef]
25. Smith, J.J.; Hill, J.M.; Little, M.J.; Nicholson, G.M.; King, G.F.; Alewood, P.F. Unique scorpion toxin with a putative ancestral fold provides insight into evolution of the inhibitor cystine knot motif. *Proc. Natl. Acad. Sci. USA* **2011**, *108*, 10478–10483. [CrossRef] [PubMed]
26. Gao, B.; Harvey, P.J.; Craik, D.J.; Ronjat, M.; De Waard, M.; Zhu, S. Functional evolution of scorpion venom peptides with an inhibitor cystine knot fold. *Biosci. Rep.* **2013**, *33*, e00047. [CrossRef] [PubMed]
27. Xiao, L.; Gurrola, G.B.; Zhang, J.; Valdivia, C.R.; SanMartin, M.; Zamudio, F.Z.; Zhang, L.; Possani, L.D.; Valdivia, H.H. Structure–function relationships of peptides forming the calcin family of ryanodine receptor ligands. *J. Gen. Physiol.* **2016**, *147*, 375–394. [CrossRef] [PubMed]
28. Animal Toxins and Ion Channels—Abstract—Europe PMC. Available online: https://europepmc.org/article/med/10783702 (accessed on 12 January 2020).

29. Lanner, J.T.; Georgiou, D.K.; Joshi, A.D.; Hamilton, S.L. Ryanodine Receptors: Structure, Expression, Molecular Details, and Function in Calcium Release. *Cold Spring Harb. Perspect. Biol.* **2010**, *2*, a003996. [CrossRef] [PubMed]
30. Bers, D. *Excitation-Contraction Coupling and Cardiac Contractile Force*, 2nd ed.; Developments in Cardiovascular Medicine; Springer: Amsterdam, The Netherlands, 2001; ISBN 978-0-7923-7157-1.
31. Smith, J.J.; Vetter, I.; Lewis, R.J.; Peigneur, S.; Tytgat, J.; Lam, A.; Gallant, E.M.; Beard, N.A.; Alewood, P.F.; Dulhunty, A.F. Multiple actions of φ-LITX-Lw1a on ryanodine receptors reveal a functional link between scorpion DDH and ICK toxins. *Proc. Natl. Acad. Sci. USA* **2013**, *110*, 8906–8911. [CrossRef]
32. Boisseau, S.; Mabrouk, K.; Ram, N.; Garmy, N.; Collin, V.; Tadmouri, A.; Mikati, M.; Sabatier, J.-M.; Ronjat, M.; Fantini, J.; et al. Cell penetration properties of maurocalcine, a natural venom peptide active on the intracellular ryanodine receptor. *Biochim. Biophys. Acta (BBA) Biomembr.* **2006**, *1758*, 308–319. [CrossRef]
33. Ram, N.; Weiss, N.; Texier-Nogues, I.; Aroui, S.; Andreotti, N.; Pirollet, F.; Ronjat, M.; Sabatier, J.-M.; Darbon, H.; Jacquemond, V.; et al. Design of a disulfide-less, pharmacologically inert, and chemically competent analog of maurocalcine for the efficient transport of impermeant compounds into cells. *J. Biol. Chem.* **2008**, *283*, 27048–27056. [CrossRef]
34. De Oliveira-Mendes, B.B.R.; Horta, C.C.R.; do Carmo, A.O.; Biscoto, G.L.; Sales-Medina, D.F.; Leal, H.G.; Brandão-Dias, P.F.P.; Miranda, S.E.M.; Aguiar, C.J.; Cardoso, V.N.; et al. CPP-Ts: A new intracellular calcium channel modulator and a promising tool for drug delivery in cancer cells. *Sci. Rep.* **2018**, *8*, 1–13. [CrossRef] [PubMed]
35. King, J.V.L.; Emrick, J.J.; Kelly, M.J.S.; Herzig, V.; King, G.F.; Medzihradszky, K.F.; Julius, D. A Cell-Penetrating Scorpion Toxin Enables Mode-Specific Modulation of TRPA1 and Pain. *Cell* **2019**, *178*, 1362–1374.e16. [CrossRef] [PubMed]
36. Almaaytah, A.; Albalas, Q. Scorpion venom peptides with no disulfide bridges: A review. *Peptides* **2014**, *51*, 35–45. [CrossRef]
37. Quintero-Hernández, V.; Ramírez-Carreto, S.; Romero-Gutiérrez, M.T.; Valdez-Velázquez, L.L.; Becerril, B.; Possani, L.D.; Ortiz, E. Transcriptome Analysis of Scorpion Species Belonging to the *Vaejovis* Genus. *PLoS ONE* **2015**, *10*, e0117188. [CrossRef] [PubMed]
38. Zeng, X.-C.; Corzo, G.; Hahin, R. Scorpion Venom Peptides without Disulfide Bridges. *IUBMB Life* **2005**, *57*, 13–21. [CrossRef] [PubMed]
39. Pucca, M.B.; Cerni, F.A.; Pinheiro-Junior, E.L.; Zoccal, K.F.; Bordon, K.d.C.F.; Amorim, F.G.; Peigneur, S.; Vriens, K.; Thevissen, K.; Cammue, B.P.A.; et al. Non-disulfide-bridged peptides from *Tityus serrulatus* venom: Evidence for proline-free ACE-inhibitors. *Peptides* **2016**, *82*, 44–51. [CrossRef]
40. Bordon, K.C.F.; Wiezel, G.A.; Amorim, F.G.; Arantes, E.C. Arthropod venom Hyaluronidases: Biochemical properties and potential applications in medicine and biotechnology. *J. Venom. Anim. Toxins Incl. Trop. Dis.* **2015**, *21*, 43. [CrossRef] [PubMed]
41. Girish, K.S.; Kemparaju, K. The magic glue hyaluronan and its eraser hyaluronidase: A biological overview. *Life Sci.* **2007**, *80*, 1921–1943. [CrossRef]
42. De Oliveira-Mendes, B.B.R.; Miranda, S.E.M.; Sales-Medina, D.F.; de Magalhães, B.F.; Kalapothakis, Y.; de Souza, R.P.; Cardoso, V.N.; de Barros, A.L.B.; Guerra-Duarte, C.; Kalapothakis, E.; et al. Inhibition of *Tityus serrulatus* venom hyaluronidase affects venom biodistribution. *PLoS Negl. Trop. Dis.* **2019**, *13*, e0007048. [CrossRef]
43. Schwartz, E.F.; Camargos, T.S.; Zamudio, F.Z.; Silva, L.P.; Bloch, C.; Caixeta, F.; Schwartz, C.A.; Possani, L.D. Mass spectrometry analysis, amino acid sequence and biological activity of venom components from the Brazilian scorpion *Opisthacanthus cayaporum*. *Toxicon* **2008**, *51*, 1499–1508. [CrossRef]
44. Incamnoi, P.; Patramanon, R.; Thammasirirak, S.; Chaveerach, A.; Uawonggul, N.; Sukprasert, S.; Rungsa, P.; Daduang, J.; Daduang, S. Heteromtoxin (HmTx), a novel heterodimeric phospholipase A_2 from *Heterometrus laoticus* scorpion venom. *Toxicon* **2013**, *61*, 62–71. [CrossRef]
45. Fletcher, P.L.; Fletcher, M.D.; Weninger, K.; Anderson, T.E.; Martin, B.M. Vesicle-associated Membrane Protein (VAMP) Cleavage by a New Metalloprotease from the Brazilian Scorpion *Tityus serrulatus*. *J. Biol. Chem.* **2010**, *285*, 7405–7416. [CrossRef]
46. Brazón, J.; Guerrero, B.; D'Suze, G.; Sevcik, C.; Arocha-Piñango, C.L. Fibrin(ogen)olytic enzymes in scorpion (*Tityus discrepans*) venom. *Comp. Biochem. Physiol. Part B Biochem. Mol. Biol.* **2014**, *168*, 62–69. [CrossRef]

47. Kazemi, S.M.; Sabatier, J.-M. Venoms of Iranian Scorpions (Arachnida, Scorpiones) and Their Potential for Drug Discovery. *Molecules* **2019**, *24*, 2670. [CrossRef] [PubMed]
48. Almeida, F.M.; Pimenta, A.M.C.; De Figueiredo, S.G.; Santoro, M.M.; Martin-Eauclaire, M.F.; Diniz, C.R.; De Lima, M.E. Enzymes with gelatinolytic activity can be found in *Tityus bahiensis* and *Tityus serrulatus* venoms. *Toxicon* **2002**, *40*, 1041–1045. [CrossRef]
49. Cordeiro, F.A.; Coutinho, B.M.; Wiezel, G.A.; de Bordon, K.C.F.; Bregge-Silva, C.; Rosa-Garzon, N.G.; Cabral, H.; Ueberheide, B.; Arantes, E.C.; Cordeiro, F.A.; et al. Purification and enzymatic characterization of a novel metalloprotease from *Lachesis muta rhombeata* snake venom. *J. Venom. Anim. Toxins Incl. Trop. Dis.* **2018**, *24*, 32. [CrossRef] [PubMed]
50. Gutiérrez, J.M.; Rucavado, A. Snake venom metalloproteinases: Their role in the pathogenesis of local tissue damage. *Biochimie* **2000**, *82*, 841–850. [CrossRef]
51. Tiwari, A.K.; Mandal, M.B.; Deshpande, S.B. Role of serotonergic mechanism in gastric contractions induced by Indian Red Scorpion (*Mesobuthus tamulus*) venom. *Indian J. Pharm.* **2009**, *41*, 255–257. [CrossRef]
52. Al-Asmari, A.K.; Kunnathodi, F.; Al Saadon, K.; Idris, M.M. Elemental analysis of scorpion venoms. *J. Venom Res.* **2016**, *7*, 16–20. [PubMed]
53. Carcamo-Noriega, E.N.; Sathyamoorthi, S.; Banerjee, S.; Gnanamani, E.; Mendoza-Trujillo, M.; Mata-Espinosa, D.; Hernández-Pando, R.; Veytia-Bucheli, J.I.; Possani, L.D.; Zare, R.N. 1,4-Benzoquinone antimicrobial agents against *Staphylococcus aureus* and *Mycobacterium tuberculosis* derived from scorpion venom. *Proc. Natl. Acad. Sci. USA* **2019**, *116*, 12642–12647. [CrossRef]
54. Thien, T.V.; Anh, H.N.; Trang, N.T.T.; Trung, P.V.; Khoa, N.C.; Osipov, A.V.; Dubovskii, P.V.; Ivanov, I.A.; Arseniev, A.S.; Tsetlin, V.I.; et al. Low-molecular-weight compounds with anticoagulant activity from the scorpion *Heterometrus laoticus* venom. *Dokl. Biochem. Biophys.* **2017**, *476*, 316–319. [CrossRef]
55. Tran, T.V.; Hoang, A.N.; Nguyen, T.T.T.; Phung, T.V.; Nguyen, K.C.; Osipov, A.V.; Ivanov, I.A.; Tsetlin, V.I.; Utkin, Y.N. Anticoagulant Activity of Low-Molecular Weight Compounds from *Heterometrus laoticus* Scorpion Venom. *Toxins* **2017**, *9*, 343. [CrossRef]
56. Cupo, P.; Cupo, P. Clinical update on scorpion envenoming. *Rev. Soc. Bras. Med. Trop.* **2015**, *48*, 642–649. [CrossRef]
57. Pucca, M.B.; Cerni, F.A.; Pinheiro Junior, E.L.; Bordon, K.d.C.F.; Amorim, F.G.; Cordeiro, F.A.; Longhim, H.T.; Cremonez, C.M.; Oliveira, G.H.; Arantes, E.C. *Tityus serrulatus* venom—A lethal cocktail. *Toxicon* **2015**, *108*, 272–284. [CrossRef] [PubMed]
58. Zoccal, K.F.; Sorgi, C.A.; Hori, J.I.; Paula-Silva, F.W.G.; Arantes, E.C.; Serezani, C.H.; Zamboni, D.S.; Faccioli, L.H. Opposing roles of LTB4 and PGE2 in regulating the inflammasome-dependent scorpion venom-induced mortality. *Nat. Commun.* **2016**, *7*, 10760. [CrossRef] [PubMed]
59. Aksel, G.; Güler, S.; Doğan, N.Ö.; Çorbacioğlu, Ş.K. A randomized trial comparing intravenous paracetamol, topical lidocaine, and ice application for treatment of pain associated with scorpion stings. *Hum. Exp. Toxicol.* **2015**, *34*, 662–667. [CrossRef] [PubMed]
60. Gupta, V. Prazosin: A Pharmacological Antidote for Scorpion Envenomation. *J. Trop. Pediatr.* **2006**, *52*, 150–151. [CrossRef]
61. Al Abri, S.; Al Rumhi, M.; Al Mahruqi, G.; Shakir, A.S. Scorpion Sting Management at Tertiary and Secondary Care Emergency Departments. *Oman Med. J.* **2019**, *34*, 9–13. [CrossRef]
62. Mesquita, M.B.S.; Moraes-Santos, T.; Moraes, M.F.D. Phenobarbital blocks the lung edema induced by centrally injected tityustoxin in adult Wistar rats. *Neurosci. Lett.* **2002**, *332*, 119–122. [CrossRef]
63. Ahmed, H.O.; Ranj, A.H. Clinical-demographic aspects of scorpion sting in al sulaimaneyah province: How frequent is hypocalcaemia in the victims? *Eur. Sci. J.* **2013**, *9*, 276–288.
64. Rodrigo, C.; Gnanathasan, A. Management of scorpion envenoming: A systematic review and meta-analysis of controlled clinical trials. *Syst. Rev.* **2017**, *6*, 74. [CrossRef]
65. León, G.; Segura, A.; Herrera, M.; Otero, R.; França, F.O.d.S.; Barbaro, K.C.; Cardoso, J.L.C.; Wen, F.H.; de Medeiros, C.R.; Prado, J.C.L.; et al. Human heterophilic antibodies against equine immunoglobulins: Assessment of their role in the early adverse reactions to antivenom administration. *Trans. R. Soc. Trop. Med. Hyg.* **2008**, *102*, 1115–1119. [CrossRef]
66. Laustsen, A. Toxin-centric development approach for next-generation antivenoms. *Toxicon* **2018**, *150*, 195–197. [CrossRef]

67. Laustsen, A.H.; María Gutiérrez, J.; Knudsen, C.; Johansen, K.H.; Bermúdez-Méndez, E.; Cerni, F.A.; Jürgensen, J.A.; Ledsgaard, L.; Martos-Esteban, A.; Øhlenschlæger, M.; et al. Pros and cons of different therapeutic antibody formats for recombinant antivenom development. *Toxicon* **2018**, *146*, 151–175. [CrossRef] [PubMed]
68. Laustsen, A.H.; Engmark, M.; Clouser, C.; Timberlake, S.; Vigneault, F.; Gutiérrez, J.M.; Lomonte, B. Exploration of immunoglobulin transcriptomes from mice immunized with three-finger toxins and phospholipases A_2 from the Central American coral snake, *Micrurus nigrocinctus*. *PeerJ* **2017**, *5*, e2924. [CrossRef] [PubMed]
69. Pucca, M.B.; Cerni, F.A.; Janke, R.; Bermúdez-Méndez, E.; Ledsgaard, L.; Barbosa, J.E.; Laustsen, A.H. History of Envenoming Therapy and Current Perspectives. *Front. Immunol.* **2019**, *10*, 1598. [CrossRef] [PubMed]
70. Sifi, A.; Adi-Bessalem, S.; Laraba-Djebari, F. Development of a new approach of immunotherapy against scorpion envenoming: Avian IgYs an alternative to equine IgGs. *Int. Immunopharmacol.* **2018**, *61*, 256–265. [CrossRef] [PubMed]
71. Navarro, D.; Vargas, M.; Herrera, M.; Segura, Á.; Gómez, A.; Villalta, M.; Ramírez, N.; Williams, D.; Gutiérrez, J.M.; León, G. Development of a chicken-derived antivenom against the taipan snake (*Oxyuranus scutellatus*) venom and comparison with an equine antivenom. *Toxicon* **2016**, *120*, 1–8. [CrossRef]
72. Leiva, C.L.; Cangelosi, A.; Mariconda, V.; Farace, M.; Geoghegan, P.; Brero, L.; Fernández-Miyakawa, M.; Chacana, P. IgY-based antivenom against *Bothrops alternatus*: Production and neutralization efficacy. *Toxicon* **2019**, *163*, 84–92. [CrossRef]
73. Liu, J.; He, Q.; Wang, W.; Zhou, B.; Li, B.; Zhang, Y.; Luo, C.; Chen, D.; Tang, J.; Yu, X. Preparation and neutralization efficacy of IgY antibodies raised against *Deinagkistrodon acutus* venom. *J. Venom. Anim. Toxins Incl. Trop. Dis.* **2017**, *23*, 22. [CrossRef]
74. Alvarez, A.; Montero, Y.; Jimenez, E.; Zerpa, N.; Parrilla, P.; Malavé, C. IgY antibodies anti-*Tityus caripitensis* venom: Purification and neutralization efficacy. *Toxicon* **2013**, *74*, 208–214. [CrossRef]
75. Aguilar, I.; Sánchez, E.E.; Girón, M.E.; Estrella, A.; Guerrero, B.; Rodriguez-Acosta, F.A. Coral snake antivenom produced in chickens (*Gallus domesticus*). *Rev. Inst. Med. Trop. São Paulo* **2014**, *56*, 61–66. [CrossRef]
76. Sevcik, C.; Díaz, P.; D'Suze, G. On the presence of antibodies against bovine, equine and poultry immunoglobulins in human IgG preparations, and its implications on antivenom production. *Toxicon* **2008**, *51*, 10–16. [CrossRef]
77. Laustsen, A.H. Recombinant Antivenoms. Ph.D. Thesis, Faculty of Health and Medical Science, University of Copenhagen, Copenhagen, Denmark, 2016.
78. Pucca, M.B.; Zoccal, K.F.; Roncolato, E.C.; Bertolini, T.B.; Campos, L.B.; Cologna, C.T.; Faccioli, L.H.; Arantes, E.C.; Barbosa, J.E. Serrumab: A human monoclonal antibody that counters the biochemical and immunological effects of *Tityus serrulatus* venom. *J. Immunotoxicol.* **2012**, *9*, 173–183. [CrossRef]
79. Riaño-Umbarila, L.; Gómez-Ramírez, I.V.; Ledezma-Candanoza, L.M.; Olamendi-Portugal, T.; Rodríguez-Rodríguez, E.R.; Fernández-Taboada, G.; Possani, L.D.; Becerril, B. Generation of a Broadly Cross-Neutralizing Antibody Fragment against Several Mexican Scorpion Venoms. *Toxins* **2019**, *11*, 32. [CrossRef]
80. Knudsen, C.; Ledsgaard, L.; Dehli, R.I.; Ahmadi, S.; Sørensen, C.V.; Laustsen, A.H. Engineering and design considerations for next-generation snakebite antivenoms. *Toxicon* **2019**, *167*, 67–75. [CrossRef] [PubMed]
81. Laustsen, A.H.; Dorrestijn, N. Integrating Engineering, Manufacturing, and Regulatory Considerations in the Development of Novel Antivenoms. *Toxins* **2018**, *10*, 309. [CrossRef] [PubMed]
82. Goldman, E.R.; Liu, J.L.; Zabetakis, D.; Anderson, G.P. Enhancing Stability of Camelid and Shark Single Domain Antibodies: An Overview. *Front. Immunol.* **2017**, *8*, 865. [CrossRef] [PubMed]
83. Yardehnavi, N.; Behdani, M.; Pooshang Bagheri, K.; Mahmoodzadeh, A.; Khanahmad, H.; Shahbazzadeh, D.; Habibi-Anbouhi, M.; Ghassabeh, G.H.; Muyldermans, S. A camelid antibody candidate for development of a therapeutic agent against *Hemiscorpius lepturus* envenomation. *FASEB J.* **2014**, *28*, 4004–4014. [CrossRef]
84. Debie, P.; Lafont, C.; Defrise, M.; Hansen, I.; van Willigen, D.M.; van Leeuwen, F.W.B.; Gijsbers, R.; D'Huyvetter, M.; Devoogdt, N.; Lahoutte, T.; et al. Size and affinity kinetics of nanobodies influence targeting and penetration of solid tumours. *J. Control. Release* **2020**, *317*, 34–42. [CrossRef]

85. Alirahimi, E.; Kazemi-Lomedasht, F.; Shahbazzadeh, D.; Habibi-Anbouhi, M.; Hosseininejad Chafi, M.; Sotoudeh, N.; Ghaderi, H.; Muyldermans, S.; Behdani, M. Nanobodies as novel therapeutic agents in envenomation. *Biochim. Biophys. Acta (BBA) Gen. Subj.* **2018**, *1862*, 2955–2965. [CrossRef]
86. Hmila, I.; Saerens, D.; Ben Abderrazek, R.; Vincke, C.; Abidi, N.; Benlasfar, Z.; Govaert, J.; El Ayeb, M.; Bouhaouala-Zahar, B.; Muyldermans, S. A bispecific nanobody to provide full protection against lethal scorpion envenoming. *FASEB J.* **2010**, *24*, 3479–3489. [CrossRef]
87. Hmila, I.; Cosyns, B.; Tounsi, H.; Roosens, B.; Caveliers, V.; Abderrazek, R.B.; Boubaker, S.; Muyldermans, S.; El Ayeb, M.; Bouhaouala-Zahar, B.; et al. Pre-clinical studies of toxin-specific nanobodies: Evidence of in vivo efficacy to prevent fatal disturbances provoked by scorpion envenoming. *Toxicol. Appl. Pharm.* **2012**, *264*, 222–231. [CrossRef]
88. Darvish, M.; Behdani, M.; Shokrgozar, M.A.; Pooshang-Bagheri, K.; Shahbazzadeh, D. Development of protective agent against *Hottentotta saulcyi* venom using camelid single-domain antibody. *Mol. Immunol.* **2015**, *68*, 412–420. [CrossRef] [PubMed]
89. Kerkis, I.; de Brandão, P.; da Silva, A.R.; Pompeia, C.; Tytgat, J.; de Sá Junior, P.L. Toxin bioportides: Exploring toxin biological activity and multifunctionality. *Cell. Mol. Life Sci.* **2017**, *74*, 647–661. [CrossRef] [PubMed]
90. 131-I-TM-601 Study in Adults with Recurrent High-Grade Glioma—Phase 2. Available online: https://clinicaltrials.gov/ct2/show/NCT00114309 (accessed on 23 June 2019).
91. Pennington, M.W.; Czerwinski, A.; Norton, R.S. Peptide therapeutics from venom: Current status and potential. *Bioorg. Med. Chem.* **2018**, *26*, 2738–2758. [CrossRef]
92. Jackson, N.; Czaplewski, L.; Piddock, L.J.V. Discovery and development of new antibacterial drugs: Learning from experience? *J. Antimicrob. Chemother.* **2018**, *73*, 1452–1459. [CrossRef] [PubMed]
93. Bontems, F.; Roumestand, C.; Gilquin, B.; Ménez, A.; Toma, F. Refined structure of charybdotoxin: Common motifs in scorpion toxins and insect defensins. *Science* **1991**, *254*, 1521–1523. [CrossRef] [PubMed]
94. Wang, X.; Wang, G. Insights into Antimicrobial Peptides from Spiders and Scorpions. *Protein Pept. Lett.* **2016**, *23*, 707–721. [CrossRef]
95. Harrison, P.L.; Abdel-Rahman, M.A.; Miller, K.; Strong, P.N. Antimicrobial peptides from scorpion venoms. *Toxicon* **2014**, *88*, 115–137. [CrossRef]
96. Du, Q.; Hou, X.; Wang, L.; Zhang, Y.; Xi, X.; Wang, H.; Zhou, M.; Duan, J.; Wei, M.; Chen, T.; et al. AaeAP1 and AaeAP2: Novel Antimicrobial Peptides from the Venom of the Scorpion, *Androctonus aeneas*: Structural Characterisation, Molecular Cloning of Biosynthetic Precursor-Encoding cDNAs and Engineering of Analogues with Enhanced Antimicrobial and Anticancer Activities. *Toxins* **2015**, *7*, 219–237. [CrossRef]
97. Dueñas-Cuellar, R.A.; Kushmerick, C.; Naves, L.A.; Batista, I.F.C.; Guerrero-Vargas, J.A.; Pires, O.R.; Fontes, W.; Castro, M.S. Cm38: A new antimicrobial peptide active against *Klebsiella pneumoniae* is homologous to Cn11. *Protein Pept. Lett.* **2015**, *22*, 164–172. [CrossRef]
98. De Melo, E.T.; Estrela, A.B.; Santos, E.C.G.; Machado, P.R.L.; Farias, K.J.S.; Torres, T.M.; Carvalho, E.; Lima, J.P.M.S.; Silva-Júnior, A.A.; Barbosa, E.G.; et al. Structural characterization of a novel peptide with antimicrobial activity from the venom gland of the scorpion *Tityus stigmurus*: Stigmurin. *Peptides* **2015**, *68*, 3–10. [CrossRef]
99. Kaya, M.; Baran, T.; Asan-Ozusaglam, M.; Cakmak, Y.S.; Tozak, K.O.; Mol, A.; Mentes, A.; Sezen, G. Extraction and characterization of chitin and chitosan with antimicrobial and antioxidant activities from cosmopolitan Orthoptera species (Insecta). *Biotechnol. Bioproc. E* **2015**, *20*, 168–179. [CrossRef]
100. Harrison, P.L.; Abdel-Rahman, M.A.; Strong, P.N.; Tawfik, M.M.; Miller, K. Characterisation of three alpha-helical antimicrobial peptides from the venom of *Scorpio maurus palmatus*. *Toxicon* **2016**, *117*, 30–36. [CrossRef] [PubMed]
101. Miyashita, M.; Kitanaka, A.; Yakio, M.; Yamazaki, Y.; Nakagawa, Y.; Miyagawa, H. Complete de novo sequencing of antimicrobial peptides in the venom of the scorpion *Isometrus maculatus*. *Toxicon* **2017**, *139*, 1–12. [CrossRef] [PubMed]
102. Marques-Neto, L.M.; Trentini, M.M.; das Neves, R.C.; Resende, D.P.; Procopio, V.O.; da Costa, A.C.; Kipnis, A.; Mortari, M.R.; Schwartz, E.F.; Junqueira-Kipnis, A.P. Antimicrobial and Chemotactic Activity of Scorpion-Derived Peptide, ToAP2, against *Mycobacterium massiliensis*. *Toxins* **2018**, *10*, 219. [CrossRef]
103. Gao, B.; Dalziel, J.; Tanzi, S.; Zhu, S. Meucin-49, a multifunctional scorpion venom peptide with bactericidal synergy with neurotoxins. *Amino Acids* **2018**, *50*, 1025–1043. [CrossRef]

104. Liu, G.; Yang, F.; Li, F.; Li, Z.; Lang, Y.; Shen, B.; Wu, Y.; Li, W.; Harrison, P.L.; Strong, P.N.; et al. Therapeutic Potential of a Scorpion Venom-Derived Antimicrobial Peptide and Its Homologs Against Antibiotic-Resistant Gram-Positive Bacteria. *Front. Microbiol.* **2018**, *9*, 1159. [CrossRef]
105. Juichi, H.; Ando, R.; Ishido, T.; Miyashita, M.; Nakagawa, Y.; Miyagawa, H. Chemical synthesis of a two-domain scorpion toxin LaIT2 and its single-domain analogs to elucidate structural factors important for insecticidal and antimicrobial activities. *J. Pept. Sci.* **2018**, *24*, e3133. [CrossRef]
106. Parente, A.M.S.; Daniele-Silva, A.; Furtado, A.A.; Melo, M.A.; Lacerda, A.F.; Queiroz, M.; Moreno, C.; Santos, E.; Rocha, H.A.O.; Barbosa, E.G.; et al. Analogs of the Scorpion Venom Peptide Stigmurin: Structural Assessment, Toxicity, and Increased Antimicrobial Activity. *Toxins* **2018**, *10*, 161. [CrossRef]
107. Luna-Ramirez, K.; Tonk, M.; Rahnamaeian, M.; Vilcinskas, A. Bioactivity of Natural and Engineered Antimicrobial Peptides from Venom of the Scorpions *Urodacus yaschenkoi* and *U. manicatus*. *Toxins* **2017**, *9*, 22. [CrossRef]
108. Cesa-Luna, C.; Muñoz-Rojas, J.; Saab-Rincon, G.; Baez, A.; Morales-García, Y.E.; Juárez-González, V.R.; Quintero-Hernández, V. Structural characterization of scorpion peptides and their bactericidal activity against clinical isolates of multidrug-resistant bacteria. *PLoS ONE* **2019**, *14*, e0222438. [CrossRef]
109. De Jesus Oliveira, T.; de Oliveira, U.C.; da Silva, P.I., Jr. Serrulin: A Glycine-Rich Bioactive Peptide from the Hemolymph of the Yellow *Tityus serrulatus* Scorpion. *Toxins* **2019**, *11*, 517. [CrossRef] [PubMed]
110. Zerouti, K.; Khemili, D.; Laraba-Djebari, F.; Hammoudi-Triki, D. Nontoxic fraction of scorpion venom reduces bacterial growth and inflammatory response in a mouse model of infection. *Toxin Rev.* **2019**, 1–15. [CrossRef]
111. Luna-Ramirez, K.; Skaljac, M.; Grotmann, J.; Kirfel, P.; Vilcinskas, A. Orally Delivered Scorpion Antimicrobial Peptides Exhibit Activity against Pea Aphid (*Acyrthosiphon pisum*) and Its Bacterial Symbionts. *Toxins* **2017**, *9*, 261. [CrossRef] [PubMed]
112. Pedron, C.N.; Torres, M.D.T.; Lima, J.A.; da Silva, P.I.; Silva, F.D.; Oliveira, V.X. Novel designed VmCT1 analogs with increased antimicrobial activity. *Eur. J. Med. Chem.* **2017**, *126*, 456–463. [CrossRef]
113. Amorim-Carmo, B.; Daniele-Silva, A.; Parente, A.M.S.; Furtado, A.A.; Carvalho, E.; Oliveira, J.W.F.; Santos, E.C.G.; Silva, M.S.; Silva, S.R.B.; Silva, A.A., Jr.; et al. Potent and Broad-Spectrum Antimicrobial Activity of Analogs from the Scorpion Peptide Stigmurin. *Int. J. Mol. Sci.* **2019**, *20*, 623. [CrossRef]
114. Cao, Z.-Y.; Mi, Z.-M.; Cheng, G.-F.; Shen, W.-Q.; Xiao, X.; Liu, X.-M.; Liang, X.-T.; Yu, D.-Q. Purification and characterization of a new peptide with analgesic effect from the scorpion *Buthus martensi* Karch. *J. Pept. Res.* **2004**, *64*, 33–41. [CrossRef]
115. Zeng, X.-C.; Wang, S.-X.; Zhu, Y.; Zhu, S.-Y.; Li, W.-X. Identification and functional characterization of novel scorpion venom peptides with no disulfide bridge from *Buthus martensii* Karsch. *Peptides* **2004**, *25*, 143–150. [CrossRef]
116. Garcia, F.; Villegas, E.; Espino-Solis, G.P.; Rodriguez, A.; Paniagua-Solis, J.F.; Sandoval-Lopez, G.; Possani, L.D.; Corzo, G. Antimicrobial peptides from arachnid venoms and their microbicidal activity in the presence of commercial antibiotics. *J. Antibiot.* **2013**, *66*, 3–10. [CrossRef]
117. Pal, M. Morbidity and Mortality Due to Fungal Infections. *J. Appl. Microbiol. Biochem.* **2017**, *1*, 1–3. [CrossRef]
118. Cabezas-Quintario, M.A.; Guerrero, C.; Gomez, P.; Perez-Fernandez, E. Prevalence of invasive fungal infections detected at necropsy in a medium-sized hospital: A 15-year review of autopsy findings. *Rev. Esp. Patol.* **2016**, *49*, 76–80. [CrossRef]
119. Kullberg, B.J.; Arendrup, M.C. Invasive Candidiasis. *N. Engl. J. Med.* **2015**, *373*, 1445–1456. [CrossRef]
120. Arendrup, M.C.; Patterson, T.F. Multidrug-Resistant Candida: Epidemiology, Molecular Mechanisms, and Treatment. *J. Infect. Dis.* **2017**, *216*, S445–S451. [CrossRef] [PubMed]
121. Machado, R.J.A.; Estrela, A.B.; Nascimento, A.K.L.; Melo, M.M.A.; Torres-Rêgo, M.; Lima, E.O.; Rocha, H.A.O.; Carvalho, E.; Silva-Junior, A.A.; Fernandes-Pedrosa, M.F. Characterization of TistH, a multifunctional peptide from the scorpion *Tityus stigmurus*: Structure, cytotoxicity and antimicrobial activity. *Toxicon* **2016**, *119*, 362–370. [CrossRef] [PubMed]
122. Guilhelmelli, F.; Vilela, N.; Smidt, K.S.; de Oliveira, M.A.; da Cunha Morales Álvares, A.; Rigonatto, M.C.L.; da Silva Costa, P.H.; Tavares, A.H.; de Freitas, S.M.; Nicola, A.M.; et al. Activity of Scorpion Venom-Derived Antifungal Peptides against Planktonic Cells of *Candida* spp. and *Cryptococcus neoformans* and *Candida albicans* Biofilms. *Front. Microbiol.* **2016**, *7*, 1844. [CrossRef] [PubMed]

123. Santussi, W.M.; Bordon, K.C.F.; Rodrigues Alves, A.P.N.; Cologna, C.T.; Said, S.; Arantes, E.C. Antifungal Activity against Filamentous Fungi of Ts1, a Multifunctional Toxin from *Tityus serrulatus* Scorpion Venom. *Front. Microbiol.* **2017**, *8*, 984. [CrossRef]
124. Woolhouse, M.; Scott, F.; Hudson, Z.; Howey, R.; Chase-Topping, M. Human viruses: Discovery and emergence. *Philos. Trans. R. Soc. Lond. B Biol. Sci.* **2012**, *367*, 2864–2871. [CrossRef]
125. Da Mata, É.C.G.; Mourão, C.B.F.; Rangel, M.; Schwartz, E.F. Antiviral activity of animal venom peptides and related compounds. *J. Venom. Anim. Toxins Incl. Trop. Dis.* **2017**, *23*, 3. [CrossRef]
126. Li, Q.; Zhao, Z.; Zhou, D.; Chen, Y.; Hong, W.; Cao, L.; Yang, J.; Zhang, Y.; Shi, W.; Cao, Z.; et al. Virucidal activity of a scorpion venom peptide variant mucroporin-M1 against measles, SARS-CoV and influenza H5N1 viruses. *Peptides* **2011**, *32*, 1518–1525. [CrossRef]
127. Zhao, Z.; Hong, W.; Zeng, Z.; Wu, Y.; Hu, K.; Tian, X.; Li, W.; Cao, Z. Mucroporin-M1 Inhibits Hepatitis B Virus Replication by Activating the Mitogen-activated Protein Kinase (MAPK) Pathway and Down-regulating HNF4α in Vitro and in Vivo. *J. Biol. Chem.* **2012**, *287*, 30181–30190. [CrossRef]
128. Li, F.; Lang, Y.; Ji, Z.; Xia, Z.; Han, Y.; Cheng, Y.; Liu, G.; Sun, F.; Zhao, Y.; Gao, M.; et al. A scorpion venom peptide Ev37 restricts viral late entry by alkalizing acidic organelles. *J. Biol. Chem.* **2018**, *294*, 182–194. [CrossRef]
129. Zeng, Z.; Zhang, R.; Hong, W.; Cheng, Y.; Wang, H.; Lang, Y.; Ji, Z.; Wu, Y.; Li, W.; Xie, Y.; et al. Histidine-rich Modification of a Scorpion-derived Peptide Improves Bioavailability and Inhibitory Activity against HSV-1. *Theranostics* **2018**, *8*, 199–211. [CrossRef]
130. Yu, Y.; Deng, Y.-Q.; Zou, P.; Wang, Q.; Dai, Y.; Yu, F.; Du, L.; Zhang, N.-N.; Tian, M.; Hao, J.-N.; et al. A peptide-based viral inactivator inhibits Zika virus infection in pregnant mice and fetuses. *Nat. Commun.* **2017**, *8*, 1–12. [CrossRef] [PubMed]
131. Ji, Z.; Li, F.; Xia, Z.; Guo, X.; Gao, M.; Sun, F.; Cheng, Y.; Wu, Y.; Li, W.; Ali, S.A.; et al. The Scorpion Venom Peptide Smp76 Inhibits Viral Infection by Regulating Type-I Interferon Response. *Virol. Sin.* **2018**, *33*, 545–556. [CrossRef] [PubMed]
132. Yu, J.-S.; Tseng, C.-K.; Lin, C.-K.; Hsu, Y.-C.; Wu, Y.-H.; Hsieh, C.-L.; Lee, J.-C. Celastrol inhibits dengue virus replication via up-regulating type I interferon and downstream interferon-stimulated responses. *Antivir. Res.* **2017**, *137*, 49–57. [CrossRef] [PubMed]
133. Simner, P.J. Medical Parasitology Taxonomy Update: January 2012 to December 2015. *J. Clin. Microbiol.* **2017**, *55*, 43–47. [CrossRef] [PubMed]
134. Gockel-Blessing, E.A. *Clinical Parasitology: A Practical Approach*, 2nd ed.; Elsevier Saunders: St. Louis, MO, USA, 2013; ISBN 978-1-4160-6044-4.
135. Kappagoda, S.; Singh, U.; Blackburn, B.G. Antiparasitic Therapy. *Mayo Clin. Proc.* **2011**, *86*, 561–583. [CrossRef]
136. Frearson, J.A.; Wyatt, P.G.; Gilbert, I.H.; Fairlamb, A.H. Target assessment for antiparasitic drug discovery. *Trends Parasitol.* **2007**, *23*, 589–595. [CrossRef]
137. Conde, R.; Zamudio, F.Z.; Rodríguez, M.H.; Possani, L.D. Scorpine, an anti-malaria and anti-bacterial agent purified from scorpion venom. *FEBS Lett.* **2000**, *471*, 165–168. [CrossRef]
138. Carballar-Lejarazú, R.; Rodríguez, M.H.; de la Cruz Hernández-Hernández, F.; Ramos-Castañeda, J.; Possani, L.D.; Zurita-Ortega, M.; Reynaud-Garza, E.; Hernández-Rivas, R.; Loukeris, T.; Lycett, G.; et al. Recombinant scorpine: A multifunctional antimicrobial peptide with activity against different pathogens. *Cell. Mol. Life Sci.* **2008**, *65*, 3081–3092. [CrossRef]
139. Gao, B.; Xu, J.; Rodriguez, M.d.C.; Lanz-Mendoza, H.; Hernández-Rivas, R.; Du, W.; Zhu, S. Characterization of two linear cationic antimalarial peptides in the scorpion *Mesobuthus eupeus*. *Biochimie* **2010**, *92*, 350–359. [CrossRef]
140. Symeonidou, I.; Arsenopoulos, K.; Tzilves, D.; Soba, B.; Gabriël, S.; Papadopoulos, E. Human taeniasis/cysticercosis: A potentially emerging parasitic disease in Europe. *Ann. Gastroenterol.* **2018**, *31*, 406–412. [CrossRef]
141. Taeniasis/Cysticercosis. Available online: https://www.who.int/news-room/fact-sheets/detail/taeniasis-cysticercosis (accessed on 22 January 2020).
142. Toledo, A.; Larralde, C.; Fragoso, G.; Gevorkian, G.; Manoutcharian, K.; Hernández, M.; Acero, G.; Rosas, G.; López-Casillas, F.; Garfias, C.K.; et al. Towards a *Taenia solium* Cysticercosis Vaccine: An Epitope Shared by *Taenia crassiceps* and *Taenia solium* Protects Mice against Experimental Cysticercosis. *Infect. Immun.* **1999**, *67*, 2522–2530. [CrossRef] [PubMed]

143. Flores-Solis, D.; Toledano, Y.; Rodríguez-Lima, O.; Cano-Sánchez, P.; Ramírez-Cordero, B.E.; Landa, A.; de la Vega, R.C.R.; del Rio-Portilla, F. Solution structure and antiparasitic activity of scorpine-like peptides from *Hoffmannihadrurus gertschi*. *FEBS Lett.* **2016**, *590*, 2286–2296. [CrossRef] [PubMed]
144. Chagas Disease. Available online: https://www.who.int/news-room/fact-sheets/detail/chagas-disease-(american-trypanosomiasis) (accessed on 22 January 2020).
145. Borges, A.; Silva, S.; Op den Camp, H.J.M.; Velasco, E.; Alvarez, M.; Alfonzo, M.J.M.; Jorquera, A.; De Sousa, L.; Delgado, O. In vitro leishmanicidal activity of *Tityus discrepans* scorpion venom. *Parasitol. Res.* **2006**, *99*, 167–173. [CrossRef] [PubMed]
146. Golias, C.; Charalabopoulos, A.; Stagikas, D.; Charalabopoulos, K.; Batistatou, A. The kinin system—Bradykinin: Biological effects and clinical implications. Multiple role of the kinin system—Bradykinin. *Hippokratia* **2007**, *11*, 124–128. [PubMed]
147. Riordan, J.F. Angiotensin-I-converting enzyme and its relatives. *Genome Biol.* **2003**, *4*, 225. [CrossRef]
148. Camargo, A.C.M.; Ianzer, D.; Guerreiro, J.R.; Serrano, S.M.T. Bradykinin-potentiating peptides: Beyond captopril. *Toxicon* **2012**, *59*, 516–523. [CrossRef]
149. Zeng, X.-C.; Wang, S.; Nie, Y.; Zhang, L.; Luo, X. Characterization of BmKbpp, a multifunctional peptide from the Chinese scorpion *Mesobuthus martensii* Karsch: Gaining insight into a new mechanism for the functional diversification of scorpion venom peptides. *Peptides* **2012**, *33*, 44–51. [CrossRef]
150. Rocha-Resende, C.; Leão, N.M.; de Lima, M.E.; Santos, R.A.; Pimenta, A.M.d.C.; Verano-Braga, T. Moving pieces in a cryptomic puzzle: Cryptide from *Tityus serrulatus* Ts3 Nav toxin as potential agonist of muscarinic receptors. *Peptides* **2017**, *98*, 70–77. [CrossRef]
151. Ferreira, L.A.F.; Alves, E.W.; Henriques, O.B. Peptide T, a novel bradykinin potentiator isolated from *Tityus serrulatus* scorpion venom. *Toxicon* **1993**, *31*, 941–947. [CrossRef]
152. Verano-Braga, T.; Figueiredo-Rezende, F.; Melo, M.N.; Lautner, R.Q.; Gomes, E.R.M.; Mata-Machado, L.T.; Murari, A.; Rocha-Resende, C.; Elena de Lima, M.; Guatimosim, S.; et al. Structure-function studies of *Tityus serrulatus* Hypotensin-I (TsHpt-I): A new agonist of B(2) kinin receptor. *Toxicon* **2010**, *56*, 1162–1171. [CrossRef]
153. Machado, R.J.A.; Junior, L.G.M.; Monteiro, N.K.V.; Silva-Júnior, A.A.; Portaro, F.C.V.; Barbosa, E.G.; Braga, V.A.; Fernandes-Pedrosa, M.F. Homology modeling, vasorelaxant and bradykinin-potentiating activities of a novel hypotensin found in the scorpion venom from *Tityus stigmurus*. *Toxicon* **2015**, *101*, 11–18. [CrossRef] [PubMed]
154. Begg, A.C.; Stewart, F.A.; Vens, C. Strategies to improve radiotherapy with targeted drugs. *Nat. Rev. Cancer* **2011**, *11*, 239–253. [CrossRef] [PubMed]
155. Elshater, A.-E.; Salman, M.; Abd-Elhady, A. Physiological studies on the effect of a bradykinin potentiating factor (BPF) isolated from scorpion venom on the burnt skin of alloxan-induced diabetic Guinea pigs. *Egypt. Acad. J. Biol. Sci. C Physiol. Mol. Biol.* **2011**, *3*, 5–15. [CrossRef]
156. Mohan, G.; Hamna, T.P.A.; Jijo, A.J.; Devi, S.K.M.; Narayanasamy, A.; Vellingiri, B. Recent advances in radiotherapy and its associated side effects in cancer—A review. *J. Basic Appl. Zool.* **2019**, *80*, 14. [CrossRef]
157. Hasan, H.F.; Radwan, R.R.; Galal, S.M. Bradykinin-potentiating factor isolated from *Leiurus quinquestriatus* scorpion venom alleviates cardiomyopathy in irradiated rats via remodelling of the RAAS pathway. *Clin. Exp. Pharm. Physiol.* **2020**, *47*, 263–273. [CrossRef]
158. Adi-Bessalem, S.; Hammoudi-Triki, D.; Laraba-Djebari, F. Scorpion Venom Interactions with the Immune System. In *Scorpion Venoms*; Gopalakrishnakone, P., Possani, L.D.F., Schwartz, E., Rodríguez de la Vega, R.C., Eds.; Springer: Dordrecht, The Netherlands, 2015; pp. 87–107, ISBN 978-94-007-6403-3.
159. Bertazzi, D.T.; de Assis-Pandochi, A.I.; Caleiro Seixas Azzolini, A.E.; Talhaferro, V.L.; Lazzarini, M.; Arantes, E.C. Effect of *Tityus serrulatus* scorpion venom and its major toxin, TsTX-I, on the complement system in vivo. *Toxicon* **2003**, *41*, 501–508. [CrossRef]
160. Adi-Bessalem, S.; Hammoudi-Triki, D.; Laraba-Djebari, F. Pathophysiological effects of *Androctonus australis* hector scorpion venom: Tissue damages and inflammatory response. *Exp. Toxicol. Pathol.* **2008**, *60*, 373–380. [CrossRef]
161. Magalhães, M.M.; Pereira, M.E.; Amaral, C.F.; Rezende, N.A.; Campolina, D.; Bucaretchi, F.; Gazzinelli, R.T.; Cunha-Melo, J.R. Serum levels of cytokines in patients envenomed by *Tityus serrulatus* scorpion sting. *Toxicon* **1999**, *37*, 1155–1164. [CrossRef]

162. Fukuhara, Y.D.M.; Reis, M.L.; Dellalibera-Joviliano, R.; Cunha, F.Q.C.; Donadi, E.A. Increased plasma levels of IL-1beta, IL-6, IL-8, IL-10 and TNF-alpha in patients moderately or severely envenomed by *Tityus serrulatus* scorpion sting. *Toxicon* **2003**, *41*, 49–55. [CrossRef]
163. Petricevich, V.L. Balance between pro- and anti-inflammatory cytokines in mice treated with *Centruroides noxius* scorpion venom. *Mediat. Inflamm.* **2006**, *2006*, 54273. [CrossRef]
164. Abdoon, N.A.; Fatani, A.J. Correlation between blood pressure, cytokines and nitric oxide in conscious rabbits injected with *Leiurus quinquestriatus quinquestriatus* scorpion venom. *Toxicon* **2009**, *54*, 471–480. [CrossRef] [PubMed]
165. Petricevich, V.L. Cytokine and nitric oxide production following severe envenomation. *Curr. Drug. Targets Inflamm. Allergy* **2004**, *3*, 325–332. [CrossRef] [PubMed]
166. Zhao, Y.; Huang, J.; Yuan, X.; Peng, B.; Liu, W.; Han, S.; He, X. Toxins Targeting the KV1.3 Channel: Potential Immunomodulators for Autoimmune Diseases. *Toxins* **2015**, *7*, 1749–1764. [CrossRef] [PubMed]
167. Oliveira, I.S.; Ferreira, I.G.; Alexandre-Silva, G.M.; Cerni, F.A.; Cremonez, C.M.; Arantes, E.C.; Zottich, U.; Pucca, M.B.; Oliveira, I.S.; Ferreira, I.G.; et al. Scorpion toxins targeting $K_V1.3$ channels: Insights into immunosuppression. *J. Venom. Anim. Toxins Incl. Trop. Dis.* **2019**, *25*. [CrossRef]
168. Lam, J.; Wulff, H. The Lymphocyte Potassium Channels $K_V1.3$ and KCa3.1 as Targets for Immunosuppression. *Drug Dev. Res.* **2011**, *72*, 573–584. [CrossRef]
169. Pucca, M.B.; Bertolini, T.B.; Cerni, F.A.; Bordon, K.C.F.; Peigneur, S.; Tytgat, J.; Bonato, V.L.; Arantes, E.C. Immunosuppressive evidence of *Tityus serrulatus* toxins Ts6 and Ts15: Insights of a novel K(+) channel pattern in T cells. *Immunology* **2016**, *147*, 240–250. [CrossRef]
170. Xiao, M.; Ding, L.; Yang, W.; Chai, L.; Sun, Y.; Yang, X.; Li, D.; Zhang, H.; Li, W.; Cao, Z.; et al. St20, a new venomous animal derived natural peptide with immunosuppressive and anti-inflammatory activities. *Toxicon* **2017**, *127*, 37–43. [CrossRef]
171. Cardoso, F.C.; Lewis, R.J. Sodium channels and pain: From toxins to therapies. *Br. J. Pharmacol.* **2018**, *175*, 2138–2157. [CrossRef]
172. Catterall, W.A.; Goldin, A.L.; Waxman, S.G. International Union of Pharmacology. XLVII. Nomenclature and structure-function relationships of voltage-gated sodium channels. *Pharm. Rev.* **2005**, *57*, 397–409. [CrossRef]
173. Deuis, J.R.; Zimmermann, K.; Romanovsky, A.A.; Possani, L.D.; Cabot, P.J.; Lewis, R.J.; Vetter, I. An animal model of oxaliplatin-induced cold allodynia reveals a crucial role for $Na_V1.6$ in peripheral pain pathways. *Pain* **2013**, *154*, 1749–1757. [CrossRef]
174. Osteen, J.D.; Herzig, V.; Gilchrist, J.; Emrick, J.J.; Zhang, C.; Wang, X.; Castro, J.; Garcia-Caraballo, S.; Grundy, L.; Rychkov, G.Y.; et al. Selective spider toxins reveal a role for $Na_V1.1$ channel in mechanical pain. *Nature* **2016**, *534*, 494–499. [CrossRef] [PubMed]
175. Cox, J.J.; Reimann, F.; Nicholas, A.K.; Thornton, G.; Roberts, E.; Springell, K.; Karbani, G.; Jafri, H.; Mannan, J.; Raashid, Y.; et al. An SCN9A channelopathy causes congenital inability to experience pain. *Nature* **2006**, *444*, 894–898. [CrossRef] [PubMed]
176. Phatarakijnirund, V.; Mumm, S.; McAlister, W.H.; Novack, D.V.; Wenkert, D.; Clements, K.L.; Whyte, M.P. Congenital insensitivity to pain: Fracturing without apparent skeletal pathobiology caused by an autosomal dominant, second mutation in SCN11A encoding voltage-gated sodium channel 1.9. *Bone* **2016**, *84*, 289–298. [CrossRef]
177. Peigneur, S.; Cologna, C.T.; Cremonez, C.M.; Mille, B.G.; Pucca, M.B.; Cuypers, E.; Arantes, E.C.; Tytgat, J. A gamut of undiscovered electrophysiological effects produced by *Tityus serrulatus* toxin 1 on NaV-type isoforms. *Neuropharmacology* **2015**, *95*, 269–277. [CrossRef] [PubMed]
178. Cologna, C.T.; Peigneur, S.; Rustiguel, J.K.; Nonato, M.C.; Tytgat, J.; Arantes, E.C. Investigation of the relationship between the structure and function of Ts2, a neurotoxin from *Tityus serrulatus* venom. *FEBS J.* **2012**, *279*, 1495–1504. [CrossRef]
179. Motin, L.; Durek, T.; Adams, D.J. Modulation of human $Na_V1.7$ channel gating by synthetic α-scorpion toxin OD1 and its analogs. *Channels* **2016**, *10*, 139–147. [CrossRef]
180. Da Mata, D.O.; Tibery, D.V.; Campos, L.A.; Camargos, T.S.; Peigneur, S.; Tytgat, J.; Schwartz, E.F. Subtype Specificity of β-Toxin Tf1a from *Tityus fasciolatus* in Voltage Gated Sodium Channels. *Toxins* **2018**, *10*, 339. [CrossRef]

181. Chow, C.Y.; Chin, Y.K.-Y.; Walker, A.A.; Guo, S.; Blomster, L.V.; Ward, M.J.; Herzig, V.; Rokyta, D.R.; King, G.F. Venom Peptides with Dual Modulatory Activity on the Voltage-Gated Sodium Channel $Na_V1.1$ Provide Novel Leads for Development of Antiepileptic Drugs. *ACS Pharm. Transl. Sci.* **2020**, *3*, 119–134. [CrossRef]
182. Pucca, M.B.; Cerni, F.A.; Cordeiro, F.A.; Peigneur, S.; Cunha, T.M.; Tytgat, J.; Arantes, E.C. Ts8 scorpion toxin inhibits the $K_V4.2$ channel and produces nociception in vivo. *Toxicon* **2016**, *119*, 244–252. [CrossRef]
183. Hakim, M.A.; Jiang, W.; Luo, L.; Li, B.; Yang, S.; Song, Y.; Lai, R. Scorpion Toxin, BmP01, Induces Pain by Targeting TRPV1 Channel. *Toxins* **2015**, *7*, 3671–3687. [CrossRef]
184. Hoang, A.N.; Vo, H.D.M.; Vo, N.P.; Kudryashova, K.S.; Nekrasova, O.V.; Feofanov, A.V.; Kirpichnikov, M.P.; Andreeva, T.V.; Serebryakova, M.V.; Tsetlin, V.I.; et al. Vietnamese *Heterometrus laoticus* scorpion venom: Evidence for analgesic and anti-inflammatory activity and isolation of new polypeptide toxin acting on $K_V1.3$ potassium channel. *Toxicon* **2014**, *77*, 40–48. [CrossRef] [PubMed]
185. Liu, X.; Li, C.; Chen, J.; Du, J.; Zhang, J.; Li, G.; Jin, X.; Wu, C. AGAP, a new recombinant neurotoxic polypeptide, targets the voltage-gated calcium channels in rat small diameter DRG neurons. *Biochem. Biophys. Res. Commun.* **2014**, *452*, 60–65. [CrossRef] [PubMed]
186. Martin-Eauclaire, M.-F.; Abbas, N.; Sauze, N.; Mercier, L.; Berge-Lefranc, J.-L.; Condo, J.; Bougis, P.E.; Guieu, R. Involvement of endogenous opioid system in scorpion toxin-induced antinociception in mice. *Neurosci. Lett.* **2010**, *482*, 45–50. [CrossRef] [PubMed]
187. Guan, R.-J.; Wang, C.-G.; Wang, M.; Wang, D.-C. A depressant insect toxin with a novel analgesic effect from scorpion *Buthus martensii* Karsch. *Biochim. Biophys. Acta (BBA) Protein Struct. Mol. Enzymol.* **2001**, *1549*, 9–18. [CrossRef]
188. Zhang, Y.; Xu, J.; Wang, Z.; Zhang, X.; Liang, X.; Civelli, O. BmK-YA, an Enkephalin-Like Peptide in Scorpion Venom. *PLoS ONE* **2012**, *7*, e40417. [CrossRef]
189. Li, Z.; Hu, P.; Wu, W.; Wang, Y. Peptides with therapeutic potential in the venom of the scorpion *Buthus martensii* Karsch. *Peptides* **2019**, *115*, 43–50. [CrossRef]
190. Renata, M.; Siqueira Cunh, A.O. New Perspectives in Drug Discovery Using Neuroactive Molecules from the Venom of Arthropods. In *An Integrated View of the Molecular Recognition and Toxinology—From Analytical Procedures to Biomedical Applications*; InTech: London, UK, 2013; Volume I, p. 13.
191. Rigo, F.K.; Bochi, G.V.; Pereira, A.L.; Adamante, G.; Ferro, P.R.; Dal-Toé De Prá, S.; Milioli, A.M.; Damiani, A.P.; da Silveira Prestes, G.; Dalenogare, D.P.; et al. TsNTxP, a non-toxic protein from *Tityus serrulatus* scorpion venom, induces antinociceptive effects by suppressing glutamate release in mice. *Eur. J. Pharmacol.* **2019**, *855*, 65–74. [CrossRef]
192. Chen, B.; Ji, Y. Antihyperalgesia effect of BmK AS, a scorpion toxin, in rat by intraplantar injection. *Brain Res.* **2002**, *952*, 322–326. [CrossRef]
193. Chen, J.; Feng, X.-H.; Shi, J.; Tan, Z.-Y.; Bai, Z.-T.; Liu, T.; Ji, Y.-H. The anti-nociceptive effect of BmK AS, a scorpion active polypeptide, and the possible mechanism on specifically modulating voltage-gated Na+ currents in primary afferent neurons. *Peptides* **2006**, *27*, 2182–2192. [CrossRef]
194. Cui, Y.; Song, Y.-B.; Ma, L.; Liu, Y.-F.; Li, G.-D.; Wu, C.-F.; Zhang, J.-H. Site-directed Mutagenesis of the Toxin from the Chinese Scorpion *Buthus martensii* Karsch (BmKAS): Insight into Sites Related to Analgesic Activity. *Arch. Pharm. Res.* **2010**, *33*, 1633–1639. [CrossRef]
195. Liu, Z.R.; Tao, J.; Dong, B.Q.; Ding, G.; Cheng, Z.J.; He, H.Q.; Ji, Y.H. Pharmacological kinetics of BmK AS, a sodium channel site 4-specific modulator on $Na_V1.3$. *Neurosci. Bull.* **2012**, *28*, 209–221. [CrossRef] [PubMed]
196. Tan, Z.-Y.; Xiao, H.; Mao, X.; Wang, C.-Y.; Zhao, Z.-Q.; Ji, Y.-H. The inhibitory effects of BmK IT2, a scorpion neurotoxin on rat nociceptive flexion reflex and a possible mechanism for modulating voltage-gated Na+ channels. *Neuropharmacology* **2001**, *40*, 352–357. [CrossRef]
197. Xiong, Y.M.; Lan, Z.D.; Wang, M.; Liu, B.; Liu, X.Q.; Fei, H.; Xu, L.G.; Xia, Q.C.; Wang, C.G.; Da-Cheng, W.; et al. Molecular characterization of a new excitatory insect neurotoxin with an analgesic effect on mice from the scorpion Buthus martensi Karsch. *Toxicon* **1999**, *37*, 1165–1180. [CrossRef]
198. Maatoug, R.; Jebali, J.; Guieu, R.; De Waard, M.; Kharrat, R. BotAF, a new *Buthus occitanus tunetanus* scorpion toxin, produces potent analgesia in rodents. *Toxicon* **2018**, *149*, 72–85. [CrossRef]
199. Song, Y.; Liu, Z.; Zhang, Q.; Li, C.; Jin, W.; Liu, L.; Zhang, J.; Zhang, J. Investigation of Binding Modes and Functional Surface of Scorpion Toxins ANEP to Sodium Channels 1.7. *Toxins* **2017**, *9*, 387. [CrossRef]
200. Zhang, F.; Wu, Y.; Zou, X.; Tang, Q.; Zhao, F.; Cao, Z. BmK AEP, an Anti-Epileptic Peptide Distinctly Affects the Gating of Brain Subtypes of Voltage-Gated Sodium Channels. *Int. J. Mol. Sci.* **2019**, *20*, 729. [CrossRef]

201. Tan, Z.-Y.; Mao, X.; Xiao, H.; Zhao, Z.-Q.; Ji, Y.-H. *Buthus martensi* Karsch agonist of skeletal-muscle RyR-1, a scorpion active polypeptide: Antinociceptive effect on rat peripheral nervous system and spinal cord, and inhibition of voltage-gated Na+ currents in dorsal root ganglion neurons. *Neurosci. Lett.* **2001**, *297*, 65–68. [CrossRef]
202. Mao, Q.; Ruan, J.; Cai, X.; Lu, W.; Ye, J.; Yang, J.; Yang, Y.; Sun, X.; Cao, J.; Cao, P. Antinociceptive Effects of Analgesic-Antitumor Peptide (AGAP), a Neurotoxin from the Scorpion *Buthus martensii* Karsch, on Formalin-Induced Inflammatory Pain through a Mitogen-Activated Protein Kinases–Dependent Mechanism in Mice. *PLoS ONE* **2013**, *8*, e78239. [CrossRef]
203. Ruan, J.-P.; Mao, Q.-H.; Lu, W.-G.; Cai, X.-T.; Chen, J.; Li, Q.; Fu, Q.; Yan, H.-J.; Cao, J.-L.; Cao, P. Inhibition of spinal MAPKs by scorpion venom peptide BmK AGAP produces a sensory-specific analgesic effect. *Mol. Pain* **2018**, *14*, 1–11. [CrossRef]
204. Zhao, F.; Wang, J.-L.; Ming, H.-Y.; Zhang, Y.-N.; Dun, Y.-Q.; Zhang, J.-H.; Song, Y.-B. Insights into the binding mode and functional components of the analgesic-antitumour peptide from *Buthus martensii* Karsch to human voltage-gated sodium channel 1.7 based on dynamic simulation analysis. *J. Biomol. Struct. Dyn.* **2019**, *38*, 1–12. [CrossRef]
205. Xu, Y.; Meng, X.; Hou, X.; Sun, J.; Kong, X.; Sun, Y.; Liu, Z.; Ma, Y.; Niu, Y.; Song, Y.; et al. A mutant of the *Buthus martensii* Karsch antitumor-analgesic peptide exhibits reduced inhibition to $hNa_V1.4$ and $hNa_V1.5$ channels while retaining analgesic activity. *J. Biol. Chem.* **2017**, *292*, 18270–18280. [CrossRef] [PubMed]
206. Guan, R.-J.; Wang, M.; Wang, D.-C.; Wang, D.-C. A new insect neurotoxin AngP1 with analgesic effect from the scorpion *Buthus martensii* Karsch: Purification and characterization. *J. Pept. Res.* **2001**, *58*, 27–35. [CrossRef] [PubMed]
207. Sun, Y.-M.; Liu, W.; Zhu, R.-H.; Wang, D.-C.; Goudet, C.; Tytgat, J. Roles of disulfide bridges in scorpion toxin BmK M1 analyzed by mutagenesis. *J. Pept. Res.* **2002**, *60*, 247–256. [CrossRef]
208. Wang, Y.; Hao, Z.; Shao, J.; Song, Y.; Li, C.; Li, C.; Zhao, Y.; Liu, Y.; Wei, T.; Wu, C.; et al. The role of Ser54 in the antinociceptive activity of BmK9, a neurotoxin from the scorpion *Buthus martensii* Karsch. *Toxicon* **2011**, *58*, 527–532. [CrossRef] [PubMed]
209. Yang, F.; Liu, S.; Zhang, Y.; Qin, C.; Xu, L.; Li, W.; Cao, Z.; Li, W.; Wu, Y. Expression of recombinant α-toxin BmKM9 from scorpion *Buthus martensii* Karsch and its functional characterization on sodium channels. *Peptides* **2018**, *99*, 153–160. [CrossRef] [PubMed]
210. Wang, Y.; Wang, L.; Cui, Y.; Song, Y.-B.; Liu, Y.-F.; Zhang, R.; Wu, C.-F.; Zhang, J.-H. Purification, characterization and functional expression of a new peptide with an analgesic effect from Chinese scorpion *Buthus martensii* Karsch (BmK AGP-SYPU1). *Biomed. Chromatogr.* **2011**, *25*, 801–807. [CrossRef]
211. Zhang, R.; Cui, Y.; Zhang, X.; Yang, Z.; Zhao, Y.; Song, Y.; Wu, C.; Zhang, J. Soluble expression, purification and the role of C-terminal glycine residues in scorpion toxin BmK AGP-SYPU2. *BMB Rep.* **2010**, *43*, 801–806. [CrossRef]
212. Zhao, Y.-S.; Zhang, R.; Xu, Y.; Cui, Y.; Liu, Y.-F.; Song, Y.-B.; Zhang, H.-X.; Zhang, J.-H. The role of glycine residues at the C-terminal peptide segment in antinociceptive activity: A molecular dynamics simulation. *J. Mol. Model.* **2013**, *19*, 1295–1299. [CrossRef]
213. Shao, J.-H.; Cui, Y.; Zhao, M.-Y.; Wu, C.-F.; Liu, Y.-F.; Zhang, J.-H. Purification, characterization, and bioactivity of a new analgesic-antitumor peptide from Chinese scorpion *Buthus martensii* Karsch. *Peptides* **2014**, *53*, 89–96. [CrossRef]
214. Lin, S.; Wang, X.; Hu, X.; Zhao, Y.; Zhao, M.; Zhang, J.; Cui, Y. Recombinant Expression, Functional Characterization of Two Scorpion Venom Toxins with Three Disulfide Bridges from the Chinese Scorpion *Buthus martensii* Karsch. *Protein Pept. Lett.* **2017**, *24*, 235–240. [CrossRef]
215. Anh, H.N.; Hoang, V.D.M.; Kudryashova, K.S.; Nekrasova, O.V.; Feofanov, A.V.; Andreeva, T.V.; Tsetlin, V.I.; Utkin, Y.N. Hetlaxin, a new toxin from the *Heterometrus laoticus* scorpion venom, interacts with voltage-gated potassium channel $K_V1.3$. *Dokl. Biochem. Biophys.* **2013**, *449*, 109–111. [CrossRef] [PubMed]
216. Srairi-Abid, N.; Othman, H.; Aissaoui, D.; BenAissa, R. Anti-tumoral effect of scorpion peptides: Emerging new cellular targets and signaling pathways. *Cell Calcium* **2019**, *80*, 160–174. [CrossRef] [PubMed]
217. Gómez Rave, L.J.; Muñoz Bravo, A.X.; Sierra Castrillo, J.; Román Marín, L.M.; Corredor Pereira, C. Scorpion Venom: New Promise in the Treatment of Cancer. *Acta Biológica Colomb.* **2019**, *24*, 213–223. [CrossRef]
218. Akef, H.M. Anticancer and antimicrobial activities of scorpion venoms and their peptides. *Toxin Rev.* **2019**, *38*, 41–53. [CrossRef]

219. Uzair, B.; Bint-e-Irshad, S.; Khan, B.A.; Azad, B.; Mahmood, T.; Rehman, M.U.; Braga, V.A. Scorpion Venom Peptides as a Potential Source for Human Drug Candidates. *Protein Pept. Lett.* **2018**, *25*, 702–708. [CrossRef] [PubMed]
220. Bernardes-Oliveira, E.; Farias, K.J.S.; Gomes, D.L.; de Araújo, J.M.G.; da Silva, W.D.; Rocha, H.A.O.; Donadi, E.A.; de Fernandes-Pedrosa, M.F.; de Crispim, J.C.O. *Tityus serrulatus* Scorpion Venom Induces Apoptosis in Cervical Cancer Cell Lines. *Evid. Based Complementary Altern. Med.* **2019**, *2019*, 1–8. [CrossRef]
221. Wang, J.; Peng, Y.; Wang, Z.; Chai, X.; Lv, Z.; Song, Q. Venom from the scorpion *Heterometrus liangi* inhibits HeLa cell proliferation by inducing p21 expression. *Biologia* **2018**, *73*, 1099–1108. [CrossRef]
222. Al-Asmari, A.K.; Riyasdeen, A.; Islam, M. Scorpion Venom Causes Apoptosis by Increasing Reactive Oxygen Species and Cell Cycle Arrest in MDA-MB-231 and HCT-8 Cancer Cell Lines. *J. Evid. Based Integr. Med.* **2018**, *23*, 215658721775179. [CrossRef]
223. Giovannini, C.; Baglioni, M.; Baron Toaldo, M.; Cescon, M.; Bolondi, L.; Gramantieri, L. Vidatox 30 CH has tumor activating effect in hepatocellular carcinoma. *Sci. Rep.* **2017**, *7*, 44685. [CrossRef]
224. Díaz-García, A.; Ruiz-Fuentes, J.L.; Rodríguez-Sánchez, H.; Fraga Castro, J.A. *Rhopalurus junceus* scorpion venom induces apoptosis in the triple negative human breast cancer cell line MDA-MB-231. *J. Venom Res.* **2017**, *8*, 9–13. [PubMed]
225. Li, B.; Lyu, P.; Xi, X.; Ge, L.; Mahadevappa, R.; Shaw, C.; Kwok, H.F. Triggering of cancer cell cycle arrest by a novel scorpion venom-derived peptide—Gonearrestide. *J. Cell. Mol. Med.* **2018**, *22*, 4460–4473. [CrossRef] [PubMed]
226. BenAissa, R.; Othman, H.; Villard, C.; Peigneur, S.; Mlayah-Bellalouna, S.; Abdelkafi-Koubaa, Z.; Marrakchi, N.; Essafi-Benkhadir, K.; Tytgat, J.; Luis, J.; et al. AaHIV a sodium channel scorpion toxin inhibits the proliferation of DU145 prostate cancer cells. *Biochem. Biophys. Res. Commun.* **2019**, *521*, 340–346. [CrossRef] [PubMed]
227. Liu, Y.-F.; Ma, R.-L.; Wang, S.-L.; Duan, Z.-Y.; Zhang, J.-H.; Wu, L.-J.; Wu, C.-F. Expression of an antitumor–analgesic peptide from the venom of Chinese scorpion *Buthus martensii* karsch in *Escherichia coli*. *Protein Expr. Purif.* **2003**, *27*, 253–258. [CrossRef]
228. Kampo, S.; Ahmmed, B.; Zhou, T.; Owusu, L.; Anabah, T.W.; Doudou, N.R.; Kuugbee, E.D.; Cui, Y.; Lu, Z.; Yan, Q.; et al. Scorpion Venom Analgesic Peptide, BmK AGAP Inhibits Stemness, and Epithelial-Mesenchymal Transition by Down-Regulating PTX3 in Breast Cancer. *Front. Oncol.* **2019**, *9*, 21. [CrossRef]
229. Tang, D.; Yang, Y.; Xiao, Z.; Xu, J.; Yang, Q.; Dai, H.; Liang, S.; Tang, C.; Dong, H.; Liu, Z. Scorpion toxin inhibits the voltage-gated proton channel using a Zn^{2+}-like long-range conformational coupling mechanism. *Br. J. Pharmacol.* **2020**, *177*, 2351–2364. [CrossRef]
230. Fernández, A.; Pupo, A.; Mena-Ulecia, K.; Gonzalez, C. Pharmacological modulation of proton channel hv1 in cancer therapy: Future perspectives. *Mol. Pharmacol.* **2016**, *90*, 385–402. [CrossRef]
231. Tong-ngam, P.; Roytrakul, R.; Hathaitip, S. BmKn-2 scorpion venom peptide for killing oral cancer cells by apoptosis. *Asian Pac. J. Cancer Prev.* **2015**, *16*, 2807–2811. [CrossRef]
232. Satitmanwiwat, S.; Changsangfa, C.; Khanuengthong, A.; Promthep, K.; Roytrakul, S.; Arpornsuwan, T.; Saikhun, K.; Sritanaudomchai, H. The scorpion venom peptide BmKn2 induces apoptosis in cancerous but not in normal human oral cells. *Biomed. Pharm.* **2016**, *84*, 1042–1050. [CrossRef]
233. Khamessi, O.; Ben Mabrouk, H.; ElFessi-Magouri, R.; Kharrat, R. RK1, the first very short peptide from *Buthus occitanus tunetanus* inhibits tumor cell migration, proliferation and angiogenesis. *Biochem. Biophys. Res. Commun.* **2018**, *499*, 1–7. [CrossRef]

biomedicines

MDPI

Article

Characterization of Synthetic Tf2 as a $Na_V1.3$ Selective Pharmacological Probe

Mathilde R. Israel [1], Thomas S. Dash [1], Stefanie N. Bothe [2,3], Samuel D. Robinson [1], Jennifer R. Deuis [1], David J. Craik [1], Angelika Lampert [2,3,4], Irina Vetter [1,5,*] and Thomas Durek [1,*]

1 Institute for Molecular Bioscience, The University of Queensland, St. Lucia, QLD 4072, Australia; mathilde.israel@uqconnect.edu.au (M.R.I.); thomasdash123@gmail.com (T.S.D.); s.robinson@imb.uq.edu.au (S.D.R.); j.deuis@uq.edu.au (J.R.D.); d.craik@imb.uq.edu.au (D.J.C.)
2 Institute of Physiology, Medical Faculty, RWTH Aachen University, 52074 Aachen, Germany; stbothe@ukaachen.de (S.N.B.); alampert@ukaachen.de (A.L.)
3 Research Training Group 2416 MultiSenses-MultiScales, RWTH Aachen University, 52074 Aachen, Germany
4 Research Training Group 2415 ME3T, RWTH Aachen University, 52074 Aachen, Germany
5 School of Pharmacy, The University of Queensland, Woolloongabba, QLD 4102, Australia
* Correspondence: i.vetter@uq.edu.au (I.V.); t.durek@uq.edu.au (T.D.); Tel.: +61-7-3346-2660 (I.V.); +61-7-3346-2021 (T.D.)

Received: 15 May 2020; Accepted: 5 June 2020; Published: 11 June 2020

Abstract: $Na_V1.3$ is a subtype of the voltage-gated sodium channel family. It has been implicated in the pathogenesis of neuropathic pain, although the contribution of this channel to neuronal excitability is not well understood. Tf2, a β-scorpion toxin previously identified from the venom of *Tityus fasciolatus*, has been reported to selectively activate $Na_V1.3$. Here, we describe the activity of synthetic Tf2 and assess its suitability as a pharmacological probe for $Na_V1.3$. As described for the native toxin, synthetic Tf2 (1 μM) caused early channel opening, decreased the peak current, and shifted the voltage dependence of $Na_V1.3$ activation in the hyperpolarizing direction by −11.3 mV, with no activity at $Na_V1.1$, $Na_V1.2$, and $Na_V1.4$-$Na_V1.8$. Additional activity was found at $Na_V1.9$, tested using the hNav1.9_C4 chimera, where Tf2 (1 μM) shifted the voltage dependence of activation by −6.3 mV. In an attempt to convert Tf2 into an $Na_V1.3$ inhibitor, we synthetized the analogue Tf2[S14R], a mutation previously described to remove the excitatory activity of related β-scorpion toxins. Indeed, Tf2[S14R](10 μM) had reduced excitatory activity at $Na_V1.3$, although it still caused a small −5.8 mV shift in the voltage dependence of activation. Intraplantar injection of Tf2 (1 μM) in mice caused spontaneous flinching and swelling, which was not reduced by the $Na_V1.1/1.3$ inhibitor ICA-121431 nor in $Na_V1.9^{-/-}$ mice, suggesting off-target activity. In addition, despite a loss of excitatory activity, intraplantar injection of Tf2[S14R](10 μM) still caused swelling, providing strong evidence that Tf2 has additional off-target activity at one or more non-neuronal targets. Therefore, due to activity at $Na_V1.9$ and other yet to be identified target(s), the use of Tf2 as a selective pharmacological probe may be limited.

Keywords: Tf2; sodium channel; $Na_V1.3$; $Na_V1.9$; scorpion; toxin

1. Introduction

Voltage-gated sodium channels (VGSCs) are large pore-forming transmembrane-spanning proteins with four homologous domains (I-IV) that regulate the influx of Na^+ ions across neuronal membranes in response to local changes in voltage [1]. This Na^+ influx is essential for action potential initiation and propagation in electrically excitable cells and crucial for the physiological function of neurons. In humans, nine different isoforms with relatively high sequence homology have been identified ($Na_V1.1$–$Na_V1.9$), each with discrete expression profiles and distinctive biophysical properties [2].

While several VGSC isoforms expressed in peripheral sensory neurons, such as $Na_V1.7$, $Na_V1.8$, and $Na_V1.9$, have a well-established role in somatosensation and nociception, the contribution of $Na_V1.3$ to peripheral neuronal excitability is less well understood.

$Na_V1.3$ is a tetrodotoxin (TTX)-sensitive channel with fast-activating and fast-inactivating currents capable of rapid repriming and sustaining repetitive firing [3]. Interestingly, $Na_V1.3$ is expressed at very low levels in adult rodent dorsal root ganglion (DRG) neurons but is upregulated in DRGs following nerve injury or streptozotocin-induced diabetes, suggesting the channel may contribute to the development and maintenance of neuropathic pain [4–6]. Indeed, shRNA-mediated knockdown of $Na_V1.3$ in DRG neurons attenuates the development of mechanical allodynia in rodent models of spared nerve injury (SNI) and diabetic neuropathy [7,8], while global $Na_V1.3$ knockout has confounding results, with minimal effect on the development of mechanical allodynia following chronic constriction injury (CCI), spinal nerve transection (SNT), and spinal nerve ligation (SNL) [9,10]. Therefore, selective pharmacological modulators of $Na_V1.3$ are required to further elucidate the contribution of the channel to neuronal excitability in physiological and pathological pain states.

Venoms from scorpions, spiders, and cone snails are a rich source of novel bioactive peptides with activity at ion channels. Many venom-derived peptides have high potency and selectivity for VGSCs and have provided us with unique insights into VGSC gating, structure, and function [11]. Scorpion peptides that act on VGSCs can be functionally distinguished as α- or β-scorpion toxins, depending on how they modulate channel opening or closing. α-Scorpion toxins cause a marked delay in fast inactivation, resulting in prolonged Na^+ influx; whereas, β-scorpion toxins shift the voltage dependence of activation to more hyperpolarized potentials, resulting in toxin-bound channels that open closer to the resting membrane potential [12,13]. Tf2 is a β-scorpion toxin originally identified from the venom of *Tityus fasciolatus* that, at a concentration of 1 μM, selectively activates $Na_V1.3$, with no effect at the other Na_V subtypes ($Na_V1.1$, $Na_V1.2$, and $Na_V1.4$–$Na_V1.8$ tested) expressed in *Xenopus* oocytes [14]. We therefore hypothesized that Tf2 could be used as a pharmacological tool to assess the contribution of $Na_V1.3$ to the excitability of peripheral sensory neurons. The remaining sodium channel subtype Nav1.9 is historically hard to express, but recent progress showed that the chimera of the human Nav1.9 with the C-terminus of Nav1.4 (hNav1.9_C4) reveals reasonable currents in HEK293 cells [8]. As Tf2 is not thought to interact with the C-terminus, this chimera is a valuable tool for testing its influences on Nav1.9 gating.

Here, we report the chemical synthesis of Tf2 and the mutant Tf2[S14R], along with previously undescribed β-scorpion activity of Tf2 at $hNa_V1.9\_C4$ in vitro. We show for the first time that Tf2 causes Ca^{2+} influx in small, medium, and large diameter mammalian sensory neurons and explore the activity of Tf2 on the peripheral somatosensory system in vivo.

2. Experimental Section

2.1. Peptide Synthesis

Tf2 was synthesized in two segments consisting of Tf2(1–26)-α-thioester and Tf2(27–62), which were linked by native chemical ligation. Tf2(1–26)-α-thioester was synthesized via Boc chemistry on trityl-associated mercaptopropionic acid lysine resin to yield the C-terminal α-thioester upon hydrogen fluoride (HF, BOC Australia, Sydney, NSW, Australia) cleavage. Tf2(27–62) was synthesized using Fmoc chemistry on Rink amide resin to yield the C-terminally amidated peptide segment after trifluoroacetic acid (TFA, Auspep, Melbourne, VIC, Australia) cleavage. The cleaved crude peptides were precipitated and washed twice with cold diethyl ether. The peptides were then dissolved in 50% acetonitrile, 0.1% TFA (*v*/*v*) in water and lyophilized. Peptides were purified by preparative reverse-phase (RP) HPLC on a Shimadzu Prominence system (Sydney, NSW, Australia). HPLC fractions containing the desired peptide (judged by HPLC/MS) of similar purity were pooled, lyophilized, and stored at −20 °C.

Tf2(1–26)-α-thioester: KEGYAMDHEGCKFSCFIRPSGFCDGY-[COS-CH2-CH2-CO]-Lys, expected MW (assuming average isotope composition): 3164.5 Da, observed MW: 3164.4 ± 0.5 Da. Tf2(27–62): CKTHLKASSGYCAWPACYCYGVPSNIKVWDYATNKC-NH_2, expected MW (assuming average isotope composition): 4031.7 Da, observed MW: 4031.2 ± 0.5 Da.

Native chemical ligation was done as previously described [11]. Briefly, 8.7 μmol (35.3 mg) of peptide Tf2(27–62) and 8.7 μmol (27.6 mg) of Tf2(1–26)-α-thioester were dissolved in 8.7 mL of ligation buffer consisting of 6 M guanidine hydrochloride, 0.2 M Na_2HPO_4, 40 mM Tris(2-carboxyethyl)phosphine hydrochloride (TCEP), and 50 mM 4-mercaptophenylacetic acid (MPAA), pH 7.25. The solution was stirred under nitrogen for 16 h and the reaction progress was monitored by HPLC-UV. The reduced full-length Tf2 (1–62) ligation product was isolated via RP-HPLC on an Agilent Zorbax 300SB, C3 column (9.4 × 250 mm, 5 μm Phenomenex Australia, Sydney, NSW, Australia). Yield: 42.5 mg; expected MW (assuming average isotope composition): 6963.0 Da, observed MW: 6962.8 ± 1.0 Da.

For oxidative folding of Tf2, 1.7 μmol (15 mg) of reduced Tf2 were dissolved in 3.75 mL of 6 M guanidine hydrochloride. Folding was initiated by diluting the peptide solution with 150 mL of folding buffer (0.1 M Tris, 0.5 M arginine, 1 M urea, 10 mM reduced glutathione, 1 mM oxidized glutathione, pH 8.0) and stirring for 72 h at 4 °C. Oxidized Tf2 was then purified by RP-HPLC on a Agilent Zorbax 300SB, C3 column (9.4 × 250 mm, 5 μm, Phenomenex Australia, Sydney, NSW, Australia). Yield: 2.2 mg. Calculated MW (assuming most abundant isotope composition): 6949.03 Da, observed MW: 6949.12 ± 0.20 Da. All reagents were obtained from Sigma-Aldrich (St Louis, MI, USA) unless otherwise stated.

2.2. Cell Culture

Human embryonic kidney (HEK) 293 cells that constitutively express the human VGSC channel α subunits Na_V1.1–1.7/β1 (SB Drug Discovery, Glasgow, UK) were maintained in minimum essential media (MEM) supplemented with 10% fetal bovine serum (FBS) and 2 mM L-glutamine, along with the selection antibiotics blasticidin, geneticin, and zeocin as recommended by the manufacturer. Chinese hamster ovary (CHO) cells expressing hNa_V1.8/β3 via a tetracycline inducible system (ChanTest, Cleveland, OH, USA) were maintained in MEM, 10% FBS, and 2 mM L-glutamine. Tetracycline (1 μg mL^{-1}) was added to culture media 48–72 h prior to assay to induce hNa_V1.8 expression. Cells were passaged every 3–4 days after reaching 70–80% confluence with TrypLE Express (Thermo Fisher Scientific, Scoresby, VIC, Australia) and grown in an incubator at 37 °C with 5% CO_2.

ND7/23 cells (Sigma-Aldrich, St. Louis, MO, USA) were maintained in high glucose Dulbecco's Modified Eagle Medium (DMEM; Gibco, Thermo Fisher Scientific, Waltham, MA, USA) with a glucose level of 4.5 g/L and supplemented with 10% FBS (Biochrom AG, Berlin, Germany). ND7/23 cells were transiently transfected with 2.75 μg hNa_V1.9_C4 plasmid (chimera of human Na_V1.9 and the C-terminus of rat Na_V1.4; pCDNA3 vector [8]), 0.25 μg of green fluorescent protein (GFP) DNA (Lonza, Basel, Switzerland), and 6 μL of JetPEI reagent (Polyplus Transfection, Illkirch, France). GFP was co-transfected to detect transfected cells via green fluorescence. Then, 24 h after transfection, cells were split either onto glass coverslips coated with poly-D-lysine (PDL) hydrobromide (Sigma-Aldrich) for treatment with 1 μM Tf2, or split into plastic petri dishes for control conditions. After recovering for 2–3 h, the cells were recorded with whole-cell patch clamp. Cells were passaged every 3–4 days after reaching 70–80% confluence with TrypLE Express (Thermo Fisher Scientific, Scoresby, VIC, Australia) in the case of HEK and CHO cells, and with accutase (Sigma-Aldrich) in the case of the ND7/23 cells. All cells were grown in an incubator at 37 °C with 5% CO_2.

2.3. Fluorescent Membrane Potential Assay

To rapidly assess the activity of Tf2 and Tf2[S14R] at hNa_V1.1–1.7, we utilized the $FLIPR^{Tetra}$ fluorescent imaging plate reader (Molecular Devices, Sunnyvale, CA, USA). Cells were plated in 384-well black-walled plates at a density of 10,000–15,000 per well in normal growth media 24–48 h before membrane potential experiments. Cells were loaded with red membrane potential dye (Molecular Devices) diluted in physiological salt solution (PSS; 140 mM NaCl, 11.5 mM glucose, 5.9 mM KCl, 1.4 mM $MgCl_2$, 1.2 mM NaH_2PO_4, 5 mM $NaHCO_3$, 1.8 mM $CaCl_2$, 10 mM HEPES) and incubated for 30 min at 37 °C as per the manufacturer's instructions. All synthetic toxins were diluted in PSS and 0.1% bovine serum albumin (BSA) to avoid adsorption to plastic surfaces. Changes in membrane potential (excitation/emission 510–545 nm/565–625 nm) were recorded each second for 5 min after the addition of toxin and the area under the curve (AUC) was computed using ScreenWorks (Molecular Devices, Version 3.2.0.14).

2.4. *Whole Cell Patch-Clamp Electrophysiology*

Whole cell patch-clamp experiments on $hNa_V1.3$, $hNa_V1.7$, and $hNa_V1.8$ cell lines were performed using the QPatch-16 automated electrophysiology platform (Sophion, Ballerup, Denmark). This set-up utilizes 16-well planar chips plates (QPlates, Sophion) with a standard resistance of 2 ± 0.02 mΩ. Cells were expanded in T-175 flasks and maintained in 37 °C and 5% CO_2 48–72 h prior to assay. On the day of experiment, cells were harvested with TrypLE Express and resuspended in DMEM with 25 mM HEPES, 100 U/mL penicillin-streptomycin, and 0.04 mg/mL trypsin inhibitor from *Glycine max* (soybean) and stirred for 30–60 min prior to use.

The external solution (ECS) for all automated VGSC recordings contained (in mM): NaCl (140), KCl (4), $CaCl_2$ (2), $MgCl_2$ (1), HEPES (10), TEA-Cl (20), and glucose (10) containing 0.1% BSA. The pH was adjusted to 7.4 with NaOH and osmolarity adjusted to 305 mOsm with sucrose. The intracellular solution (ICS) consisted of (in mM): CsF (140), EGTA/CsOH (1/5), HEPES (10), and NaCl (10) adjusted to pH 7.4 with CsOH and 320 mOsm with sucrose. The cell positioning pressure was set to −60 mbar, minimum seal resistance 0.1 GΩ, holding pressure −20 mbar, and currents were filtered at 25 kHz (8th order Bessel, cut off 5 kHz). A standard P/4 leak subtraction protocol was included, and as such, leak subtracted and non-leak subtracted currents were acquired in parallel.

After obtaining the stable whole-cell configuration, voltage clamp experiments proceeded as follows from a holding potential of −90 mV. All protocols included a brief (15 ms) pre-conditioning pulse to 0 mV followed by a 120 ms recovery to allow voltage-sensor trapping by β-scorpion toxins [15]. Current–voltage (IV) relationships were determined using a series of 500 ms pulses ranging from −90 to +55 mV (in 5 mV steps), followed by a 20 ms pulse to −20 mV for $hNa_V1.3$ and $hNa_V1.7$ or +10 mV for $hNa_V1.8$ to assess the voltage dependence of fast inactivation. Peak current values were normalized to a buffer control. Toxins were diluted in ECS with 0.1% BSA and incubated for 5 min prior to recording.

Whole-cell patch-clamp experiments on ND7/23 cells transfected with hNav1.9_C4 were performed at room temperature, using an EPC-10 USB amplifier and PatchMaster software (HEKA Elektronik, Lambrecht, Germany) and analysis was done using Igor Pro 6.3 (WaveMetrics, Lake Oswego, OR, USA). Glass pipettes were prepared with a DMZ puller (Zeitz Instruments, Martinsried, Germany) to a resistance of 0.9 to 2.5 MΩ and filled with ICS. The ICS for hNav1.9_C4 recordings consisted of (in mM): CsF (140), EGTA (1), HEPES (10) and NaCl (10), sucrose (18) adjusted to pH 7.33 with CsOH, and 310 mOsm with additional sucrose. The ECS for hNav1.9_C4 recordings contained (in mM): NaCl (140), KCl (3), $CaCl_2$ (1), $MgCl_2$ (1), HEPES (10), glucose (20), and 0.1 % BSA. The pH was adjusted to 7.4 with NaOH and osmolarity adjusted to 305 mOsm with glucose. TTX (500 nM) was added to the ECS to block endogenous Na^+ currents in ND7/23 cells. Tf2 (1 μM) was diluted in ECS with 0.1% BSA and incubated for 5 min prior to recording. Capacitive transients were cancelled and series resistance (≤6 MΩ) was compensated by at least 70%. Leak current was subtracted online using a P/4 procedure following each test pulse. Signals were sampled with 100 kHz and filtered at 10 kHz for activation and fast inactivation protocols and at 30 kHz for the deactivation protocol. Recording protocols were started 5 min after establishing the whole-cell configuration to allow for current stabilization. The holding potential for all recordings was −120 mV. The voltage dependence of activation was measured using a series of 40 ms pulses ranging from −120 mV to 30 mV in 10 mV steps at an interval of 5 s. The voltage dependence of steady-state fast inactivation was measured using a series of 500 ms pre-pulses ranging from −160 to −20 mV, in steps of 10 mV, followed by a 40 ms depolarizing test pulse at −40 mV. The voltage dependence of deactivation was measured using a series of 1.5 ms depolarizing pre-pulses to −20 mV. This was followed by a repolarization test pulse ranging from −130 to −20 mV, in 10 mV steps, at an interval of 5 s.

2.5. Ca^{2+} *Imaging of Isolated Dorsal Root Ganglion Neurons*

Primary cultures of mouse DRG neurons were prepared as previously described [16,17]. Briefly, DRG ganglia, removed from all spinal levels of 4-week-old male C57BL/6 mice, were incubated in DMEM (Gibco, Waltham, MD, USA) with 1 mg mL^{-1} Collagenase IV (Gibco, Life Technologies, NY, USA) for 90 min at 37 °C, then triturated with fire-polished Pasteur pipettes and plated in 96-well plates coated with PDL (Corning, ME, USA). After 1 h, wells were flooded with DMEM supplemented with 10% FBS and pencillin/streptomycin (Gibco, Waltham, MD, USA) and maintained for 16–24 h before assay. Cells were loaded with Fluo-4 AM calcium indicator, according to the manufacturer's instructions (ThermoFisher Scientific, MA, USA). After loading (1 h), the dye-containing solution was replaced with assay solution (1 x Hanks' balanced salt solution, 20 mM HEPES). Fluorescence corresponding to $[Ca^{2+}]_i$ of 100–200 DRG cells per experiment was monitored in parallel using a Nikon Ti-E Deconvolution inverted microscope (Nikon, Tokyo, Japan), equipped with a Lumencor Spectra LED Lightsource (Lumencor, Beavertown, OR, USA). Images were acquired at 10× objective at 1 frame/s (excitation 485 nm, emission 521 nm). For each experiment, baseline fluorescence was monitored for 30 s. At 30 s, 60 s, and 180 s, assay solution was replaced with fresh assay solution (as a negative control), Tf2 (1 μM in assay solution), and KCl (30 mM in assay solution), respectively. Experiments with TTX and Tf2[S14R] were performed in the same way. Cells responding to KCl and/or Tf2 were considered neuronal and grouped according to size: Large (>600 μm^2), medium (300–600 μm^2), and small diameter (<300 μm^2). Experiments involving the use of mouse tissue were approved by The University of Queensland Animal Ethics Committee. Data were derived from 2–3 independent experiments, and plotted using GraphPad Prism 8. Where differences were tested, unpaired *t*-tests were used.

2.6. *Animals*

For behavioral assessment, we used adult male wildtype or homozygous $Na_V1.9$-deficient ($Na_V1.9^{-/-}$) mice aged 6–8 weeks (~25g) on a C57BL/6J background. Homozygous Nav1.9 knockout mice on a C57BL/6J background were generated using CRISPR/Cas9 technology by the Queensland Facility for Advanced Genome Editing (The University of Queensland, Australia). In brief, two sgRNAs were designed to target exon 2 of the *Scn11a* gene. The deletion of exon 2 generated a frame shift mutation resulting in the introduction of stop codons in exon 3. The guide sgRNAs were microinjected together with Cas9 mRNA into fertilized eggs collected from C57BL/6J mice and transferred into pseudopregnant surrogate CD1 female mice. Offspring born to the foster mothers were genotyped by PCR (see below) and DNA sequencing. One F0 male mouse was bred to C57BL/6J female mice to generate F1 heterozygous mice, and F1 heterozygous mice were inbred to obtain homozygous mice. Genomic DNA was extracted from ear clippings and mice were genotyped by PCR using the following primers (forward: 5′-GCTGCTCAGACACTCACAGT-3′) and (reverse: 5′ATTCTGCCACCAGAGACTGC-3′) by the AEGRC genotyping and sequencing facility (The University of Queensland). Animals were housed in groups of 3 or 4 per cage, under 12-h light-dark cycles, and had standard rodent chow and water ad libitum. Age-matched controls were used for studies involving knockout animals. All behavioral assessment was performed by a blinded observer unaware of the genotype and/or treatments received.

Ethical approval for in vivo experiments was obtained from The University of Queensland Animal Ethics Committee prior to experimentation. All animals experiments were conducted in accordance with local and national regulations, including the International Association for the Study of Pain Guidelines for the Use of Animals in Research in agreement with the Animal Care and Protection Regulation Qld (2012), and the Australian Code of Practice for the Care and Use of Animals for Scientific Purposes, 8th edition (2013) (TRI/IMB/093/17, 31 March 2017; IMB/PACE/421/18, 18 October 2018).

2.7. Behavioral Assessment

First, Tf2 (1 µM), Tf2[S14R] (10 µM), or ICA-121431 (500 nM) were diluted in saline with 0.1% *w*/*v* BSA and administered either alone or in combination by intraplantar (i.pl) injection into the left hind paw in a volume of 40 µL under light isoflurane (3 %) anesthesia. Mice were then placed individually into polyvinyl boxes (10 × 10 × 10 cm) and recorded by video for 20 min post-injection. The number of spontaneous pain behaviors, including licks, shakes, and flinches, were counted later by a blinded observer. Once spontaneous pain behavior had ceased, mechanical thresholds were assessed using an electronic von Frey apparatus (MouseMet Electronic von Frey, TopCat Metrology, Ely, UK), heat thresholds were assessed using the thermal probe test (MouseMet Thermal), and weight bearing was assessed using the Catwalk XT (Noldus Information Technology, Wageningen, The Netherlands) as previously described [18,19]. To quantify weight bearing, the parameter 'mean intensity of the 15 most intense pixels' was used as a surrogate measure.

2.8. Paw Thickness

In a separate cohort of animals, paw thickness was measured along the distal–proximal axis at the metatarsal level using a digital vernier caliper (Kincrome, Vic, Australia) 10 min after i.pl. injection of Tf2 (1 µM) or Tf2[S14R] (10 µM).

2.9. Data Analysis

Data were plotted and analyzed by GraphPad Prism, versions 8.2.0 and 8.4.2. Statistical significance was defined as $p < 0.05$ and was determined by *t*-test or one-way ANOVA with Dunnett's post-test, as indicated. In case of deactivation, multiple *t*-tests (one per row) were used without assuming equal standard deviation and with the Holm–Sidak method for correcting *p*-values for multiple comparisons. Concentration–response curves were fitted with a four-parameter Hill equation with a variable Hill coefficient. Conductance–voltage relationships for activation were calculated for each voltage step using $G = \frac{I}{(V - V_{rev})}$ where V_{rev} is the reversal potential. Resulting data were fitted using a Boltzmann equation: $G_{Na} = \frac{G_{Na,max}}{1 + e^{[(Vm - V\frac{1}{2})]/k}}$; G_{Na} is the voltage-dependent sodium conductance, $G_{Na,max}$ is the maximal sodium conductance, V_m is the membrane potential, $V_{1/2}$ is the membrane potential at half-maximal activation, and k is the slope factor. Current–voltage relationships for inactivation were fitted using a Boltzmann equation: $I_{Na} = \frac{I_{Na,max}}{1 + e^{[(Vm - V\frac{1}{2})]/k}}$ I_{Na} is the voltage-dependent sodium current, $I_{Na,max}$ is the maximal sodium current, V_m is the membrane potential, $V_{1/2}$ is the half-maximal inactivation, and k is the slope factor. The time course of current decay at deactivating voltages over 10 ms was fitted by the double-exponential equation, $y = y_0 + amp_1 * e^{-\frac{x}{\tau_1}} + amp_2 * e^{-\frac{x}{\tau_2}}$, where y_0 is the current amplitude at steady state, amp_1 and amp_2 are the amplitude coefficient for the fast and slow time constants, and τ_1 and τ_2 are the fast and slow time constants. Data are expressed as the mean ± standard error of the mean (SEM).

3. Results

3.1. Chemical Synthesis of Tf2

We used chemical synthesis to prepare multi-milligram quantities of Tf2. This toxin is a relatively large (62 amino acid residues) and post-translationally modified protein, whose 3-D structure is stabilized by four disulfide crosslinks. The target polypeptide chain was split into two segments of manageable size (26 and 36 residues), which were assembled individually by solid-phase peptide synthesis and purified. The full-length polypeptide chain was obtained in good yield by native chemical ligation of the two segments. Folding of the 62 amino acid peptide chain and oxidation of the eight cysteines required extensive optimization and allowed the isolation of synthetic Tf2 in acceptable yields and excellent purity for further functional studies. Functional equivalence with venom-derived Tf2 was established through activity testing (see below) as well as partial assignment of NMR data, which are in agreement with the expected cysteine-stabilized αβ fold that is characteristic for this class of scorpion toxins (Figure S1).

3.2. *Synthetic β-Scorpion Tf2 Causes Early Channel Opening at $Na_V1.3$ and $Na_V1.9$*

To examine the potency and selectivity of synthetic Tf2, we used a high-throughput fluorescence-based assay to measure changes in the membrane potential at $hNa_V1.1$–1.7 expressed heterologously in HEK293 cells. Synthetic Tf2 potently activated $hNa_V1.3$, with an EC_{50} of 213 ± 57 nM (Figure 1A). Consistent with the activity previously reported for venom-derived Tf2 [14], synthetic Tf2 retained selectivity for $hNa_V1.3$, with no effect on $hNa_V1.1$, $hNa_V1.2$, or $hNa_V1.4$–1.7 up to 10 μM (Figure 1A), making it more than 50-fold selective over these isoforms. To assess the mechanism of action of synthetic Tf2, we used whole-cell patch-clamp electrophysiology in HEK293 cells expressing $hNa_V1.3$. Consistent with the β-scorpion activity previously reported for the native toxin, synthetic Tf2 (hereafter Tf2) at 1 μM caused a decrease in the peak current and a hyperpolarizing shift (Δ −11.3 mV) in the voltage dependence of activation (V_{50} control: −29.5 ± 0.7 mV; V_{50} Tf2: −40.8 ± 1.3 mV; $p < 0.05$; Figure 1B,C). The slope factor of the conductance–voltage curve also significantly increased in the presence of Tf2 at 1 μM, indicating a higher conductance at more hyperpolarizing membrane potentials (control: 3.6 ± 0.6 mV; Tf2: 8.0 ± 1.1 mV; $p < 0.05$; Figure 1C).

It has previously been shown that Tf2 does not alter the voltage dependence of activation of $hNa_V1.7$ or $hNa_V1.8$ expressed in *Xenopus* oocytes [14]. We thus sought to confirm this in mammalian cells and extend these studies to include the human $Na_V1.9$ isoform. For this, we utilized the previously described hNav1.9_C4 construct in which the C-terminus from $rNa_V1.4$ replaces the C-terminus of $hNa_V1.9$, enabling trafficking of the channel to the cell surface [8,20]. Consistent with previous reports, 1 μM Tf2 does not shift the voltage dependence of activation at $hNa_V1.7$ (V_{50} control: −23.1 ± 0.6 mV; V_{50} Tf2: −24.3 ± 0.7 mV; $p > 0.05$; Figure 1D) or $hNa_V1.8$ (V_{50} control: −1.1 ± 0.3 mV; V_{50} Tf2: −1.2 ± 0.4 mV; $p > 0.05$; Figure 1E). Interestingly, 1 μM Tf2 was active at hNav1.9_C4, causing a hyperpolarizing shift (Δ −6.3 mV) in the voltage dependence of activation (V_{50} control: −55.1 ± 1.9 mV; V_{50} Tf2 −61.4 ± 1.2 mV; $p < 0.05$, Figure 1F) and a change (Δ −1.3) in the slope factor (control: 8.8 ± 0.4; Tf2: 7.6 ± 0.2; $p < 0.05$, Figure 1F). Given the novel activity at hNav1.9_C4, we also assessed whether Tf2 affects any other parameters of hNav1.9_C4 channel kinetics. Tf2 did not change the current density (control: 61.8 ± 12.6 pA/pF; Tf2: 68.1 ± 10.3 pA/pF; $p > 0.05$), or the voltage dependence of fast inactivation (V_{50} control: −98.16 ± 1.9 mV; V_{50} Tf2 −98.16 ± 1.5 mV; $p > 0.05$) or deactivation (see Figure S2A–C).

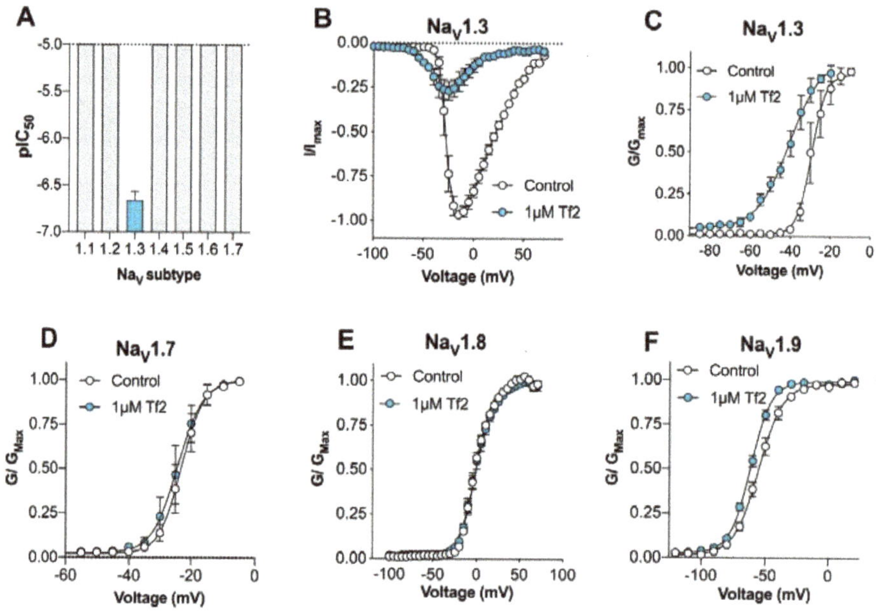

Figure 1. Synthetic Tf2 shifts the voltage dependence of activation at hNa$_V$1.3 and hNa$_V$1.9_C4. (**A**) Synthetic Tf2 retains selectivity for hNa$_V$1.3, with no effect on hNa$_V$1.1, hNa$_V$1.2, or hNa$_V$1.4–1.7 up to 10 μM in the FLIPR^{Tetra} membrane potential assay (n = 4–6 wells) (**B**) hNa$_V$1.3 current–voltage relationship before (white circles) and after the addition of 1 μM Tf2 (blue circles). Tf2 causes early channel opening and an overall decrease in the peak current (n = 5 cells). (**C**) hNa$_V$1.3 conductance–voltage relationship before (white circles) and after the addition of 1 μM Tf2 (blue circles). Tf2 causes a significant (Δ −11.3 mV) hyperpolarizing shift in the voltage dependence of activation and increases the slope factor (n = 4 cells). (**D**) hNa$_V$1.7 conductance–voltage relationship before (white circles) and after the addition of 1 μM Tf2 (blue circles) (n = 4 cells). (**E**) hNa$_V$1.8 conductance–voltage relationship before (white circles) and after addition of 1 μM Tf2 (blue circles) (n = 12 cells). (**F**) hNav1.9_C4 conductance–voltage relationship incubated with vehicle (0.1% BSA, white circles) or with 1 μM Tf2 (blue circles). Tf2 causes a significant hyperpolarizing (Δ −6.3 mV) shift in the voltage dependence of activation and decreased the slope factor (Δ −1.3) (n = 11–14 cells). Data presented as mean ± SEM.

3.3. *Tf2[S14R] has Reduced Excitatory Activity at Na$_V$1.3*

It has been demonstrated for several β-scorpion toxins that a single amino acid residue replacement of S14 (in Ts1) or E15 (in Cn2 and Css4) with an arginine can uncouple the 'excitatory' activity from the 'inhibitory' activity, producing β-scorpion toxin mutants that inhibit the peak current without causing early channel opening [11,20,21]. We therefore synthesized a Tf2[S14R] mutant and assessed activity at hNa$_V$1.3. Unlike Tf2, the S14R mutant, at concentrations up to 10 μM, did not activate hNa$_V$1.3 in a fluorescence-based membrane potential assay (Figure 2A). In patch-clamp electrophysiology, 10 μM Tf2[S14R] caused a reduction in peak current, although a small hyperpolarizing shift (Δ −5.8 mV) in the voltage dependence of activation remained (control: −24.3 ± 0.4 mV; Tf2[S14R]: −30.1 ± 0.7 mV; $p < 0.05$; Figure 2B,C). However, unlike wildtype Tf2, the slope factor of the conductance–voltage curve was not significantly different in the presence of Tf2[S14R] at 10 μM, indicating the S14R mutant had lost significant excitatory activity (control: 3.9 ± 0.4; Tf2[S14R]: 4.0 ± 0.6; $p > 0.05$; Figure 2C).

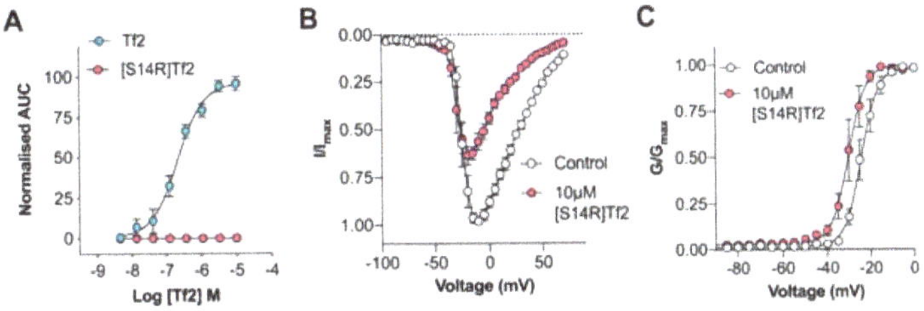

Figure 2. Tf2[S14R] loses excitatory activity at hNa$_V$1.3. (**A**) Comparative activity of Tf2 and Tf2[S14R] on hNa$_V$1.3 assessed using the FLIPR^{Tetra} membrane potential assay. Tf2 (blue circles) concentration-dependently increased the membrane potential (EC_{50} 213 ± 57 nM) while Tf2[S14R] (pink circles) had no effect up to 10 µM (n = 3–4 wells). (**B**) hNa$_V$1.3 current–voltage relationship before (white circles) and after the addition of 10 µM Tf2[S14R] (pink circles). Tf2[S14R] decreased the peak current with a smaller effect on early channel opening compared to Tf2 (n = 5 cells). (**C**) hNa$_V$1.3 conductance–voltage relationship before (white circles) and after the addition of 10 µM Tf2[S14R] (pink circles). Tf2[S14R] causes a smaller but significant (Δ −5.8 mV) hyperpolarizing shift in the voltage dependence of activation without affecting the slope factor (n = 5 cells). Data presented as mean ± SEM.

3.4. *Tf2 Induces Calcium Influx in DRG Neurons*

It has been reported that Na$_V$1.3 is expressed at low levels in the adult rodent peripheral nervous system [4]. Application of 1 µM Tf2 to isolated mouse DRG neurons caused an immediate, rapid, and sustained increase in the intracellular Ca^{2+} concentration ($[Ca^{2+}]_i$) in a subset of neurons (Figure 3A,B). Small, medium, and large diameter neurons were activated (Figure 3C). Activation was completely blocked ($p < 0.05$) in the presence of 1 µM TTX (Figure 3D), indicating that the effects of Tf2 on Ca^{2+} influx in mouse DRG neurons is dependent on the expression of TTX-sensitive VGSCs. At the same concentration (1 µM), Tf2[S14R] was not significantly different to cells treated with the negative control (p = 0.71), indicating that this analogue lacks the capacity to activate DRG neurons, consistent with its reduced excitatory activity of Na$_V$1.3.

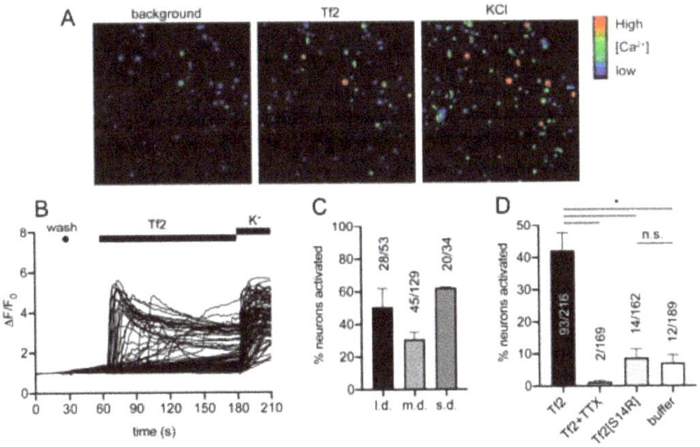

Figure 3. Tf2 activates mouse dorsal root ganglion neurons. (**A**) DRG cells before (background) and after the addition of 1 µM Tf2 and 30 mM KCl. (**B**) Traces from all neurons (defined as cells responding to 30 mM KCl and/or 1 µM Tf2) of one representative experiment. (**C**) Percentage of large (>600 µm^2), medium (300–600 µm^2), and small diameter (<300 µm^2) neurons activated in the presence of 1 µM Tf2. (**D**) Percentage of neurons (total) activated in the presence of 1 µM Tf2, 1 µM Tf2 + 1 µM TTX, 1 µM Tf2[S14R], or buffer (negative control). Data are presented as SEM with the total number of neurons from 2–3 independent experiments; l.d., large diameter, m.d., medium diameter; s.d., small diameter; K^+, 30 mM KCl; *, $p < 0.05$ using unpaired t-test; n.s., not significant.

3.5. Tf2 Causes Spontaneous Pain and Swelling In Vivo

Intraplantar injection of 1 μM (40 μL) Tf2 in mice caused a rapid induction of spontaneous pain behaviors, including flinching, licking, and shaking of the injected hind paw, that slowly subsided over 20 min (Figure 4A,B). In contrast, 10 μM Tf2[S14R] caused no spontaneous pain behaviors, consistent with the loss of excitatory activity at $Na_V1.3$ and in DRG neurons seen in vitro (flinches/10 min: control, 5 ± 3; Tf2, 102 ± 12; Tf2[S14R], 5 ± 1; $p < 0.05$, Figure 4B). To assess if 10 μM (40 μL) Tf2[S14R] could compete with wild-type toxin for $Na_V1.3$ binding in vivo, we co-administered it with 1 μM (40 μL) Tf2; however, it had no effect on Tf2-induced spontaneous flinching (flinches/10 min: Tf2 + Tf2[S14R] 101 ± 11; Figure 4B). In addition, the $Na_V1.1/1.3$ inhibitor ICA-121431 (500 nM) had no effect on Tf2-induced spontaneous flinching (flinches/10 min: Tf2 + ICA-121431 88 ± 6; $p > 0.05$; Figure 4B), suggesting the flinching is not mediated via $Na_V1.3$. Spontaneous pain was accompanied by erythema (redness) and swelling (Figure 4C), which occurred immediately after injection of Tf2 and also unexpectedly after Tf2[S14R], suggesting that this inflammatory response is not mediated via activation of $Na_V1.3$ but instead through an additional target (paw thickness: control, 2.5 ± 0.2 mm; Tf2, 3.2 ± 0.1 mm; Tf2[S14R], 3.5 ± 0.1 mm; $p < 0.05$; Figure 4D). As Tf2 also activated $hNa_V1.9$_C4, we assessed whether activation of $Na_V1.9$ contributed to Tf2-induced spontaneous pain and swelling in vivo using $Na_V1.9^{-/-}$ mice. Compared to wildtype (WT) controls, $Na_V1.9^{-/-}$ mice did not exhibit a significant reduction in spontaneous pain behaviors (flinches/10 min: WT, 197 ± 25; $Na_V1.9^{-/-}$, 218 ± 32; $p > 0.05$) or paw swelling (paw thickness: WT, 3.3 ± 0.1 mm; $Na_V1.9^{-/-}$, 3.3 ± 0.1 mm; $p > 0.05$) after injection of Tf2 (Figure 4E,F). Once spontaneous pain subsided (~40 min post injection), we also assessed the effect of intraplantar Tf2 on mechanical thresholds, thermal thresholds, and weight bearing behavior in WT mice. Tf2 had no significant effect on mechanical thresholds (paw withdrawal threshold (PWT): control, 2.7 ± 0.4 g; Tf2, 1.9 ± 0.4 g; $p > 0.05$; Figure 4G) or paw thermal thresholds (PWT: control, 49.0 ± 0.5 °C; Tf2, 48.2 ± 0.3 °C; $p > 0.05$; Figure 4H) but did cause a significant reduction in weight bearing (arbitrary fluorescent unit (AFU): control, 108.9 ± 1.7; Tf2, 97.5 ± 1.9; $p < 0.05$; Figure 4I).

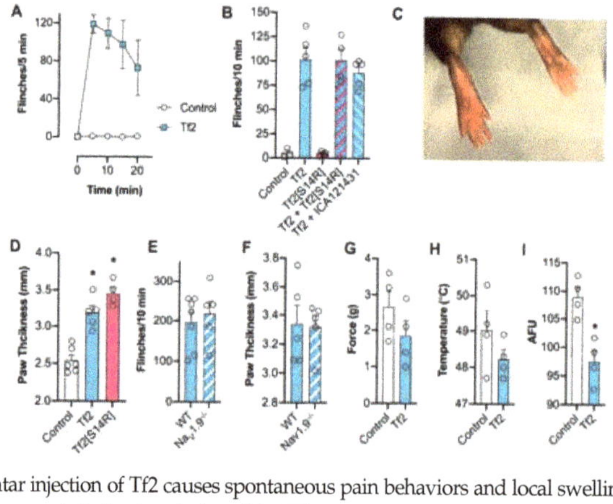

Figure 4. Intraplantar injection of Tf2 causes spontaneous pain behaviors and local swelling in mice (**A**) Time course of spontaneous pain behaviors induced by Tf2 (1 μM i.pl.). (**B**) Intraplantar injection of Tf2 (1 μM) causes spontaneous pain behaviors while intraplantar injection of Tf2[S14R] (10 μM) does not. Co-injection of Tf2[S14R] (10 μM) with Tf2 (1 μM) or ICA-121431 (500 nM) causes no reduction in spontaneous pain behaviors. (**C**) Intraplantar injection of Tf2 (left hind paw) causes local erythema (redness) and swelling. (**D**) Intraplantar injection of both Tf2 (1 μM) and Tf2[S14R] (10 μM) causes a significant increase in paw swelling. (**E**) Tf2-induced spontaneous pain behaviors are not attenuated in $Na_V1.9^{-/-}$ mice. (**F**) Tf2-induced swelling is not attenuated in $Na_V1.9^{-/-}$ mice. (**G**) Intraplantar injection of Tf2 (1 μM) has no effect on mechanical thresholds. (**H**) Intraplantar injection of Tf2 (1 μM) has no effect on heat thresholds. (**I**) Intraplantar injection of Tf2 (1 μM) causes a reduction in weight bearing (as measured by arbitrary fluorescence units; AFU). Data are presented as mean ± SEM with individual values plotted (n = 3–7 mice). Statistical significance was determined using t-test or one-way ANOVA with Dunnett's post-test as appropriate, * $p < 0.05$ compared to control or WT.

4. Discussion

Here, we describe for the first time the activity of synthetic β-scorpion toxin Tf2 on the full panel of human VGSCs ($Na_V1.1$–1.9) constitutively expressed in mammalian cells, on the calcium influx in primary sensory DRG neurons, and on nociceptive behaviors in mice in vivo, with the overall aim to investigate its suitability as a selective $Na_V1.3$ pharmacological probe. Modern chemical peptide synthesis strategies applied to α- and β-long chain scorpion toxins have allowed the production of these molecules on the multi-milligram scale and have allowed structural and functional studies that are difficult to perform with the small quantities usually isolated from scorpion venom [22–25]. Synthetic Tf2 faithfully reproduced the activity and mode-of-action of venom-derived Tf2 reported previously, strongly suggesting that both samples are also structurally identical. Whilst previously described as a selective $Na_V1.3$ activator [14], we found that Tf2 had additional activity at $hNa_V1.9$_C4, which is a TTX-resistant isoform preferentially expressed on small diameter DRG neurons that is associated with both 'painless' and 'painful' channelopathies [26,27].

The pharmacology of scorpion toxins at $Na_V1.9$ remains largely unexplored, partly due to difficulties in the functional expression of $Na_V1.9$ in heterologous systems. However, the β-scorpion toxin Ts1 (also known as TsVII), which has 73.4% sequence identity to Tf2, is also active on $Na_V1.9$ [28]. This suggests that activity at $Na_V1.9$ may be broadly conserved amongst other related β-scorpion toxins, but this remains to be assessed. Despite shifting the voltage dependence of activation at $Na_V1.9$ (Δ −6.3 mV), Tf2-induced spontaneous pain and swelling developed normally in $Na_V1.9^{-/-}$ mice, indicating that this isoform had a minimal contribution to in vivo activity. This result was somewhat surprising, given the mutation L1158P in human $Na_V1.9$ causes a similar hyperpolarizing shift in activation (Δ −6.7 mV), and has been linked to increased excitability of DRG neurons and painful peripheral neuropathy [29]. However, this mutation also slows deactivation, which was a channel parameter unaffected by Tf2, suggesting that changes in $Na_V1.9$ deactivation may be important for neuronal excitability.

Selective VGSC modulators remain useful tool compounds for delineating the contribution of particular isoforms to the excitability of neurons in both physiological and pathological states [17,30]. Despite being implicated in neuropathic pain and epilepsy, there is a lack of highly potent and selective inhibitors of $Na_V1.3$ available. The small molecule ICA-121431 is the most potent $Na_V1.3$ inhibitor described to the date, but off-target activity at $Na_V1.1$, which is also expressed on peripheral and central neurons, limits its use as a research tool in vivo [31]. In an attempt to rationally design a selective $Na_V1.3$ inhibitor, we synthesized Tf2[S14R], where we mutated the serine at position 14 to a positively charged arginine. In the homologous β-scorpion toxin Ts1, mutation of S14 to an arginine resulted in a toxin that could still bind to $Na_V1.4$ but no longer shifted the voltage dependence of activation [32]. In line with this observation, Tf2[S14R] inhibited the peak current of $Na_V1.3$ without causing the same early channel opening as the native Tf2; however, it was unable to reverse Tf2-induced spontaneous pain behaviors in vivo. This is possibly due to the mutation causing a loss in potency, as the related toxin Cn2[E15R] required application at a concentration 200 times higher than the native to inhibit $Na_V1.6$ in vivo [11]. Unfortunately, because the potency of Tf2 is already relatively weak, and Tf2[S14R] caused paw swelling at 10 μM, higher concentrations could not be assessed.

Tf2 caused Ca^{2+} influx in both small and large mouse adult DRG neurons, which was surprising given $Na_V1.3$ is only expressed at significant levels in embryonic sensory neurons or in adult neurons after axotomy [4]. Interestingly, colonic neurons isolated from mouse thoracolumbar (T10-L1) and lumbosacral (L5-S2) DRGs express $Na_V1.3$ mRNA transcripts at similar levels to $Na_V1.1$ and $Na_V1.2$ [33]. As DRG neurons in this study were isolated from all spinal levels, we cannot rule out the presence of these $Na_V1.3$-expressing neurons in culture. However, given the definitive lack of proteomic evidence for $Na_V1.3$ expression in adult uninjured DRG neurons, and that Tf2 activated a large proportion of all DRG neurons, it is more likely that the observed effect on Ca^{2+} influx is due to activity at other neuronal targets. This is consistent with Tf2-induced spontaneous flinching not being reversed by the $Na_V1.1/1.3$ inhibitor ICA-121431 in vivo. Indeed, it is not uncommon for scorpion toxins to have promiscuous activity on both VGSCs and voltage-gated potassium (K_V) channels, and blockade of a K_V channel could also result in Ca^{2+} influx [34,35]. Furthermore, there are scorpion toxins that modulate members of the family of voltage-gated calcium channels (Ca_V), such as kurtoxin from *Parabuthus transvaalicus* [36]; however, the activity of Tf2 at voltage-gated potassium and calcium channels in heterologous expression systems remains to be tested. Inhibition of Tf2-induced Ca^{2+} influx by TTX could also be explained by a global depression of neuronal excitability rather than direct opposition of Tf2-induced $Na_V1.3$ activation. The observation that Tf2[S14R], which lost activity at $Na_V1.3$, also lost excitatory activity in DRG neurons suggests that the pharmacophore of Tf2 at this other neuronal target(s) overlaps at least partially with that of $Na_V1.3$. In addition, the observation that Tf2[S14R], which lost excitatory activity in DRG neurons, still caused swelling in vivo suggests that Tf2-induced inflammation is mediated by an additional non-neuronal target. Scorpion venom- or toxin-induced inflammatory responses have been described previously and have been linked to the activation of innate immune cells via interaction with pattern recognition receptors [37]. The use of global and sensory neuron-specific $Na_V1.3$ knockout mice would be required to tease out what contribution, if any, $Na_V1.3$ has to Tf2-induced pain and inflammation.

In summary, Tf2 does not appear to be a suitable tool to study the effects of Nav1.3 channel activation in sensory neurons. This is due to additional activity at $Na_V1.9$ and the probability of other neuronal and non-neuronal targets. Results from in vivo experiments that use Tf2 should be interpreted accordingly. There is, however, scope to use Tf2 in studying the activity of $Na_V1.9$ in vitro, particularly in heterologous expression systems. Indeed, very few toxins to date are known to modulate the $Na_V1.9$ isoform. Finally, the somewhat surprising finding that Tf2 and Tf2[S14R] cause inflammation in vivo could be explored further to understand how scorpion toxin envenomation affects inflammatory processes in humans.

Supplementary Materials: Supplementary materials can be found at http://www.mdpi.com/2227-9059/8/6/155/s1. Figure S1: NMR secondary Hα chemical shift analysis of synthetic Tf2. Figure S2: Activity of Tf2 on other channel parameters of $hNa_V1.9\_C4$.

Author Contributions: M.R.I., A.L., T.D. and I.V. conceived of and designed the experiments. M.R.I., J.R.D., T.S.D., S.D.R., S.N.B. and T.D. performed the experiments. M.R.I., J.R.D., T.D., D.J.C., S.D.R. and S.N.B. analyzed the data. M.R.I. and J.R.D. wrote the paper. All authors have read and agreed to the published version of the manuscript.

Funding: This work was supported by an Australian National Health and Medical Research Council (NMHRC) Career Development Fellowship (APP1162503, I.V.), an NHMRC Early Career Fellowship (APP1139961, J.R.D.), funded by the Deutsche Forschungsgemeinschaft (DFG, German Research Foundation, LA2740/3-1; 363055819/GRK2415; 368482240/GRK2416, A.L.) and supported by a grant from the Interdisciplinary Centre for Clinical Research within the faculty of Medicine at the RWTH Aachen University (IZKF TN1-8/IA 532008). DJC is an Australian Research Council Australian Laureate Fellow (FL150100146).

Conflicts of Interest: The authors declare no conflict of interest. The funders had no role in the design of the study; in the collection, analyses, or interpretation of data; in the writing of the manuscript, or in the decision to publish the results.

References

1. Shen, H.; Zhou, Q.; Pan, X.; Li, Z.; Wu, J.; Yan, N. Structure of a eukaryotic voltage-gated sodium channel at near-atomic resolution. *Science* **2017**, *355*. [CrossRef]
2. Catterall, W.A.; Goldin, A.L.; Waxman, S.G. International Union of Pharmacology. XLVII. Nomenclature and structure-function relationships of voltage-gated sodium channels. *Pharm. Rev.* **2005**, *57*, 397–409. [CrossRef] [PubMed]
3. Cummins, T.R.; Aglieco, F.; Renganathan, M.; Herzog, R.I.; Dib-Hajj, S.D.; Waxman, S.G. Nav1.3 sodium channels: Rapid repriming and slow closed-state inactivation display quantitative differences after expression in a mammalian cell line and in spinal sensory neurons. *J. Neurosci.* **2001**, *21*, 5952–5961. [CrossRef] [PubMed]
4. Waxman, S.G.; Kocsis, J.D.; Black, J.A. Type III sodium channel mRNA is expressed in embryonic but not adult spinal sensory neurons, and is reexpressed following axotomy. *J. Neurophysiol.* **1994**, *72*, 466–470. [CrossRef] [PubMed]

5. Craner, M.J.; Klein, J.P.; Renganathan, M.; Black, J.A.; Waxman, S.G. Changes of sodium channel expression in experimental painful diabetic neuropathy. *Ann. Neurol.* **2002**, *52*, 786–792. [CrossRef]
6. Black, J.A.; Cummins, T.R.; Plumpton, C.; Chen, Y.H.; Hormuzdiar, W.; Clare, J.J.; Waxman, S.G. Upregulation of a silent sodium channel after peripheral, but not central, nerve injury in DRG neurons. *J. Neurophysiol.* **1999**, *82*, 2776–2785. [CrossRef]
7. Samad, O.A.; Tan, A.M.; Cheng, X.; Foster, E.; Dib-Hajj, S.D.; Waxman, S.G. Virus-mediated shRNA knockdown of Na(v)1.3 in rat dorsal root ganglion attenuates nerve injury-induced neuropathic pain. *Mol. Ther.* **2013**, *21*, 49–56. [CrossRef]
8. Goral, R.O.; Leipold, E.; Nematian-Ardestani, E.; Heinemann, S.H. Heterologous expression of Na1.9 chimeras in various cell systems. *Pflug. Arch.* **2015**. [CrossRef]
9. Minett, M.S.; Falk, S.; Santana-Varela, S.; Bogdanov, Y.D.; Nassar, M.A.; Heegaard, A.M.; Wood, J.N. Pain without nociceptors? Nav1.7-independent pain mechanisms. *Cell Rep.* **2014**, *6*, 301–312. [CrossRef]
10. Nassar, M.A.; Baker, M.D.; Levato, A.; Ingram, R.; Mallucci, G.; McMahon, S.B.; Wood, J.N. Nerve injury induces robust allodynia and ectopic discharges in Nav1.3 null mutant mice. *Mol. Pain* **2006**, *2*, 33. [CrossRef]
11. Israel, M.R.; Morgan, M.; Tay, B.; Deuis, J.R. Toxins as tools: Fingerprinting neuronal pharmacology. *Neurosci. Lett.* **2018**, *679*, 4–14. [CrossRef] [PubMed]
12. Bosmans, F.; Tytgat, J. Voltage-gated sodium channel modulation by scorpion alpha-toxins. *Toxicon* **2007**, *49*, 142–158. [CrossRef] [PubMed]
13. Pedraza Escalona, M.; Possani, L.D. Scorpion beta-toxins and voltage-gated sodium channels: Interactions and effects. *Front. Biosci. (Landmark Ed.)* **2013**, *18*, 572–587. [CrossRef]
14. Camargos, T.S.; Bosmans, F.; Rego, S.C.; Mourao, C.B.; Schwartz, E.F. The Scorpion Toxin Tf2 from Tityus fasciolatus Promotes Nav1.3 Opening. *PLoS ONE* **2015**, *10*, e0128578. [CrossRef]
15. Cestele, S.; Qu, Y.; Rogers, J.C.; Rochat, H.; Scheuer, T.; Catterall, W.A. Voltage sensor-trapping: Enhanced activation of sodium channels by beta-scorpion toxin bound to the S3-S4 loop in domain II. *Neuron* **1998**, *21*, 919–931.
16. Robinson, S.D.; Mueller, A.; Clayton, D.; Starobova, H.; Hamilton, B.R.; Payne, R.J.; Vetter, I.; King, G.F.; Undheim, E.A.B. A comprehensive portrait of the venom of the giant red bull ant, Myrmecia gulosa, reveals a hyperdiverse hymenopteran toxin gene family. *Sci. Adv.* **2018**, *4*, eaau4640. [CrossRef]
17. Israel, M.R.; Tanaka, B.S.; Castro, J.; Thongyoo, P.; Robinson, S.D.; Zhao, P.; Deuis, J.R.; Craik, D.J.; Durek, T.; Brierley, S.M.; et al. NaV 1.6 regulates excitability of mechanosensitive sensory neurons. *J. Physiol.* **2019**, *597*, 3751–3768. [CrossRef]
18. Deuis, J.R.; Vetter, I. The thermal probe test: A novel behavioral assay to quantify thermal paw withdrawal thresholds in mice. *Temperature* **2016**, *3*, 199–207. [CrossRef]
19. Yin, K.; Deuis, J.R.; Lewis, R.J.; Vetter, I. Transcriptomic and behavioural characterisation of a mouse model of burn pain identifies the cholecystokinin 2 receptor as an analgesic target. *Mol. Pain* **2016**, *12*, 1–13. [CrossRef]
20. Sizova, D.V.; Huang, J.; Akin, E.J.; Estacion, M.; Gomis-Perez, C.; Waxman, S.G.; Dib-Hajj, S.D. A 49-residue sequence motif in the C terminus of Nav1.9 regulates trafficking of the channel to the plasma membrane. *J. Biol. Chem.* **2020**, *295*, 1077–1090. [CrossRef]
21. Karbat, I.; Ilan, N.; Zhang, J.Z.; Cohen, L.; Kahn, R.; Benveniste, M.; Scheuer, T.; Catterall, W.A.; Gordon, D.; Gurevitz, M. Partial agonist and antagonist activities of a mutant scorpion beta-toxin on sodium channels. *J. Biol. Chem.* **2010**, *285*, 30531–30538. [CrossRef] [PubMed]
22. Kubota, T.; Durek, T.; Dang, B.; Finol-Urdaneta, R.K.; Craik, D.J.; Kent, S.B.; French, R.J.; Bezanilla, F.; Correa, A.M. Mapping of voltage sensor positions in resting and inactivated mammalian sodium channels by LRET. *Proc. Natl. Acad. Sci. USA* **2017**, *114*, E1857–E1865. [CrossRef] [PubMed]
23. Dang, B.; Kubota, T.; Mandal, K.; Correa, A.M.; Bezanilla, F.; Kent, S.B. Elucidation of the Covalent and Tertiary Structures of Biologically Active Ts3 Toxin. *Angew. Chem. Int. Ed. Engl.* **2016**, *55*, 8639–8642. [CrossRef] [PubMed]
24. Durek, T.; Vetter, I.; Wang, C.I.; Motin, L.; Knapp, O.; Adams, D.J.; Lewis, R.J.; Alewood, P.F. Chemical engineering and structural and pharmacological characterization of the alpha-scorpion toxin OD1. *ACS Chem. Biol.* **2013**, *8*, 1215–1222. [CrossRef]
25. Israel, M.R.; Thongyoo, P.; Deuis, J.R.; Craik, D.J.; Vetter, I.; Durek, T. The E15R Point Mutation in Scorpion Toxin Cn2 Uncouples Its Depressant and Excitatory Activities on Human NaV1.6. *J. Med. Chem.* **2018**, *61*, 1730–1736. [CrossRef]

26. Dib-Hajj, S.D.; Tyrrell, L.; Black, J.A.; Waxman, S.G. NaN, a novel voltage-gated Na channel, is expressed preferentially in peripheral sensory neurons and down-regulated after axotomy. *Proc. Natl. Acad. Sci. USA* **1998**, *95*, 8963–8968. [CrossRef]
27. Dib-Hajj, S.D.; Black, J.A.; Waxman, S.G. NaV1.9: A sodium channel linked to human pain. *Nat. Rev. Neurosci.* **2015**, *16*, 511–519. [CrossRef] [PubMed]
28. Bosmans, F.; Puopolo, M.; Martin-Eauclaire, M.F.; Bean, B.P.; Swartz, K.J. Functional properties and toxin pharmacology of a dorsal root ganglion sodium channel viewed through its voltage sensors. *J. Gen. Physiol.* **2011**, *138*, 59–72. [CrossRef]
29. Huang, J.; Han, C.; Estacion, M.; Vasylyev, D.; Hoeijmakers, J.G.; Gerrits, M.M.; Tyrrell, L.; Lauria, G.; Faber, C.G.; Dib-Hajj, S.D.; et al. Gain-of-function mutations in sodium channel Na(v)1.9 in painful neuropathy. *Brain J. Neurol.* **2014**, *137*, 1627–1642. [CrossRef]
30. Deuis, J.R.; Dekan, Z.; Wingerd, J.S.; Smith, J.J.; Munasinghe, N.R.; Bhola, R.F.; Imlach, W.L.; Herzig, V.; Armstrong, D.A.; Rosengren, K.J.; et al. Pharmacological characterisation of the highly NaV1.7 selective spider venom peptide Pn3a. *Sci. Rep.* **2017**, *7*, 40883. [CrossRef]
31. McCormack, K.; Santos, S.; Chapman, M.L.; Krafte, D.S.; Marron, B.E.; West, C.W.; Krambis, M.J.; Antonio, B.M.; Zellmer, S.G.; Printzenhoff, D.; et al. Voltage sensor interaction site for selective small molecule inhibitors of voltage-gated sodium channels. *Proc. Natl. Acad. Sci. USA* **2013**, *110*, E2724–E2732. [CrossRef] [PubMed]
32. Kubota, T.; Dang, B.; Carvalho-de-Souza, J.L.; Correa, A.M.; Bezanilla, F. Nav channel binder containing a specific conjugation-site based on a low toxicity beta-scorpion toxin. *Sci. Rep.* **2017**, *7*, 16329. [CrossRef] [PubMed]
33. Hockley, J.R.; Gonzalez-Cano, R.; McMurray, S.; Tejada-Giraldez, M.A.; McGuire, C.; Torres, A.; Wilbrey, A.L.; Cibert-Goton, V.; Nieto, F.R.; Pitcher, T.; et al. Visceral and somatic pain modalities reveal NaV 1.7-independent visceral nociceptive pathways. *J. Physiol.* **2017**, *595*, 2661–2679. [CrossRef] [PubMed]
34. Liu, P.; Jo, S.; Bean, B.P. Modulation of neuronal sodium channels by the sea anemone peptide BDS-I. *J. Neurophysiol.* **2012**, *107*, 3155–3167. [CrossRef]
35. Klint, J.K.; Senff, S.; Rupasinghe, D.B.; Er, S.Y.; Herzig, V.; Nicholson, G.M.; King, G.F. Spider-venom peptides that target voltage-gated sodium channels: Pharmacological tools and potential therapeutic leads. *Toxicon* **2012**, *60*, 478–491. [CrossRef]
36. Sidach, S.S.; Mintz, I.M. Kurtoxin, a gating modifier of neuronal high- and low-threshold ca channels. *J. Neurosci.* **2002**, *22*, 2023–2034. [CrossRef]
37. Reis, M.B.; Zoccal, K.F.; Gardinassi, L.G.; Faccioli, L.H. Scorpion envenomation and inflammation: Beyond neurotoxic effects. *Toxicon* **2019**, *167*, 174–179. [CrossRef]

biomedicines

Article

Small Molecules in the Venom of the Scorpion *Hormurus waigiensis*

Edward R. J. Evans [1], Lachlan McIntyre [2], Tobin D. Northfield [3], Norelle L. Daly [1] and David T. Wilson [1,*]

[1] Centre for Molecular Therapeutics, AITHM, James Cook University, Cairns, QLD 4878, Australia; edwardrobertjonathan.evans@my.jcu.edu.au (E.R.J.E.); norelle.daly@jcu.edu.au (N.L.D.)
[2] Independent Researcher, P.O. Box 78, Bamaga, QLD 4876, Australia; lach.mcintyre@gmail.com
[3] Department of Entomology, Tree Fruit Research and Extension Center, Washington State University, Wenatchee, WA 98801, USA; TNORTHFIELD@WSU.EDU
* Correspondence: david.wilson4@jcu.edu.au; Tel.: +61-7-4232-1707

Received: 30 June 2020; Accepted: 28 July 2020; Published: 31 July 2020

Abstract: Despite scorpion stings posing a significant public health issue in particular regions of the world, certain aspects of scorpion venom chemistry remain poorly described. Although there has been extensive research into the identity and activity of scorpion venom peptides, non-peptide small molecules present in the venom have received comparatively little attention. Small molecules can have important functions within venoms; for example, in some spider species the main toxic components of the venom are acylpolyamines. Other molecules can have auxiliary effects that facilitate envenomation, such as purines with hypotensive properties utilised by snakes. In this study, we investigated some non-peptide small molecule constituents of *Hormurus waigiensis* venom using LC/MS, reversed-phase HPLC, and NMR spectroscopy. We identified adenosine, adenosine monophosphate (AMP), and citric acid within the venom, with low quantities of the amino acids glutamic acid and aspartic acid also being present. Purine nucleosides such as adenosine play important auxiliary functions in snake venoms when injected alongside other venom toxins, and they may have a similar role within *H. waigiensis* venom. Further research on these and other small molecules in scorpion venoms may elucidate their roles in prey capture and predator defence, and gaining a greater understanding of how scorpion venom components act in combination could allow for the development of improved first aid.

Keywords: venom; scorpion; adenosine; purine; nucleoside; nucleotide; citric acid; glutamic acid; aspartic acid

1. Introduction

Scorpion envenomation poses a significant public health issue in certain areas of the world, particularly in northern Saharan Africa, South and East Africa, the Near- and Middle-East, southern India, Mexico, Brazil, and within the Amazonian basin [1]. Although the effects of scorpion venom can be severe when injected by a scorpion, individual venom components can have a wide range of positive applications in medicine when administered in a controlled way [2]. Past research into scorpion venoms has primarily focused on peptide constituents, as these molecules display the greatest diversity within the venom, are often responsible for the greatest toxic effects, and have the largest potential for development of therapeutics or bioinsecticides [3–6]. However, scorpions possess complex venom containing a mixture of proteins, peptides, small molecules, and salts [7]. Whilst non-peptide small molecules are often reported to be present within scorpion venom, and despite being known to play important roles in the venom of different taxa [8–10], the identities and functions of small molecules in scorpion venom remain poorly described. Identifying the small molecules present in scorpion venoms may allow a greater understanding of how scorpion venoms function, have evolved, and may help improve treatment of stings. Additionally, certain venom-derived small molecules may have applications as therapeutics [11]. At present, only a very small number of non-peptide small molecules (<1 kDa) have been confidently characterised from scorpion venoms, including an alkaloid described from *Megacormus gertschi* [12], two 1,4-benzoquinone derivatives from *Diplocentrus melici* [13], adenosine from *Heterometrus laoticus* [14,15], and citric acid from *Centruroides sculpturatus* [16]. Other published material identified the presence of spermidine in the venom of *Palamneus phipsoni* (*Heterometrus phipsoni*) [17,18] and 5-hydroxytryptamine (serotonin) in *Leiurus quinquestriatus* and *Buthotus minax* (*Hottentotta minax*) [17,19]; however, no definitive data were collected, and therefore re-examination of these venoms with modern analytical techniques would help to confirm their presence. Furthermore, free amino acids, nucleotides, lipids, amines, heterocyclic compounds, and inorganic salts are reportedly present in scorpion venoms [4,20,21], but their specific molecular compositions and functions remain generally unknown.

Venomous organisms commonly possess low-molecular weight non-peptide molecules within their venom [9,10]. The identities and functions of the low-molecular weight non-peptide molecules found in different organisms may provide insights into those that may be found in scorpions. Spiders are one of the most closely related groups of venomous organisms to scorpions, and are also one of the most widely studied groups of venomous animals. Different spider species possess a large range of small molecules within their venom, including acylpolyamines and polyamines [11,22–26]; alkaloids [27–29]; nucleosides, nucleotides, and analogues [30–35]; and free-amino acids [33,36], alongside other molecules that have been subject to less intensive study [37–39]. Given that scorpions use their venom against similar predators and prey to spiders, the small molecules they possess may be similar to those found in spiders.

Small molecules can act directly as toxins within venom, have facilitatory roles that increase the overall toxicity or effectiveness of the venom, or alternatively have functional roles linked to the maintenance of toxins within the venom gland [8,40–42]. For example, polyamines in the venom of spiders in the genus *Nephila* are sufficiently toxic towards insects to directly aid in the incapacitation of prey [42]. Alternatively, nigriventrine from the Brazilian armed spider (*Phoneutria nigriventer*) can induce convulsions in mammals, and therefore help the spider to defend against predators [40]. Whilst such molecules directly contribute to venom toxicity when targeting prey or potential predators, some small-molecule venom constituents do not induce a toxic effect when injected into a target organism, but can still play an important role within venom by acting in conjunction with toxins to facilitate envenomation or incapacitation of the target [8,43]. For example, purine nucleosides such as adenosine, guanosine, and inosine are present within a wide range of elapid and viperine snake venoms, and whilst these molecules generally have very low toxicity and are naturally present within the target organism, injection of high concentrations alongside other toxins can improve the overall effectiveness of the venom by facilitating envenomation and incapacitation [8,43]. Aird [8] explains that snake venom has three primary modes of action against prey—immobilisation by hypotension, immobilisation by paralysis, and digestion—and that the suite of small molecules injected have key roles in all three functions. As the body of research investigating the small molecule constituents of snake venoms is expanding, there is growing understanding that non-toxic small molecules can play important auxiliary roles within venoms, and future research should aim to elucidate the complex interactions that occur during envenomation [10]. In addition to these functions as toxins or facilitators of toxins, small molecules can have functions within the venom gland associated with maintenance and production of toxins. For example, citrate, which can inhibit the action of venom proteins within the gland, may be in the venom to prevent self-harm [16,41,44]. As scorpion venoms contain a suite of uncharacterised small molecules, it is possible that some may induce toxicity directly, have auxiliary effects that increase overall venom toxicity, or have functions associated with the production and storage of toxins.

In this study, we investigated some of the small molecule compositions of Australian rainforest scorpion (*Hormurus waigiensis*) venom using reversed-phase high-performance liquid chromatography (RP-HPLC), liquid chromatography/mass spectrometry (LC/MS), and nuclear magnetic resonance (NMR) spectroscopy. *H. waigiensis* is a burrowing scorpion that is widely distributed across Southeast Asia, the Pacific, New Guinea, and Australia [45]. Within Australia, it is found in tropical and sub-tropical forests along the eastern coast from northern New South Wales to Cape York, with reports of populations also present in the Northern Territory and Western Australia [46]. Stings from this species are considered mild, with the venom causing moderate pain and swelling [47]. Presently just one toxin, φ-liotoxin-Lw1a (φ-LITX-Lw1a), has been characterised from *H. waigiensis* [48,49]. The toxin φ-LITX-Lw1a was the first scorpion toxin reported to adopt a disulfide-directed β-hairpin (DDH) structure and may provide a missing link explaining how the three-disulfide inhibitor cystine knot (ICK) motif has evolved in scorpions [48,49]. The remaining constituents of *H. waigiensis* venom have not been characterised. Scorpion venom research has historically been skewed towards medically significant species, all of which belong to the family Buthidae [50]. *H. waigiensis* is a member of the family Hormuridae, which has been subject to far fewer investigations by toxinologists. Given the structural novelty of φ-LITX-Lw1a, *H. waigiensis* venom may contain other molecules with significant structural differences to those present in more thoroughly studied Buthid venoms.

2. Materials and Methods

2.1. Scorpion Collection

Scorpions were collected from rainforest sites in the vicinity of Kuranda (QLD, Australia), and kept on the premises of Minibeast Wildlife, Kuranda. The scorpions were housed in plastic food containers with substrate and a piece of bark, and kept at ambient temperature. Prior to milking, individuals had been maintained in captivity for less than one year.

2.2. Venom Extraction and Purification

Venom samples were collected from *H. waigiensis* using a square-wave stimulator (Arthur H. T. Thomas Co. Scientific Apparatus, Philadelphia, PA, USA) to electrostimulate the venom gland at 25V DC, 0.5 ms pulse duration, at a frequency of 1 pulse/sec. The samples were pooled into 20 μL of MilliQ water and stored at −20 °C. Pooled samples collected on two separate dates were further pooled prior to analysis. A further five scorpions (two male and three female) were milked and the samples were stored separately in 30 μL of MilliQ water for LC/MS analysis.

Crude pooled venom was fractionated by reversed-phase HPLC (RP-HPLC) using a Phenomenex Jupiter® C_{18} column (250 × 10 mm, 10 μm, 100 Å; Phenomenex, Torrence, CA, USA). Fractionation of the venom components was achieved using a linear gradient of two mobile phases: H_2O/0.05% trifluoroacetic acid (TFA; Auspep, Tullamarine, VIC, Australia) (solvent A) and 90% acetonitrile (ACN; Sigma-Aldrich, St. Louis, MO, USA)/H_2O/0.045% TFA (solvent B). Separation used a gradient of 0–60% solvent B in 120 min, 60–90% solvent B in 5 min, 90% solvent B for 10 min, and 90–0% solvent B in 5 min, at a flow rate of 3 mL/min. The venom component elution was monitored at 214 nm and 280 nm, and 0.5 min fractions were collected.

2.3. Liquid Chromatography/Mass Spectrometry (LC/MS)

Five individual scorpion venom samples and serial dilutions of adenosine and adenosine monophosphate (AMP) standards were analysed by liquid chromatography/mass spectrometry (LC/MS) using a Shimadzu LCMS-2020 mass spectrometer coupled to a Shimadzu Prominence HPLC system (Shimadzu, Kyoto, Japan) to allow quantitation of these molecules within the venom. A small amount of pooled venom was also analysed by LC/MS to observe the composition and determine the molecular weights of the molecules present. Then, 8 μL of the individually stored venom samples were injected in triplicate, 5 μL of the adenosine and AMP serial dilutions were injected in triplicate, and 10 μL of pooled venom (3 μL in 7 μL MilliQ water) was injected. The samples were injected via an autosampler (Shimadzu SIL-20AC$_{HT}$) onto a reversed-phase high-performance liquid chromatography (HPLC) column (Phenomonex Aeris 3.6 μm PEPTIDE XB-C18 100 Å; Phenomenex, Torrence, CA, USA) at 30 °C. Solvent delivery (solvent A: 0.1% formic acid (FA; Sigma-Aldrich, St. Louis, MO, USA)/water; solvent B: 90% acetonitrile (ACN; OPTIMA LCMS grade, Thermo Fisher Scientific, Scoresby, VIC, Australia)/0.09% formic acid/water) was via Shimadzu LC-20AD pumps at a flow rate of 0.250 mL/min. Samples were eluted with a 1% gradient (0–60% solvent B, 60 min; 60–90% solvent B, 5 min; 90% solvent B, 5 min; 90—0% solvent B, 5 min; 0% solvent B, 10 min), and the UV absorbance was observed at 214 nm and 280 nm on a Shimadzu SPD-20A detector. Mass spectra were collected in positive ion mode over a scan range of *m*/*z* 130–2000 and negative mode with a scan range of *m*/*z* 200–2000, with a detector voltage of 1.15 kV, nebulizing gas flow of 1.5 L/min, and drying gas flow of 3.0 L/min. Data were collected and analysed using the Shimadzu LabSolutions v5.96 software (Shimadzu, Kyoto, Japan). The 280 nm peak areas for the peaks containing adenosine and AMP, both in the individual venom samples and serial dilutions, were exported and analysed further in R version 3.6.1 [51]. The peak areas for standard samples and venom samples run in triplicate were averaged prior to further analysis. A linear model was fit to the serial dilution data to produce a standard curve, which was used to predict the quantity of adenosine and AMP in the 8 μL injection of each venom sample. These quantities were then divided by eight and multiplied by thirty to provide an estimate of the quantity contained within the whole venom samples. As the crude venoms were suspended in 30 μL of water, the total volume would be slightly greater than 30 μL; therefore, we calculated a slight underestimate of the quantity of adenosine and AMP contained within the venom.

2.4. Mass Spectrometry and NMR Analysis

NMR spectra were recorded at 290 K on a Bruker Avance III 600 MHz spectrometer (Bruker, Billerica, MA, USA) equipped with a cryoprobe. Samples were dissolved in 90% H_2O/10% D_2O (*v*/*v*) (100 μM). D_2O (99.9%) was obtained from Cambridge Isotope Laboratories, Woburn, MA, USA, for ^1H NMR measurements. Spectra were referenced to the water signal. Two-dimensional spectra included TOCSY, NOESY, DQF-COSY, HSQC, HMBC, and HSQC-TOCSY. TOCSY and NOESY mixing times of 80 ms and 500 ms, respectively, were used. Spectra were analysed using Topspin v3.6.1(Bruker, Billerica, MA, USA).

High-resolution mass spectrometry (MS) was performed using a SCIEX TOF/TOF™ 5800 MALDI (SCIEX, Framingham, MA, USA) and a SCIEX TripleTOF 6600 (SCIEX, Framingham, MA, USA) mass spectrometers. Matrix-assisted laser desorption ionisation mass spectrometry (MALDI-MS) samples were spotted on 384-well stainless steel target plates using 0.5 μL of sample and 0.5 μL of either α–cyano-4-hydroxycinnamic acid (CHCA; Sigma-Aldrich, St. Louis, MO, USA) matrix (7.5 mg/mL in 50% ACN/0.1% TFA) or a 2,5-dihydroxybenzoic acid (DHB; Sigma-Aldrich, St. Louis, MO, USA) matrix (10 mg/mL in 50% ethanol/0.1% TFA). Calibration was performed before spectra collection for each sample using Calibration Mix Solution 2 (SCIEX, Framingham, MA, USA). Spectra were acquired in reflector positive ion mode from *m*/*z* 200 to 400, and averaged over 2000 laser shots. Tandem-MS (MS/MS) was performed in 1 kV positive ion mode with collision-induced dissociation (CID) and averaged over 2000 shots. Samples were manually infused to the SCIEX TripleTOF 6600 mass spectrometer equipped with a DuoSpray Ion Source using the syringe pump and a 1 mL 4.61 mm i.d. Hamilton syringe (Reno, NV, USA) at a flow rate of 5 μL/min. Data acquisition was performed with Analyst® TF 1.7.1 software (SCIEX, Framingham, MA, USA). Product ion mass spectra were collected in positive ion mode with an accumulation time of 500 ms and a mass range of *m*/*z* 100 to 400. The source temperature was 470 °C, the curtain gas was set to 45 psi, the ion source gas 1 and 2 were set to 40 and 50 psi respectively, and the ion-spray voltage floating set to 4.9 kV. MS/MS data were collected on manually selected product ions under the same conditions with an accumulation time of 250 ms and a mass range of *m*/*z* 20 to 350.

3. Results

3.1. Venom Collection and Fractionation

Crude venom pooled from ~15 venom extractions of *H. waigiensis* scorpions was fractionated using RP-HPLC with a C_{18} semi-preparative RP-HPLC column, and 30 s fractions were collected (see Figure 1). A small sample of the pooled venom (3 μL) was also subjected to liquid chromatography/mass spectrometry (LC/MS) analysis, which provided a venom mass profile and identified the presence of a number of small molecules in early eluting peaks.

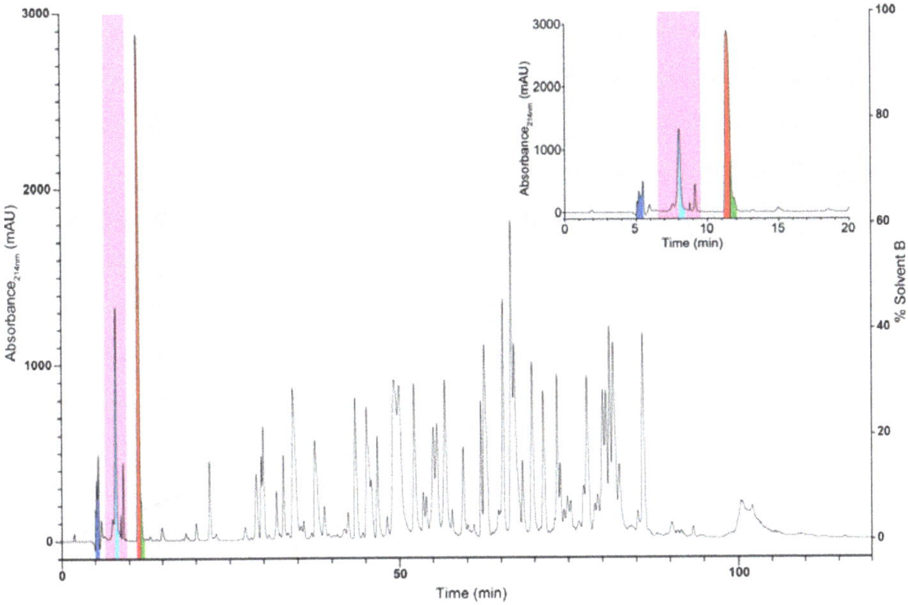

Figure 1. Reversed-phase high performance liquid chromatography (RP-HPLC) chromatogram of pooled crude *H. waigiensis* venom (Phenomenex Jupiter® C_{18} column; 250 × 10 mm, 10 μm, 100 Å; 3 mL/min flow rate; solvent A H_2O/0.05% TFA, solvent B 90% ACN/H_2O/0.045% TFA; 0–60% solvent B in 120 min, 60–90% solvent B in 5 min, 90% solvent B for 10 min, and 90–0% solvent B in 5 min; absorbance at 214 nm). The inset shows an expanded view of the highlighted area in the full chromatogram. The fractions of interest and corresponding peaks in the chromatogram are highlighted in dark blue (glutamic acid and aspartic acid), red (adenosine), and light blue (adenosine monophosphate), respectively. The pink section shows the fractions containing citric acid. The fraction highlighted in green is likely to be inosine. The dashed line shows the solvent B gradient.

3.2. NMR Analysis of RP-HPLC Fractions

Fractions collected from 5.5 to 23 min were analysed by one-dimensional ^{1}H NMR spectroscopy to observe the presence of small molecules, typified by sharp peaks and an absence of or minimal peaks in the amide region (see Figures 2–5). Fractions corresponding to the RP-HPLC peaks highlighted in dark blue and red in Figure 1 appeared to be relatively clean and produced good signal-to-noise ratios in the ^{1}H NMR spectra. Therefore, these fractions were selected for further analysis by two-dimensional NMR spectroscopy and the structures were elucidated based on correlations observed in the HMBC, HSQC, and COSY spectra. The dark blue peak highlighted in Figure 1 represented 1.28% of the total peak area within the 214 nm RP-HPLC chromatogram and was shown to contain glutamic acid and aspartic acid (see Figure 2). The red peak (Figure 1) represented 7.68% of the total peak area within the

214 nm RP-HPLC chromatogram and contained adenosine (see Figure 3). AMP (see Figure 4) was present within the light blue peak, which represented 2.42% of the total peak area of the RP-HPLC chromatogram (Figure 1). Fractions collected in the pink coloured region (Figure 1) contained citric acid, although as it does not have an absorbance profile at 214 nm nor 280 nm, it was not observed in the RP-HPLC chromatogram and was characterised based on NMR data (Figure 5). The green peak representing 0.33% of the total peak area of the 214 nm RP-HPLC chromatogram (Figure 1) contained a molecule with a mass 1 Da greater than adenosine, suggesting it may be inosine; however, we were unable to confirm its identity due to its low abundance and coelution with adenosine. A molecule was also observed with the mass of inosine monophosphate (IMP); however, low abundance and coelution with AMP on the RP-HPLC system prevented us from confirming its identity. Full 1D NMR spectra of RP-HPLC fractions and standards labelled with peak integration values used for molecular characterisation are contained within the Supplementary Materials.

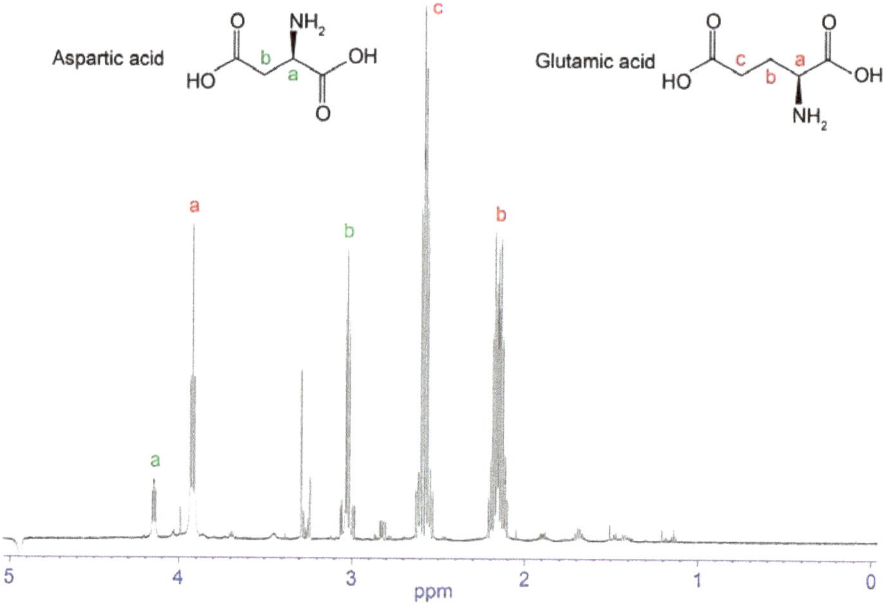

Figure 2. Chemical structure and 1D NMR spectrum of a fraction from *H. waigiensis* venom containing aspartic acid and glutamic acid. The assignments were derived based on two-dimensional NMR spectra and one-dimensional NMR spectra of glutamic acid and aspartic acid standards.

3.3. High-Resolution Mass Spectrometry

High-resolution mass spectrometry data collected using a SCIEX TripleTOF 6600 (SCIEX, Framingham, MA, USA) and SCIEX TOF/TOF™ 5800 MALDI (SCIEX, Framingham, MA, USA) were consistent with and confirmed the elucidated structures. For the dark blue peak fraction, $[M + H]^+$ ions were observed at m/z 148.0350 and m/z 134.0187, confirming the presence of glutamic acid (147.053158 Da) and aspartic acid (133.037508 Da). For the red peak fraction, a $[M + H]^+$ ion was observed at m/z 268.0783, confirming the presence of adenosine (267.096741 Da). Using a precursor ion of m/z 268.1, the red peak fraction showed a strong ion at m/z 136.0827 corresponding to adenine following fragmentation and cleavage of the ribose. For the light blue peak fraction, an $[M + H]^+$ ion was observed at m/z 348.0649, confirming the presence of AMP (347.063084 Da). Using a precursor ion of m/z 348.06 on this fraction showed an ion at m/z 136.1006, which also corresponded to adenine following fragmentation and cleavage of the ribose.

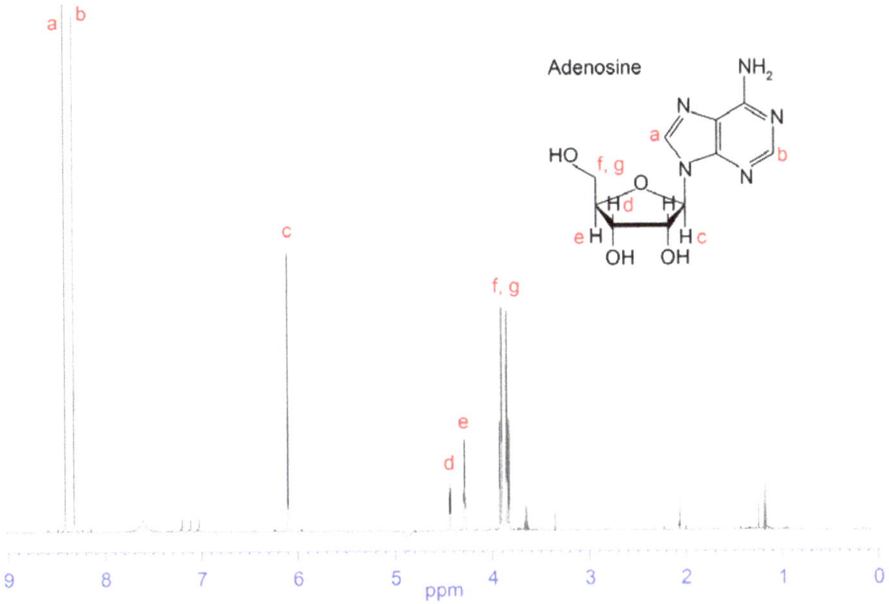

Figure 3. Chemical structure and 1D NMR spectrum of a fraction from *H. waigiensis* venom containing adenosine. The assignments were derived based on one-dimensional NMR spectra of an adenosine standard.

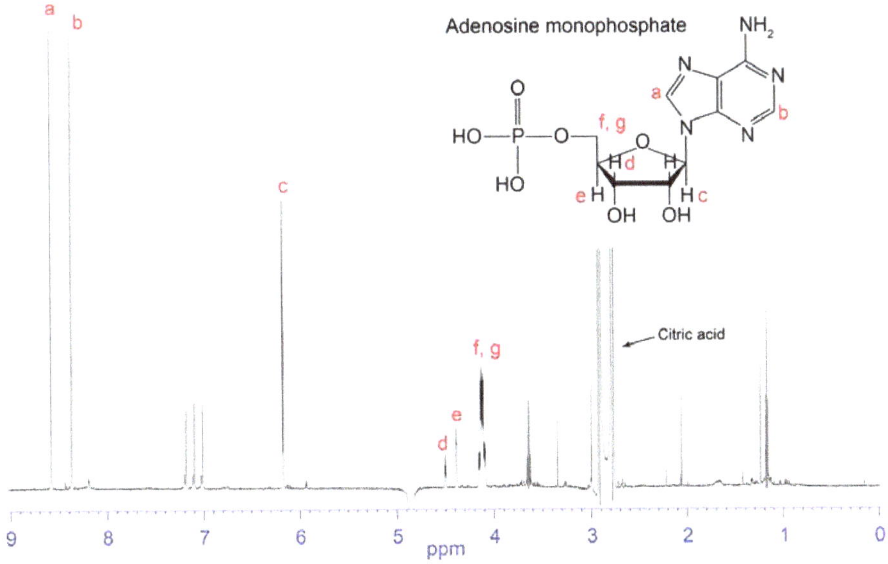

Figure 4. Chemical structure and 1D NMR spectrum of a fraction from *H. waigiensis* venom containing adenosine monophosphate. The assignments were derived based on one-dimensional NMR spectra of an adenosine monophosphate standard. The presence of citric acid is also highlighted.

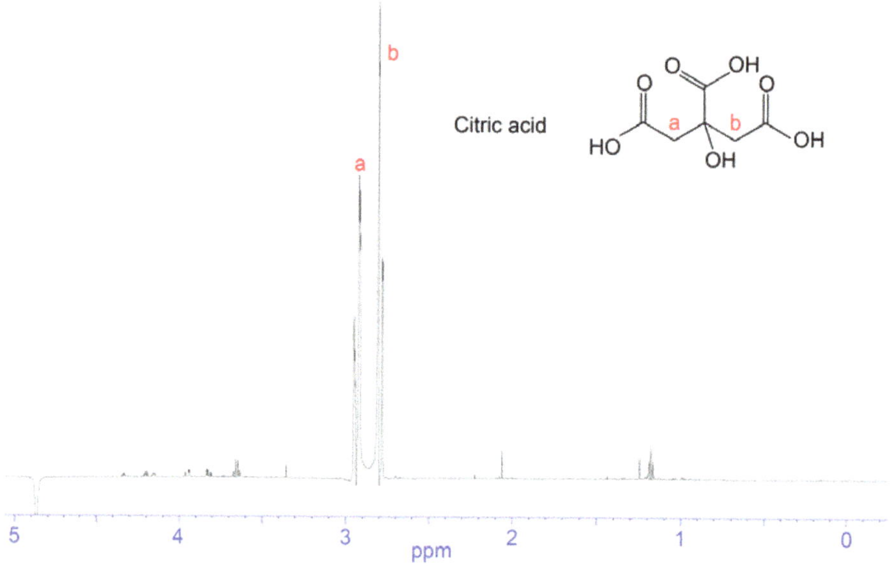

Figure 5. Chemical structure and 1D NMR spectrum of a fraction from *H. waigiensis* venom containing citric acid. The assignments were derived based on one-dimensional NMR spectra of a citric acid standard.

3.4. Adenosine Quantitation by LC/MS

Five adult scorpions were milked individually to estimate the quantities of adenosine and AMP contained within the total venom by comparing the LC/MS 280 nm absorbance peak areas against those of a serial dilution of standards run under identical chemical conditions. All five scorpion venoms contained adenosine. Quantities of approximately 4.462 µg and 2.448 µg were present within the two male venoms; and 4.555 µg, 2.016 µg, and 5.808 µg were present within the female venoms. The abundance of AMP displayed greater variation between individuals and was absent from two of the female scorpions at detectable levels. The estimated quantity of AMP within the whole venoms of the two males were 0.682 µg and 2.778 µg, while the single female venom contained 0.318 µg. It is important to note that these values are slight underestimates of the true quantity contained within the venom gland. By comparing the volumes of venom collected in the pipette tip against set volumes of water, we estimated that each scorpion produced between 1.5 µL and 3.5 µL during milking, and therefore an average milking contained roughly 2.5 µL of venom. This indicates that the values calculated from 30 µL of the sample are slight underestimates of the true total, but this variation is small in comparison to the large differences observed between individuals.

4. Discussion

Adenosine, AMP, citric acid, glutamic acid, and aspartic acid were all found to be present within the venom of *H. waigiensis*. Molecules were also observed with masses corresponding to inosine and IMP; however, we were unable to confirm their identity due to low abundances and coelution with adenosine and AMP, respectively.

4.1. Adenosine

Adenosine has been previously identified within the venom of the scorpion *Heterometrus laoticus* [14,15], and is a known constituent of other arthropod venoms, including those belonging to the spiders *Haplopelma lividum* and *Latrodectus menavodi* [31,52], the wasp *Cyphononyx dorsalis* [53], and the ant *Pseudomyrmex triplarinus* [54]. Inosine was also found to be present within the venom of *L. menavodi* [31] and other spider species, including *Parawixia bistriata* [32], *Cyriopagopus hainanus* (*Selenocosmia huwena*) [55], *Loxosceles reclusa* [56], and six more species [57]. Purine nucleosides such as adenosine and inosine are common constituents of elapid and viperine snake venoms and are thought to play important accessory roles in helping snakes envenomate and incapacitate their prey [8,10,43,58]. Adenosine has a wide range of physiological effects in mammalian targets, including inducing vasodilation, causing increased vascular permeability, increasing blood coagulation time, and inhibiting neurotransmitter release [8,14]. The effects of inosine are not so well understood, but it is also known to increase vascular permeability and induce hypotension through selective binding with mast cell A_3 receptors [59], as well as having vasodilatory properties ([60]; reviewed in [8]). Aird [8] provides an overview of the large body of literature studying the physiological effects of adenosine and inosine in mammalian targets, and summarises how these properties may translate to a functional role within a venom. For example, by inducing vasodilation and increasing vascular permeability venomous organisms may improve their systemic envenomation of the target [8,10,43,58].

Whilst the effects of adenosine and inosine in mammalian targets are relatively well understood, scorpions do not solely utilise their venom to defend against mammals [61]. Unlike elapid and viperid snakes, which frequently target vertebrates, scorpions predominantly hunt invertebrates, although in certain environments they are known to take small vertebrates such as blind snakes [62]. Whilst Aird [8] discusses the role of adenosine and inosine in snake venoms that target mammalian prey, it is unclear how closely this translates to scorpions aiming to incapacitate invertebrate prey. Purinoreceptors evolved at an early date, and therefore structural similarities exist between the receptors that vertebrates and invertebrates possess [63]. It is, therefore, possible that adenosine will interact with invertebrate and vertebrate purinoreceptors in similar ways [8,63], but morphological differences between them may lead to different overall effects. For example, insects and mammals have distinctly different circulatory systems, and therefore the hypotensive effects induced by adenosine in mammals may not directly translate to an insect model. It is, however, likely that other effects of adenosine, such as reducing the release of neurotransmitters, may be more closely paralleled between insects and mammals [43]. IMP induces delayed paralysis when injected into termites, but it remains untested whether inosine would have the same effect [32]. Because *H. waigiensis* scorpions generally attack invertebrate prey but have to defend themselves against vertebrates, their venom contains components effective specifically against vertebrates and invertebrates, as well as components against both [64]. It is currently unclear whether adenosine facilitates the envenomation and incapacitation of invertebrate prey when injected alongside other venom components, or whether it is more heavily involved in defence against vertebrates. It could also function within the venom to aid capture of small vertebrate prey in environments with low invertebrate prey abundance [62].

4.2. AMP

In addition to adenosine, we identified AMP within the venom of *H. waigiensis*. Similar to adenosine, AMP has hypotensive properties, and therefore could act in a similar way to facilitate envenomation in mammalian aggressors [43,65]. Aird [43] found that only a small number of snake venoms contained AMP compared with adenosine, but stated that the presence of purine monophosphates within venoms is unsurprising due to the hypotensive effects they share with free purines. We are unaware of previous reports of AMP, adenosine diphosphate (ADP), or adenosine triphosphate (ATP) from scorpion venoms; however, they are present within different tarantula venoms, including those belonging to *H. lividum*, *Lasiodora* sp., *Aphonopelma* sp., and *Aphonopelma hentzi* (*Dugesiella hentzi* and *Eurypelma californicum*) [30,33,52,66,67]. Unlike adenosine, which binds to

P1 receptors, ADP and ATP bind to P2 receptors [68], with evidence suggesting that they also have auxiliary roles alongside toxins within venom [30,66]. As with adenosine, ADP and AMP possess hypotensive properties and may fulfil a similar auxiliary function within the venom [8,66]. On the other hand, ATP is less vasodilatory and can lead to hypertension [8,65], and therefore may function differently within the venom. However, Chan, Geren, Howell, and Odell [30] showed that ATP works synergistically with the specific toxins to increase toxicity towards mice. It is possible that adenosine and AMP may act in a similar way to increase the overall toxicity of scorpion venom. To test this, future work could perform a bioassay injecting adenosine and AMP alongside other venom toxins, looking for synergistic or auxiliary effects. Of the five scorpions we tested, the whole venoms contained between 2.016 μg and 5.808 μg of adenosine. Intravenous injection of much lower quantities (0.1 μg) in mice induced hypotension [65], while topically applied 10^{-5} M adenosine solution increased vascular permeability in hamster cheek pouches [69]. This suggests that it is likely that the quantity of adenosine contained within the venom is large enough to elicit such effects at the site of injection.

4.3. Citric Acid/Citrate

Citric acid or citrate is a common constituent of venoms, present within spider, snake, bee, wasp, ant, and scorpion venoms [16,38,41]. Its presence within spider venoms is particularly well documented, having been recorded from at least 48 species belonging to 16 families [38]. Despite the common occurrence of citrate within venoms, its role is not fully understood, and it may serve multiple functions. One proposed function of venom citrate is the inhibition of toxins within the venom gland, thereby preventing self-harm [44]. As citrate can act as a chelator and form strong complexes with divalent metal ions such as Ca^{2+}, Mg^{2+}, and Zn^{2+}, it can inhibit venom proteins that are dependent on these metal ions [44]. Citrate, therefore, inhibits venom proteins such as calcium-ion-dependant phospholipase A_2 (PLA_2) neurotoxins and myotoxins, as well as zinc-ion-dependant venom metalloprotease haemorrhagic toxins [38,41]. For example, it has been demonstrated experimentally that honey bee (*Apis mellifera*) venom PLA_2 is at least partially inhibited by citrate [16], and that the citrate concentration present within the fer-de-lance snake (*Bothrops asper*) venom is high enough to likely completely inhibit PLA_2 and 5′-nucleotidase activity, whilst partially inhibiting (75%) phosphodiesterase activity [44]. Scorpion venoms can contain both PLA_2 proteins [70] and metalloproteases [71] within their venom; therefore, citrate may act as an inhibitor of these toxins within the venom gland. One study found that dried Arizona bark scorpion (*Centruroides sculpturatus*) venom contained 7.77 ± 1.2% citrate, but the extent that citrate is present in the venoms of different scorpion species remains unknown [16]. It is, therefore, important to test more scorpion venoms for the presence of citrate, particularly those well known to contain PLA_2 or metalloproteases, to identify if this is its primary function within scorpion venom. Other proposed functions of citric acid within the venom gland include having direct antimicrobial effects or enhancing the effects of antimicrobial molecules [38,72]. Furthermore, it has been suggested that in spiders citric acid may be present to counter cationic peptides and acylpolyamines within the venom gland [38]. At the time of writing no acylpolyamines have been characterised from scorpion venoms, but cationic peptides are present [73–75]. It is likely that citrate has multiple functions within the venom gland of scorpions, but additionally it may have a role once injected into the target organism. An example of this has been demonstrated with the cardiotoxin A3 (CTX A3) from the Taiwan cobra (*Naja atra*), where heparin-sulphate-mediated cell retention of CTX A3 is citrate dependant [76]. However, it is currently unknown if citrate acts in conjunction with any scorpion toxins within an envenomated organism.

4.4. Free Amino Acids

Free amino acids have been widely reported from snake venoms [10,77] and spider venoms [33,36,78], but to our knowledge their possible functions within the venoms remain unknown. We found aspartic acid and glutamic acid to be present within *H. waigiensis* venom, but these molecules were only present in low abundance (Figure 1). The fraction containing glutamic acid and aspartic acid contained other small molecules at lower abundance, indicated by the presence of extra peaks within the NMR spectra (Figure 2), but we were unable to characterise these molecules. A cocktail of amino acids is naturally found in body fluids and can be released from degrading cells, and these molecules may not have a function contributing to the toxicity of the venom. However, if this was the case we might expect to see a more diverse range of amino acids present within the venom. It is possible that other amino acids are present within the venom of *H. waigiensis* and we were only able to identify aspartic acid and glutamic acid as we were able to attain the cleanest NMR spectra for these molecules, but the presence of these same amino acids in spider venoms suggests they may have some specific function. In tarantulas, glutamic acid has been found in the venom of *H. lividum*, and in two separate studies both aspartic acid and glutamic acid were identified from *A. hentzi* [33,36]. Furthermore, NMR screening has shown that aspartic acid is found within the venom of the spider *Pisaura mirabilis*, while glutamic acid is a common component of many different araneomorph spider venoms [34]. Glutamic acid, or the conjugate base glutamate, is an important neurotransmitter in the central nervous system [79], and injection in certain parts of the body will likely disrupt the nervous system. More work is required to explain the presence of these molecules in venom.

4.5. Conclusions

Whilst scorpion venoms have been subject to intensive study, research has been heavily skewed to focus on peptide venom constituents. Members of the family Buthidae have also been subject to more intensive study than other scorpion families, as Buthidae contains all medically significant species [50]. *H. waigiensis* belongs to the family Hormuridae [80], which has received comparatively little attention from researchers. It may be that members of this family and other neglected families also utilise small molecules within their venom arsenals. To our knowledge, adenosine has previously been reported from just one other scorpion species, *H. laoticus*, which belongs to the family Scorpionidae [15]. Scorpions show great toxin diversity between species, and the presence of adenosine in two scorpion species belonging to different families suggests that it may be more commonly utilised by other species. Furthermore, to our knowledge this study provides the first direct evidence of nucleotides (AMP) and specific amino acids within a scorpion venom. Our investigation highlights that the small molecules contained within *H. waigiensis* venom are similar to those found in other closely and distantly related venomous organisms, suggesting that such molecules may have important functions in the venoms of a wide range of organisms. Future work should aim to investigate the extent that small molecules are utilised by different scorpion species, paying particular attention to understudied families. Characterising the suite of small molecules within scorpion venoms will help us gain a greater understanding of the biochemical mechanisms involved in scorpion envenomation. This understanding may allow for the development of improved and optimised treatment of scorpion envenomation, or allow facilitation or modulation of the action of developed scorpion-venom-derived therapeutics and bioinsecticides. Furthermore, the abundance and diversity of small-molecule venom constituents in different species of scorpions remains largely unstudied, and uncharacterised bioactive molecules could have potential applications in pharmacology.

Supplementary Materials: The following are available online at http://www.mdpi.com/2227-9059/8/8/259/s1.

Author Contributions: E.R.J.E, D.T.W., and N.L.D. designed the study. E.R.J.E. and D.T.W. carried out the experiments. E.R.J.E., D.T.W., and L.M. analysed the results. E.R.J.E., D.T.W., and N.L.D. wrote the paper. T.D.N. edited the paper. All authors analysed the results and approved the final version of the manuscript.

Funding: This research received no external funding. The Northcote Trust supports E.R.J.E. with a Northcote Graduate Scholarship.

Acknowledgments: This work was supported in part by an Australian Research Council Linkage Infrastructure, Equipment and Facilities (LIEF) grant (#LE160100218). The authors are grateful to Jeremy Potriquet and Yide Wong for assistance with the SCIEX 6600 TripleTOF mass spectrometry and Alan Henderson (Minibeast Wildlife, QLD) for providing scorpion specimens.

Conflicts of Interest: The authors declare no conflict of interest.

References

1. Chippaux, J.-P.; Goyffon, M. Epidemiology of scorpionism: A global appraisal. *Acta Trop.* **2008**, *107*, 71–79. [CrossRef] [PubMed]
2. Ahmadi, S.; Knerr, J.M.; Argemi, L.; Bordon, K.C.; Pucca, M.B.; Cerni, F.A.; Arantes, E.C.; Çalışkan, F.; Laustsen, A.H. Scorpion venom: Detriments and benefits. *Biomedicines* **2020**, *8*, 118. [CrossRef] [PubMed]
3. King, G.F. Venoms as a platform for human drugs: Translating toxins into therapeutics. *Expert Opin. Biol. Ther.* **2011**, *11*, 1469–1484. [CrossRef] [PubMed]
4. Ortiz, E.; Gurrola, G.B.; Schwartz, E.F.; Possani, L.D. Scorpion venom components as potential candidates for drug development. *Toxicon* **2015**, *93*, 125–135. [CrossRef] [PubMed]
5. Possani, L.D.; Becerril, B.; Delepierre, M.; Tytgat, J. Scorpion toxins specific for Na+-channels. *Eur. J. Biochem.* **1999**, *264*, 287–300. [CrossRef]
6. Smith, J.J.; Herzig, V.; King, G.F.; Alewood, P.F. The insecticidal potential of venom peptides. *Cell. Mol. Life Sci.* **2013**, *70*, 3665–3693. [CrossRef]
7. Inceoglu, B.; Lango, J.; Jing, J.; Chen, L.; Doymaz, F.; Pessah, I.N.; Hammock, B.D. One scorpion, two venoms: Prevenom of *Parabuthus transvaalicus* acts as an alternative type of venom with distinct mechanism of action. *Proc. Natl. Acad. Sci. USA* **2003**, *100*, 922–927. [CrossRef]
8. Aird, S.D. Ophidian envenomation strategies and the role of purines. *Toxicon* **2002**, *40*, 335–393. [CrossRef]
9. Daly, N.L.; Wilson, D. Structural diversity of arthropod venom toxins. *Toxicon* **2018**, *152*, 46–56. [CrossRef]
10. Villar-Briones, A.; Aird, S. Organic and peptidyl constituents of snake venoms: The picture is vastly more complex than we imagined. *Toxins (Basel)* **2018**, *10*, 392. [CrossRef]
11. Wilson, D.; Boyle, G.; McIntyre, L.; Nolan, M.; Parsons, P.; Smith, J.; Tribolet, L.; Loukas, A.; Liddell, M.; Rash, L. The aromatic head group of spider toxin polyamines influences toxicity to cancer cells. *Toxins (Basel)* **2017**, *9*, 346. [CrossRef]
12. Banerjee, S.; Gnanamani, E.; Lynch, S.R.; Zuñiga, F.Z.; Jiménez-Vargas, J.M.; Possani, L.D.; Zare, R.N. An alkaloid from scorpion venom: Chemical structure and synthesis. *J. Nat. Prod.* **2018**, *81*, 1899–1904. [CrossRef] [PubMed]
13. Carcamo-Noriega, E.N.; Sathyamoorthi, S.; Banerjee, S.; Gnanamani, E.; Mendoza-Trujillo, M.; Mata-Espinosa, D.; Hernández-Pando, R.; Veytia-Bucheli, J.I.; Possani, L.D.; Zare, R.N. 1,4-Benzoquinone antimicrobial agents against *Staphylococcus aureus* and *Mycobacterium tuberculosis* derived from scorpion venom. *Proc. Natl. Acad. Sci. USA* **2019**, *116*, 12642–12647. [CrossRef] [PubMed]
14. Thien, T.V.; Anh, H.N.; Trang, N.T.T.; Van Trung, P.; Khoa, N.C.; Osipov, A.; Dubovskii, P.; Ivanov, I.; Arseniev, A.; Tsetlin, V. Low-molecular-weight compounds with anticoagulant activity from the scorpion *Heterometrus laoticus* venom. *Dokl. Biochem. Biophys.* **2017**, *476*, 316–319. [CrossRef] [PubMed]
15. Tran, T.; Hoang, A.; Nguyen, T.; Phung, T.; Nguyen, K.; Osipov, A.; Ivanov, I.; Tsetlin, V.; Utkin, Y. Anticoagulant activity of low-molecular weight compounds from *Heterometrus laoticus* scorpion venom. *Toxins (Basel)* **2017**, *9*, 343. [CrossRef]
16. Fenton, A.W.; West, P.R.; Odell, G.V.; Hudiburg, S.M.; Ownby, C.L.; Mills, J.N.; Scroggins, B.T.; Shannon, S.B. Arthropod venom citrate inhibits phospholipase A2. *Toxicon* **1995**, *33*, 763–770. [CrossRef]
17. Francke, O.F. Conspectus Genericus Scorpionorum 1758–1985 (Arachnida: Scorpiones) updated through 2018. *Zootaxa* **2019**, *4657*, 1–56. [CrossRef]
18. Arjunwadkar, A.; Reddy, S.R.R. Spermidine in the venom of the scorpion, *Palamneus phipsoni*. *Toxicon* **1983**, *21*, 321–325. [CrossRef]
19. Adam, K.; Weiss, C. Distribution of 5-hydroxytryptamine in scorpion venoms. *Nature* **1959**, *183*, 1398–1399. [CrossRef]
20. Dai, L.; Corzo, G.; Naoki, H.; Andriantsiferana, M.; Nakajima, T. Purification, structure–function analysis, and molecular characterization of novel linear peptides from scorpion *Opisthacanthus madagascariensis*. *Biochem. Biophys. Res. Commun.* **2002**, *293*, 1514–1522. [CrossRef]
21. Luna-Ramírez, K.; Quintero-Hernandez, V.; Juárez-González, V.R.; Possani, L.D. Whole transcriptome of the venom gland from *Urodacus yaschenkoi* scorpion. *PLoS ONE* **2015**, *10*, e0127883. [CrossRef] [PubMed]
22. Hisada, M.; Fujita, T.; Naoki, H.; Itagaki, Y.; Irie, H.; Miyashita, M.; Nakajima, T. Structures of spider toxins: Hydroxyindole-3-acetylpolyamines and a new generalized structure of type-E compounds obtained from the venom of the Joro spider, *Nephila clavata*. *Toxicon* **1998**, *36*, 1115–1125. [CrossRef]

23. Itagaki, Y.; Fujita, T.; Naoki, H.; Yasuhara, T.; Andriantsiferana, M.; Nakajima, T. Detection of new spider toxins from a *Nephilengys borbonica* venom gland using on-line μ-column HPLC continuous flow (FRIT) FAB LC/MS and MS/MS. *Nat. Toxins* **1997**, *5*, 1–13. [CrossRef]
24. McCormick, K.D.; Meinwald, J. Neurotoxic acylpolyamines from spider venoms. *J. Chem. Ecol.* **1993**, *19*, 2411–2451. [CrossRef]
25. Palma, M.S.; Nakajima, T. A natural combinatorial chemistry strategy in acylpolyamine toxins from nephilinae orb-web spiders. *Toxin Rev.* **2005**, *24*, 209–234. [CrossRef]
26. Skinner, W.S.; Dennis, P.A.; Lui, A.; Carney, R.L.; Quistad, G.B. Chemical characterization of acylpolyamine toxins from venom of a trap-door spider and two tarantulas. *Toxicon* **1990**, *28*, 541–546. [CrossRef]
27. Cesar, L.M.; Mendes, M.A.; Tormena, C.F.; Marques, M.R.; De Souza, B.M.; Saidemberg, D.M.; Bittencourt, J.C.; Palma, M.S. Isolation and chemical characterization of PwTx-II: A novel alkaloid toxin from the venom of the spider *Parawixia bistriata* (Araneidae, Araneae). *Toxicon* **2005**, *46*, 786–796. [CrossRef]
28. Marques, M.R.; Mendes, M.A.; Tormena, C.F.; Souza, B.M.; Marcondes Cesar, L.M.; Rittner, R.; Palma, M.S. Structure determination of a tetrahydro-β-carboline of arthropod origin: A novel alkaloid-toxin subclass from the web of spider *Nephila clavipes*. *Chem. Biodivers.* **2005**, *2*, 525–534. [CrossRef]
29. Saidemberg, D.M.; Ferreira, M.A.; Takahashi, T.N.; Gomes, P.C.; Cesar-Tognoli, L.M.; da Silva-Filho, L.C.; Tormena, C.F.; da Silva, G.V.; Palma, M.S. Monoamine oxidase inhibitory activities of indolylalkaloid toxins from the venom of the colonial spider *Parawixia bistriata*: Functional characterization of PwTX-I. *Toxicon* **2009**, *54*, 717–724. [CrossRef]
30. Chan, T.K.; Geren, C.; Howell, D.; Odell, G. Adenosine triphosphate in tarantula spider venoms and its synergistic effect with the venom toxin. *Toxicon* **1975**, *13*, 61–66. [CrossRef]
31. Horni, A.; Weickmann, D.; Hesse, M. The main products of the low molecular mass fraction in the venom of the spider *Latrodectus menavodi*. *Toxicon* **2001**, *39*, 425–428. [CrossRef]
32. Rodrigues, M.C.A.; Guizzo, R.; Gobbo-Neto, L.; Ward, R.J.; Lopes, N.P.; dos Santos, W.F. The biological activity in mammals and insects of the nucleosidic fraction from the spider *Parawixia bistriata*. *Toxicon* **2004**, *43*, 375–383. [CrossRef] [PubMed]
33. Savel-Niemann, A. Tarantula (*Eurypelma californicum*) venom, a multicomponent system. *Biol. Chem. Hoppe Seyler* **1989**, *370*, 485–498. [CrossRef] [PubMed]
34. Schroeder, F.C.; Taggi, A.E.; Gronquist, M.; Malik, R.U.; Grant, J.B.; Eisner, T.; Meinwald, J. NMR-spectroscopic screening of spider venom reveals sulfated nucleosides as major components for the brown recluse and related species. *Proc. Natl. Acad. Sci. USA* **2008**, *105*, 14283–14287. [CrossRef] [PubMed]
35. Taggi, A.E.; Meinwald, J.; Schroeder, F.C. A new approach to natural products discovery exemplified by the identification of sulfated nucleosides in spider venom. *J. Am. Chem. Soc.* **2004**, *126*, 10364–10369. [CrossRef]
36. Schanbacher, F.; Lee, C.; Hall, J.; Wilson, I.; Howell, D.; Odell, G. Composition and properties of tarantula *Dugesiella hentzi* (Girard) venom. *Toxicon* **1973**, *11*, 21–29. [CrossRef]
37. Escoubas, P.; Diochot, S.; Corzo, G. Structure and pharmacology of spider venom neurotoxins. *Biochimie* **2000**, *82*, 893–907. [CrossRef]
38. Kuhn-Nentwig, L.; Stöcklin, R.; Nentwig, W. Venom composition and strategies in spiders: Is everything possible? *Adv. Insect Physiol.* **2011**, *40*, 1–86.
39. Vassilevski, A.; Kozlov, S.; Grishin, E. Molecular diversity of spider venom. *Biochemistry (Moscow)* **2009**, *74*, 1505–1534. [CrossRef]
40. Gomes, P.C.; de Souza, B.M.; Dias, N.B.; Cesar-Tognoli, L.M.; Silva-Filho, L.C.; Tormena, C.F.; Rittner, R.; Richardson, M.; Cordeiro, M.N.; Palma, M.S. Nigriventrine: A low molecular mass neuroactive compound from the venom of the spider *Phoneutria nigriventer*. *Toxicon* **2011**, *57*, 266–274. [CrossRef]
41. Odell, G.; Fenton, A.; Ownby, C.; Doss, M.; Schmidt, J. The role of venom citrate. *Toxicon* **1999**, *37*, 407–409. [PubMed]
42. Yoshioka, M.; Narai, N.; Teshima, T.; Matsumoto, T.; Wakamiya, T.; Shiba, T.; Tokoro, N.; Okauchi, T.; Kono, Y. Characterization of a new insecticide, clavamine, from the venom of a spider, *Nephila clavata* by use of a synthetic compound. *Chem. Pharm. Bull. (Tokyo)* **1992**, *40*, 3005–3008. [CrossRef]
43. Aird, S.D. Taxonomic distribution and quantitative analysis of free purine and pyrimidine nucleosides in snake venoms. *Comp. Biochem. Physiol. B Biochem. Mol. Biol.* **2005**, *140*, 109–126. [CrossRef] [PubMed]
44. Francis, B.; Seebart, C.; Kaiser, I.I. Citrate is an endogenous inhibitor of snake venom enzymes by metal-ion chelation. *Toxicon* **1992**, *30*, 1239–1246. [CrossRef]

45. Koch, L. The taxonomy, geographic distribution and evolutionary radiation of Australo-Papuan scorpions. *Rec. West. Aust. Mus.* **1977**, *5 Pt 2*, 83–367.
46. Monod, L.; Volschenk, E. *Liocheles litodactylus* (Scorpiones: Liochelidae): An unusual new *Liocheles* species from the Australian wet tropics (Queensland). *Mem. Qld. Mus.* **2004**, *49*, 675–690.
47. Isbister, G.; Volschenk, E.; Seymour, J. Scorpion stings in Australia: Five definite stings and a review. *Intern. Med. J.* **2004**, *34*, 427–430. [CrossRef]
48. Smith, J.J.; Hill, J.M.; Little, M.J.; Nicholson, G.M.; King, G.F.; Alewood, P.F. Unique scorpion toxin with a putative ancestral fold provides insight into evolution of the inhibitor cystine knot motif. *Proc. Natl. Acad. Sci. USA* **2011**, *108*, 10478–10483. [CrossRef]
49. Smith, J.J.; Vetter, I.; Lewis, R.J.; Peigneur, S.; Tytgat, J.; Lam, A.; Gallant, E.M.; Beard, N.A.; Alewood, P.F.; Dulhunty, A.F. Multiple actions of φ-LITX-Lw1a on ryanodine receptors reveal a functional link between scorpion DDH and ICK toxins. *Proc. Natl. Acad. Sci. USA* **2013**, *110*, 8906–8911. [CrossRef]
50. Santos, M.S.; Silva, C.G.; Neto, B.S.; Júnior, C.R.G.; Lopes, V.H.; Júnior, A.G.T.; Bezerra, D.A.; Luna, J.V.; Cordeiro, J.B.; Júnior, J.G. Clinical and epidemiological aspects of scorpionism in the world: A systematic review. *Wilderness Environ. Med.* **2016**, *27*, 504–518. [CrossRef]
51. R Core Team. *R: A Language and Environment for Statistical Computing*; R Foundation for Statistical Computing: Vienna, Austria, 2019.
52. Moore, S.; Smyth, W.F.; Gault, V.A.; O'Kane, E.; McClean, S. Mass spectrometric characterisation and quantitation of selected low molecular mass compounds from the venom of *Haplopelma lividum* (Theraphosidae). *Rapid Commun. Mass Spectrom.* **2009**, *23*, 1747–1755. [CrossRef] [PubMed]
53. Konno, K.; Hisada, M.; Naoki, H.; Itagaki, Y.; Yasuhara, T.; Juliano, M.A.; Juliano, L.; Palma, M.S.; Yamane, T.; Nakajima, T. Isolation and sequence determination of peptides in the venom of the spider wasp (*Cyphononyx dorsalis*) guided by matrix-assisted laser desorption/ionization time of flight (MALDI-TOF) mass spectrometry. *Toxicon* **2001**, *39*, 1257–1260. [CrossRef]
54. Hink, W.; Romstedt, K.; Burke, J.; Doskotch, R.; Feller, D. Inhibition of human platelet aggregation and secretion by ant venom and a compound isolated from venom. *Inflammation* **1989**, *13*, 175–184. [CrossRef] [PubMed]
55. Yimin, S.; Bingkun, X.; Songping, L.; Shunyi, L. Separation and identification of inosine in the *Selenocosmia huwena* spider. *Chin. J. Anal. Chem.* **1995**, *9*, 25.
56. Geren, C.R.; Chan, T.K.; Howell, D.E.; Odell, G.V. Partial characterization of the low molecular weight fractions of the extract of the venom apparatus of the brown recluse spider and of its hemolymph. *Toxicon* **1975**, *13*, 233–238. [CrossRef]
57. venoMS. Available online: https://www.venoms.ch/ (accessed on 30 June 2020).
58. Laustsen, A.H. Toxin synergism in snake venoms. *Toxin Rev.* **2016**, *35*, 165–170. [CrossRef]
59. Tilley, S.L.; Wagoner, V.A.; Salvatore, C.A.; Jacobson, M.A.; Koller, B.H. Adenosine and inosine increase cutaneous vasopermeability by activating A3 receptors on mast cells. *J. Clin. Investig.* **2000**, *105*, 361–367. [CrossRef]
60. Juhasz-Nagy, A.; Aviado, D.M. Inosine as a cardiotonic agent that reverses adrenergic beta blockade. *J. Pharmacol. Exp. Ther.* **1977**, *202*, 683–695.
61. Evans, E.R.J.; Northfield, T.D.; Daly, N.L.; Wilson, D.T. Venom costs and optimization in scorpions. *Front. Ecol. Evol.* **2019**, *7*, 196. [CrossRef]
62. McCormick, S.; Polis, G.A. Arthropods that prey on vertebrates. *Biol. Rev. Camb. Philos. Soc.* **1982**, *57*, 29–58. [CrossRef]
63. Burnstock, G. Purinoceptors: Ontogeny and phylogeny. *Drug Dev. Res.* **1996**, *39*, 204–242. [CrossRef]
64. Gangur, A.N.; Smout, M.; Liddell, M.J.; Seymour, J.E.; Wilson, D.; Northfield, T.D. Changes in predator exposure, but not in diet, induce phenotypic plasticity in scorpion venom. *Proc. R. Soc. Lond. B Biol. Sci.* **2017**, *284*, 20171364. [CrossRef] [PubMed]
65. Gillespie, J. The biological significance of the linkages in adenosine triphosphoric acid. *J. Physiol.* **1934**, *80*, 345. [CrossRef] [PubMed]
66. Horta, C.; Rezende, B.; Oliveira-Mendes, B.; Carmo, A.; Capettini, L.; Silva, J.; Gomes, M.; Chávez-Olórtegui, C.; Bravo, C.; Lemos, V. ADP is a vasodilator component from *Lasiodora* sp. mygalomorph spider venom. *Toxicon* **2013**, *72*, 102–112. [CrossRef]

67. Nentwig, W. The species referred to as Eurypelma californicum (Theraphosidae) in more than 100 publications is likely to be *Aphonopelma hentzi*. *J. Arachnol.* **2012**, *40*, 128–131. [CrossRef]
68. Burnstock, G. Purine and pyrimidine receptors. *Cell. Mol. Life Sci.* **2007**, *64*, 1471. [CrossRef]
69. Gawlowski, D.M.; Duran, W.N. Dose-related effects of adenosine and bradykinin on microvascular permselectivity to macromolecules in the hamster cheek pouch. *Circ. Res.* **1986**, *58*, 348–355. [CrossRef]
70. Krayem, N.; Gargouri, Y. Scorpion venom phospholipases A2: A minireview. *Toxicon* **2020**, *184*, 48–54. [CrossRef]
71. Ortiz, E.; Rendón-Anaya, M.; Rego, S.C.; Schwartz, E.F.; Possani, L.D. Antarease-like Zn-metalloproteases are ubiquitous in the venom of different scorpion genera. *Biochim. Biophys. Acta* **2014**, *1840*, 1738–1746. [CrossRef]
72. Lee, Y.L.; Thrupp, L.; Owens, J.; Cesario, T.; Shanbrom, E. Bactericidal activity of citrate against Gram-positive cocci. *Lett. Appl. Microbiol.* **2001**, *33*, 349–351. [CrossRef]
73. Gao, B.; Xu, J.; del Carmen Rodriguez, M.; Lanz-Mendoza, H.; Hernández-Rivas, R.; Du, W.; Zhu, S. Characterization of two linear cationic antimalarial peptides in the scorpion *Mesobuthus eupeus*. *Biochimie* **2010**, *92*, 350–359. [CrossRef] [PubMed]
74. Moerman, L.; Bosteels, S.; Noppe, W.; Willems, J.; Clynen, E.; Schoofs, L.; Thevissen, K.; Tytgat, J.; Van Eldere, J.; Van Der Walt, J. Antibacterial and antifungal properties of α-helical, cationic peptides in the venom of scorpions from southern Africa. *Eur. J. Biochem.* **2002**, *269*, 4799–4810. [CrossRef] [PubMed]
75. Willems, J.; Noppe, W.; Moerman, L.; van der Walt, J.; Verdonck, F. Cationic peptides from scorpion venom can stimulate and inhibit polymorphonuclear granulocytes. *Toxicon* **2002**, *40*, 1679–1683. [CrossRef]
76. Lee, S.-C.; Guan, H.-H.; Wang, C.-H.; Huang, W.-N.; Tjong, S.-C.; Chen, C.-J.; Wu, W.-G. Structural basis of citrate-dependent and heparan sulfate-mediated cell surface retention of cobra cardiotoxin A3. *J. Biol. Chem.* **2005**, *280*, 9567–9577. [CrossRef]
77. Bieber, A. Metal and nonprotein constituents in snake venoms. In *Snake Venoms*; Springer: Berlin, Germany, 1979; pp. 295–306.
78. Kuhn-Nentwig, L.; Schaller, J.; Nentwig, W. Biochemistry, toxicology and ecology of the venom of the spider *Cupiennius salei* (Ctenidae). *Toxicon* **2004**, *43*, 543–553. [CrossRef]
79. Olive, M.F.; Powell, G.; McClure, E.; Gipson, C.D. Neurotransmitter Systems: Glutamate. In *The Therapeutic Use of N-Acetylcysteine (NAC) in Medicine*; Springer: Berlin, Germany, 2019; pp. 19–28.
80. Monod, L.; Prendini, L. Evidence for Eurogondwana: The roles of dispersal, extinction and vicariance in the evolution and biogeography of Indo-Pacific Hormuridae (Scorpiones: Scorpionoidea). *Cladistics* **2015**, *31*, 71–111. [CrossRef]

biomedicines

Article

Addition of K22 Converts Spider Venom Peptide Pme2a from an Activator to an Inhibitor of $Na_V1.7$

Kathleen Yin [1,2,†], Jennifer R. Deuis [2,†], Zoltan Dekan [2], Ai-Hua Jin [2], Paul F. Alewood [2], Glenn F. King [2], Volker Herzig [2,3,*] and Irina Vetter [2,4,*]

1. Centre for Health Informatics, Australian Institute of Health Innovation, Macquarie University, North Ryde, NSW 2109, Australia; kathleen.yin@mq.edu.au
2. Institute for Molecular Bioscience, The University of Queensland, St. Lucia, QLD 4072, Australia; j.deuis@uq.edu.au (J.R.D.); z.dekan@imb.uq.edu.au (Z.D.); a.jin@imb.uq.edu.au (A-H.J.); p.alewood@imb.uq.edu.au (P.F.A.); glenn.king@imb.uq.edu.au (G.F.K.)
3. School of Science & Engineering, University of the Sunshine Coast, Sippy Downs, QLD 4556, Australia
4. School of Pharmacy, The University of Queensland, Woolloongabba, QLD 4102, Australia

* Correspondence: vherzig@usc.edu.au (V.H.); i.vetter@uq.edu.au (I.V.); Tel.: +61-7-5456-5382 (V.H.); +61-7-3346-2660 (I.V.)

† These authors contributed equally to this work.

Received: 22 January 2020; Accepted: 17 February 2020; Published: 19 February 2020

Abstract: Spider venom is a novel source of disulfide-rich peptides with potent and selective activity at voltage-gated sodium channels (Na_V). Here, we describe the discovery of μ-theraphotoxin-Pme1a and μ/δ-theraphotoxin-Pme2a, two novel peptides from the venom of the Gooty Ornamental tarantula *Poecilotheria metallica* that modulate Na_V channels. Pme1a is a 35 residue peptide that inhibits $Na_V1.7$ peak current (IC_{50} 334 ± 114 nM) and shifts the voltage dependence of activation to more depolarised membrane potentials ($V_{1/2}$ activation: $\Delta = +11.6$ mV). Pme2a is a 33 residue peptide that delays fast inactivation and inhibits $Na_V1.7$ peak current ($EC_{50} > 10$ μM). Synthesis of a [+22K]Pme2a analogue increased potency at $Na_V1.7$ (IC_{50} 5.6 ± 1.1 μM) and removed the effect of the native peptide on fast inactivation, indicating that a lysine at position 22 (Pme2a numbering) is important for inhibitory activity. Results from this study may be used to guide the rational design of spider venom-derived peptides with improved potency and selectivity at Na_V channels in the future.

Keywords: sodium channel; $Na_V1.7$; $Na_V1.8$; venom; spider; peptide

1. Introduction

Voltage-gated sodium channels (Na_V) are pore-forming transmembrane proteins that regulate the influx of Na^+ ions across excitable cell membranes, making them essential for the initiation and propagation of action potentials. In humans, nine different subtypes have been described ($Na_V1.1$-1.9), each with unique biophysical properties and tissue-specific expression profiles [1]. Several subtypes, including $Na_V1.7$ and $Na_V1.8$, are highly expressed in peripheral sensory neurons and are therefore critical for somatosensation and nociception.

$Na_V1.7$ and $Na_V1.8$ are almost exclusively expressed in the peripheral nervous system, with preferential expression in small-diameter unmyelinated nociceptive or "pain-sensing" neurons [2–4]. In humans, loss-of-function mutations in *SCN9A*, the gene encoding $Na_V1.7$, leads to congenital insensitivity to pain, while several gain-of-function mutations in *SCN9A* and *SCN10A* (the gene encoding $Na_V1.8$) are associated with painful peripheral neuropathies [5–7]. This is consistent with studies in rodents, whereby knockout of *Scn9a* or *Scn10a* leads to deficits in mechanical, thermal and inflammatory pain [8,9], making both $Na_V1.7$ and $Na_V1.8$ promising therapeutic targets of interest for the treatment of pain.

While many small-molecule Na_V inhibitors are used in the clinic, non-selective activity over other Na_V subtypes, including the central isoforms $Na_V1.1$ and $Na_V1.2$ and the cardiac specific isoform $Na_V1.5$ [10,11], limits their widespread use as analgesics. Therefore, there has been a push to develop novel Na_V inhibitors with improved subtype selectivity that target the less conserved voltage-sensing domains of the channel [12]. One source of novel Na_V modulators is venoms from spiders, cone snails and scorpions, from which many peptides with exquisite Na_V subtype selectivity have been described [13,14]. However, compared to tetrodotoxin (TTX)-sensitive Na_V subtypes, relatively few venom-derived peptides with sub-micromolar potency at $Na_V1.8$ have been characterised [15].

Therefore, the aim of this study was to use a high-throughput screen at $Na_V1.8$ to identify novel bioactives from spider venom. Here, we describe the isolation and characterisation of two novel peptides from the Gooty Ornamental tarantula *Poecilotheria metallica* that modulate sodium channels.

2. Experimental Section

2.1. Cell Culture

Human Embryonic Kidney (HEK) 293 cells stably expressing human $Na_V1.7/\beta1$ (SB Drug Discovery, Glasgow, UK) were cultured in Minimum Essential Medium (MEM) supplemented with 10% fetal bovine serum (FBS), 2 mM L-glutamine, and the selection antibiotics G-418 (0.6 mg/mL) and blasticidin (4 µg/mL), as recommended by the manufacturer. Chinese Hamster Ovary (CHO) cells stably expressing human $Na_V1.8/\beta3$ in a tetracycline-inducible system (ChanTest, Cleveland, OH, USA) were cultured in MEM supplemented with 10% FBS and 2 mM L-glutamine. Expression of $hNa_V1.8$ was induced by the addition of tetracycline (1 µg/mL) for 48–72 h prior to assays. HEK293 cells stably expressing rat transient receptor potential vanilloid 1 (TRPV1) were cultured in Dulbecco's Modified Eagle Medium (DMEM) containing 10% FBS under selection with hygromycin B (100 µg/mL), generated as previously described [16]. Cells were grown in an incubator at 37 °C with 5% CO_2 and passaged every 3–4 days (at 70%–80% confluency) using TrypLE Express (Thermo Fisher Scientific, Scoresby, VIC, Australia).

2.2. Venom Collection

Venom of female *P. metallica* spiders was extracted by weak electrical stimulation as previously described [17] and dried and stored at −20 °C, before being pooled and redissolved in milliQ water for further analysis.

2.3. Membrane Potential Assay at $Na_V1.8$

CHO cells stably expressing $hNa_V1.8/\beta3$ were plated 48 h before the assay on 384-well black-walled imaging plates coated with CellBIND (Corning, MA, USA) at a density of 10,000–15,000 cells/well and loaded with red membrane potential dye (Molecular Devices, Sunnyvale, CA, USA) plus TTX (1 µM) diluted in physiological salt solution (PSS; 140 mM NaCl, 11.5 mM glucose, 5.9 mM KCl, 1.4 mM $MgCl_2$, 1.2 mM NaH_2PO_4, 5 mM $NaHCO_3$, 1.8 mM $CaCl_2$, 10 mM HEPES) and incubated for 30 min at 37 °C. Crude dried venom (10 µg/well) was diluted in PSS with 0.1% bovine serum albumin (BSA) and added using the FLIPR^{TETRA} (Molecular Devices) and incubated for 5 min before activation of $Na_V1.8$ by addition of deltamethrin (150 µM). Changes in membrane potential were assessed using the FLIPR^{TETRA} (excitation, 515–545 nm; emission, 565–625 nm) every 2 s for 25 min after adding the agonist. To quantify the activity of crude venom at $Na_V1.8$, the area under the curve (AUC) after the addition of deltamethrin was computed using ScreenWorks (Molecular Devices, Version 3.2.0.14).

2.4. Isolation of Pme1a and Pme2a

Crude *P. metallica* venom (1 mg dried mass) was dissolved in 5% acetonitrile (ACN)/0.1% trifluoroacetic acid (TFA) and loaded onto an analytical C_{18} Reversed-Phase (RP) High-Pressure Liquid

Chromatography (HPLC) column (Vydac 4.6 × 250 mm, 5 μm; Grace, Columbia, MD, USA) attached to an UltiMate 3000 HPLC system (Dionex, Sunnyvale, CA, USA). Venom fractions were collected in 1 min intervals eluting at a flow rate of 0.7 mL/min with solvent A (0.1% formic acid in H_2O) and solvent B (90% ACN, 0.1% formic acid in H_2O) using the gradient: 5% solvent B over 5 min, followed by 5%–50% solvent B over 45 min followed by 50%–100% solvent B over 25 min.

Venom fractions were assessed for activity at $hNa_V1.8$ using the $FLIPR^{TETRA}$ membrane potential assay as described above. The active fraction was further fractionated to near-purity and peptide masses were determined using matrix-assisted laser desorption/ionization time-of-flight (MALDI-TOF) mass spectrometry (MS) using a Model 4700 Proteomics Analyser (Applied Biosystems, Foster City, CA, USA) with α-cyano-4-hydroxycinnamic acid (7 mg/mL in 50% ACN + 5% formic acid in H_2O) as the matrix. Peptide sequences were determined by Edman degradation performed by the Australian Proteome Analysis Facility (Macquarie University, NSW, Australia). Sequence ambiguity was clarified by MS/MS sequencing.

2.5. Peptide Synthesis

Peptides (Pme1a, Pme2a and [+K22]Pme2a) were assembled using a Symphony (Protein Technologies Inc., Tuscon, AZ, USA) automated peptide synthesizer on Fmoc-Rink-amide polystyrene resin on 0.1 mmol scale. Amino acid sidechains were protected as Asn(Trt), Arg(Pbf), Asp(OtBu), Cys(Trt), Gln(Trt), Glu(OtBu), His(Trt), Lys(Boc), Ser(tBu), Thr(tBu), Trp(Boc) and Tyr(tBu). Fluorenylmethyloxycarbonyl (Fmoc) removal was achieved using successive treatments with 30% piperidine/dimethylformamide (DMF) of 1 min then 3 min. Couplings were performed using 5 equivalents of HCTU/Fmoc-amino acid/N,N-diisopropylethylamine (DIEA) (1:1:1) in DMF, repeated twice (4 min then 8 min). Peptide-resins were cleaved using 3% triisopropylsilane (TIPS)/3% H_2O/TFA for 2 h. Following evaporation of TFA under a stream of nitrogen, peptides were precipitated and washed with cold diethyl ether, dissolved in 50% ACN/0.1 % TFA/H_2O and lyophilised. Crude peptides were purified by preparative RP-HPLC. Oxidative folding was performed in the presence of oxidised and reduced glutathione for 2 day at 4 °C, and the major folded products of correct mass were isolated by preparative RP-HPLC.

2.6. Calcium Responses in TRPV1-HEK Cells

HEK cells stably expressing rTRPV1 were plated 48 h before the assay on 384-well black-walled imaging plates coated with poly D-lysine (ViewPlate-384, Perkin Elmer, Victoria, Australia) at a density of 10,000–15,000 cells/well and loaded with Calcium 4 no-wash dye (Molecular Devices) diluted in PSS and incubated for 30 min at 37 °C. Capsaicin and Pme1a were diluted in PSS with 0.1% bovine serum albumin (BSA) at the concentrations stated and added using the $FLIPR^{TETRA}$. Changes in fluorescence were assessed using the $FLIPR^{TETRA}$ (excitation 470–495 nm, emission 515–575 nm) every 1 s for 300 s after the addition of compounds. Fluorescence responses were quantified by the maximum increase in fluorescence calculated using ScreenWorks 3.2.0.14.

2.7. Electrophysiology

Whole-cell patch-clamp experiments in $Na_V1.7$-HEK cells and $Na_V1.8$-CHO cells were performed on a QPatch-16 automated electrophysiology platform (Sophion Bioscience, Ballerup, Denmark) as previously described [18]. The extracellular solution contained in mM: NaCl 140, KCl 4, $CaCl_2$ 2, $MgCl_2$ 1, HEPES 10 and glucose 10; pH 7.4; osmolarity 305 mOsm. The intracellular solution contained in mM: CsF 140, EGTA/CsOH 1/5, HEPES 10 and NaCl 10; pH 7.3 with CsOH; osmolarity 320 mOsm. Concentration–response curves were acquired using a holding potential of −90 mV and a 50 ms pulse to −20 mV (for $Na_V1.7$) or +10 mV (for $Na_V1.8$) every 20 s (0.05 Hz). Peptides were diluted in extracellular solution with 0.1% BSA and each peptide concentration was incubated for 5 min. Peak current was normalized to buffer control. The time constant of fast inactivation (τ) was computed by fitting the current decay traces with a single exponential function using the QPatch Assay Software

5.6 (Sophion). *I-V* curves were obtained with a holding potential of −90 mV followed by a series of 500 ms step pulses that ranged from −110 to +55 mV in 5 mV increments (repetition interval 5 s) before and after 5 min incubation or Pme1a (1 μM). Conductance-voltage curves were obtained by calculating the conductance (G) at each voltage (V) using the equation $G = I/(V - V_{rev})$, where V_{rev} is the reversal potential and were fitted with a Boltzmann equation.

2.8. Data Analysis

Data were plotted and analysed using GraphPad Prism, version 8.2.0. For concentration–response curves, a four-parameter Hill equation with variable Hill coefficient was fitted to the data. Data are presented as the mean ± SEM.

3. Results

3.1. Isolation of the Novel Spider Venom Peptides μ-TRTX-Pme1a and μ/δ-TRTX-Pme2a from *P. metallica*

Crude venom isolated from *P. metallica* (Figure 1A) inhibited deltamethrin-induced membrane potential changes in CHO cells stably expressing $hNa_V1.8$, with activity guided fractionation isolating this activity to a single peak eluting at ~35% solvent B (Figure 1A). Matrix-assisted laser desorption/ionization time-of-flight mass spectrometry (MALDI-TOF MS) indicated that this fraction was dominated by two masses $(M + H)^+$ of 3911.6 *m/z* and 3808.5 *m/z* (Figure 1B). N-terminal sequencing revealed two novel 35 and 33 residue peptides that we named μ-TRTX-Pme1a (hereafter Pme1a) and μ/δ-TRTX-Pme2a (hereafter Pme2a) based on the rational nomenclature for peptide toxins (Figure 1C) [19]. The calculated masses and observed masses differed by −1 Da, indicating both Pme1a and Pme2a have an amidated C-terminus. Synthetic Pme1a and Pme2a with C-terminal amidation were used for all further experiments.

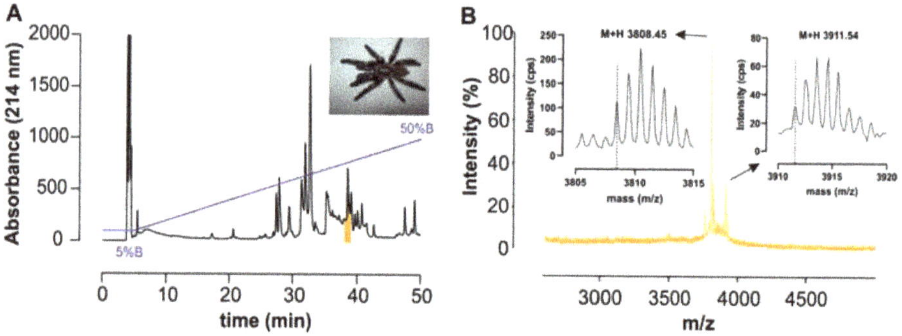

C

Toxin name	Sequence	Observed mass (Da)	Calculated mass (Da)*
μ-TRTX-Pme1a	GGCRYFLGGCSEHSDCCEHLRCKMGLNYCAWDGTF*	3910.6	3910.6
μ/δ-TRTX-Pme2a	-GCTKFMGSCKTDADCCEHLEC-YKYKWCGWDGTF*	3807.5	3807.5

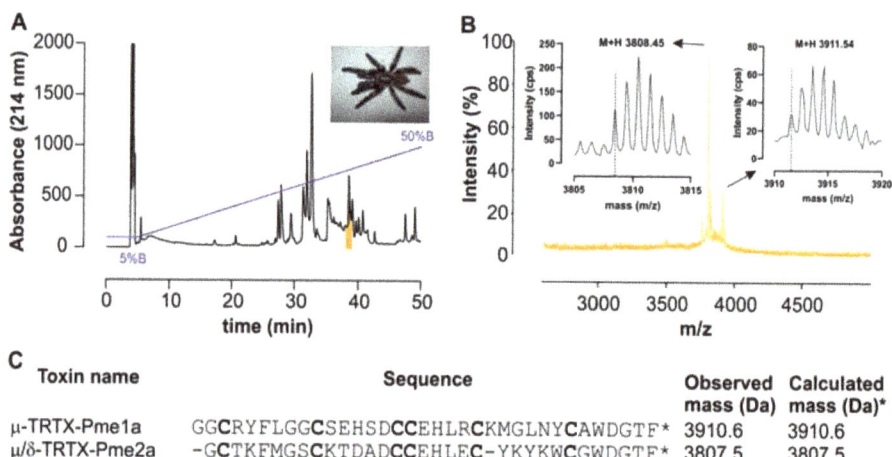

Figure 1. Isolation of novel spider peptides μ-TRTX-Pme1a and μ/δ-TRTX-Pme2a from the venom of *P. metallica*. (**A**) Chromatogram resulting from fractionation of the crude venom using RP-HPLC. Blue line indicates gradient of solvent B. Colour indicates the active peak that was further purified using activity guided fraction. (**B**) MALDI-TOF MS spectrum showing the $M + H^+$ ions for the dominant masses present in the active peak. (**C**) Sequences of μ-TRTX-Pme1a and δ-TRTX-Pme2a identified by N-terminal sequencing and their observed (uncharged) and calculated (uncharged) monoisotopic masses. The calculated mass was −1 Da due to the amidated C-terminus (as indicated by *).

3.2. Pharmacological Activity of Pme1a

Alignment of Pme1a to peptide sequences from the Universal Protein Resource (www.uniprot.org) revealed that the peptide shares high sequence homology (56%–80%) with the vanillotoxins (Figure 2), a family of peptides from *Psalmopoeus cambridgei* that activate TRPV1 with EC_{50}s ranging between 0.32 and 12 μM [20]. We therefore tested the activity of Pme1a on TRPV1 heterologously expressed in HEK293 cells. In comparison to the TRPV1 activator capsaicin (EC_{50} 83 nM), Pme1a (up to 30 μM) had no activity on TRPV1, suggesting that amino acid residue(s) crucial for TRPV1 activity are missing from this peptide (Figure 3A). As Pme1a was discovered using a Na_V channel screen, we next characterised its activity on Na_V channels using automated whole-cell patch-clamp electrophysiology.

Name	Sequence	Target	(%)
μ-TRTX-Pme1a	----GGC-RYFLGGCSEHSDCCEHLRCKMGLNYCAWDGTF-*	Na_V	100
Pf32	----AGC-RYFLGGCTEHSDCCEHLSCKMGLNYCAWDGTF-	Unknown	91
Pf29	------CSRYFLGGCTEHSDCCEHLSCKMGLNYCAWDGTF-	Unknown	86
τ-TRTX-Pc1b	----GAC-RWFLGGCKSTSDCCEHLSCKMGLDYCAWDGTF-*	TRPV1	80
δ-TRTX-Cg2a	-----EC-TKFLGGCSEDSECCPHLGCKDVLYYCAWDGTF-*	Na_V	77
τ/κ-TRTX-Pc1a	----SEC-RWFMGGCDSTLDCCKHLSCKMGLYYCAWDGTF-*	TRPV1/K_V2.1	73
κ-TRTX-Cg1a	-----EC-RKMFGGCSVDSDCCAHLGCKPTLKYCAWDGTF-*	K_V2.1	70
δ-TRTX-Hm1a	-----EC-RYLFGGCSSTSDCCKHLSCRSDWKYCAWDGTFS	Na_V1.1	67
μ-TRTX-Pn3a	-----DC-RYMFGDCEKDEDCCKHLGCKRKMKYCAWDFTFT	Na_V1.7	58
τ-TRTX-Pc1c	-----EC-RWYLGGCKEDSECCEHLQCHSYWEWCLWDGSF-*	TRPV1	56
β-TRTX-Cm2a	GVDKEGC-RKLLGGCTIDDDCCPHLGCNKKYWHCGWDGTF-*	Na_V1.5	56
μ/δ-TRTX-Pme2a	-----GC-TKFMGSCKTDADCCEHLEC-YKYKWCGWDGTF-*	Na_V	51

!

Figure 2. Sequence alignment of Pme1a and Pme2a. Sequence alignment of Pme1a and Pme2a with % sequence identity (to Pme1a) to selected mature spider peptides with a known target from Universal Protein Resource (www.uniprot.org) and two sequences identified from the venom gland of the related species *P. formosa* with unknown activity. Cysteine residues are shown in bold and * indicates amidated C-terminus. Pme1a and Pme2a align to spider peptides belonging to NaSpTx2 family 2.

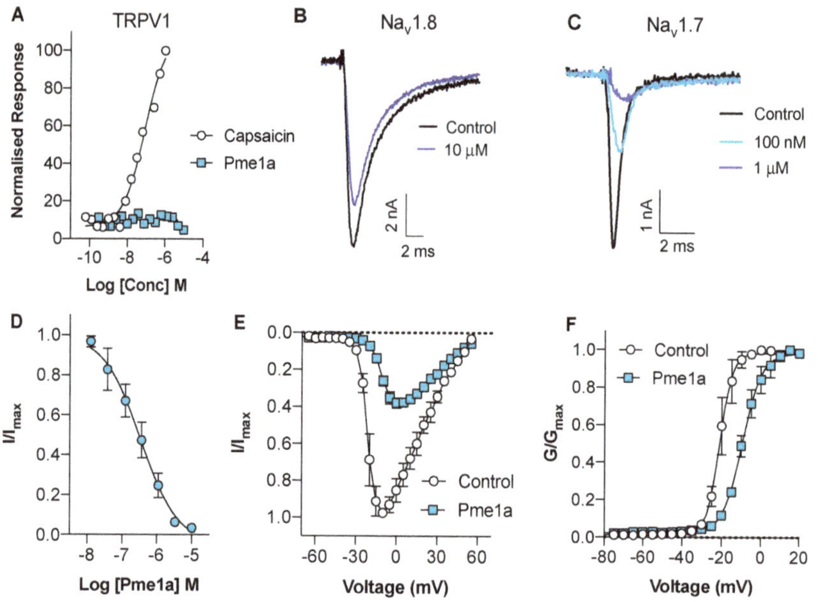

Figure 3. Activity of synthetic Pme1a on TRPV1, $Na_V1.8$ and $Na_V1.7$. (**A**) Concentration–response curves for capsaicin and Pme1a at rTRPV1 assessed by calcium dye. Data are presented as the mean ± SEM, with $n = 3$–5 wells per data point. (**B**) Representative $hNa_V1.8$ current trace before (black) and after addition of Pme1a (blue). Currents were elicited by a 50 ms pulse to +10 mV from a holding potential of −90 mV. (**C**) Representative $hNa_V1.7$ current trace before (black) and after addition of Pme1a (blue). Currents were elicited by a 50 ms pulse to −20 mV from a holding potential of −90 mV. (**D**) Concentration–response curve for Pme1a at $hNa_V1.7$ (IC_{50} 334 ± 114 nM). (**E**) Current-voltage relationship before (white circles) and after addition of 1 μM Pme1a (blue squares). (**F**) Conductance-voltage curve before (white circles) and after addition of 1 μM Pme1a (blue squares). Pme1a shifted the $V_{1/2}$ of voltage dependence of activation by +11.6 mV. Data are presented as the mean ± SEM, with $n = 3$–6 cells per data point.

Despite being isolated as an inhibitor of $Na_V1.8$ using a fluorescent screen, Pme1a only had modest activity on Nav1.8, inhibiting 21 ± 2 % of the peak current at a concentration of 10 μM (Figure 3B). In contrast, Pme1a was more potent at $Na_V1.7$, inhibiting peak current with an IC_{50} of 334 ± 114 nM (Figure 3C,D). Activity at other Na_V channel subtypes is not unexpected, given the high-sequence homology between Na_V subtypes [12]. To examine the mechanism of channel block, we next assessed the effect of Pme1a on the voltage-current relationship at $Na_V1.7$ (Figure 3E). Pme1a (1 μM) shifted the voltage dependence of activation at $Na_V1.7$ to more depolarised membrane potentials ($V_{1/2}$ activation: $\Delta = +11.6$ mV), confirming it binds to the voltage-sensing domain(s) to modify channel gating (Figure 3F).

3.3. *Pharmacological Activity of Pme2a*

Alignment of Pme2a to peptide sequences from the Universal Protein Resource (www.uniprot.org) revealed that the peptide shares sequence homology (<65%) to Pme1a and other peptides with activity at Na_V channels (Figure 2). Similar to Pme1a, Pme2a had no activity at TRPV1 (data not shown), and only modest activity at Nav1.8, with the highest concentration tested (10 μM) inhibiting 22 ± 4 % of peak current (Figure 4A). Pme2a also had modest activity at $Na_V1.7$, concentration-dependently delaying-fast inactivation, albeit not potently, with an estimated EC_{50} > 10 μM (Figure 4B,C). Due to low potency at $Na_V1.7$, no further pharmacological characterisation was performed.

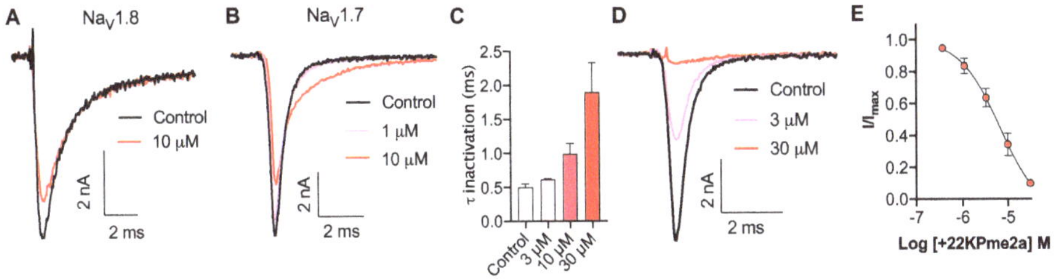

Figure 4. Activity of synthetic Pme2a and [+22K]Pme2a on $Na_V1.8$ and $Na_V1.7$. (**A**) Representative $hNa_V1.8$ current trace before (black) and after addition of Pme2a (red). Currents were elicited by a 50 ms pulse to +10 mV from a holding potential of −90 mV. (**B**) Representative $hNa_V1.7$ current trace before (black) and after addition of Pme2a (red). Currents were elicited by a 50 ms pulse to −20 mV from a holding potential of −90 mV. (**C**) Pme2a concentration-dependently increases the time constant of fast inactivation (τ) at $hNa_V1.7$. (**D**) Representative $hNa_V1.7$ current trace before (black) and after addition of [+22K]Pme2a (red). Currents were elicited by a 50 ms pulse to −20 mV from a holding potential of −90 mV. (**E**) Concentration–response curve for [+22K]Pme2a at $hNa_V1.7$ (IC_{50} 5.6 ± 1.1 μM). Data are presented as the mean ± SEM, with $n = 4$ cells per data point.

Sequence alignment revealed that loop 4 of Pme2a is one amino acid residue shorter compared to others in the family, and peptides with activity on TTX-sensitive Na_V channels generally contain a positively charged amino acid at the equivalent position, most often a lysine (Figure 2). We therefore synthesised a [+22K]Pme2a mutant and assessed how the addition of a lysine affected activity at $Na_V1.7$. [+22K]Pme2a concentration-dependently inhibited $Na_V1.7$ peak current, without the delay in fast activation seen with the native peptide, with a more potent IC_{50} of 5.6 ± 1.1 μM (Figure 4D,E).

4. Discussion

Here, we describe the isolation and Na_V activity of two novel spider venom-derived peptides, which are the first peptides to be isolated and functionally characterised from the venom of the species *P. metallica*, as well as the entire *Poecilotheria* genus [21]. A transcriptome and proteome from the venom gland of the related species *P. formosa* identified two related, but not identical peptide sequences (Pf29 and Pf32) [22], indicating that the entire *Poecilotheria* genus is likely to be a rich source of novel Na_V modulators (Figure 2). Indeed, crude venom from several species of the *Poecilotheria* genus, including *P. metallica*, has previously been shown to modulate $Na_V1.7$ [23], consistent with activity of Pme1a and Pme2a at both $Na_V1.7$ and $Na_V1.8$ described here. The two peptides isolated here were only moderately potent at $Na_V1.7$ and $Na_V1.8$, indicating that there may still be additional peptides in the crude venom with more potent activity.

Specifically, both Pme1a and Pme2a align with NaSpTx family 2, which is a large family of spider venom peptides that have promiscuous activity on Na_V, K_V and Ca_V channels [24]. Interestingly, this family also contains members that have high selectivity for Na_V channels of therapeutic interest, including the $Na_V1.7$ inhibitor μ-TRTX-Pn3a and the $Na_V1.1$ activator δ-TRTX-Hm1a. However, little is known about the structure–activity relationships that define the pharmacology of this family [25,26]. Here, we describe the importance of a lysine (K) at position "22" (using Pme2a numbering) for Na_V channel activity. The presence of the positively charged amino acid residue lysine is often important for facilitating membrane interactions in venom-based peptides [18,27]. Addition of K22 altered the pharmacology of Pme2a, converting the native peptide from being a $Na_V1.7$ channel activator to a more potent $Na_V1.7$ channel inhibitor. This is a significant finding, indicating that the amino acid residue(s) present at or around this site can dictate whether family 2 peptides function as Na_V activators or inhibitors. It is also possible that extending loop 4 of Pme2a by one amino acid residue contributed to the change in activity by slightly altering the overall structure of the peptide. Future studies elucidating the full Na_V selectivity of Pme1a and Pme2a will further define which amino acid residues are important for Na_V channel potency and subtype selectivity.

In conclusion, we have identified two novel spider venom-derived peptides that modulate Na_V channels. Results from this study provide structure–activity relationship information that may guide the future rational design of spider venom-derived peptides with improved activity and selectivity at Na_V channels.

Author Contributions: K.Y., J.R.D., Z.D. and I.V. conceived of and designed the experiments. K.Y, J.R.D., Z.D., A.-H.J., V.H. and I.V. performed the experiments. K.Y. and J.R.D. analysed the data. G.F.K. and P.F.A. contributed reagents/materials/analysis tools. J.R.D., V.H. and I.V. wrote the paper. All authors have read and agreed to the published version of the manuscript.

Funding: This work was supported by an Australian National Health and Medical Research Council (NMHRC) Career Development Fellowship (APP1162503, I.V.), an NHMRC Early Career Fellowship (APP1139961, J.R.D.), NHMRC Principal Research Fellowships (APP1080593, P.F.A.; APP1136889 G.F.K.) and a University of Queensland Research Scholarship (K.Y.).

Acknowledgments: This research was facilitated by access to the Australian Proteome Analysis Facility, which is supported under the Australian Government's National Collaborative Research Infrastructure Strategy. We thank the members of the Deutsche Arachnologische Gesellschaft (DeArGe) for providing *P. metallica* spiders for milking, particularly Henrik Krehenwinkel, Arnd Schlosser, Ralf Lühr, Michelle Lüscher, Bastian Rast and Patrick Meyer.

Conflicts of Interest: The authors declare no conflict of interest.

References

1. Catterall, W.A.; Goldin, A.L.; Waxman, S.G. International Union of Pharmacology. XLVII. Nomenclature and structure-function relationships of voltage-gated sodium channels. *Pharmacol. Rev.* **2005**, *57*, 397–409. [CrossRef] [PubMed]
2. Shields, S.D.; Ahn, H.S.; Yang, Y.; Han, C.; Seal, R.P.; Wood, J.N.; Waxman, S.G.; Dib-Hajj, S.D. Nav1.8 expression is not restricted to nociceptors in mouse peripheral nervous system. *Pain* **2012**, *153*, 2017–2030. [CrossRef] [PubMed]
3. Djouhri, L.; Fang, X.; Okuse, K.; Wood, J.N.; Berry, C.M.; Lawson, S.N. The TTX-resistant sodium channel Nav1.8 (SNS/PN3): Expression and correlation with membrane properties in rat nociceptive primary afferent neurons. *J. Physiol.* **2003**, *550*, 739–752. [CrossRef] [PubMed]
4. Black, J.A.; Frezel, N.; Dib-Hajj, S.D.; Waxman, S.G. Expression of $Na_V1.7$ in DRG neurons extends from peripheral terminals in the skin to central preterminal branches and terminals in the dorsal horn. *Mol. Pain* **2012**, *8*, 82. [CrossRef] [PubMed]
5. Faber, C.G.; Lauria, G.; Merkies, I.S.; Cheng, X.; Han, C.; Ahn, H.S.; Persson, A.K.; Hoeijmakers, J.G.; Gerrits, M.M.; Pierro, T.; et al. Gain-of-function $Na_V1.8$ mutations in painful neuropathy. *Proc. Natl. Acad. Sci. USA* **2012**, *109*, 19444–19449. [CrossRef] [PubMed]
6. Xiao, Y.; Barbosa, C.; Pei, Z.; Xie, W.; Strong, J.A.; Zhang, J.M.; Cummins, T.R. Increased resurgent sodium currents in Nav1.8 contribute to nociceptive sensory neuron hyperexcitability associated with peripheral neuropathies. *J. Neurosci.* **2019**, *39*, 1539–1550. [CrossRef]
7. Waxman, S.G.; Dib-Hajj, S.D. The two sides of NaV1.7: Painful and painless channelopathies. *Neuron* **2019**, *101*, 765–767. [CrossRef]
8. Abrahamsen, B.; Zhao, J.; Asante, C.O.; Cendan, C.M.; Marsh, S.; Martinez-Barbera, J.P.; Nassar, M.A.; Dickenson, A.H.; Wood, J.N. The cell and molecular basis of mechanical, cold, and inflammatory pain. *Science* **2008**, *321*, 702–705. [CrossRef]
9. Gingras, J.; Smith, S.; Matson, D.J.; Johnson, D.; Nye, K.; Couture, L.; Feric, E.; Yin, R.; Moyer, B.D.; Peterson, M.L.; et al. Global $Na_V1.7$ knockout mice recapitulate the phenotype of human congenital indifference to pain. *PLoS ONE* **2014**, *9*, e105895. [CrossRef]
10. Rogart, R.B.; Cribbs, L.L.; Muglia, L.K.; Kephart, D.D.; Kaiser, M.W. Molecular cloning of a putative tetrodotoxin-resistant rat heart Na^+ channel isoform. *Proc. Natl. Acad. Sci. USA* **1989**, *86*, 8170–8174. [CrossRef]

11. Whitaker, W.R.; Faull, R.L.; Waldvogel, H.J.; Plumpton, C.J.; Emson, P.C.; Clare, J.J. Comparative distribution of voltage-gated sodium channel proteins in human brain. *Brain Res. Mol. Brain Res.* **2001**, *88*, 37–53. [CrossRef]
12. Vetter, I.; Deuis, J.R.; Mueller, A.; Israel, M.R.; Starobova, H.; Zhang, A.; Rash, L.D.; Mobli, M. $Na_V1.7$ as a pain target—From gene to pharmacology. *Pharmacol. Ther.* **2017**, *172*, 73–100. [CrossRef] [PubMed]
13. Israel, M.R.; Morgan, M.; Tay, B.; Deuis, J.R. Toxins as tools: Fingerprinting neuronal pharmacology. *Neurosci. Lett.* **2018**, *679*, 4–14. [CrossRef] [PubMed]
14. Israel, M.R.; Tay, B.; Deuis, J.R.; Vetter, I. Sodium channels and venom peptide pharmacology. *Adv. Pharmacol.* **2017**, *79*, 67–116. [CrossRef] [PubMed]
15. Gilchrist, J.; Bosmans, F. Animal toxins can alter the function of $Na_V1.8$ and $Na_V1.9$. *Toxins (Basel)* **2012**, *4*, 620–632. [CrossRef]
16. Vetter, I.; Wyse, B.D.; Monteith, G.R.; Roberts-Thomson, S.J.; Cabot, P.J. The μ opioid agonist morphine modulates potentiation of capsaicin-evoked TRPV1 responses through a cyclic AMP-dependent protein kinase a pathway. *Mol. Pain* **2006**, *2*, 22. [CrossRef]
17. Herzig, V.; Hodgson, W.C. Neurotoxic and insecticidal properties of venom from the Australian theraphosid spider *Selenotholus foelschei*. *Neurotoxicology* **2008**, *29*, 471–475. [CrossRef]
18. Deuis, J.R.; Dekan, Z.; Inserra, M.C.; Lee, T.H.; Aguilar, M.I.; Craik, D.J.; Lewis, R.J.; Alewood, P.F.; Mobli, M.; Schroeder, C.I.; et al. Development of a μO-Conotoxin analogue with improved lipid membrane interactions and potency for the analgesic sodium channel $Na_V1.8$. *J. Biol. Chem.* **2016**, *291*, 11829–11842. [CrossRef]
19. King, G.F.; Gentz, M.C.; Escoubas, P.; Nicholson, G.M. A rational nomenclature for naming peptide toxins from spiders and other venomous animals. *Toxicon* **2008**, *52*, 264–276. [CrossRef]
20. Siemens, J.; Zhou, S.; Piskorowski, R.; Nikai, T.; Lumpkin, E.A.; Basbaum, A.I.; King, D.; Julius, D. Spider toxins activate the capsaicin receptor to produce inflammatory pain. *Nature* **2006**, *444*, 208–212. [CrossRef]
21. Pineda, S.S.; Chaumeil, P.A.; Kunert, A.; Kaas, Q.; Thang, M.W.C.; Le, L.; Nuhn, M.; Herzig, V.; Saez, N.J.; Cristofori-Armstrong, B.; et al. ArachnoServer 3.0: An online resource for automated discovery, analysis and annotation of spider toxins. *Bioinformatics* **2018**, *34*, 1074–1076. [CrossRef] [PubMed]
22. Oldrati, V.; Koua, D.; Allard, P.M.; Hulo, N.; Arrell, M.; Nentwig, W.; Lisacek, F.; Wolfender, J.L.; Kuhn-Nentwig, L.; Stocklin, R. Peptidomic and transcriptomic profiling of four distinct spider venoms. *PLoS ONE* **2017**, *12*, e0172966. [CrossRef] [PubMed]
23. Klint, J.K.; Smith, J.J.; Vetter, I.; Rupasinghe, D.B.; Er, S.Y.; Senff, S.; Herzig, V.; Mobli, M.; Lewis, R.J.; Bosmans, F.; et al. Seven novel modulators of the analgesic target $Na_V1.7$ uncovered using a high-throughput venom-based discovery approach. *Br. J. Pharmacol.* **2015**, *172*, 2445–2458. [CrossRef] [PubMed]
24. Klint, J.K.; Senff, S.; Rupasinghe, D.B.; Er, S.Y.; Herzig, V.; Nicholson, G.M.; King, G.F. Spider-venom peptides that target voltage-gated sodium channels: Pharmacological tools and potential therapeutic leads. *Toxicon* **2012**, *60*, 478–491. [CrossRef]
25. Deuis, J.R.; Dekan, Z.; Wingerd, J.S.; Smith, J.J.; Munasinghe, N.R.; Bhola, R.F.; Imlach, W.L.; Herzig, V.; Armstrong, D.A.; Rosengren, K.J.; et al. Pharmacological characterisation of the highly $Na_V1.7$ selective spider venom peptide Pn3a. *Sci. Rep.* **2017**, *7*, 40883. [CrossRef]
26. Osteen, J.D.; Herzig, V.; Gilchrist, J.; Emrick, J.J.; Zhang, C.; Wang, X.; Castro, J.; Garcia-Caraballo, S.; Grundy, L.; Rychkov, G.Y.; et al. Selective spider toxins reveal a role for the $Na_V1.1$ channel in mechanical pain. *Nature* **2016**, *534*, 494–499. [CrossRef]
27. Lin King, J.V.; Emrick, J.J.; Kelly, M.J.S.; Herzig, V.; King, G.F.; Medzihradszky, K.F.; Julius, D. A Cell-penetrating scorpion toxin enables mode-specific modulation of TRPA1 and pain. *Cell* **2019**, *178*, 1362–1374. [CrossRef]

biomedicines

MDPI

Review

Caterpillar Venom: A Health Hazard of the 21st Century

Andrea Seldeslachts, Steve Peigneur and Jan Tytgat *

Toxicology and Pharmacology, KU Leuven, Campus Gasthuisberg, O & N2, Herestraat 49, P.O. Box 922, 3000 Leuven, Belgium; andrea.seldeslachts@kuleuven.be (A.S.); steve.peigneur@kuleuven.be (S.P.)

* Correspondence: jan.tytgat@kuleuven.be

Received: 30 April 2020; Accepted: 24 May 2020; Published: 30 May 2020

Abstract: Caterpillar envenomation is a global health threat in the 21st century. Every direct or indirect contact with the urticating hairs of a caterpillar results in clinical manifestations ranging from local dermatitis symptoms to potentially life-threatening systemic effects. This is mainly due to the action of bioactive components in the venom that interfere with targets in the human body. The problem is that doctors are limited to relieve symptoms, since an effective treatment is still lacking. Only for *Lonomia* species an effective antivenom does exist. The health and economical damage are an underestimated problem and will be even more of a concern in the future. For some caterpillar species, the venom composition has been the subject of investigation, while for many others it remains unknown. Moreover, the targets involved in the pathophysiology are poorly understood. This review aims to give an overview of the knowledge we have today on the venom composition of different caterpillar species along with their pharmacological targets. Epidemiology, mode of action, clinical time course and treatments are also addressed. Finally, we briefly discuss the future perspectives that may open the doors for future research in the world of caterpillar toxins to find an adequate treatment.

Keywords: caterpillar venom; venomics; pathophysiology; antivenom; treatments

1. Introduction

Envenomation by caterpillars constitutes an emerging public health issue of international concern. Caterpillars belong to the order Lepidoptera, the second largest order of insects in the phylum Arthropoda. This order comprises approximately 160,000 species organized in 43 superfamilies with 133 families, distributed around the globe [1]. Many species are recognized by their beautiful and colorful patterning scales and hairs (called setae or spines) on the body [2]. Of the 133 families, nine families (Erebidae, Euclidae, Lasiocampidae, Limacodidae, Megalopygidae, Notodontidae, Nymphalidae, Saturniidae and Zygaenidae) cause severe pathophysiological conditions and are commonly involved in human and animal intoxications [3,4].

These accidents are reported throughout the world and, in some communities, this has even reached epidemic records which underscores the high burden [5]. Often, accidental contact involves a single caterpillar or, more severely, a colony with a dangerous number of caterpillars camouflaged in the trees [6]. However, in some countries, the reactions are even seen over a considerable distance from the origin. This is due to the capacity of some caterpillar species to release the setae into the air as part of their defense system, comparable with the problem caused by pollen. Contact with the airborne setae is sufficient to cause local and/or systemic reactions [7]. Among caterpillar species, the most dangerous species are classified within the family Saturniidae and are responsible for severe and fatal accidents, occurring mainly in the tropical climate zones. In these countries, caterpillar envenomation is relatively more common but still remains an underestimated problem with considerable health and economical damage.

Most of the health symptoms are consequences of a direct, usually under accidental circumstances, or indirect (air) contact with the urticating setae/spines. In some cases, the hemolymph or other droplets produced by the poisonous larvae of the caterpillar can have toxic properties [8,9]. This means that caterpillars can be both poisonous (via hemolymph or other droplets) and venomous (i.e., toxins delivered via setae or spines). These substances are used as a defense system and allow the caterpillar to respond actively against predators. For example, after physical irritation, the chitin-rich tips at the distal end of the setae readily break and release a complex venomous cocktail [10].

As a result of positive evolutionary pressure, this venomous cocktail offers a wide spectrum of biochemical and toxicological diversity that interferes with important physiological functions for humans and animals [11]. Despite multiple studies already being performed on the content and interaction of venom components of, e.g., snakes, conus, spiders and scorpions, caterpillar species have been somewhat neglected. The already investigated mixtures consist of components such as proteins, enzymes, peptides, allergens and/or low molecular molecules that determine a wide range of clinical manifestations. Depending on the family and species involved, some toxins provoke local urticating dermatitis, a burning sensation, allergic reactions, respiratory system problems and/or opthalmia nodosa, whereas others cause systemic effects, including hemorrhagic syndrome, acute kidney injury and/or phalangeal periarthritis [3].

With recent advances in cutting-edge technologies such as genomics, transcriptomics and proteomics, the venom of caterpillar species can be explored in unprecedented detail. In this way, a collection of diverse molecules involved in the pathology has been surmised. Despite state-of-the-art advancements in the qualitative and quantitative characterization of venom toxins, the target(s) of the venom component(s) in many species remain poorly understood. Hence, it is difficult to make a clear correlation between the identified components and the reactions seen. Additionally, for many species, the venom composition is still not well known and often displays a variability between species [12].

This review summarizes the main issues of caterpillar envenoming, including the epidemiology, mechanism of action and the diversity of molecules involved in the clinical manifestations. In this way, the review aims to enhance our knowledge of the already identified bioactive component(s), their role on human body target(s) and finally combine this information into an integrated framework for future research. The diagnosis and current treatments are highlighted, together with the future perspectives to better understand and confront caterpillar envenomation with a true selective medicine.

2. Evolving Global Epidemiology

Every year, thousands of people worldwide are affected either after direct contact with a caterpillar or indirectly via air or objects on which a caterpillar has moved. In the 21st century, envenomation by caterpillars is still clinically challenging owing to their potential to provoke a diverse array of symptoms. Nowadays, doctors have limited means at their disposal to relieve symptoms caused by many caterpillar species. Treatments are mainly supportive and not efficient. The only specific treatment on the market is the *Lonomia* antivenom. It is used to address the intoxication by the extremely venomous *Lonomia obliqua* from the Saturniidae family, commonly known as Taturana or fire caterpillar, and predominantly found in southern Brazil (Table 1) [13]. Despite the introduction of an antivenom therapy in 1994, mortality rates due to *Lonomia* species continue to occur [14]. The high morbidity and lethality are mainly induced by the development of an acute kidney injury [15]. In Brazil from 2000 to 2018, the Ministry of Health reported 60,588 caterpillar envenomation cases, of which there were 33 mortalities, and an incidence rate of 3.2 envenomations per 100,000 inhabitants [16]. From the same family, Saturniidae, several cases of envenomation by *Hylesia metabus* and *Leucanella memusae* (Figure 1A) were also reported as indicated in Table 1 [17,18].

In the United States, *Megalopyge opercularis* from the family Megalopygidae, known as woolly slug or puss caterpillar, has gained a foothold (Figure 1B, Table 2) [19]. A recent study by the Texas Department of State Health Service described 3484 *M. opercularis* caterpillar envenomations reported by the Texas Poison centers between 2000 and 2016 [20]. Although envenomation by *M. opercularis* can occur throughout the year, the levels of envenomation reach their peak in July and in the period from October to November. In Asia, epidemic peaking outbreaks of *Dendrolimus pini* and *Euproctis* species were reported and are indicated in Table 1 [3,4,21].

Currently, not only humans suffer from the intoxication. Animals such as domestic pets, grazers and horses experience serious health effects. In Australia, for example, the setae produced by *Ochrogaster lunifer* (Table 2), from the family Notodontidae, cause equine amnionitis and fetal loss on horse farms. The abortions caused by these caterpillars cost horse owners approximately AUD 27–43 million every year [22].

In Europe, other Lepidoptera caterpillars sharing a similar setae-based defense system include *O. Lunifer*, causing plagues. In particular, wider public health implications in France and Italy are caused by the pine processionary caterpillar from the family Notodontidae (*Thaumetopoea pityocampa*) (Figure 1C, Table 2). In France, the incidence rates were 18%, and 60% from veterinary practitioners experiencing symptoms caused by the setae [22]. Other species of the genus *Thaumetopoea* also cause epidemic spreads of the airborne disease. In the summer of 2019, the oak processionary caterpillar (*Thaumetopoea processionea*) was responsible for a major impact on public health, with a soaring number of itchy dermatitis in Belgium, Netherlands, the United Kingdom, Germany and Austria (Figure 1D, Table 2) [3,23].

An important fact is that caterpillar envenoming is seen as an occupational disease. The specific populations at risk are chainsaw operators, people that need to climb in trees, and forestry and agricultural workers [22]. For example, in the rubber tree areas of Brazil, latex collectors are forced to stop their job because of a repeatable contact with *Premolis semirufa* of the family Erebidae (Table 1). This caterpillar is known to cause chronic symptoms similar to rheumatoid arthritis. Due to these devastating effects, the caterpillar was added in the "Manual of diagnosis and treatment of envenomation", released by the Brazilian Ministry of Health [24].

In fact, everyone can be intoxicated, not only in the near vicinity of the caterpillar but also during outdoor activities and social events. As often as not, it seems that young children are more vulnerable because they play on the ground or in trees and the beautiful caterpillar colors attract curious children [25]. For some species, it is even known that the setae remain active for several years [26]. This means that at any time of the year, there is a risk for intoxication, thus posing a long-term threat to humans and animals [27].

Despite the various reported health problems, caterpillar envenomation remains an underestimated problem. The true number of accidents due to caterpillars worldwide is unknown. The World Health Organization does not report epidemiological data by all classes of venomous animals [28]. It is thus considered that the incidence rate of caterpillar envenomation is under-reported [14]. Moreover, there is a trend towards increased reporting of caterpillar envenomation cases. The rise in outbreaks is likely to continue and will be even of greater concern in the near future due to the triangle relationship between climate, international trade and local factors which can be explained further as follows. Global warming and international trade are greatly favoring the survival and distribution range of caterpillar species [23]. For instance, *T. processionea* has expanded its distribution northward. The main cause for this distribution is the observed warmer temperatures during winter and spring [23]. In Brazil, *L. obliqua* has traveled to neighboring countries, such as the province of Misiones in Argentina [14]. It is believed that this change in distribution is the result of human interventions to deforest the natural habitat. This forces the caterpillar to live in other regions with trees located in close proximity of people [15]. Hence, caterpillar–human contact is becoming more frequently reported. Also, local factors are playing a role in the increase in caterpillar envenomation. Regarding local effects, we refer to the extensive use of pesticides in recent years. This causes the death of many natural enemies of the caterpillar. Not only beneficial insects (wasps, stink bug and ants), but also valuable birds, such great tits, starlings, woodpeckers and *Anairetes alpinus* disappeared [29]. The worldwide incidence rates and the rise in the outbreaks emphasize the importance of recognizing caterpillar envenomation as an emerging health hazard.

Table 1. Occurrence, cases and venom effects from caterpillars of moths described in this review. The table shows seven of the nine venomous caterpillar families. For the Eucliedae and Nymphalidae family, no reference in the literature was found of envenomation incidences.

Superfamily	Family	Species	Occurrence	Cases		Venom Effects	References
				Year	Number		
Bombycoidea	Saturniidae	*Hylesia metabus*	Venezuela, French, Guiana	-	Epidemic outbreaks Number not defined	Pruriginous dermatitis Edema and Erythema Local tissue damage Pain	[17,30–32]
		Leucanella memusae	Argentina	-	Not defined	Local tissue damage Pain	[18]
		Lonomia achelous	Argentina	-	Not defined	Edema and Erythema Haemostatic disturbances Acute kidney injury Pain	[8,33,34]
		Lonomia obliqua	Southern Brazil	2000–2018	60.588 cases 33 mortalities incidence rate of 3,2 envenomations per 100,000 inhabitants	Edema and Erythema Local tissue damage Pain Haemostatic disturbances Acute kidney injury	[8,13–15] [16,18,35,36]
Lasiocampoidea	Lasiocampidae	*Dendrolimus pini*	Eastern Europe, Central Asia, Northern Asia, Northern Africa	-	Not defined	Dendrolimiasis: Urticating dermatitis Edema and Erythema Osteoarthritis Pain	[3,4]
Noctuoidea	Erebidae	*Euproctis chrysorrhea*	Japan, China	-	Hundred thousand persons Exact number not defined	Contact dermatitis Edema and Erythema Conjunctivitis Allergic reactions Pain	[4,21]
	Erebidae Subfamily: Arctiidae	*Premolis semirufa*	Brazil	-	Not defined	Local tissue damage Edema and Erythema Pain Joint immobilization Loss of cartilage	[24,34,37–39]

Table 2. Occurrence, cases and venom effects from caterpillars of moths described in this review. The table shows seven of the nine venomous caterpillar families. For the Eucliedae and Nymphalidae family, no reference in the literature was found of envenomation incidences.

Superfamily	Family	Species	Occurrence	Cases		Venom effects	References
				Year	Number		
Noctuoidea	Notodontidae	*Ochrogaster lunifer*	Australia	-	Endemic to Australia Number not defined	Equine Amnionitis Fetal Loss of horses Contact dermatitis Ophthalmia Severe allergic reaction Pain	[22,25]
	Notodontidae Subfamily Thaumetopoeinae	*Thaumetopoea pityocampa* *Thaumetopoea processionea*	Europe: France, Italy, Belgium, Netherlands, United Kingdom, Germany	-	18% of humans infected in outbreak areas 60% of veterinary practitioners in France experience symptoms Epidemic outbreaks Number not defined	Contact dermatitis Edema and Erythema Severe allergic reaction Burning pain Conjunctivitis	[3,21,22,40] [3,23,40]
Papilionoidea	Nymphalidae	*Morpheis ehrenbergii*	Mexico	-	Not defined	Contact dermatitis Pain	[53]
Zygaenoidea	Megalopygidae	*Megalopyge lanata*	Argentina	-	Not defined	Edema and Erythema Pain	[41]
		Megalopyge opercularis	Virginia, Texas	2000–2016	3484 cases	Contact dermatitis Edema and Erythema Local tissue damage Pain	[20]
		Lagoa crispate	Oklahoma	-	Not defined	Edema and Erythema Pain	[42]
		Podalia ca. fuscescens	Argentina	-	Not defined	Edema and Erythema Pain	[18]
		Podalia orsilochus	Argentina	-	Not defined	Edema and Erythema Pain	[18]
	Limacodidae	*Latoia consocia*	China, Taiwan	-	Not defined	Pain	[43]

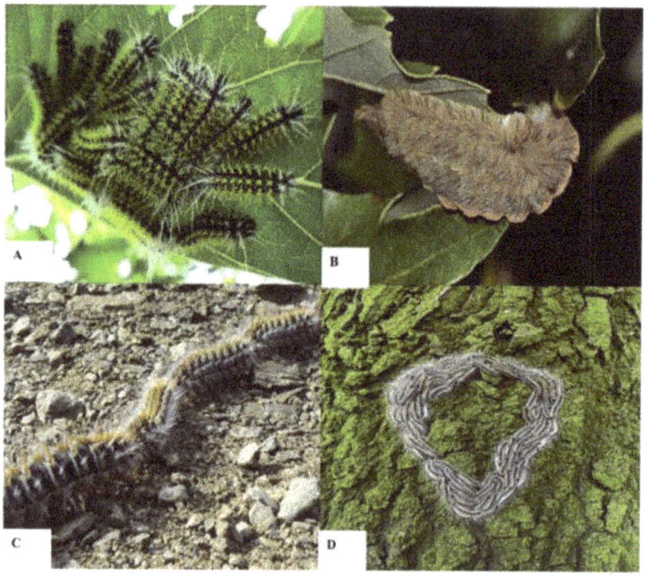

Figure 1. Representation of different venomous caterpillar species. (**A**) *Leucanella memusae*, (**B**) *Megalopyge opercularis*, (**C**) pine processionary caterpillar (*Thaumetopoea pityocampa*), (**D**) oak processionary caterpillar (*Thaumetopoea processionea*).

3. Mechanism of Action

Caterpillars inject their venom through a specialized delivery system that includes harpoon-shaped setae or spines located all over the body and are more prominent on the integument of abdominal tergites, as shown in Figure 2A,B. As perfectly reviewed by Battisti et al. (2011) [44] and Villas-Boas et al. (2018) [4], the morphology, size and color vary depending on the family and species [4,44]. Different from other venomous insects, the larvae of a caterpillar lack a specialized venom gland [45]. Instead, venom is synthesized by secretory epithelial cells and stored inside the hollow canal of the setae [43]. The harpoon-shaped setae/spines have chitin-rich tips that easily break and thus serve as an injection needle for the venom. Once the venom is released from the hollow canal, the bioactive components can exert local and/or systemic pathological effects, acting on various organs in humans and animals.

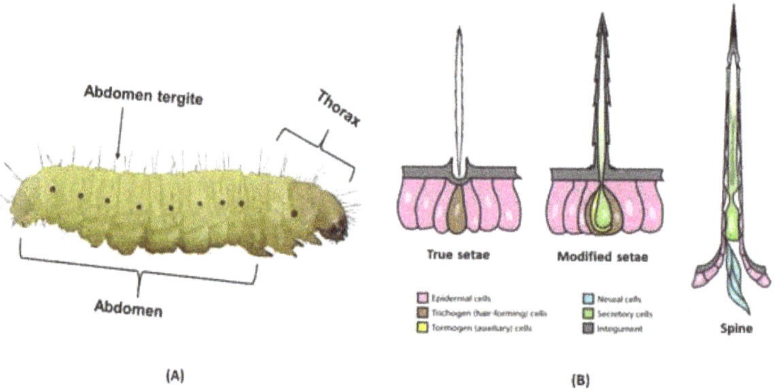

Figure 2. (**A**) Caterpillar morphology. (**B**) Schematic representation of setae/spine copied with permission from [44].

4. Technologies to Analyze Caterpillar Venom Composition and Function

Classically, a gel-based strategy is applied to investigate the venom components inside the setae [46]. In this strategy, the complex mixture is first separated into different fractions by reversed-phase liquid-chromatography (HPLC). Venom components are then quantified with the results of sodium dodecyl sulfate polyacrylamide gel electrophoresis (SDS-PAGE). In this way, the researchers were able to visualize the complexity of the venomous mixture, but usually overlooked the low abundant components [47]. This limitation has sparked the development of refined methods to determine the venomous composition in more detail. Advances were provided by proteomics, transcriptomics and genomics. For proteomics, the gel-based strategy was combined with liquid chromatography tandem mass spectrometry (LC-MS) [22]. If the symptoms indicate an allergic reaction, an immune-proteome analysis may be performed to identify possible immunogenic components [48]. Immunoproteomics is a domain where immunoblotting is combined with mass spectrometry. Transcriptomic analysis (cDNA libraries, micro arrays and next generation sequencing) gives profiles of expressed genes in cells and tissues. It is a powerful tool to unravel the functional effects of toxins on cells and tissue. Above all, it also gives a better understanding of the pathways involved in the pathophysiology. For the genomic part, genomes are used to study gene function. However, big steps still need to be made for caterpillar species. For the majority of Lepidoptera superfamilies, there is no genomic database. So far, for six of the 43 Lepidoptera superfamilies (Bombycoidea, Geometroidea, Noctuoidea, Papilionoidea, Pyraloidea and Yponomeutoidea), at least one genome with a functional gene annotation is available [49]. For two superfamilies (Gracillarioidea and Hepialoidea), only a single genome without functional annotation exists [49].

All these analytical techniques are necessary for purification and preliminary characterization of the venom components. In addition to the characterization of the structure of the toxins, both primary and secondary, knowledge regarding the functional aspect is also required. A functional analysis could be investigated with a bioassay. An example of such a potent bioassay is an electrophysiological assay where the ligands are brought into contact with a molecular target in a heterological expression system. Figure 3 illustrates a typical example of such an electrophysiological bioassay in which a G-protein coupled receptor (GPCR) can be coupled to an effector channel. It enables researchers to investigate the bioactivity of venom components, for example from a caterpillar, in a specific and accurate way.

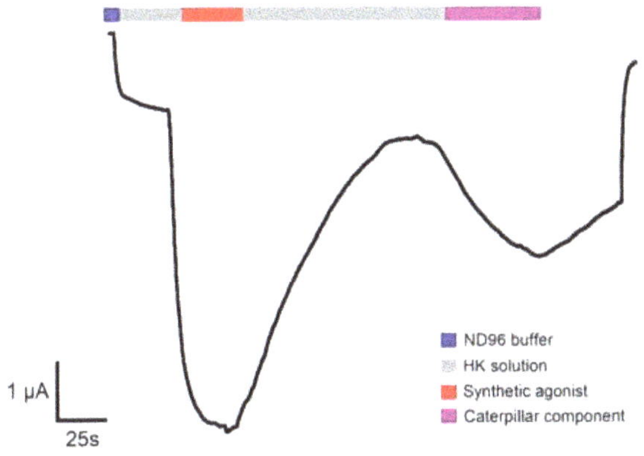

Figure 3. Electrophysiology-based bioassay with a two-electrode voltage clamp technique, as measured in *Xenopus laevis* oocytes. Shown is a validation trace experiment where a G-protein coupled receptor (GPCR) is coupled to an effector channel, an inward rectifier potassium channel via a $G_{i/o}$ cascade. Currents were induced by exchanging a control saline low potassium solution (ND96 buffer = blue) with a measuring solution with elevated potassium (HK solution = grey). The trace reveals the agonistic activity of a bioactive component originating from a caterpillar (pink). A synthetic agonist was used as control.

5. Venom Induced Pathophysiology and Diagnosis

In this part, identified bioactive components of different caterpillar species and their role on human body targets in pathophysiology are reviewed, summarized and illustrated in Figure 4.

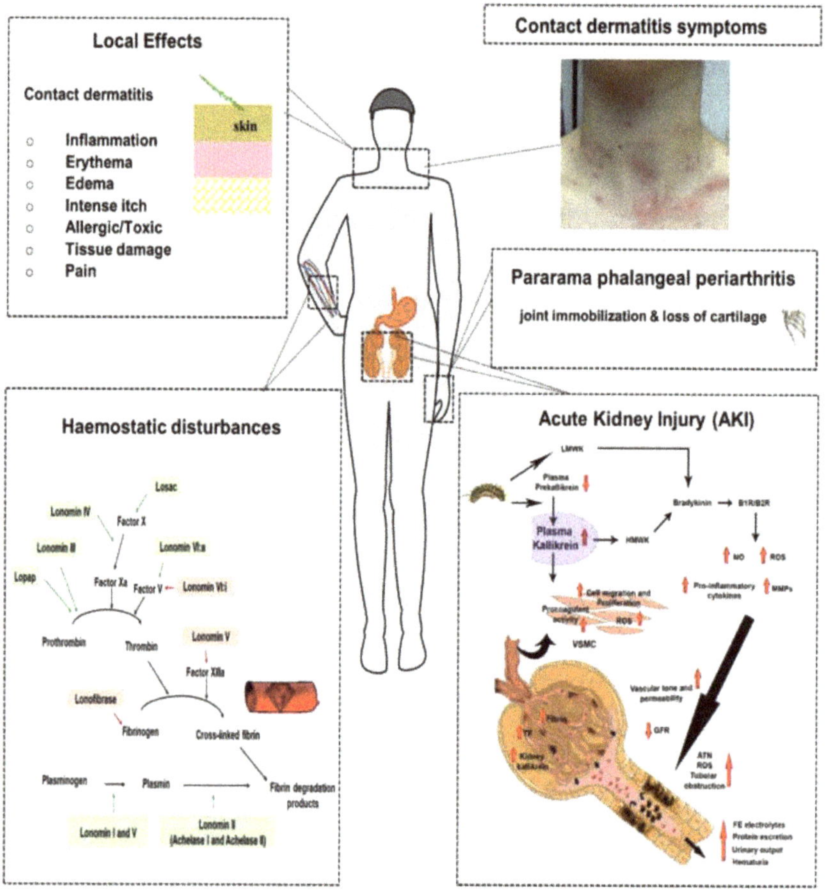

Figure 4. Venom components of different caterpillar species and their role on human body targets in the pathophysiology. Caterpillar venoms contain pharmacologically active components that are able to interfere with targets in the normal human cellular physiology. Some components are responsible for the local effects such as inflammation, erythema, edema, intense itch, tissue damage, pain and may exert an allergic reaction. Others affect the hemostasis by acting on the coagulation cascade or on the fibrinolytic pathway. Venom components colored in green activate a step in the cascade, while the components colored in red are able to inhibit a step. In some cases, this can lead to the development of an acute kidney injury (AKI). The venom-induced AKI cascade in the figure is copied with permission from [50].

5.1. Local Effects

Local effects are a hallmark physiological response to envenomation by many caterpillar species. Progress has been made in unraveling the underlying mechanism that causes the local effects. Different researchers identified venom components of several species and tried to link this information with the reactions seen in humans.

5.1.1. Contact Dermatitis

5.1.1.1. Allergic/Toxic Reaction

The most frequent clinical manifestation caused by caterpillar envenomation is the development of contact dermatitis, characterized by an extensive local inflammatory process with swelling, redness and an itch at the site of envenomation. This inflammatory environment is often initiated by an external trigger, a toxic compound, on a target in the human body. Therefore, several researchers looked at the venom composition of different caterpillar species and their target(s) to unravel the mechanism responsible for the provoked contact dermatitis symptoms.

One of the targets of caterpillar venom component(s) are mast cells. Mast cells are known to cause adverse skin reactions and play an important role in the pathogenesis of allergy, dermatitis, psoriasis and arthritis [51,52]. They are mainly disturbed in parts that are commonly exposed to the external environment, such as the skin, respiratory system and gastrointestinal tract [53]. Galicia-Curiel et al. (2014) [53] were the first to indicate that substances present in the setae of the Mexican caterpillar *Morpheis ehrenbergii*, from the family Nymphalidae, activate mast cells *in vitro* (Table 2). Once activated, mast cells release histamine which causes a rapid urticarial reaction. No massive degranulation was observed. Furthermore, the authors confirmed that no histamine was found in the crude venom extract. Moreover, no urticarial reaction was seen *in vivo* when the extract was preheated. This reinforces the hypothesis that a protein inside the setae is involved in an urticarial reaction since heat denatures proteins and does not affect histamine [53]. This is an interesting observation but certainly not a conclusive answer. Some targets are intrinsically temperature-dependent (e.g., TRPV1) and the binding of a ligand can alter the range of their temperature-dependence. Even in the absence of a ligand (setae extract), a change in temperature is sufficient in order to desensitize the targets and thereby stop the targets from responding [54].

Earlier, the same findings were also found in a study of the European caterpillar *T. pityocampa* of the family Notodontidae [55]. In this research, an abnormal permeability of surface blood vessels following the injection of venom was observed. This suggests an action of histamine, kinins and prostaglandins which are released after the activation of mast cells. Furthermore, dermal mast cell degranulation takes place 12 to 24 h after exposure to *T. pityocampa* venom extract. However, again, no excessive dermal mast cell degranulation was observed after contact with *T. pityocampa* setae. Thus, there remains the possibility that toxic substances inside the venom can either induce an inflammation process directly or indirectly via the activation of mast cells.

In the light of the research conducted by Lamy et al. (1983) [55], further investigations were performed on the venom content of *T. pityocampa* and other species in the family Notodontidae in order to gain more insight into the pathogenesis. The family Notodontidae is widely distributed in Europe (*T. processionea, T. pinivora, T. pityocampa and T. wilkinsoni*), Australia (*O. lunifer*), Africa (*H. semifusca*) and Asia (*Gazalina* sp.) [21]. Almost all species in this family are known as the leading cause of caterpillar epidemic airborne diseases, diagnosed with symptoms such as erythema, edema, papules, intense itch; swallowing can lead to a sore throat or difficulties with swallowing and contact with the eyes can lead to conjunctivitis [3]. The reaction may evolve to general malaise, fever or even an anaphylactic reaction [56]. This is mainly due to the ability to release urticaria setae as part of their protection mechanism. Such reactions were also seen in *Euproctis chrysorrhea* of the family Erebidae [57].

The European *T. pityocampa* is by far the most studied caterpillar in the family Notodontidae. Until now, three major proteins with allergenic activity have been identified and named thaumetopoein, Tha p 1 and Tha p 2. Thaumetopoein was the first specific protein fraction isolated from the setae of *T. pityocampa* with urticating properties. Electrophoretic techniques revealed two bands at 13 and 15 kDa [58]. Functionally, thaumetopoein has a direct non IgE-dependent effect on the mast cells [59–61]. However, an IgE-dependent effect via an immediate hypersensitivity reaction, responsible for more severe reactions (anaphylactic reactions), cannot be ruled out [27,59]. It is important to note is that Werno et al. (1993) [60] warned us to consider this protein as an important insect allergen. Unfortunately, thaumetopoein was never sequenced. As a consequence, researchers were not able to find homologies with other proteins or compare it. Tha p 1 is the second allergen found in the venom of *T. pityocampa,* with a molecular weight of 15 kDa and a N-terminal amino acid sequence GETYSDKYDTIDVNEVLQ [46]. This partial sequence does not show any homologies to other known proteins. Because of this, it is difficult to derive the biological function from the N-terminal amino acid sequence, which further increases the interest to study this protein in the future. Immunoblotting experiments could recognize the allergen in nine out of the 11 sera from patients sensitive to *T. pityocampa* [46]. Therefore, Tha p 1 is recognized as a major caterpillar allergen by the World Health Organization and International Union of Immunological Societies [62]. A third protein, unrelated to Tha p 1, with a molecular weight of 13 kDa and 115 amino acids, was successfully isolated and sequenced by Rodriguez-Mahillo et al. (2012) [48]. This third protein was called Tha p 2 [22]. In total, the researchers characterized 70 proteins, among them seven allergens, in the venom by using SDS-PAGE and immunoblotting techniques [48].

In 2015, Berardi et al. [40] added additional information about the structure of Tha p 2. They discovered that Tha p 2 is a glycine-, serine- and cysteine-rich protein that is present in the genome of all Notodontidae species investigated in the study (*T. bonjeani T. herculeana, T. ispartaensis, T. libanotic, T. pinivora, T. pityocampa, T. processionea, T. solitaria and T. wilkinsoni*) [22,40].

Cutting-edge technologies such as genomics, transcriptomics and proteomics made it possible to explore the venom of *T. pityocampa* in more detail [63]. By applying SDS-PAGE together with LC-MS/MS analysis, Berardi et al. (2017) [22] could identify 353 proteins in the complex mixture of *T. pityocampa*. The large amount of proteins found by LC-MS/MS compared to the study by Rodriguez-Mahillo et al. (2012) [48] is amazing. This shows even more how efficient and sensitive this technique is. Despite this, the characterization of Tha p 1 is still incomplete. The authors suggest that the isolation and full sequencing of the Tha p 1 could shed light on the function/nature of Tha p 1 [22]. In addition, serine proteases are found in the proteome with similarities to proteins in *Bombyx*, *Helicoverpa* and *Mamestra* [22]. Also, enzymes involved in chitin synthesis are noticed. It is known that chitin has a role in immune reactions. In any case, the role of a chitin-induced immune reaction due to contact with setae of caterpillars is not yet known. Furthermore, in clinical studies, it was noted that the majority of patients developed symptoms after 2-8 h. This suggests that the IgE-mediated immune pathway is relevant but does not explain in full the symptoms in patients [21]. Other mechanisms than those mediated by IgE must be at play. Some researchers, for example, refer to a toxic mechanism [64]. There is also no evidence for IgG antibodies participation [48]. Although a collection of diverse proteins has been identified in the venom of *T. pityocampa*, the targets of the venom component(s) are poorly understood. At this moment, there is no clear evidence of a correlation between an allergenic/toxic reaction and the already identified proteins. This information is necessary to unravel the mechanism of action.

In contrast with the amount of scientific literature on *T. pityocampa*, little is known about other processionary caterpillars. More research on the venom components of these species will undoubtedly shed light on the mechanism and may help to find a selective treatment options to adequately address the symptoms.

5.1.1.2. Edema and Erythema

For *L. obliqua,* the greatest advancement has been made to understand the formation of edema and erythema. In the research conducted by De Castro Bastos et al. (2004) [35], the data revealed a significant inhibition of edema formation by the G protein-coupled histamine 1 receptor (H1R) antagonist, loratadine [35]. This suggests the involvement of histamine (released after activation of a target or due to a histamine-like component) in the formation of edema as response on the envenomation. The presence of histamine or histamine analogues was also found in other caterpillar species such as in *Dendrolimus pini* (family Lasiocampidae), *Euproctis chrysorrhoea* (family Erebidae), *Lymantria dispar* (gypsy moth, family Erebidae), *Doratifera oxleyi* (family Limacodidae), and *Latoia consocia* (family Limacodidae) [4]. Thanks to the contemporary knowledge we have of other isoforms (H2R, H3R and

H4R), it is of course very interesting to gain scientific insight into whether the toxins or components of these caterpillar species can also interact with other histamine receptors and, if so, with what specificity.

On the other hand, it is also essential to note that for some caterpillar species, such as in *M. ehrenbergii* and *H. metabus*, no histamine was found in the venom [30,42,53]. In addition, many patients envenomed by setae of Lepidoptera species show a delayed onset of the dermal reactions. This suggests that rapid reactants such as histamine are not likely responsible for the effects observed [30,44]. Unfortunately, there is not much information about this mode of action yet.

Several years after the research by De Castro Bastos et al. (2004) [35], Bohrer et al. (2007) [65] added important information on the mechanism of the formation of edema. The researchers investigated the effects of the venom extract of *L. obliqua* on the kallikrein-kinin system (KKS). It was shown that the venom extract releases a kinin, kallidin, from low molecular weight kininogens (LMWK) and activates plasma pre-kallikrein. By the activation of plasma pre-kallikrein, the venom induces an indirect release of bradykinin from the high molecular weight kininogens (HMWK). Both bradykinin and kallidin are peptides that exert their biological effects by the activation of a G-protein coupled bradykinin receptor (B1/B2 receptor) [66]. In these experiments, it was observed that the rats developed edema and erythema in the peripheral tissues as a result of the activation of the B2 receptor (B2R). In this way, they could prove that the edematogenic action is not only mediated by histamine but also by the release of kinins. The same mechanism of KKS activation and resulting edema was also seen in other venomous animals, such as snakes, wasps and spiders [65].

Another study of the toxic content was performed on the female *H. metabus*. The female *H. metabus* from the family Saturniidae is mainly known in Venezuela, where a great number of envenomation accidents (Caripito itch) take place [31,32]. In the study conducted by Cabrera et al. (2015) [30], the researchers noticed that the edema generation by *H. metabus* was caused by the proteolytic activity of a fraction isolated by ammonium sulfate precipitation. In SDS-PAGE, two bands of 29 and 40 kDa were noticed [30]. Mass spectrometry revealed the presence of the same protein in the two bands. Moreover, a sequences alignment search of peptides yielded a significant homology with serine proteases of the S1A subfamily. The peptide, HM-PT60, was thus annotated as a S1 serine protease with a structural N-glycosylation by ESI-MS/MS. Next, the function of the N-glycosylated S1A serine protease was investigated in animal experiments. In these experiments, guinea pigs were inoculated with the toxin, which resulted in edema formation, massive fibrin deposition and hemorrhages. Also, an inflammatory process was activated since a leukocyte flux was observed. Histological analysis revealed that edema was formed as a result of the proteolytic activity of the toxin found in the venom. In fact, it seems that the optimal proteolytic activity of the toxin depends on the N-glycans present in the structure [30]. N-glycans are able to stabilize the 3D structure and/or optimize the enzyme-substrate binding by ionic interaction. In a subsequent research by Cabrera et al. (2017) [67], the authors could identify that the protein content of the setae is dominated by enzymes. More specifically, using SDS-PAGE analysis, they could identify that 65% of the venom content is represented by five proteases with homology to S1A serine proteases [67]. The function of these S1A serine proteases still needs more investigation, although for one of the proteases, HM-PT60, the function was already described as mentioned above [30]. Additionally, the data indicate the presence of a chitinase. Chitinases can break down chitins into small chitin fragments that may potentiate an inflammatory response. Moreover, the authors suggested that the combination of proteases and chitin can damage the exoskeleton of predatory arthropods. Slightly less important in causing the symptoms in humans, the caterpillar also contains vitellogenin, a bacteriostatic protein, which is important in the protection mechanism against pathogens. The observed tissue damage with hemorrhages induced by *H. metabus* will be further explained in the next topic about local tissue damage.

5.1.1.3. Local Tissue Damage

Local tissue damage can appear at the site of envenomation as result of the action of some venom components. This favors the spread of toxins into the body which can lead to actions on the systemic level [36]. These actions are often provoked by the presence of hyaluronidases in the venom. Hyaluronidases are able to hydrolyze hyaluronan from the extracellular matrix which disturbs the extracellular matrix of tissue and blood vessel wall [37]. This disturbance facilitates the toxins to diffuse into the tissue. For that reason, these enzymes are known as toxin spreading factors for many venomous animals (snakes, wasps, scorpions, bees, spiders and caterpillars) [37]. For caterpillars, the presence of hyaluronidases has been reported in the venom of *L. obliqua, P. semirufa, M. urens* (Family Megalopygidae), *L. memusae*, and *Podalia* ca. *fuscescens* (Family Megalopygidae) [18,24,36,37]. For *L. obliqua*, the presence of hyaluronidases was proven by a zymogram experiment conducted by Gouveia et al. (2005) [36]. In this experiment, two hyaluronidases, lonoglyases, with a molecular mass of 49 and 53 kDa, were able to degrade hyaluronic acid. Specifically, they show an β-endohexosaminidase activity which enables them to produce terminal N-acetylglucosamine sugar residues after cleaving hyaluronic acid. In addition to hyaluronic acid, they can also cleave chondroitin sulfate residues linked to the extracellular matrix (ECM). The most optimal activity was observed within the pH range 6–7 [36]. No activity was detected below pH 5 and above pH 8. This means that the hyaluronidases are active under normal physiological conditions. All these observations may explain the disturbances of cell adhesion and migration events that are seen after envenomation [36]. Moreover, the authors speculate that there is a synergy with other toxins in the venom, a phenomena also seen in other venomous animals [68]. This could explain the formation of local hemorrhaging, characterized by a disruption of the subendothelial extracellular matrix causing blood vessel wall instability [36]. It is important to emphasize that the activity of hyaluronidases of many caterpillar venoms may lie at the root of the development of local tissue damage that evolves to a systemic effect.

In contrast, very low activity towards hyaluronic acid was found in the venom from *Megalopyge lanata* and *Podalia orsilochus* (Table 2) [41]. In *Lagoa crispate*, no hyaluronidases were found (Table 2) [42]. The listed caterpillars belong to the family of Megalopygidae. The first two are widely distributed in the Neotropics, whereas *L. crispate* accidents are mainly reported in Oklahoma. Envenomation by these caterpillar species is mainly characterized by the appearance of cutaneous reactions such as pain, edema and erythema. Systemic troubles are not really attributed to these caterpillars.

Furthermore, Berger et al. (2013) [69] confirmed the occurrence of myotoxins in the venom of *L. obliqua*. Using *in vivo* experiments, the authors saw an increase in creatine kinase and histologically muscle damage in subcutaneous tissue (at the contact site) and myocardial necrosis [69]. For *L. obliqua*, the toxins responsible for this myotoxic activity are still unknown. Contrarily, for many snake venoms, these myotoxins have been identified. Here, phospholipase A_2 enzymes are accountable for the damage to the muscles and the development of necrosis [70]. Phospholipases A were also found in the venom of *E. chrysorrhoea* and *E. subflava* caterpillars and are presumably responsible for the cutaneous reactions seen in patients envenomed by these species.

It is important to highlight is that the venom-induced local tissue injury caused by *P. orsilochus* is quite similar to the one observed after *L. obliqua* envenomation. In the research of Sánchez et al. (2019) [41], they noticed the presence of serine proteases in the venom by applying a gel electrophoresis technique. This type of enzyme could perhaps explain the observation that the venom is able to hydrolyze both fibrinogen and fibrin with a specificity towards the α chain of both molecules and which may lead to the observed vascular lesion [41]. Furthermore, skin microscopy revealed not only the presence of vascular lesions, but also an inflammation reaction, hemorrhage and necrosis [41]. Some researchers proposed that the cell necrosis in the epidermis results from the reaction with lepidopteran toxin(s). Furthermore, no muscle necrosis could be determined. This perhaps can be explained by the fact that no phospholipase A_2 enzyme activity was detected. In addition, hemorrhaging started several hours after the start of necrosis. The toxin(s) or molecules that are responsible for the development of necrosis are still under investigation but the scientists suggest a mechanism where the toxin(s) or components act directly on the cell membrane [41].

Tissue damage, such as erosion of capillary vessels and focal hemorrhage, was also observed after envenomation by *H. metabus* [30]. The action is most likely caused by the proteolytic activity of S1A serine proteases found in the venom, as described previously. Furthermore, an inflammatory process was observed. The activation of the innate immune system was mediated by the structural presence of sulfate groups linked to the N-glycans [30]. Above all, it is believed that antigens are recognized, which results in the influx of leukocytes, fibrin deposition and activation of blood coagulation cascade by neutrophils.

5.1.1.4. Pain

When a venomous extract of setae/spines comes into contact with human skin, it can induce an intense (burning) pain sensation (Tables 1 and 2). In more severe cases, patients describe this pain as similar to having "a hot coal applied to the skin" or "being hit on the arm with a baseball bat" [71]. A pain signal, in general, is generated by increasing the sensitivity of nociceptor. This activation results in the release of chemical factors from nociceptors or non-neural cells (e.g., mast cells, basophils, platelets, macrophages, neutrophils, endothelial cells, keratinocytes and fibroblast) [72,73]. The chemical factors such as serotonin, histamine, glutamate, ATP, adenosine, bradykinin, prostaglandins, interleukin 1β (IL-1β), extracellular proteases and tumor necrosis factor α (TNF-α) interact directly with the nociceptor by binding with one or more cell surface receptors (G-protein coupled receptor, transient receptor potential (TRP), acid-sensitive ion channels (ASIC), voltage-gated ion channels (VGICs), two-pore potassium channels (K2P), and receptor tyrosine kinases (RTK)) [72,73]. This information is necessary to understand and to link the role of some venom components with the pathogenesis of pain.

For *L. obliqua*, de Castro Bastos et al. (2004) [35] studied the nociceptive responses elicited by a crude extract *in vivo* in rats. Pain was assessed by investigating the change in shaking and lifting of the injected hind paw. Surprisingly, they saw that the shaking and lifting was strongly inhibited after treatment with indomethacin. Indomethacin is a pain medicine that works by inhibiting the production of prostaglandins [74]. The nociceptive responses were thus elicited by prostaglandins. Therefore, the authors proposed that prostaglandins were formed by the phospholipase A_2 activity found in the spine extract of *L. obliqua* [8,35]. Phospholipase A_2 is a low molecular mass enzyme (15 kDa) that produces arachidonic acids which can be converted into prostaglandin by cyclooxygenase [75]. Other researchers suggested that the KKS mechanism, which was also involved in the formation of edema, may play an important role in the pain response that humans experience after envenomation. The KKS mechanism releases bradykinin, which is a powerful pain mediator. It namely sensitizes nociceptors following the release of prostaglandins and cytokines [65].

It seems that not only the KKS mechanism may be involved. Both genetic and electrophysiological studies with whole-cell patch clamp have, in fact, shown that transient receptor potential vanilloid 1 channel (TRPV1) is one of the primary targets of the *L. consocia* venom (Figure 5) [43].

L. consocia is a caterpillar found in South-West China that induces an intense burning pain sensation. By targeting the sensory nerve endings of the TRPV1 channel, it mediates nociceptive triggers from the peripheral nervous system to the central nervous system where it is received as pain. Additionally, Yao et al. (2019) [43] did not rule out that more pain-related receptors are involved in the pathway. In their *in vivo* experiments, they saw that the paw licking behavior of the mice was not completely eliminated by a specific TRPV1 antagonist, capsazepine (Figure 6). According to the observations, they mainly believe that there is a possibility that other targets work synergistically with the TRPV1 channel to induce pain. Additionally, the authors investigated the venom composition of the caterpillar. They were able to identify 126,670 universal genes, 162 of which are related to the defense mechanism. Overall, they could demonstrate that the venom is rich in peptide fragments. Although more research still needs to be performed to indicate the bioactive components and their target in the pain pathway of *L. consocia*, it appears that venomous animals that induce pain usually have venom components acting on TRP channels. For example, the DkTx toxin of the Chinese bird spider, *Ornithoctonus huwena*, activates TRPV1 channels and causes severe pain [76]. Also, the Chinese red-headed centipede (*Scolopendra subspinipes*) and some scorpion venoms induce pain by the same pathway [43].

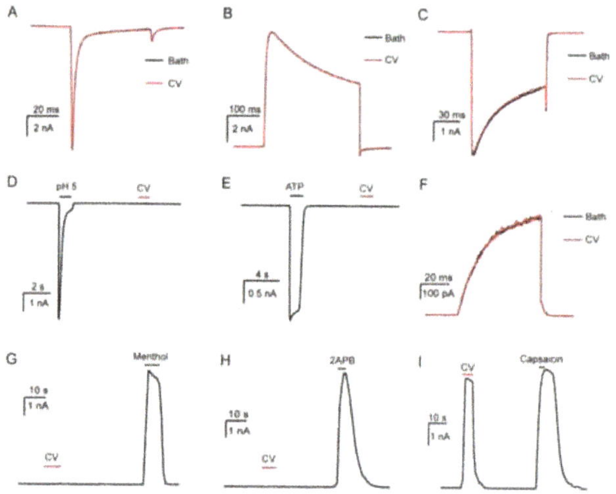

Figure 5. In these experiments, Yao et al. (2019) [43] tested the response of the crude *L. consocia* venom (CV) extract on pain-related ion channels: (**A**) dorsal root ganglion sodium channel (DRG-Na); (**B**) dorsal root ganglion potassium channel (DRG-K); (**C**) dorsal root ganglion calcium channel (DRG-Ca); (**D**) acid-sensing ion channel 2a (mASIC2a); (**E**) P2X ligand-gated ion channel 3 (hP2X3); (**F**) mKCNQ4; (**G**) transient receptor-potential M8 (mTRPM8); (**H**) transient receptor-potential vanilloid 2 (mTRPV2) (**I**) TRPV1. The electrophysiological profiles of *L. consocia* venom reveals a potent and specificity towards the TRPV1 channel with similar amplitude to the agonist, capsaicin, evoked current (**I**). No evoked currents were seen for the other channels (**A–H**). The figure was copied with permission from [43].

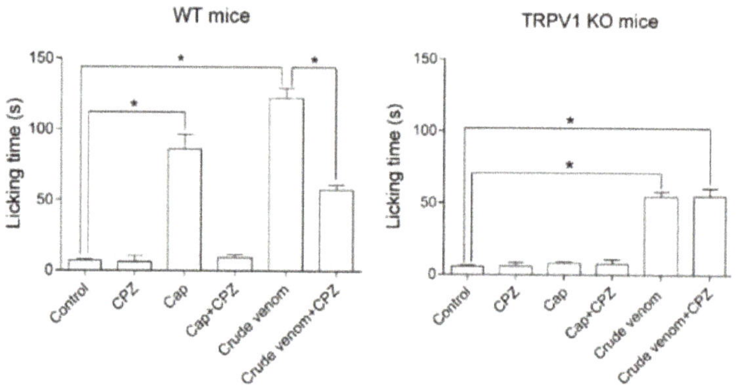

Figure 6. The TRPV1 antagonist, capsazepine, could not completely eliminate the paw licking behavior. Paw licking duration was monitored by Yao et al. (2019) [43] using the following experimental conditions. (A) Ten microliters of saline (control), capsazepine (CPZ, 2 mM), capsaicin (Cap, 500 μM), crude venom (100 μg/mL), capsaicin (500 μM)/capsazepine (2 mM) mixture, and crude venom (100 μg/mL)/capsazepine (2 mM) mixture injected into the left hind paw of WT mice. Two-sided *t*-test: *, $p < 0.05$; n = 6. (B) Mean durations of paw licking induced by 10 μL of saline (control), capsazepine (2 mM), capsaicin (500 μM), crude venom (100 μg/mL), capsaicin (500 μM)/capsazepine (2 mM) mixture, and crude venom (100 μg/mL)/capsazepine (2 mM) mixture injected into the paw of TRPV1 KO mice. The figure was copied with permission from [43].

5.2. Systemic Effect

Just as beauty is not inherent in a visual image, envenomation by caterpillars is a complex clinical manifestation that often not only involves local effects but also systemic effects. Frequently, the clinical profile after envenomation by some caterpillar species, e.g., *Lonomia* species, begins with burning pain, dermatitis, headache and nausea symptoms but evolves rapidly into a hemorrhagic syndrome accompanied by acute kidney injury (AKI) [10].

5.2.1. Haemostatic Disturbances

Hemostatic disturbances are a major consequence of envenomation by some caterpillar species and, more specifically, by *Lonomia* species. They not only occur at the site of the accident but may manifest at the systemic level and consequently lead to abdominal or brain hemorrhage. Also, consumptive coagulopathy can occur [36]. For two *Lonomia* species, *L. obliqua* and *L. achelous*, some responsible mechanisms are well described, but still a lot of information remains not entirely elucidated. Although the pathophysiologic processes are not completely known, it seems that depending on the species, another mechanism is involved in this hemostatic disturbance. The effect of some toxins from *L. obliqua* and *L. achelous* are highlighted in Figure 4 and further explored below.

For *L. obliqua*, important information was derived from the proteome and transcriptome analysis. Researchers found sequences from 1278 independent clones assembled into 702 clusters of genes coding for putative toxins such as lipocalins, blood coagulation factors, phospholipase A_2 hemolins, cystein-proteases, serine-protease inhibitors, serpins and hyaluronidases [5]. Firstly, the most abundantly studied toxin was found in the lipocalin protein family, called Lopap (*Lonomia obliqua* prothrombin activator protease) [77]. Lopap is a 69 kDa toxin and the first lipocalin described with proteolytic activity. Hence, it activates prothrombin through hydrolysis of Arg^{284}-$Thr^{285}$and Arg^{320}-Ile^{321} peptide bonds, which leads to the generation of thrombin [8]. It is surprising that Lopap did not show any similarity with other prothrombin activators or serine proteases but only with lipocalins. As a result of the thrombin formation, Lopap may indirectly induce a platelet aggregation. In contrast, Lopap could also inhibit platelet aggregation [77]. This inhibition results from the release of cell platelet aggregation inhibitors from endothelial cells such as nitric oxide (NO) and prostacyclin (PGI_2). Besides the inhibition of platelet activation, NO and PGI_2 display potent vasodilation properties [5]. All these factors play an important role in the venom-induced consumption coagulopathy, extended defibrinogenation and incoagulability [78]. Clinically, it will result in an alteration of blood clotting tests after the *in vivo* administration of Lopap. The resulting condition may evolve into systemic bleeding, especially when the integrity of blood vessels is disrupted [33]. Secondly, a 35 kDa enzyme (Lonofibrase) isolated from the hemolymph with fibrin(ogen)olytic activity was found. Lonofibrase cleaves Aα and Bβ chains of fibrinogen. The specificity of Lonofibrase against the α- and β-chains of fibrin is sufficient to prevent the clotting reaction, which explains the severe hemorrhagic clinical profile seen. Next, a 45 kDa Factor X activator, known as Losac (*Lonomia obliqua* stuart factor activator), was found. When Factor X is activated, it will integrate the prothrombinase complex (phospholipids and calcium ions) to produce thrombin. Consequently, a fibrin clot is formed [79]. For many snake venoms, it is known that they contain enzymes that activate Factor X [80]. The only difference with Losac from *L. obliqua* is that these enzymes critically depend on the presence of calcium ions. Losac is able to activate Factor X in the absence of calcium ions. It seems clear that proteolytic activation of Factor X is made possible due to the serine like protease activity of Losac since its action can be abolished by a serine protease inhibitor, diisopropyl fluorosphosphate[8]. Interestingly, Losac does not show homology to known proteases, but instead it has a high similarity with the hemolin group. Hemolin is an immunoglobulin-like peptide with an important role in insect immunity and cell adhesion properties [79]. It is exclusively expressed in Lepidoptera species. Moreover, experimental thrombosis studies showed that Losac has no effect on fibrin or fibrinogen [79]. This again reinforces the evidence that Losac has an important and specific roll in inducing blood coagulation. Beyond the role in coagulation, Losac is also able to induce proliferation and inhibit apoptosis [79,80]. Moreover, the occurrence of intravascular hemolysis was confirmed by *in vivo* experiments in rats [8]. This hemolytic process is most likely initiated by the deposition of hemoglobin in the renal tubes which is highly nephrotoxic [69]. One important contributor to the hemolytic activity is a 15 kDA group III phospholipase A_2 found in the venom of *L. obliqua*. Furthermore, proteomic data of *L. obliqua* venom demonstrated the presence of elements that modulate cell adhesion and signaling. This is probably mediated by the activation of RAC1 signaling pathway. RAC1 is a member of the Rho GTPase family and promotes actin assembly, which influences the cell function due to changes in cell adhesion and migration [81]. Finally, physicians often note a sudden drop in blood pressure in the patient. Bohrer et al. (2007) [65] revealed that this hypotension was mediated by the activation of the KKS system. This was proven by the inhibition of hypotension by aprotinin, a plasma kallikrein inhibitor, and HOE-14, a bradykinin B2 antagonist [35].

While *L. obliqua* venom predominantly acts on the coagulation cascade, *L. achelous* mainly affects fibrinolysis [8,33]. Several studies of *L. achelous* hemolyph supported the hypotheses that different venom fractions play a role in haemostatic disturbance, including Lonomin I, Lonomin II (Achelase I and Achelase II), Lonomin III, Lonomin IV, Lonomin V, Lonomin VI:a, Lonomin VI:I, and Lonomin VII [8,82]. The actions of these venom components are visualized in Figure 4 and further explained below.

Two venom fractions, Lonomin I and Lonomin II (Achelase I and Achelase II), have an intense fibrinolytic activity and can induce lysis of whole blood clots and fibrin plates. Lonomin I is a 16 kDa venom toxin with urokinase plasminogen activator-like activity and Achelase I (22.4 kDa) and Achelase II (22.7 kDa) have a plasmin-like activity. Furthermore, two prothrombin activators are found. Lonomin III can activate prothrombin independently from calcium ions and phospholipids (prothrombinase complex). Meanwhile, Lonomin IV is a factor Xa activator, since its activity increases in the presence of factor V, phospholipids and calcium ions. Next, *L. achelous* venom contains a Factor V activator, Lonomin VI:a, and inhibitors, including Lonomin VI:I [83]. Lonomin VI:a appears to be a thermostable metalloprotease, since its activity is inhibited by metalloprotease inhibitors. For a variety of snake venoms, it is known that they have Factor V activators in their venom, mainly responsible for the progression of hemorrhaging. In contrast, the venom also contains a Factor V inhibitor, Lonomin VI:i, which is a serine or cysteine protease. Besides Lonomin II, Lonomin V is the second most important enzyme, with intense fibrinolytic activity. Lonomin V is a 25 kDa factor XIII proteolytic urokinase-like enzyme that degrades the extracellular matrix proteins such as laminin, vitronectin and fibronectin [8]. The adhesion and aggregation inhibition in platelets destroy the capillaries and contributes to the hemorrhagic syndrome. Additionally, its activity is inhibited by serine protease inhibitors, suggesting that it is a serine protease. At last, thrombosis experiments on the whole venom indicate that Lonomin V not only inhibits thrombus growth but also induces lysis of preformed thrombi [8].

Besides their presence in *Lonomia* species, proteins related to the haemostatic disturbance were also identified in other species from the same or different family. Quintana et al. (2017) [18] investigated the protein content of *L. obliqua*, *L. memusae* and *P.* ca. *fuscescens* and compared it. In a one-dimensional electrophoretic profile, shown in Figure 7, it is clearly visible that the venom of Saturniidae species (*L. obliqua* and *L. memusae*) are more complex compared to the venom of *P.* ca. *fuscescens* from the Megalopygidae family. Notably, the same coagulation disturbance proteins such as serpins and serine proteases from *L. obliqua* were also found in *L. memusae*. In contrast with the intense presence of Achelase 2 (anticoagulant protein) and serine proteases in *L. obliqua* venom, lower intense bands were noticed in *L. memusae* venom. Clinically, the patients showed a prolonged activated partial thromboplastin time of the normal human plasma (APTT). This is a blood test that characterizes the coagulation of blood. The authors suggest that the action is caused by the proteolysis of coagulation factor(s). However, the venom did not degrade human fibrinogen [18].

Another important result of the research conducted by Quintana et al. (2017) [18] is that Losac, a hemolin of *L. obliqua*, was detected in the venom of *L. memusae*. Surprisingly, the same component, Losac, is also found in other species of the Megalopygidae family such as *Podalia* ca. *fuscescens* and *P. orsilochus* (Table 2). Just like *L. obliqua*, both species are able to hydrolyze fibrinogen and fibrin with a particular preference towards the α chain of both fibrinogen and fibrin (as described in the section

Contact Dermatitis with local tissue damage for *P. orsilochus*). Indeed, envenomated patients show a shortening of the clotting time of human plasma, similar to *L. obliqua* envenomed patients [18,41]. Of note, *P.* ca. *fuscescens* needs more time to act on the plasma protein. This action may be due to a weak coagulant component in the venom. Serine proteases and serpins are also found in both species. The only strange observation which is important to emphasize is that for *L. memusae*, *P. orsilochus* and *P.* ca. *fuscescens*, no clinical symptoms of hemostatic disturbance have been reported yet [41]. Overall, it was hereby again shown that enzymes are one of the most common toxic components found in caterpillar species [67,84].

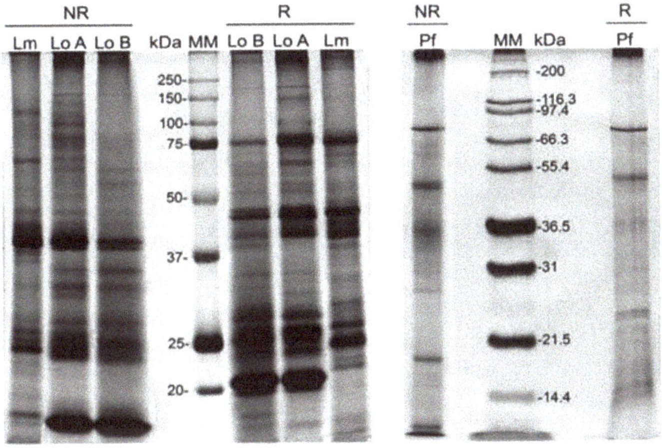

Figure 7. One-dimensional electrophoretic profile of (**A**) Saturniidae and (**B**) Megalopygidae venom extract under reducing (R) and non-reducing (NR) conditions. Lo A: *Lonomia obliqua* from Argentina; Lo B: *Lonomia obliqua* from Brazil; Lm: *Leucanella memusae*; Pf: *Podalia* ca. *fuscescens*; MM: molecular mass markers. The figure was copied from Quintana et al. (2017) [18] with permission from Elsevier.

5.2.2. Acute Kidney Injury

The development of an acute kidney injury (AKI) is associated with a high morbidity and mortality. Envenomed patients experience a sudden loss of basic renal function, such as filtration and excretion capacities and the maintenance of homeostasis [15,50,85]. Berger et al. (2019) [50] were the first to expose the mechanisms associated with the pathogenesis of renal damage by *L. obliqua*. The results are summarized in Figure 4.

Firstly, they discovered that bradykinin, released from LMWK (directly) and HMWK (indirectly), as described previously in the section Contact Dermatitis with Edema and Erythema, contributes to kidney injury mainly by the activation of its two receptors, B1R and B2R [50]. Both receptors belong to the G-protein-coupled receptor group. It is important to note that under normal physiological conditions, B1R is not expressed, but may be upregulated by an inflammatory stimulus [66,85]. When B2R is stimulated with bradykinin, a vasorelaxant effect was observed, while the activation of B1R by the bradykinin metabolite, Arg^9-bradykinin, resulted in a renal vasoconstrictor response. The renal vasoconstrictor response induces a decrease in glomerular filtration rate and electrolyte balance. Additionally, it was observed that *L. obliqua* venom induces the production of several cytokines, increased the expression of matrix metalloproteinases (MMPs) and increased the levels of nitric oxide (NO). As a consequence, these alterations resulted in tubular lesions and hereby the role of the activation of kininogen-kallikrein-BK-B1R/B2R in *L. obliqua* envenomation was shown [50]. Moreover, this work pointed out that cytokines and coagulation factors are produced in the plasma during the envenomation. Also, activation of vascular smooth muscle cell (VSMC) procoagulant activity, increased reactive oxygen species production (ROS), and cell proliferation and migration were observed [50].

The venom can also act directly on the VSCMC and thus cause the same cascade of events as plasma [6]. At last, researchers have asserted that renal obstruction or reduced filtration capacity is caused by activation of the VSMC by the venom components that lead to fibrin formation and deposition in glomerular capillaries. All these findings and their role in the pathogenesis of AKI are summarized and presented in Figure 4. Other species of the Saturniidae family, such as *Dirphia* species and *L. achelous*, are also known to induce AKI [34].

5.2.3. Pararama-Associated Phalangeal Periarthritis

Pararama-associated phalangeal periarthritis is an occupational and serious health disease in the Brazilian Amazon region. The name of disease is derived from the caterpillar causing the disease, i.e., *P. semirufa* or pararama. *Premolis* species belongs to the Erebidae family and are found in South America, where they feed on the *Heyea brasiliensis*, the rubber trees (*P. semirufa* in Brazil, French Guiana, Ecuador, Peru and Panama; *P. excavata* in Panama; *P. rhyssa* in Peru and *P. amaryllis* in French Guiana) [24]. The disease is a unique form of erucism that begins with symptoms such as pain, itch, heat and redness but may rapidly escalate to pararamose or joint immobilization, loss of cartilage and bone structure when repeated contact with the setae of the caterpillar occurs (Figure 4) [38]. In fact, one can compare this chronic situation with the symptoms caused by an inflammation joint disease such as rheumatoid arthritis. The envenomation by *Premolis* species is not only seen as an occupational disease, but it can also have a serious social impact [39].

Villas-Boas et al. (2012) [24] took the first steps to investigate the venom composition of *P. semirufa* in order to gain more insight into the mechanism. Soon it became clear that the venom has a complex composition with different enzymes acting alone or together to generate and develop the clinical symptoms. Firstly, they found hyaluronidases in the venom. As described in the section Contact Dermatitis with Local Tissue Damage, these enzymes degrade the extracellular matrix of the tissue, which facilitates the systemic influx of toxins. The link with the loss of cartilage and joint immobility can be found in the important function of hyaluronic acid. Hyaluronic acids are essential substances of the intercellular matrix of the skin, cartilage and synovial fluid that stabilize the joints and acts as lubricant [24]. A degradation of these hyaluronic acids results in the pararama-induced loss of cartilage and bone structure. Thus, the authors suggested that hyaluronidases are important factors behind pararama-associated phalangeal periarthritis.

Secondly, a serine protease with gelatinase activity was found. The gelatinase activity is often related with degradation of type IV, V, VII and XI collagens that are present in bone and cartilage. This protein is also related with a serine protease activity [24]. As described in a previous section about hemostatic disturbance, these serine proteases have diverse pharmacological activities. Some of them work on coagulation cascade by activating Factor V, whereas others have a fibrinogenolysis activity and activate plasminogen [24]. As a result, these compounds may be involved in the clinical manifestation. In contrast with many other venomous animals and other caterpillars, *P. semirufa* venom extract does not exert a phospholipase A_2 activity.

Also, the participation of the immune system in the pathogenesis of pararama was investigated by Villas-Boas et al. (2013) [34]. Immunohistochemical and immunofluorescence research on BALB/c mouse injected with the venom revealed an elevated level of neutrophils in the connective tissue at the site of injection [34]. Besides their role in the innate immune system, neutrophils can also promote tissue injury and may be responsible for the inflammatory responses. In addition, the obtained results indicate an influx of macrophages which produce cytokines such as TNF-α, IL-1β and IL-6. In this way the inflammatory response is maintained. Moreover, the level of other cytokines, IL-6, IL-12, IL-10, IL-17 and IL-23 was increased [34]. Also, proliferation and activation of T and B lymphocytes was observed. The exact function and response of T and B lymphocytes on the venom remains to be elucidated. In a subsequent study in 2015, the same author added important information to the function of the serine proteases. According to the data, a serine protease containing fraction (Ps82) is able to activate the complement system and release anaphylatoxins [39]. This excessive complement system activation starts the development of an inflammation process. The same action is also seen in other venomous animals. For example, in many snake venoms, toxins were described to target the complementary system causing the observed pathogenesis [86].

6. Clinical Time Course

The symptoms that occur after envenomation by caterpillars can be divided into immediate, short- and long-term effects.

6.1. Immediate Effects

The immediate emerging effects appear within minutes after exposure to the setae/spines. These effects may vary depending on the type of species and the person envenomed. In many cases, a feeling of pain is experienced, which is obvious since caterpillars use their setae/spines purely as defense. In a specific case of *L. obliqua*, the victim experienced a sharp pain immediately after contact with the caterpillar [10]. Other species, more specifically, processionary caterpillars, are known to cause a direct intense itch reaction. Sometimes, patients are sensitized because of a repeatable contact with the caterpillar. In such case, the clinical pattern progressively evolves and may result in a severe life-threatening form of a systemic allergic reaction, as seen in *T. pityocampa* and *T. processionea* envenomation [26,61].

6.2. Short-Term Effects

Short-term effects are mainly the skin reactions seen at the place of the envenomation. These skin reactions are characterized by the formation of papules, pustules, swelling, acute inflammation and erythema and appear usually within 4–12 h (a delayed onset). In more rare cases, tissue necrosis in the area of contact may progress. The complete disappearance of these symptoms and restoration of the normal function takes 1–2 weeks, but may persist for up to a month [87,88]. In some cases, the setae of caterpillars are spread in the air by the wind. This can cause the setae to be inhaled. Usually, the victim will then develop a sore throat and experience difficulties with swallowing within four hours. Sometimes breathing problems, vomiting or abdominal pain may develop. Although vomiting or abdominal pain is not always related with inhalation of the setae, it is possible that these symptoms indicate a systemic envenoming resulting from the action of some specific component(s) inside the venom.

6.3. Long-Term Effects

In some caterpillars, the effect of the toxins may lead to a permanent loss of function. For example, when setae of processionary caterpillars penetrate into the mucous membrane of the eye, inflammatory signs (ophthalmia nodosa) can progress within 1–4 h [89]. If these setae are not removed, it can lead to irreversible blindness. Another example is related to the pararama caterpillar in South America. After repeated contact with this caterpillar, the patient may develop chronic symptoms similar to rheumatoid arthritis (as described in the section Venom-Induced Pathophysiology) [24]. For *L. obliqua*, the clinical profile may become even worse. Systemic effects begin with nausea and headache symptoms that become obvious after 24 h and can last about 72 h. Hemorrhagic vesicles are usually noticed four days after envenomation. Usually, blood tests show a prothrombin activity lower than 10% and undetectable plasma fibrinogen [10]. Abdominal pain, bleeding and coagulopathy also develop and may persist when the patient is not treated. If on day seven hematuria persists and the symptoms remain untreated, the patient will likely die [10]. Therefore, it is important to respond quickly and deliver the antivenom to save the patient.

7. Treatments and Limitations

Caterpillar envenomation has become a serious health problem in the world, but especially in the tropical zones, where it even can lead to fatalities. Prevention, proper management and an effective treatment option play an important role in minimizing discomfort and treat the complication after caterpillar envenomation. However, the presence of a treatment to adequately address the conditions of the envenomation by many caterpillar species is still lacking. Of course, it is obvious that the best preventive measure is to avoid any direct or indirect contact with caterpillar species. However, the real question everyone wants to get answered is what to do if one is intoxicated with the setae of a caterpillar. At this moment, doctors have limited means at their disposal and mainly propose supportive treatments to relieve symptoms provoked by many caterpillar species.

7.1. Antivenom for Management of Systemic Effects

In response to an outbreak in 1989 of *L. obliqua* species with a great number of accidents and mortalities, the Brazil institution Butantan in São Paulo developed a *Lonomia* antivenom to treat victims of *L. obliqua* envenomation [90]. For many venomous animals, an antivenom treatment is the standard-of-care to treat envenomation. However, for caterpillar species, this was the first and only antivenom manufactured in the world. The antivenom was made by immunizing horses with the venom extract from the spines of *L. obliqua* over a period of one year [90,91]. As a reaction, horses produced antibodies that were able to recognize and neutralize the coagulopathy effect of the toxic substances inside the venom. From the plasma of the horses, researchers obtained the specific purified F(ab')2 immunoglobulin which forms the basis of the antivenom. This antivenom was manufactured to treat envenomed patients and showed an ED_{50} and potency of 38.61 µl and 0.29 mg/mL, respectively [91]. It is important to note that the introduction of this antivenom on the market in 1994 in Brazil significantly reduced the mortality rate, but unfortunately it could not be reduced to zero. People continue to die after envenomation by *L. obliqua*. As mentioned in the epidemiology section, this is mainly due to the development of an acute kidney injury [15]. The reason why this happens was exposed in the research by Berger et al. (2019) [50] and described in the section Venom-Induced Pathophysiology. By an experimental model of induced AKI, the researchers could highlight that a pharmacological inhibition of kallikrein with aprotinin results in restoring the renal function. Therefore, they suggested that a kallikrein inhibitor can be used as a promising therapeutic option complementary to the antivenom therapy, thereby reducing the mortality rate.

As noticed, the *Lonomia* antivenom is made based on a *L. obliqua* venom extract. Therefore, researchers want to investigate the efficacy and possibility of using the antivenom to treat envenomation by other *Lonomia* species. Sano-Martins et al. (2018) [92] were the first to investigate this and indicated that the *Lonomia* antivenom can restore the hemostatic disturbances caused by contact with *L. orientoandensis* and *L. casanarensis* in Colombia [92]. In Venezuela, the recommended treatment of *L. achelous* is mainly based on the use of antifibrinolytic medicines or replacement therapy of the whole blood, plasma or cryoprecipitates. This is in contrast with envenomation by *L. obliqua*. Gonçalves et al. (2007) [93] observed a high death rate in rats that were envenomed with *L. obliqua* and treated with an antifibrinolytic drugs, such as epsilonaminocaproic acid (EACA). The data indicate that the use of EACA could worsen the coagulation disturbances and that the *Lonomia* antivenom is probably the only effective treatment option today [94]. The differences in pathophysiology induced by both species may explain this observation.

Lonomia antivenom is only manufactured by the Instituto Butantan in Brazil. Yearly, several vials of the antivenom are distributed to the whole country by the Ministry of Health in Brazil. This means that according to the law, there is no authorization to commercialize the *Lonomia* antivenom outside Brazil. Due to this, physicians must request a Temporary Use Authorization delivered by the National Agency of Drugs to use the *Lonomia* antivenom outside Brazil. An example of such a case occurred in 2018 [10]. In this case, a good cooperation between all parties ensured that a patient in French Guiana could be saved and recovered without complications.

Despite the life-saving effect of the *Lonomia* antivenom, it also has some therapeutic limitations [28,50]. (i) Conventional antivenom vials contain around 70% or more IgG that are not specific against the venom proteins. These are IgGs that the animal has produced against antigens encountered during its lifetime. These extra antibodies are medically not relevant and can be responsible for the occurrence of adverse effects. (ii) Furthermore, the administration of an antivenom can lead to life-threating systemic effects such as an anaphylactic reaction (IgE or non-IgE mediated). (iii) In addition, antivenoms are costly to produce, often poorly distributed in areas with a high incidence rate and, very often, trained health staff for a good healthcare are lacking.

7.2. Supportive Treatment for Management of Local Effects

Although there is a difference between caterpillar species, there seems to be a consensus on the use of the different supportive treatments to treat the local effects. The first aid treatment entails the immediately soft removal of the remaining setae on the skin and to remove the clothes that may be contaminated with the setae as soon as possible. It has been recommended to cover the area with a sticky tape or to use forceps to remove the setae. Clothes are best washed at a minimum of 60 °C to get rid of the setae [88]. After removing the setae, the affected areas need to be washed with soap and water and dried without contacting the skin to prevent crushing and further release of the venom from residual setae (do not use a towel but dry with a hair dryer).

Cutaneous reactions are often treated with oral antihistamines and application of topical corticosteroids. Notwithstanding herewith, it is known that the therapy with antihistamine shows low efficacy and the use of topical corticosteroid is associated with side effects such as skin thinning [4]. However, for many patients, the use of antihistamine or topical corticosteroid is not even enough. Anti-itching products that contain menthol or phenol may help to relieve pruritus [26]. Moreover, in some caterpillars, ice packs or cold-water compresses are used to reduce inflammation, swelling and pain sensation. Also, analgesics such as tramadol hydrochloride may be used [95]. In severe cases of pain, the combination of a local anesthesia with analgesics appear to be a good combination to manage the pain [71]. More rarely, some caterpillars can induce an anaphylactic shock. If this happens, it is recommended to urgently administer epinephrine subcutaneously [3,95].

In the case of contact with the eyes, it is important that the patients urgently consult an ophthalmologist. Often, the eyes are first rinsed thoroughly with water and examined for remaining setae. Topical anesthetic products can assist in examinations and reduce the pain in the eyes that the patients experience. Stinging setae that have penetrated deep into the eye tissue must be removed surgically in order to prevent further damage and irritation [89,96].

Finally, no effective treatment exists to help patients after an accident with the pararama caterpillar, although it is believed that systemic corticosteroids would prevent the onset of a chronic situation wherein joint immobilization, loss of cartilage and bone structure occur [24].

From the above proposed summarization of existing symptomatic and supportive treatments, we can conclude that their availability is quite low and show low efficacy. There are many people who suffer from envenomation by many caterpillars around the globe. This clearly demonstrates the necessity of further research on caterpillars in order to open new perspectives for drug development.

8. Future Perspectives

The toxin variation among some caterpillar families or even between species certainly does not make it easy to find a cure that relieves all the symptoms and does not create adverse effects. Therefore, it is important for the future that we extend the extraction of venom components inside urticating setae of different species of Lepidoptera. In the past, researchers mainly focused on the analysis of the venom via the gold standard technique, SDS-PAGE. However, as demonstrated by Berardi et al. (2017) [22], we therefore miss a lot of important information about the venom composition. It is expected that in the future, new tools, such as genomics, transcriptomics and proteomics (LC-MS/MS), that are able to sequence miniscule droplets of the venom, will reveal the presence of much more bioactive molecules or toxins. When more transcriptome and proteome databases become available, it will provide us with essential information on the venom composition of caterpillar species and the inferring function of their proteins. From the new developed genomic databases, bioinformatics tools can be used to search for open reading frames encoding new toxins and possible isoforms. On the other hand, if we really want to unravel and clarify the mechanism and find a cure, we also need to focus on functional studies. At this moment, the research data point to a possible participation of TRPV1 channels and activation of mast cells in provoking the local effects. This of course makes it particularly interesting to investigate other ion channels and receptors, such as other TRP channels, histamine receptors and sodium channels in order to find new target(s) of the toxins in the pathway. This information will enable us to make a correlation between the reactions seen in humans and the identified proteins but also extend it to other Lepidoptera sharing similar defense systems. Only in this way will we get a step closer to discovering and understanding the origin of the complex symptoms and pave the way to new treatments. The ideal treatment would be one that effectively inactivates the toxins, is readily available, easy to use and cheap. There is a great expectation to find a truly selective and potent medicine in the form of a cream, lotion or ointment. Perhaps the search for selective blockers of TRP channels can open new perspectives in finding a treatment to adequately address the conditions. Many side effects can be avoided by using a drug to be applied externally. To conclude, we think that the world of caterpillars has still many unexplored paths to walk. Further research will certainly open new perspectives to combat this 21st-century health hazard.

9. Conclusions

Even in the 21st century, caterpillars cause serious health effects, from local dermatitis symptoms to potentially fatal systemic ones. The serious health effects make us realize that, in this modern world of medicine, we urgently need to find a solution. The provoked symptoms are a testimony of a colorful resource of clinically relevant bioactive molecules inside the venom. Recent advances in technologies have provided essential information on the venom protein composition that made it possible to link the effects of the toxins with the symptoms seen in patients. However, there is still a lot of work to do in the world of caterpillar toxins. Understanding the origin of the complex symptoms in the pathogenesis of a caterpillar should pave the way to discovering an effective treatment and this knowledge might be useful to compare and to treat envenomations with caterpillars that share a similar defense mechanism. In this way, the goal shifts to help countless people worldwide.

Funding: This research was funded by grants G0E7120N, GOC2319N and GOA4919N from the F.W.O Vlaanderen awarded to J.T. S.P was supported by KU Leuven funding (PDM/19/164). A.S. was supported in part by Leuven Research & Development (LRD).

Acknowledgments: We would like to thank Andrea Battisti from the University of Padova, Italy; Markus Berger from the Laboratory Biochemistry and Pharmacology, Experimental Research Center (CPE); Jie Zheng from the University of California, USA; Lei Luo from the Institute of Zoology, Kunming, China; Yuhua Tian from University School of Pharmacy, Qingdao, China, for kindly providing and authorizing the use of images included in this review article. Additionally, we would like to thank all the photographers from Pixabay, J_Wberg, Brett Hondow, Alessandro Paiva, Marc Pascual, OpenClipart-Vectors, Clker-Free-Vector-Images and SilviaP_Design, for the use of images includes in this review article.

Conflicts of Interest: The authors declare no conflict of interest.

References

1. Mitter, C.; Davis, N.R.; Cummings, M.P. Phylogeny and Evolution of Lepidoptera. *Annu. Rev. Èntomol.* **2017**, *62*, 265–283. [CrossRef] [PubMed]
2. Kristensen, N.P.; Scoble, M.J.; Karsholt, O. Lepidoptera phylogeny and systematics: The state of inventorying moth and butterfly diversity. *Zootaxa* **2007**, *1668*, 699–747. [CrossRef]
3. Diaz, J.H. The Evolving Global Epidemiology, Syndromic Classification, Management, And Prevention of Caterpillar Envenoming. *Am. J. Trop. Med. Hyg.* **2005**, *72*, 347–57. [CrossRef] [PubMed]

4. Boas, I.V.; Bonfá, G.; Tambourgi, D.V. Venomous caterpillars: From inoculation apparatus to venom composition and envenomation. *Toxicon* **2018**, *153*, 39–52. [CrossRef] [PubMed]
5. Alvarez-Flores, M.; Zannin, M.; Chudzinski-Tavassi, A. New Insight into the Mechanism of *Lonomia obliqua* Envenoming: Toxin Involvement and Molecular Approach. *Pathophysiol. Haemost. Thromb.* **2009**, *37*, 1–16. [CrossRef]
6. Moraes, J.A.; Rodrigues, G.; Nascimento-Silva, V.; Renovato-Martins, M.; Berger, M.; Guimarães, J.A.; Barja-Fidalgo, C. Effects of *Lonomia obliqua* Venom on Vascular Smooth Muscle Cells: Contribution of NADPH Oxidase-Derived Reactive Oxygen Species. *Toxins* **2017**, *9*, 360. [CrossRef]
7. Fagrell, B.; Jörneskog, G.; Larsson, S.; Holm, G.; Salomonsson, A.-C. Skin reactions induced by experimental exposure to setae from larvae of the northern pine processionary moth (*Thaumetopoea pinivora*). *Contact Dermat.* **2008**, *59*, 290–295. [CrossRef]
8. Carrijo-Carvalho, L.C.; Chudzinski-Tavassi, A.M. The venom of the *Lonomia* caterpillar: An overview. *Toxicon* **2007**, *49*, 741–757. [CrossRef]
9. Pentzold, S.; Zagrobelny, M.; Khakimov, B.; Engelsen, S.B.; Clausen, H.; Petersen, B.L.; Borch, J.; Møller, B.L.; Bak, S. Lepidopteran defence droplets—A composite physical and chemical weapon against potential predators. *Sci. Rep.* **2016**, *6*, 22407. [CrossRef]
10. Mayence, C.; Mathien, C.; Sanna, A.; Houcke, S.; Tabard, P.; Roux, A.; Valentin, C.; Resiere, D.; Lemonnier, D.; Cho, F.N.; et al. *Lonomia* caterpillar envenoming in French Guiana reversed by the Brazilian antivenom: A successful case of international cooperation for a rare but deadly tropical hazard. *Toxicon* **2018**, *151*, 74–78. [CrossRef]
11. Walker, A.A.; Robinson, S.D.; Yeates, D.K.; Jin, J.; Baumann, K.; Dobson, J.S.; Fry, B.G.; King, G.F. Entomo-venomics: The evolution, biology and biochemistry of insect venoms. *Toxicon* **2018**, *154*, 15–27. [CrossRef] [PubMed]
12. Kuspis, D.A.; Rawlins, J.; Krenzelok, E.P. Human exposures to stinging caterpillar: *Lophocampa caryae* exposures. *Am. J. Emerg. Med.* **2001**, *19*, 396–398. [CrossRef] [PubMed]
13. Heinen, T.E.; Da Veiga, A.B.G. Arthropod venoms and cancer. *Toxicon* **2011**, *57*, 497–511. [CrossRef] [PubMed]
14. Favalesso, M.M.; Lorini, L.M.; Peichoto, M.; Guimarães, A.T.B. Potential distribution and ecological conditions of *Lonomia obliqua* Walker 1855 (Saturniidae: Hemileucinae) in Brazil. *Acta Trop.* **2019**, *192*, 158–164. [CrossRef] [PubMed]
15. Burdmann, E.; Jha, V. Acute kidney injury due to tropical infectious diseases and animal venoms: A tale of 2 continents. *Kidney Int.* **2017**, *91*, 1033–1046. [CrossRef]
16. S. Brazil Ministry of Health. Accidents by Venomous Animals: What to Do and How to Avoid. Available online: https://saude.gov.br/saude-de-a-z/acidentes-por-animais-peconhentos (accessed on 7 April 2020).
17. Ciminera, M.; Auger-Rozenberg, M.-A.; Caron, H.; Herrera, M.; Scotti-Saintagne, C.; Scotti, I.; Tysklind, N.; Roques, A. Genetic Variation and Differentiation of *Hylesia metabus* (Lepidoptera: Saturniidae): Moths of Public Health Importance in French Guiana and in Venezuela. *J. Med. Èntomol.* **2018**, *56*, 137–148. [CrossRef]
18. Quintana, M.; Sciani, J.M.; Auada, A.V.V.; Martínez, M.M.; Sánchez, M.N.; Santoro, M.L.; Fan, H.W.; Peichoto, M. Stinging caterpillars from the genera *Podalia*, *Leucanella* and *Lonomia* in Misiones, Argentina: A preliminary comparative approach to understand their toxicity. *Comp. Biochem. Physiol. Part C Toxicol. Pharmacol.* **2017**, *202*, 55–62. [CrossRef]
19. McMillan, C.W.; Purcell, W.R. The Puss Caterpillar, Alias Woolly Slug. *N. Engl. J. Med.* **1964**, *271*, 147–149. [CrossRef]
20. Forrester, M.B. *Megalopyge opercularis* Caterpillar Stings Reported to Texas Poison Centers. *Wilderness Environ. Med.* **2018**, *29*, 215–220. [CrossRef]
21. Battisti, A.; Larsson, S.; Roques, A. Processionary Moths and Associated Urtication Risk: Global Change–Driven Effects. *Annu. Rev. Èntomol.* **2017**, *62*, 323–342. [CrossRef]
22. Berardi, L.; Pivato, M.; Arrigoni, G.; Mitali, E.; Trentin, A.R.; Olivieri, M.; Kerdelhué, C.; Dorkeld, F.; Nidelet, S.; Dubois, E.; et al. Proteome Analysis of Urticating Setae From *Thaumetopoea pityocampa* (Lepidoptera: Notodontidae). *J. Med. Èntomol.* **2017**, *54*, 1560–1566. [CrossRef] [PubMed]
23. Mindlin, M.J.; Waroux, O.L.P.D.; Case, S.; Walsh, B. The arrival of oak processionary moth, a novel cause of itchy dermatitis, in the UK: Experience, lessons and recommendations. *Public Health* **2012**, *126*, 778–781. [CrossRef] [PubMed]

24. Boas, I.V.; Gonçalves-De-Andrade, R.M.; Pidde-Queiroz, G.; Assaf, S.L.M.R.; Portaro, F.C.V.; Sant'Anna, O.A.; Berg, C.W.V.D.; Tambourgi, D.V. *Premolis semirufa* (Walker, 1856) Envenomation, Disease Affecting Rubber Tappers of the Amazon: Searching for Caterpillar-Bristles Toxic Components. *PLoS Negl. Trop. Dis.* **2012**, *6*, e1531. [CrossRef]
25. E Perkins, L.; Cribb, B.W.; Pagendam, E.D.; Zalucki, M.P. Variation in Morphology and Airborne Dispersal of the Urticating Apparatus of *Ochrogaster lunifer* (Lepidoptera: Notodontidae), an Australian Processionary Caterpillar, and Implications for Livestock and Humans. *J. Insect Sci.* **2019**, *19*, 1–8. [CrossRef]
26. Vega, J.; Moneo, I. Skin Reactions on Exposure to the Pine Processionary Caterpillar (*Thaumetopoea pityocampa*). *Actas Dermo-Sifiliográficas (English Edition)* **2011**, *102*, 658–667. [CrossRef]
27. Fuentes, V.; Zapatero, R.L.; Martínez, M.M.; Alonso, L.E.; Beitia, Z.B.; Mazuecos, J.M.B. Allergy to the pine processionary caterpillar (Thaumetopoea pityocampa). *Allergol. Immunopathol.* **1999**, *29*, 1418–1423.
28. Laustsen, A.H.; Gutiérrez, J.M.; Knudsen, C.; Johansen, K.H.; Bermúdez-Méndez, E.; Cerni, F.A.; Jürgensen, J.A.; Ledsgaard, L.; Martos-Esteban, A.; Øhlenschlæger, M.; et al. Pros and cons of different therapeutic antibody formats for recombinant antivenom development. *Toxicon* **2018**, *146*, 151–175. [CrossRef]
29. Greeney, H.F.; Dyer, L.A.; Smilanich, A.M. Feeding by lepidopteran larvae is dangerous: A review of caterpillars' chemical, physiological, morphological, and behavioral defenses against natural enemies. *Invertebr. Surviv. J.* **2012**, *9*, 7–34.
30. Cabrera, G.; Salazar, V.; Montesino, R.; Tambara, Y.; Struwe, W.B.; Leon, E.; Harvey, D.J.; Lesur, A.; Rincon, M.; Domon, B.; et al. Structural characterization and biological implications of sulfated N-glycans in a serine protease from the neotropical moth *Hylesia metabus* (Cramer 1775) (Lepidoptera: Saturniidae). *Glycobiology* **2015**, *26*, cwv096. [CrossRef]
31. Jourdain, F.; Girod, R.; Vassal, J.; Chandre, F.; Lagneau, C.; Fouque, F.; Guiral, D.; Raude, J.; Robert, V. The moth *Hylesia metabus* and French Guiana lepidopterism: Centenary of a public health concern. *Parasite* **2012**, *19*, 117–128. [CrossRef]
32. Paniz-Mondolfi, A.E.; Pérez-Alvarez, A.M.; Lundberg, U.; Fornés, L.; Reyes-Jaimes, O.; Hernández-Pérez, M.; Hossler, E. Tropical medicine rounds Cutaneous lepidopterism : Dermatitis from contact with moths of Hylesia metabus (Cramer 1775) (Lepidoptera : Saturniidae), the causative agent of caripito itch. *Int. J. Dermatol.* **2011**, *50*, 535–541. [CrossRef] [PubMed]
33. Sano-Martins, I.S.; Duarte, A.C.; Guerrero, B.; Moraes, R.H.P.; Barros, E.J.G.; Arocha-Piñango, C.L. Hemostatic disorders induced by skin contact with *Lonomia obliqua* (Lepidoptera, Saturniidae) caterpillars. *Revista do Instituto de Medicina Tropical de São Paulo* **2017**, *59*, 1–9. [CrossRef] [PubMed]
34. Boas, I.V.; Gonçalves-De-Andrade, R.M.; Squaiella-Baptistão, C.C.; Sant'Anna, O.A.; Tambourgi, D.V. Characterization of Phenotypes of Immune Cells and Cytokines Associated with Chronic Exposure to *Premolis semirufa* Caterpillar Bristles Extract. *PLoS ONE* **2013**, *8*, e71938. [CrossRef]
35. Bastos, L.D.C.; Da Veiga, A.B.G.; Guimaraes, J.A.; Tonussi, C.R. Nociceptive and edematogenic responses elicited by a crude bristle extract of *Lonomia obliqua* caterpillars. *Toxicon* **2004**, *43*, 273–278. [CrossRef] [PubMed]
36. Gouveia, A.I.D.C.; Da Silveira, R.B.; Nader, H.B.; Dietrich, C.P.; Gremski, W.; Veiga, S. Identification and partial characterisation of hyaluronidases in *Lonomia obliqua* venom. *Toxicon* **2005**, *45*, 403–410. [CrossRef] [PubMed]
37. Bordon, K.C.F.; Wiezel, G.A.; Amorim, F.G.; Arantes, E.C. Arthropod venom Hyaluronidases: Biochemical properties and potential applications in medicine and biotechnology. *J. Venom. Anim. Toxins Incl. Trop. Dis.* **2015**, *21*, 43. [CrossRef] [PubMed]
38. Bala, E.; Hazarika, R.; Singh, P.; Yasir, M.; Shrivastava, R. A biological overview of Hyaluronidase: A venom enzyme and its inhibition with plants materials. *Mater. Today Proc.* **2018**, *5*, 6406–6412. [CrossRef]
39. Boas, I.V.; Pidde-Queiroz, G.; Magnoli, F.C.; Gonçalves-De-Andrade, R.M.; Berg, C.W.V.D.; Tambourgi, D.V. A Serine Protease Isolated from the Bristles of the Amazonic Caterpillar, *Premolis semirufa*, Is a Potent Complement System Activator. *PLoS ONE* **2015**, *10*, e0118615. [CrossRef]
40. Berardi, L.; Battisti, A.; Negrisolo, E. The allergenic protein Tha p 2 of processionary moths of the genus *Thaumetopoea* (Thaumetopoeinae, Notodontidae, Lepidoptera): Characterization and evolution. *Gene* **2015**, *574*, 317–324. [CrossRef]

41. Sánchez, M.N.; Sciani, J.M.; Quintana, M.A.; Martínez, M.M.; Tavares, F.L.; Gritti, M.A.; Fan, H.W.; Teibler, G.P.; Peichoto, M. Understanding toxicological implications of accidents with caterpillars *Megalopyge lanata* and *Podalia orsilochus* (Lepidoptera: Megalopygidae). *Comp. Biochem. Physiol. Part C Toxicol. Pharmacol.* **2019**, *216*, 110–119. [CrossRef]
42. Lamdin, J.; Howell, D.; Kocan, K.; Murphey, D.; Arnold, D.; Fenton, A.; Odell, G.; Ownby, C. The venomous hair structure, venom and life cycle of *Lagoa crispata*, a puss caterpillar of Oklahoma. *Toxicon* **2000**, *38*, 1163–1189. [CrossRef]
43. Yao, Z.; Kamau, P.; Han, Y.; Hu, J.; Luo, A.; Luo, L.; Zheng, J.; Tian, Y.; Lai, R. The *Latoia consocia* Caterpillar Induces Pain by Targeting Nociceptive Ion Channel TRPV1. *Toxins* **2019**, *11*, 695. [CrossRef] [PubMed]
44. Battisti, A.; Holm, G.; Fagrell, B.; Larsson, S. Urticating Hairs in Arthropods: Their Nature and Medical Significance. *Annu. Rev. Èntomol.* **2011**, *56*, 203–220. [CrossRef] [PubMed]
45. Da Veiga, A.B.G.; Blochtein, B.; Guimaraes, J.A. Structures involved in production, secretion and injection of the venom produced by the caterpillar *Lonomia obliqua* (Lepidoptera, Saturniidae). *Toxicon* **2001**, *39*, 1343–1351. [CrossRef]
46. Moneo, I.; Vega, J.; Caballero, M.L.; Vega, J.; Alday, E. Isolation and characterization of Tha p 1, a major allergen from the pine processionary caterpillar *Thaumetopoea pityocampa*. *Allergy* **2003**, *58*, 34–37. [CrossRef] [PubMed]
47. Marisa, A.; Paola, M.; Carrijo-Carvalho, L.C.; Esther, M. *Toxins from Lonomia obliqua—Recombinant Production and Molecular Approach. In An Integrated View of the Molecular Recognition and Toxinology—From Analytical Procedures to Biomedical Applications*; IntechOpen: London, UK, 2013.
48. Rodríguez-Mahillo, A.I.; Gonzalez-Muñoz, M.; Vega, J.M.; Lopez, J.A.; Yart, A.; Kerdelhué, C.; Camafeita, E.; Ortiz, J.C.G.; Vogel, H.; Toffolo, E.P.; et al. Setae from the pine processionary moth (*Thaumetopoea pityocampa*) contain several relevant allergens. *Contact Dermat.* **2012**, *67*, 367–374. [CrossRef]
49. Triant, D.A.; Cinel, S.D.; Kawahara, A.Y. Lepidoptera genomes: Current knowledge, gaps and future directions. *Curr. Opin. Insect Sci.* **2018**, *25*, 99–105. [CrossRef]
50. Berger, M.; De Moraes, J.A.; Beys-Da-Silva, W.O.; Santi, L.; Terraciano, P.B.; Driemeier, D.; Cirne-Lima, E.O.; Passos, E.P.; Vieira, M.A.R.; Barja-Fidalgo, T.C.; et al. Renal and vascular effects of kallikrein inhibition in a model of *Lonomia obliqua* venom-induced acute kidney injury. *PLoS Negl. Trop. Dis.* **2019**, *13*, e0007197. [CrossRef]
51. Munitz, A.; Piliponsky, A.M.; Levi-Schaffer, F. IgE-Independent Activation of Human Mast Cells Indicates their Role in the Late Phase Reaction of Allergic Inflammation. *Cell Tissue Bank.* **2003**, *4*, 25–28. [CrossRef]
52. Shaik-Dasthagirisaheb, Y.; Varvara, G.; Murmura, G.; Saggini, A.; Potalivo, G.; Caraffa, A.; Antinolfi, P.; Tetè, S.; Tripodi, D.; Conti, F.; et al. Vascular Endothelial Growth Factor (VEGF), Mast Cells and Inflammation. *Int. J. Immunopathol. Pharmacol.* **2013**, *26*, 327–335. [CrossRef]
53. Galicia-Curiel, M.F.; Quintanar, J.L.; Jiménez, M.; Salinas, E. Mast cells respond to urticating extract from lepidoptera larva *Morpheis ehrenbergii* in the rat. *Toxicon* **2014**, *77*, 121–124. [CrossRef] [PubMed]
54. Cuypers, E.; Yanagihara, A.; Karlsson, E.; Tytgat, J. Jellyfish and other cnidarian envenomations cause pain by affecting TRPV1 channels. *FEBS Lett.* **2006**, *580*, 5728–5732. [CrossRef] [PubMed]
55. Lamy, M.; Vincendeau, P.; Ducombs, G.; Pastureaud, M.H. Irritating substance extracted from the *Thaumetopoea pityocampa* caterpillar; mechanism of action. *Cell. Mol. Life Sci.* **1983**, *39*, 299. [CrossRef] [PubMed]
56. Gottschling, S.; Meyer, S.; Dill-Mueller, D.; Wurm, D.; Gortner, L. Outbreak Report of Airborne Caterpillar Dermatitis in a Kindergarten. *Dermatology* **2007**, *215*, 5–9. [CrossRef]
57. Faninger, A. Dermatitis erucarum (*Euproctis chrysorrhea*). *Med. Glas.* **1972**, 26.
58. Lamy, M.; Pastureaud, M.-H.; Novak, F.; Ducombs, G.; Vincedeau, P.; Maleville, J.; Texier, L. Thaumetopoein: An urticating protein from the hairs and integument of the pine processionary caterpillar (*Thaumetopoea pityocampa* schiff., Lepidoptera, Thaumetopoeidae). *Toxicon* **1986**, *24*, 347–356. [CrossRef]
59. Kalender, Y.; Kalender, S.; Uzunhisarcikli, M.; Ogutcu, A.; Açikgoz, F. Effects of *Thaumetopoea pityocampa* (Lepidoptera: Thaumetopoeidae) larvae on the degranulation of dermal mast cells in mice; an electron microscopic study. *Folia Boil.* **2004**, *52*, 13–17.
60. Werno, J.; Lamy, M.; Vincendeau, P. Caterpillar hairs as allergens. *Lancet* **1993**, *342*, 936–937. [CrossRef]
61. Lamy, M. Contact dermatitis (erucism) produced by processionary caterpillars (Genus *Thaumetopoea*). *J. Appl. Èntomol.* **1990**, *110*, 425–437. [CrossRef]

62. S.n. WHO/IUIS Allergen Nomenclature Sub-Committee. "Allergen Tha p 1," Allergen Nomenclature. 2006. Available online: http://www.allergen.org/viewallergen.php?aid=614 (accessed on 18 April 2020).
63. Gschloessl, B.; Dorkeld, F.; Berges, H.; Beydon, G.; Bouchez, O.; Branco, M.; Bretaudeau, A.; Burban, C.; Dubois, E.; Gauthier, P.; et al. Draft genome and reference transcriptomic resources for the urticating pine defoliator *Thaumetopoea pityocampa* (Lepidoptera: Notodontidae). *Mol. Ecol. Resour.* **2018**, *18*, 602–619. [CrossRef]
64. Ziprkowski, L.; Rolant, F.; Ziprkowski, F.R.L. Study of the Toxin from Poison Hairs of *Thaumetopoea Wilkinsoni* Caterpillars. *J. Investig. Dermatol.* **1972**, *58*, 274–277. [CrossRef] [PubMed]
65. Bohrer, C.; Junior, J.R.; Fernandes, D.; Sordi, R.; Guimaraes, J.A.; Assreuy, J.; Termignoni, C. Kallikrein–kinin system activation by *Lonomia obliqua* caterpillar bristles: Involvement in edema and hypotension responses to envenomation. *Toxicon* **2007**, *49*, 663–669. [CrossRef] [PubMed]
66. Calixto, J.B.; Medeiros, R.; Fernandes, E.S.; Ferreira, J.; Cabrini, A.D.; Campos, M.M. Kinin B1 receptors: Key G-protein-coupled receptors and their role in inflammatory and painful processes. *Br. J. Pharmacol.* **2004**, *143*, 803–818. [CrossRef] [PubMed]
67. Cabrera, G.; Lundberg, U.; Rodríguez, L.A.E.; Herrera, M.; Machado, W.; Portela, M.; Palomares, S.; Espinosa, L.A.; Ramos, Y.; Durán, R.; et al. Protein content of the *Hylesia metabus* egg nest setae (Cramer 1775) (Lepidoptera: Saturniidae) and its association with the parental investment for the reproductive success and lepidopterism. *J. Proteom.* **2017**, *150*, 183–200. [CrossRef]
68. Clémençon, B.; Kuhn-Nentwig, L.; Langenegger, N.; Kopp, L.; Peigneur, S.; Tytgat, J.; Nentwig, W.; Lüscher, B.P. Neurotoxin Merging: A Strategy Deployed by the Venom of the Spider *Cupiennius salei* to Potentiate Toxicity on Insects. *Toxins* **2020**, *12*, 250. [CrossRef]
69. Berger, M.; Beys-da-Silva, W.O.; Santi, L.; de Oliveira, I.M.; Jorge, P.M.; Henriques, J.A.P.; Driemeier, D.; Vieira, M.A.R.; Guimarães, J.A. Acute Lonomia obliqua caterpillar envenomation-induced physiopathological alterations in rats: Evidence of new toxic venom activities and the efficacy of serum therapy to counteract systemic tissue damage. *Toxicon* **2013**, *74*, 179–192. [CrossRef]
70. Gutiérrez, J.M.; Calvete, J.J.; Habib, A.G.; Harrison, R.A.; Williams, D.J.; Warrell, D.A. Snakebite envenoming. *Nat. Rev. Dis. Prim.* **2017**, *3*, 17063. [CrossRef]
71. Maíra, M.P.B.; Carla, F.B.-F.; Camila, C.P.; Taís, F.G.; Marcus, T.S.; Eduardo, M.D.C.; Stephen, H.; Fábio, B. Management of severe pain after dermal contact with caterpillars (erucism): A prospective case series. *Clin. Toxicol.* **2019**, *57*, 338–342.
72. Basbaum, A.I.; Bautista, D.M.; Scherrer, G.; Julius, D. Cellular and Molecular Mechanisms of Pain. *Cell* **2009**, *139*, 267–84. [CrossRef]
73. Julius, D.; Basbaum, A.I. Molecular mechanisms of nociception. *Nature* **2001**, *413*, 203–210. [CrossRef]
74. Pacifici, G.M. Clinical Pharmacology of Indomethacin in Preterm Infants: Implications in Patent Ductus Arteriosus Closure. *Pediatr. Drugs* **2013**, *15*, 363–376. [CrossRef] [PubMed]
75. Seibert, C.S.; Tanaka-Azevedo, A.M.; Santoro, M.L.; Mackessy, S.P.; Torquato, R.J.S.; Lebrun, I.; Tanaka, A.S.; Sano-Martins, I.S. Purification of a phospholipase A2 from Lonomia obliqua caterpillar bristle extract. *Biochem. Biophys. Res. Commun.* **2016**, *342*, 1027–1033. [CrossRef] [PubMed]
76. Bohlen, C.J.; Priel, A.; Zhou, S.; King, D.; Siemens, J.; Julius, D. A Bivalent Tarantula Toxin Activates the Capsaicin Receptor, TRPV1, by Targeting the Outer Pore Domain. *Cell* **2010**, *141*, 834–45. [CrossRef] [PubMed]
77. Ricci-Silva, M.E.; Valente, R.H.; León, I.R.; Tambourgi, D.V.; Ramos, O.H.P.; Perales, J.; Chudzinski-Tavassi, A.M. Immunochemical and proteomic technologies as tools for unravelling toxins involved in envenoming by accidental contact with *Lonomia obliqua* caterpillars. *Toxicon* **2008**, *51*, 1017–1028. [CrossRef]
78. Chudzinski-Tavassi, A.; Carrijo-Carvalho, L.C. Biochemical and biological properties of *Lonomia obliqua* bristle extract. *J. Venom. Anim. Toxins Incl. Trop. Dis.* **2006**, *12*, 156–171. [CrossRef]
79. Alvarez-Flores, M.; Furlin, D.; Ramos, O.H.P.; Balan, A.; Konno, K.; Chudzinski-Tavassi, A. Losac, the First Hemolin that Exhibits Procogulant Activity through Selective Factor X Proteolytic Activation. *J. Boil. Chem.* **2010**, *286*, 6918–6928. [CrossRef]
80. Alvarez-Flores, M.; Fritzen, M.; Reis, C.V.; Chudzinski-Tavassi, A.M. Losac, a factor X activator from *Lonomia obliqua* bristle extract: Its role in the pathophysiological mechanisms and cell survival. *Biochem. Biophys. Res. Commun.* **2006**, *343*, 1216–1223. [CrossRef]

81. Bernardi, L.; Pinto, A.F.M.; Mendes, E.; Yates, J.; Lamers, M.L. *Lonomia obliqua* bristle extract modulates Rac1 activation, membrane dynamics and cell adhesion properties. *Toxicon* **2019**, *162*, 32–39. [CrossRef]
82. Chan, K.; Lee, A.; Onell, R.; Etches, W.; Nahirniak, S.; Bagshaw, S.M.; Larratt, L.M. Caterpillar-induced bleeding syndrome in a returning traveller. *Can. Med Assoc. J.* **2008**, *179*, 158–161. [CrossRef]
83. Rosing, J.; Govers-Riemslag, J.W.; Yukelson, L.; Tans, G. Factor V Activation and Inactivation by Venom Proteases. *Pathophysiol. Haemost. Thromb.* **2001**, *31*, 241–246. [CrossRef]
84. Fernandes-Pedrosa, M.F.; Félix-Silva, J.; Menezes, Y.A. Toxins from Venomous Animals: Gene Cloning, Protein Expression and Biotechnological Applications. In *An Integrated View of the Molecular Recognition and Toxinology: From Analytical Procedures to Biomedical Applications*; IntechOpen: London, UK, 2012.
85. Brusco, I.; Justino, A.B.; Silva, C.R.; Fischer, S.; Cunha, T.M.; Scussel, R.; Machado-de-Ávila, R.A.; Ferreira, J.; Oliveira, S.M. Kinins and their B 1 and B 2 receptors are involved in fibromyalgia-like pain symptoms in mice. *Biochem. Pharmacol.* **2019**, *168*, 119–132. [CrossRef] [PubMed]
86. Samartin, L.G.; Luchini, G.; Pidde, C.C. Squaiella-baptistão, and D. V Tambourgi, Complement System Inhibition Modulates the Pro-Inflammatory Effects of a Snake Venom Metalloproteinase. *Front. Immunol.* **2019**, *10*, 1–11.
87. Haddad, V.; Cardoso, J.L.C.; Lupi, O.; Tyring, S.K. Tropical dermatology: Venomous arthropods and human skin: Part, I. Insecta. *J. Am. Acad. Dermatol.* **2012**, *67*, 331-e1. [CrossRef]
88. Rahlenbeck, S.I.; Utikal, J. The oak processionary moth: A new health hazard? *Br. J. Gen. Pr.* **2015**, *65*, 435–436. [CrossRef] [PubMed]
89. Saleh, S.; Brownstein, S.; Kapasi, M.; O'Connor, M.; Blanco, P. Ophthalmia nodosa secondary to caterpillar-hair-induced conjunctivitis in a child. *Can. J. Ophthalmol.* **2020**, *55*, e56–e59. [CrossRef] [PubMed]
90. Da Silva, W.D.; Campos, C.M.; Gonçalves, L.R.; Sousa-E-Silva, M.C.; Higashi, H.G.; Yamagushi, I.K.; Kelen, E.M. Development of an antivenom against toxins of *Lonomia obliqua* caterpillars. *Toxicon* **1996**, *34*, 1045–1049. [CrossRef]
91. Rocha-Campos, A.C.; Sousa-E-Silva, M.C.; Oliveira, J.E.; Da Silva, W.D.; Ribela, M.T.; Yamagushi, I.K.; Fernandes, I.; Gonçalves, L.R.; Higashi, H.G. Specific heterologous F(ab')2 antibodies revert blood incoagulability resulting from envenoming by *Lonomia obliqua* caterpillars. *Am. J. Trop. Med. Hyg.* **2001**, *64*, 283–289. [CrossRef] [PubMed]
92. Sano-Martins, I.S.; González, C.; Anjos, I.V.; Diaz, J.; Gonçalves, L.R.C. Effectiveness of *Lonomia* antivenom in recovery from the coagulopathy induced by *Lonomia orientoandensis* and *Lonomia casanarensis* caterpillars in rats. *PLoS Negl. Trop. Dis.* **2018**, *12*, e0006721. [CrossRef]
93. Gonçalves, L.R.C.; Sousa-E-Silva, M.C.C.; Tomy, S.C.; Sano-Martins, I.S. Efficacy of serum therapy on the treatment of rats experimentally envenomed by bristle extract of the caterpillar *Lonomia obliqua*: Comparison with epsilon-aminocaproic acid therapy. *Toxicon* **2007**, *50*, 349–356. [CrossRef]
94. Junior, V.H.; Lastória, J.C. Envenomation by caterpillars (erucism): Proposal for simple pain relief treatment. *J. Venom. Anim. Toxins Incl. Trop. Dis.* **2014**, *20*, 21. [CrossRef]
95. Tsai, M.K.; Yang, D.H. Caterpillar-Induced Protracted Anaphylaxis. Available online: https://www.google.com/url?sa=t&rct=j&q=&esrc=s&source=web&cd=&ved=2ahUKEwjl6YeH4eDpAhXqy6YKHVdNB3AQFjAAegQIARAB&url=http%3A%2F%2Faustinpublishinggroup.com%2Fallergy%2Fdownload.php%3Ffile%3Dfulltext%2Faja-v5-id1033.pdf&usg=AOvVaw393wKfvuACAlXDld1qf3HL (accessed on 30 May 2020).
96. Boas, I.V.; Alvarez-Flores, M.; Chudzinski-Tavassi, A.; Tambourgi, D.V. Envenomation by Caterpillars. In *Toxinology*; Springer Science and Business Media LLC: Berlin, Germany, 2018; pp. 429–449.

biomedicines

MDPI

Article

It Takes Two: Dimerization Is Essential for the Broad-Spectrum Predatory and Defensive Activities of the Venom Peptide Mp1a from the Jack Jumper Ant *Myrmecia pilosula*

Samantha A. Nixon [1,2], Zoltan Dekan [1], Samuel D. Robinson [1], Shaodong Guo [1], Irina Vetter [1,3], Andrew C. Kotze [2], Paul F. Alewood [1], Glenn F. King [1,*] and Volker Herzig [1,4,*]

1. Institute for Molecular Bioscience, The University of Queensland, St Lucia, QLD 4072, Australia; samantha.nixon@uq.net.au (S.A.N.); z.dekan@imb.uq.edu.au (Z.D.); s.robinson@imb.uq.edu.au (S.D.R.); s.guo@imb.uq.edu.au (S.G.); i.vetter@imb.uq.edu.au (I.V.); p.alewood@imb.uq.edu.au (P.F.A.)
2. CSIRO Agriculture and Food, St Lucia, QLD 4072, Australia; Andrew.Kotze@csiro.au
3. School of Pharmacy, The University of Queensland, Woolloongabba, QLD 4102, Australia
4. School of Science & Engineering, University of the Sunshine Coast, Sippy Downs, QLD 4556, Australia

* Correspondence: glenn.king@imb.uq.edu.au (G.F.K.); vherzig@usc.edu.au (V.H.); Tel.: +61-7-3346-2025 (G.F.K.); +61-7-5456-5382 (V.H.)

Received: 11 June 2020; Accepted: 24 June 2020; Published: 30 June 2020

Abstract: Ant venoms have recently attracted increased attention due to their chemical complexity, novel molecular frameworks, and diverse biological activities. The heterodimeric peptide Δ-myrtoxin-Mp1a (Mp1a) from the venom of the Australian jack jumper ant, *Myrmecia pilosula*, exhibits antimicrobial, membrane-disrupting, and pain-inducing activities. In the present study, we examined the activity of Mp1a and a panel of synthetic analogues against the gastrointestinal parasitic nematode *Haemonchus contortus*, the fruit fly *Drosophila melanogaster*, and for their ability to stimulate pain-sensing neurons. Mp1a was found to be both insecticidal and anthelmintic, and it robustly activated mammalian sensory neurons at concentrations similar to those reported to elicit antimicrobial and cytotoxic activity. The native antiparallel Mp1a heterodimer was more potent than heterodimers with alternative disulfide connectivity, as well as monomeric analogues. We conclude that the membrane-disrupting effects of Mp1a confer broad-spectrum biological activities that facilitate both predation and defense for the ant. Our structure–activity data also provide a foundation for the rational engineering of analogues with selectivity for particular cell types.

Keywords: ant; venom; venom peptide; pilosulin; heterodimer; antiparasitic; antimicrobial

1. Introduction

The Australian jack jumper ant, *Myrmecia pilosula*, is a species of bull ant within the *M. pilosula* species complex, endemic to the temperate Eastern regions of Australia [1]. These ants are well known for their jumping ability and highly painful stings that can cause severe allergic reactions [2,3]. *M. pilosula* venom is a cocktail of peptidic toxins (2–25 kDa) that is employed for both predation and defense [4]. By far the most abundant venom component is a small, antiparallel disulfide-linked heterodimeric peptide named Δ-myrtoxin-Mp1a (Mp1a) (previously referred to as 'pilosulin 3') [5–7].

Although most animal venoms have evolved to assist with predation, they are used for a variety of other roles including defense against predators (e.g., bees [8]), intraspecific competition (e.g., platypus [9]), conspecific communication (e.g., wasps [10]), chemical detoxification (e.g., formicine ants [11]), detection of envenomed prey (e.g., rattlesnakes [12]), and courtship and mating (e.g., scorpions [13]). Thus, Mp1a could play a number of roles in *M. pilosula* venom, but its ecological function is currently not clear. Intraplantar injection of Mp1a into mice induces nocifensive behavior and mechanical allodynia [5]. Mp1a also has broad-spectrum activity against a diverse range of bacteria, fungi and cell lines [5]. We hypothesized that Mp1a, as a membrane-disrupting peptide and the major venom component, might serve both defensive (i.e., pain-inducing) and predatory (i.e., insecticidal) roles.

There is also growing interest in ant venoms as a source of structurally and pharmacologically diverse peptides with potential applications in medicine, agriculture and biotechnology [14]. Mp1a and synthetic analogues have already been shown to have antibiotic activity, including against the opportunistic human pathogen *Acinetobacter baumannii* [5]. Several venom-derived antimicrobial peptides are active against a range of human parasites, including cupiennin 1a from the wandering spider *Cupiennius salei*, which is active against both trypanosomes and malaria parasites [15,16], the antimalarial peptides meucin-24 and 25 from the scorpion *Mesobuthus eupeus* [17], and the antitrypanosomal dinoponeratoxins from the giant ant *Dinoponera quadriceps* [18]. We therefore explored whether Mp1a might be active against *Haemonchus contortus*, a pathogenic blood-feeding parasitic nematode of ruminants, which serves as a model organism for anthelmintic drug discovery. While often found in ant venoms [14,19], small disulfide-bridged heterodimeric toxins are uncommon in nature. We therefore used a series of synthetic Mp1a analogues to explore the structure—activity relationships for Mp1a in relation to their insecticidal, cytotoxic, antiparasitic and algogenic properties to assess their selectivity and potential as human or veterinary therapeutics.

2. Experimental Section

2.1. Peptide Synthesis

The linear A- and B-chains of Mp1a were synthesized via Fmoc solid phase peptide synthesis (SPPS) and purified using reversed-phase high-performance liquid chromatography (RP-HPLC) [5]. Mp1a (**1a**) was formed by mixing the reduced forms of the two chains in an equimolar ratio at pH 8.0. The cysteine oxidation reaction yielded a single major product that co-eluted with the major venom toxin on RP-HPLC [5], indicating that correct disulfide pairings had been achieved and potential homodimers, cyclized monomers, parallel heterodimers or polymers were not formed [5]. The monomeric chains of Mp1a (**3a** and **4a**) were readily prepared by dimethyl sulfoxide (DMSO) oxidation. Analogue **5a** was produced using the purified reduced form of the A-chain dissolved in 6 M guanidium hydrochloride (GnHCl) and diluted with 0.2 M NH_4HCO_3 (pH 8.0) to a final concentration of 2 mM peptide and 1 M GnHCl, and then stirred in an open vessel at room temperature for 48 h. Analysis of the product using HPLC and MS revealed a predominant peak corresponding to the correct mass of the dimeric A chain (calc. avg. 1577.0 M + 4H, found 1576.9), which was isolated using preparative HPLC.

2.2. *Drosophila Melanogaster* Microinjection Assay

The insecticidal activity of the chemically synthesized **1a** and analogues thereof were determined by injection into adult female *D. melanogaster* aged 3–5 days (mass 0.7–0.9 mg) as described previously [20]. Analogues were dissolved in water and intrathoracically injected using pulled glass capillaries at a volume of 50 nL per fruit fly, and the results were compared against an equivalent injection volume of water alone. All injections were performed in the morning or early afternoon. At 24 h post-injection flies were monitored for lethality. Dose–response curves were constructed using 7–10 doses per analogue (each dose tested in eight flies) and three separate dose–response curves were constructed for each analogue. The lethality in the groups receiving the analogues were adjusted using the respective control group lethality using the Henderson-Tilton formula [20]. The median lethal dose (LD_{50}) of each analogue was calculated based on the three dose–response curves using GraphPad Prism 8.0 [21]. One-way ANOVA followed by Dunnett's multiple comparison test were used to compare LD_{50} values.

2.3. *Calcium Imaging of Mammalian Sensory Neurons*

Calcium imaging of a heterogenous population of mouse dorsal root ganglion (DRG) sensory neurons was performed as previously described [22]. In brief, dorsal root ganglion (DRG) cells isolated from 4–8-week-old male C57BL/6 mice under ethics approval TRI/IMB/093/17 (University of Queensland Animal Ethics Committee, approval date 31/03/2017) were dissociated and then plated in Dulbecco's modified Eagle's medium (Gibco, Grand Island, NY, USA) containing 10% fetal bovine serum (FBS; Assaymatrix, Melbourne, Australia) and penicillin/streptomycin (Gibco) on a 96-well poly-D-lysine–coated culture plate (Corning, Lowell, MA, USA), and maintained overnight. Cells were loaded with Fluo-4 AM calcium indicator as per the manufacturer's instructions (Thermo Fisher Scientific, Grand Island, NY, USA). After loading for 1 h, the dye solution was replaced with assay solution (Hanks' balanced salt solution and 20 mM HEPES). Fluorescence corresponding to intracellular calcium ($[Ca^{2+}]_i$) of typically 100–150 DRG cells per experiment was monitored in parallel using a Nikon Ti-E deconvolution inverted microscope, equipped with a Lumencor Spectra LED light source. Images were acquired at a 20× objective at one frame/s (excitation 485 nm; emission 521 nm). For each experiment, baseline fluorescence was monitored for 30 s and then a wash of assay solution was applied. At 60 s, the assay solution was replaced with assay solution containing individual peptides (10 μM) and the cells were observed for a further 90 s.

2.4. *FLIPR Assay*

F11 cells were cultured as previously described [23]. Cells were maintained on Ham's F12 media supplemented with 10% fetal bovine serum (FBS), 100 μM hypoxanthine, 0.4 μM aminopterin, and 16 μM thymidine (Hybri-MaxTM, Sigma Aldrich, North Ryde, Australia). Then, 384-well imaging plates (Corning) were seeded 48 h prior to imaging resulting in 90–95% confluence at imaging. Cells were incubated for 30 min with the Calcium 4 assay component A according to the manufacturer's instructions (Molecular Devices, Sunnyvale, CA, USA) in physiological salt solution (PSS; composition in mM: 140 NaCl, 11.5 D-glucose, 5.9 KCl, 1.4 $MgCl_2$, 1.2 NaH_2PO_4, 5 $NaHCO_3$, 1.8 $CaCl_2$, 10 HEPES) at 37°C. Fluorescence was measured using a fluorescent imaging plate reader ($FLIPR^{TETRA}$) equipped with a CCD camera (Excitation: 470–490 nm, Emission: 515–575 nM) (Molecular Devices, Sunnyvale, CA, USA). Signals were read every second for 10 s before, and 300 s after the addition of peptides in PSS supplemented with 0.1% bovine serum albumin. All data are the mean ± SEM of assays performed in triplicate. Maximum–minimum fluorescence in the 300 s period after peptide addition was recorded as the response. Concentration–response data were fitted with a four-parameter Hill equation (variable slope) using GraphPad Prism 8 to obtain effective concentration (EC_{50}) values.

2.5. *Haemonchus Contortus Isolation and Larval Development Assay*

Sheep were infected with *H. contortus* Kirby isolate (field isolate from the University of New England Kirby Research Farm in 1986; susceptible to all commercial anthelmintics [24]) and housed at the Commonwealth Scientific and Industrial Research Organisation (CSIRO) FD McMaster Laboratory, Armidale, NSW. All animal procedures were approved by the FD McMaster Animal Ethics Committee, CSIRO (Approval Number AEC 17/12, approval date 15.6.2017). Eggs were prepared from overnight fecal collection as described [25]. In brief, feces were filtered through mesh filters, settled, and supernatant removed by vacuum. Eggs were recovered by density centrifugation using 10 and 25% (*w*/*v*) sucrose solutions, centrifuged at 650× *g* for 7 min. Eggs were recovered from the interface of the two sucrose layers, rinsed with distilled water, sterilized with bleach, rinsed again, and diluted to 4500 eggs/mL. Tylosin tartrate (800 μg/mL) and amphotericin B (25.0 μg/mL) were added, and eggs were used immediately for larval development assays.

Assays were conducted using 96-well microtitre plates, with each well containing 50 μL of 2% agar, 20 μL of egg solution and 20 μL of peptide solution in water. The commercial anthelmintic levamisole (Sigma Aldrich) was used as a positive control (final 1% *v*/*v*). Negative controls contained equivalent volumes of water or DMSO (final 1% *v*/*v*). Plates were incubated at 26 °C for six days. After 24 h, each well was fed with 10 μL of a nutrient solution containing *Escherichia coli* XL1-Blue1 (grown overnight at 37 °C) and growth medium. The growth medium consisted of yeast extract (1% *w*/*v*), Earle's salt solution (10% *v*/*v*), saline solution (0.9% NaCl, *w*/*v*), and sodium bicarbonate (1 mM) in Luria-Bertani medium (LB). Larvae were killed and stained with Lugol's iodine solution after six days. Larvae that had developed to the infective L3 stage were counted, and the numbers in treated assay wells were expressed as a percentage of the number of infective L3 stage larvae in multiple control wells. Concentrations that caused 50% inhibition (IC50 values) were calculated from three experiments of duplicate assays. A biphasic response was observed for one peptide, and hence separate IC_{50} values were calculated for the two components of the response curve.

2.6. Cytotoxicity Assay

HEK293 (ATCC® CRL-1573, Gaithersburg, MD, USA) cells were seeded at 3000 cells/well in clear bottom 384-well plates (Corning) in a volume of 20 μL in DMEM medium (GIBCO-Invitrogen #11995-073, Grand Island, NY, USA) with 10% FBS. Cells were incubated at 37 °C in 5% CO_2 for 24 h to allow cell attachment. Compounds were dissolved in water at 1.28 mg/mL with subsequent threefold dilutions in cell culture medium, giving a final concentration range of 0.02–50 μg/mL. Tamoxifen (Sigma-Aldrich) was used as a negative cell survival control as a single point 100 μM and as a dose response with concentrations ranging from 0.18 to 400 μM. The cells were incubated with the compounds for 24 h at 37 °C, 5% CO_2. After incubation, 10 μM resazurin (Sigma-Aldrich, dissolved in PBS) was added to each well and the plates were incubated for a further 3 h at 37 °C, 5% CO_2. The fluorescence intensity was measured using a Polarstar Omega (BMG Technologies, Mornington, Australia) spectrophotometer (BMG Labtech, Mornington, Australia) with excitation/emission of 560/590 nm. The concentration required to induce 50% cell death (CC_{50}, determined as 50% reduction in absorbance relative to untreated control) was calculated using Graph Pad Prism 8.0. Cytotoxicity assays were performed as two independent experiments of duplicate assays to obtain data of $n = 4$.

2.7. Hemolysis Assay

Whole human blood (10 mL/tube) was washed in triplicate with three volumes of 0.9% NaCl, with centrifugation at 500× *g* (with reduced deceleration) for 10 min between washes. Cells were counted with a hemocytometer and then diluted to 0.5×10^8/mL in 0.9% NaCl. Cell suspension (180 μL/well) was added to assay plates and then plates were sealed and incubated at 37 °C for 1 h. Plates were then centrifuged at 1000× *g* for 10 min to pellet cells and debris and 25 μL of supernatant was recovered into a 384-well flat bottom polystyrene plate. Absorbance was read at 405 nm using a Tecan M1000 Pro monochromator plate reader. The percentage of hemolysis was calculated for each well relative to the negative control (1% DMSO in PBS) and positive control (1% Triton X-100 in PBS). Significant differences in hemolysis values were determined by fractional deviation from the mean, calculated using the average and standard deviation of the sample wells (no controls) on the same plate. The concentration required to lyse 50% of the red blood cells (HC_{50}) was determined from two independent experiments of duplicate assays to obtain data of $n = 4$.

2.8. Minimum Inhibitory Concentration (MIC) Dilution Assay

Compounds were serially diluted in cation-adjusted Mueller Hinton Broth (CaMHB) twofold across the wells of non-binding surface 96-well plates (Corning), plated in duplicate. Bacteria (strains listed in Table 1) were cultured in CaMHB at 37 °C overnight, then diluted 40-fold and incubated at 37 °C for a further 2–3 h. The resultant mid-log phase cultures were diluted in CaMHB and added to each well of the compound-containing 96-well plates to give a final cell density of 5 × 105 CFU/mL, and a final compound concentration range of 0.06–128 μg/mL. The plates were covered and incubated at 37 °C for 20 h. Inhibition of bacterial growth was determined visually, where the minimum inhibitory concentration (MIC) was recorded as the lowest compound concentration that yielded no visible growth.

Table 1. Minimum inhibitory concentrations of **5a** (A-chain homomer) and **1a** (native antiparallel heterodimer) against Gram-negative and Gram-positive bacteria from the genera *Escherichia, Klebsiella, Acinetobacter, Pseudomonas,* and *Staphylococcus*.

Strain	MIC 1a (μM) [a] (Native Antiparallel Heterodimer)	MIC 5a (μM) (A-Chain Homomer)
E. coli ATCC 25922	0.1–0.2	0.42–0.84
K. pneumoniae ATCC 700603	0.4–0.8	0.84–1.67
K. pneumoniae ATCC BAA-2146	0.1–0.2	0.84
A. baumannii ATCC 19606	0.025	0.03–0.1
P. aeruginosa ATCC 27853	0.4–0.8	0.84
P. aeruginosa FADDI-PA70	0.8	0.84–3.34
S. aureus ATCC 43300	0.8	1.67–3.34
S. aureus NRS 1	3.2	6.7
S. aureus NRS 17	0.4–0.8	1.67
S. aureus NARSA-VRS1	3.2–6.4	> 6.7
S. aureus NARSA-VRS10	0.8	1.67
S. pneumoniae ATCC 700677	0.4–0.8	1.67

[a] Minimum inhibitory concentration (MIC) (μM) values for **1a** taken from Dekan et al. [5].

2.9. Statistical Analysis

Significant differences in the insecticidal, anthelmintic and algogenic activities of Mp1a and analogues were determined using one-way ANOVA with multiple comparison followed by Tukey's post-hoc test in GraphPad Prism 8.0.

3. Results

3.1. Synthesis of Mp1a and Analogues

We synthesized Mp1a (**1a**) and analogues [5], as well as a novel A-chain homodimer with unknown disulfide connectivity (**5a**) (sequences and connectivity shown in Figure 1). Mp1a A and B-chains were produced in their reduced forms using Fmoc SPPS. Mp1a (**1a**) was formed exclusively as the antiparallel heterodimer by air oxidation of the two reduced chains without the use of orthogonal cysteine protecting groups. As no parallel heterodimer was obtained using this method, it was necessary to employ a directed strategy to prepare the non-native parallel heterodimers **2a** and **2b** as previously described [5].

3.2. Mp1a Activates Sensory Neurons

Mp1a induces spontaneous pain and mechanical allodynia when injected into the hind paw of mice [5]. We used calcium imaging to investigate the effects of Mp1a (**1a**) on mouse DRG sensory cells, and to assess how structural modifications affect cellular activation. Stimulation of nociceptive neurons can be initiated via activation of various ion channels or receptors, but it is invariably associated with an increase $[Ca^{2+}]_i$ in these neurons resulting from downstream activation of voltage-gated calcium (Ca_V) channels. Thus, increases in $[Ca^{2+}]_i$ in sensory neurons can be used as a proxy for activation [22,26,27]. The addition of 1 μM **1a** resulted in a rapid increase in $[Ca^{2+}]_i$ in all cells (both neuronal and non-neuronal). This was followed by a gradual decrease in fluorescence as dye leaked into the extracellular medium, indicating cytolysis [22] (Figure 2A). The heterodimeric analogues (**1–2**) and the A-homodimer **5a** also activated all DRG cells and caused dye leakage; however, at 1 μM, analogues **3–4** had no effect.

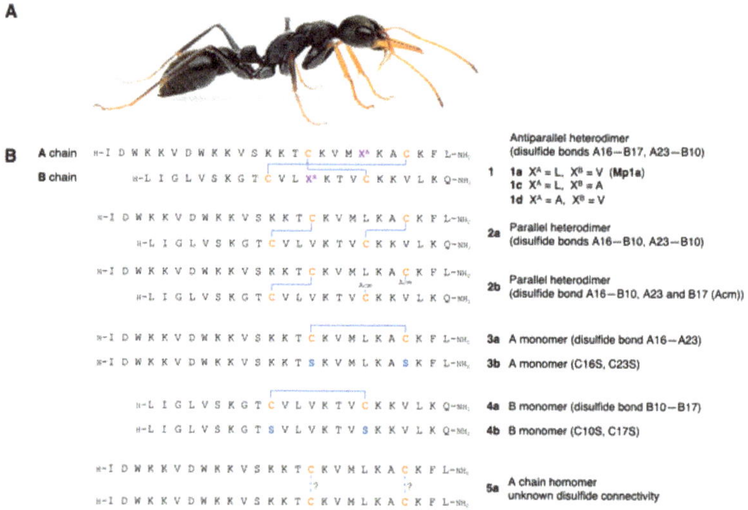

Figure 1. (**A**) Adult female *M. pilsoula* (photograph credit: Dr Alexander Wild). (**B**) Sequence and disulfide-bond connectivity of native Δ-myrtoxin-Mp1a (Mp1a) (**1a**) and synthetic analogues (**1a–4b** previously described [5]). The native peptide forms an antiparallel heterodimer comprised of one A chain and one B chain connected by two disulfide bonds (A16–B17, A23–B10). Cysteines are shown in orange, with blue lines indicating disulfide bonds. Dashed blue lines indicate unknown disulfide connectivity. Amino acid substitutions are coloured (serine in blue, miscellaneous in purple). Acetamidomethylated cysteine (Acm). Methylated cysteine (Me).

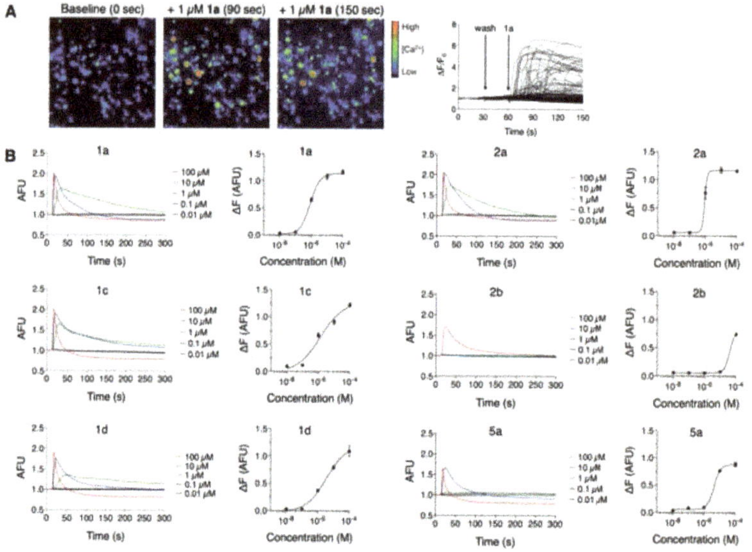

Figure 2. (**A**) Application of 1 μM Mp1a (**1a**) to dorsal root ganglion (DRG) cells induced a rapid increase in $[Ca^{2+}]_i$ followed by release of fluorescent dye into the media. The left panels (20x) show micrographs taken at baseline (0 s) and after addition of 1 μM **1a** (synthetic Mp1a. at 90 and 150 s). The graph on the right (20x) shows fluorescence responses for individual cells within the field of view. (**B**) Fluorescence responses of F11 cells after addition of **1a–1d**, **2a**, **2b** and **5a** over a range of concentrations (0.01–100 μM) recorded using a FLIPR. Changes in fluorescence (ΔF) from the maximal response less baseline fluorescence were recorded (n = 3) and used to generate concentration–response curves.

The activity of the peptides was quantified via FLIPR analysis of the effect on F11 cells (a neuroblastoma × DRG neuron hybrid cell line) (Figure 2B). The effective concentration (EC_{50}) for stimulation of these cells ranged from 0.8 to 5 μM, with the exception of **2b** which was 45-fold less active than native Mp1a (EC_{50} 38.5 μM). In F11 cells, all peptides induced a rapid increase in fluorescence followed by a decrease to or below baseline, reflecting cytolysis. This effect was observed at concentrations ≥ 1 μM for **1a**, **1c**, **1d**, and **2a**, ≥ 10 μM for **5a**, and 100 μM for **2b** (Table 2).

Table 2. Summary of bioassay data for synthetic Mp1a and analogues, including effective concentration (EC_{50}) for activation of F11 cells, concentrations that caused 50% inhibition (IC50) for inhibition of larval development of *H. contortus*; median lethal dose (LD_{50}) for lethal insecticidal effects on *D. melanogaster*; concentrations required to induce 50% cell death (CC_{50}) for effects on viability of HEK293 cells, and concentrations required to lyse 50% of the red blood cells (HC_{50}) for lysis of human red blood cells. All errors are SEM.

Peptide	Description	Neuronal Cell Activation (EC_{50}, μM)	Anthelmintic Activity (IC_{50}, μM)	Insecticidal Activity (LD_{50}, pmol/g)	Cytotoxicity (CC_{50} μM) [b]	Hemolysis (HC_{50} μM) [b]
1a	Antiparallel heterodimer (native)	0.85 ± 0.03	6.8 ± 0.5 [c]	260.1 ± 16.6	0.6	2.2
1c	Antiparallel heterodimer	1.39 ± 0.34	7.2 ± 0.1	552.7 ± 18.2 [a]	0.7	> 12
1d	Antiparallel heterodimer	3.38 ± 2.8	9.5 ± 0.3	578 ± 9.7 [a]	0.7	> 12
2a	Parallel heterodimer	0.9 ± 0.08	35.8 ± 1.9 [a]	> 600	> 10	> 10
2b	Parallel heterodimer	38.5 ± 2.3 [a]	65.6 ± 14.7 [a]	> 600	> 10	> 10
3a	A monomer (A16–A23)	inactive	46.8 ± 0.6 [a]	> 600	> 20	> 20
3b	A monomer [C16S, C23S]	inactive	64.9 ± 6.3 [a]	> 600	> 20	> 20
4a	B monomer (B10–B17)	inactive	65.5 ± 5.5 [a]	> 600	> 15	> 15
4b	B monomer [C10S, C17S]	inactive	61.3 ± 4.4 [a]	> 600	> 15	> 15
5a	A chain homomer	4.3 ± 1.3	9.2 ± 0.7	415.4 ± 29.6 [a]	2.4	> 10

[a] Significantly different relative to **1a** based on one-way ANOVA. [b] Data from Dekan et al. [5] with the exception of analogue **5a**. [c] IC_{50} value shown here represents the response observed in the majority of the nematode population (approximately 90%). The IC_{50} value for the response observed at lower concentrations (< 2 μM) was calculated at 0.2 ± 0.1 μM.

3.3. *Synthetic Mp1a Shows Insecticidal Activity against D. melanogaster*

We used a *D. melanogaster* injection model to investigate the insecticidal activity of Mp1a, as *M. pilosula* favours predation of smaller fly species [28]. The injection of synthetic Mp1a (**1a**) resulted in a rapid paralysis of the flies that was ultimately lethal over a 24 h period with an LD_{50} of 260 pmol/g (Figure 3A). Of the analogues, only the antiparallel heterodimers **1c** and **1d** and the A chain homodimer **5a** were insecticidal, but they were less active (LD_{50} values of 415–578 pmol/g) than the native heterodimer **1a** (Table 2). All other analogues were inactive in fruit flies, with LD_{50} values > 600 pmol/g, indicating that the antiparallel heterodimeric scaffold is important for the insecticidal activity of Mp1a.

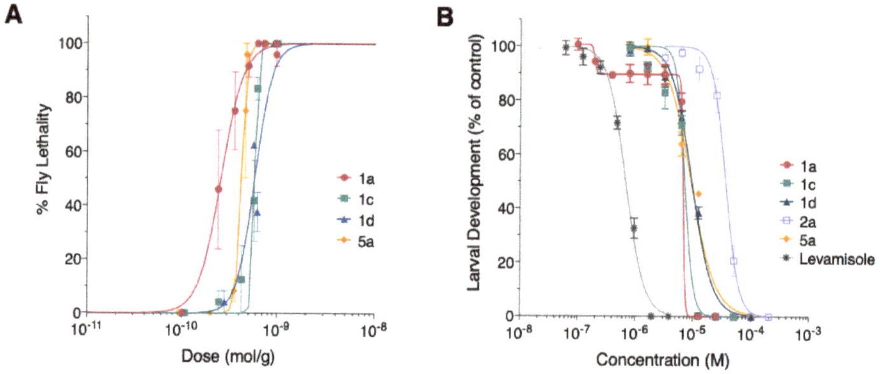

Figure 3. (**A**) Dose–response curves for insecticidal effects of Mp1a analogues **1a**, **c**, **d** and **5a** following microinjection into adult female fruit flies (*D. melanogaster*). (**B**) Concentration–response curves for anti-parasitic effects of Mp1a analogues against *H. contortus*. For both assays, data points represent the mean ± standard error of the mean (SEM) based on *n* = three experiments.

3.4. Mp1a Is Active against the Gastrointestinal Nematode H. contortus In Vitro

We investigated whether Mp1a and analogues could inhibit the larval development of *H. contortus*. Analogue **1a** and the native-like antiparallel heterodimers **1c** and **1d**, and the A-chain homodimer **5a**, inhibited larval development with IC_{50} values of 6.8–9.5 μM, approximately 10-fold higher than the commercial anthelmintic levamisole (Figure 3B). One-way ANOVA indicated that the anthelmintic activities of **1a–1d** and **5a** were not significantly different from each other. In contrast the parallel homodimer (**2a**) was fivefold less active and all other analogues were significantly less active against the parasite (between six and 10-fold, exemplified by **2a** in Figure 3B, rest not shown, $p < 0.001$). Analogue **1a** showed a biphasic response, with larval development reduced to 90% of that observed in control assays at low micromolar concentrations (< 2 μM), followed by the complete inhibition of development at higher peptide concentrations. The IC_{50} value for the response observed at low concentrations was 0.19 μM, compared to the IC_{50} of 6.8 μM observed at higher concentrations. This biphasic response was not observed with other analogues.

3.5. Cytotoxicity and Antimicrobial Activity

Analogues 1–4 were previously assayed for cytotoxicity and antimicrobial activity [5]. We screened the novel A chain homomer **5a** against the human embryonic kidney-derived cell line HEK293 and human red blood cells. Analogue **5a** was cytotoxic to HEK293 cells (CC_{50} 2.2 μM) but was less active against red blood cells (HC_{50} > 10 μM, Table 1). Analogue **5a** also had low micromolar activity against Gram-negative and Gram-positive bacterial pathogens and was most active against the important human pathogen *A. baumannii* (MIC 0.03—0.1 μM, Table 1).

4. Discussion

Recent advances in omics technologies have enabled detailed study of venoms produced only in small quantities, such as those of ants. This has revealed an unsuspected diversity of ant venom peptides [7,8,19] and has increased interest in the potential of ant venom peptides for development as biomedicines and pharmacological tools [29]. Such developments would be supported by further knowledge on the structure—activity relationships of ant toxins. We investigated the bioactivity of the antiparallel heterodimeric venom peptide Mp1a from the Australian jack jumper ant, *M. pilosula*, to explore its ecological role and to assess its potential use as a veterinary or human therapeutic. We report that synthetic Mp1a (**1a**) has broad-spectrum bioactivity, which includes moderate insecticidal activity, potent anthelmintic activity against the veterinary nematode *H. contortus*, and the robust activation of mammalian sensory neurons (summarised in Table 2).

4.1. Mp1a Shows Insecticidal and Algogenic Activities, Dependent on Dimerization

Injection of Mp1a into fruit flies resulted in rapid, irreversible paralysis leading to death. *M. pilosula* is reported to preferentially prey on small flies [28], so this finding is consistent with Mp1a serving a predatory function. The insecticidal potency of Mp1a is similar to that of the spider toxins ω/κ-hexatoxin-Hv1c (LD_{50} 210 pmol/g) and U_1-agatoxin-Ta1a (240 pmol/g), but lower than the highly potent insecticidal spider toxins ω-hexatoxin-Hv1a (9 pmol/g) and β-diguetoxin-Dc1a (59 pmol/g), in the same assay [20]. Native Mp1a was the most active of the ant peptides tested, with the antiparallel analogues **1c** and **1d** being significantly less active (LD_{50} ~550 pmol/g, $p < 0.0001$) and the A-chain homomer **5a** was 1.5-fold less active (LD_{50} 415 pmol/g, $p < 0.002$). All remaining analogues had LD_{50} values well over 600 pmol/g, indicating that the heterodimer and antiparallel orientation are important for insecticidal activity. We hypothesize that due to Mp1a's membrane-disrupting effects, this insecticidal activity likely extends to other insect species, though this remains to be tested.

The addition of low micromolar concentrations of Mp1a to cells isolated from mouse dorsal root ganglia resulted in the rapid activation of both neuronal and non-neuronal cells. This was followed by a decrease in $[Ca^{2+}]_i$ reflective of cytolysis (Figure 2a). These data are consistent with Mp1a's previously reported membrane-disrupting activity and algogenic effects in mice after intraplantar injection [5]. Similar effects were observed from each dimeric peptide analogue but, in striking contrast, the monomers were inactive up to 10 μM. Analogue **1a** activated cells at submicromolar concentrations (EC_{50} 0.85 μM) followed by rapid lysis. Analogues **1c**, **1d** and **2a** similarly activated cells at low micromolar concentrations, with **5a** being fivefold less active than **1a**. These data indicate that the dimerization of Mp1a is also critical for its algogenic activity and thus its presumed defensive role in the venom.

4.2. Mp1a Shows Antiparasitic Activity against the Veterinary Nematode H. contortus

Antimicrobial peptides with membrane-disrupting and cytolytic activities, including those from animal venoms, have previously been shown to be antiparasitic [15]. However, very few studies have reported venom peptides with activity against nematode parasites [29,30], and none from ants. *H. contortus* is a highly virulent gastrointestinal ruminant that shows widespread drug-resistance [31], and recent reports of its multidrug resistance [32] have highlighted the need for new treatments. This prompted us to screen Mp1a and its analogues for their antiparasitic activity against *H. contortus*. Synthetic Mp1a (**1a**) was found to have low micromolar anthelmintic activity against the larval stages of the nematode (6.8 μM). Analogue **1a** is about threefold more potent than the previously reported anthelmintic activity of the spider-venom peptide Hi1a in the same assay (IC_{50} 22.9 μM) [30], but 10-fold less active than the commercial anthelmintic levamisole (IC_{50} 0.68 μM, Figure 3B) in a drug-susceptible isolate. We hypothesize that Mp1a's broad-spectrum cytolytic activity will extend its anthelmintic activity to drug-resistant isolates, but this remains to be confirmed.

Interestingly, **1a** showed a biphasic response in the larval development assay (Figure 3B), which was not observed in any other analogues. One possible explanation for this phenomenon is that a small fraction of the nematodes (~10%) had greater sensitivity to the toxin. A biphasic concentration–response curve was previously observed in a monepantel-resistant isolate of *H. contortus*, with the larval development assay revealing the presence of two distinct sub-populations showing low and high levels of resistance to the anthelmintic [33]. Alternatively, there may be a secondary molecular target for Mp1a. The cause of this biphasic response remains an area for further investigation.

The other antiparallel heterodimeric analogues **1c** and **1d,** as well as the A-chain homodimer **5a,** also showed low micromolar activity against nematodes, indicating that dimerization is important for anthelmintic activity. However, the anthelmintic activity of the dimers was only observed at concentrations 10-fold higher than required for neuronal cell activation, cytotoxicity and hemolysis.

Analogues with reduced cytotoxicity, such as the parallel heterodimers **2a** and **2b**, were also less active against *H. contortus*, suggesting that the anthelmintic activity is likely due to non-specific cytolytic activity. This close link between anthelmintic activity, cytotoxicity and sensory neuron activation suggests that these analogues would also have adverse effects in vivo, similar to the known nocifensive activity of Mp1a and would, for this reason, make poor antiparasitic drug candidates. This contrasts with the broadly cytolytic peptide cupiennin-1a from the wandering spider, *C. salei*, which has > 400-fold selectivity for trypanosomes over human red blood cells [15]. Thus, further investigation into venom-derived membrane-disrupting peptides may still enable the identification or engineering of more suitable antiparasitic drug leads.

4.3. *Mp1a Analogues Show Some Selectivity Across Bioassasys*

In general, we found that the bioactivities across all assays were correlated, with the dimerization of Mp1a being critical for its insecticidal, anthelmintic and algogenic activities. Some analogues had better taxonomic selectivity; for example, the A-chain homodimer **5a** was fourfold less active than **1a** against HEK293 and red blood cells (Table 1), though this was still closely correlated with both insecticidal and anthelmintic activity. The A and B-chain monomers were essentially inactive across all assays, consistent with previous studies of Mp1a's antimicrobial activity [5]. Interestingly, the native-like antiparallel orientation of the A and B-chains was important for both anthelmintic and insecticidal activity; the parallel-oriented heterodimers **2a** and **2b** were four- to eightfold less active against *H. contortus* and completely inactive against *D. melanogaster* (Table 1). In contrast, parallel heterodimer **2a** was equipotent with synthetic Mp1a **1a** against F11 cells in a FLIPR model of sensory neuron activation, suggesting that chain orientation may be less important in neuronal membrane interactions. The exception was single disulfide-bridged heterodimer **2b** which was 45-fold less active than the native heterodimer (EC_{50} 38.5 μM, $p < 0.0001$) in the sensory neuron assay (Table 1). This peptide was similarly less active against *H. contortus* and inactive against *D. melanogaster* (LD_{50} > 600 pmol/g), which may be due to its increased flexibility because of the single disulfide bridge. Promisingly, however, this peptide has a potent activity against the Gram-negative pathogen *A. baumannii* (minimum inhibitory concentration 0.025–0.1 μM), approximately 1500-fold lower than its EC_{50} against F11 cells. These data suggest that there may be opportunities to increase the selectivity of Mp1a analogues as antimicrobials. One unexplored analogue is the B-chain homodimer, as the A-homodimer **5a** had a similar insecticidal and anthelmintic activity as the native-heterodimer **1a** (1.2- and 1.5-fold changes respectively). Future structure–activity relationship studies could explore further modifications such as N-terminal acylation, which was found to increase the affinity of the wasp venom peptide mastoparan-X for negatively charged bacterial membranes, thereby improving selectivity over host cells [34].

Based on the present and previously reported data, Mp1a shows a remarkably broad-spectrum bioactivity, with insecticidal, algogenic, cytotoxic, hemolytic, and antimicrobial activities that rely upon the dimerization of the peptide. Thus, Mp1a seems to serve both predatory and defensive roles in *M. pilosula* venom. The multifunctional nature of Mp1a may explain why it is the predominant toxin in the relatively simple *M. pilosula* venom, in contrast with spider [35], scorpion [36] and cone snail [37] venoms, which contain a rich diversity of ion channel-modulating toxins.

Author Contributions: Conceptualization, S.A.N. and Z.D.; methodology, S.A.N., Z.D., S.D.R., S.G.; formal analysis, S.A.N., S.D.R, V.H.; investigation, S.A.N., Z.D., S.D.R., S.G.; resources, P.F.A., I.V., A.C.K., G.F.K.; data curation, S.A.N., V.H.; writing—original draft preparation, S.A.N.; writing—review and editing, S.D.R, A.C.K., P.F.A., G.F.K., V.H.; visualization, S.A.N.; supervision, V.H., G.F.K., A.C.K., I.V., P.F.A.; project administration, S.A.N., V.H., G.F.K.; funding acquisition, S.A.N., G.F.K., V.H. All authors have read and agreed to the published version of the manuscript.

Funding: This research was funded by the Australian National Health & Medical Research Council (Principal Research Fellowship APP1136889 and Program Grant AP1072113 to G.F.K.; Career Development Fellowship APP1162503 to I.V.), the Australian Research Council (Future Fellowship FT190100482 to V.H.

and Discovery Grant DP190103787 to G.F.K.) and the Westpac Bicentennial Foundation (Westpac Future Leaders Scholarship to S.A.N.).

Acknowledgments: We thank Alexander Wild for sharing photographs of *M. pilosula* (Graphical Abstract and Figure 1), Phillip Skuce for the photograph of *H. contortus* (graphical abstract), Sean Millard (School of Biomedical Sciences, The University of Queensland, Brisbane, Australia) for providing *D. melanogaster*, and the Community for Open Antimicrobial Drug Discovery (Institute for Molecular Bioscience, The University of Queensland) for performing cytotoxicity, hemolysis and antibacterial assays.

Conflicts of Interest: The authors declare no conflict of interest.

References

1. Taylor, R.W. Ants with attitude: Australian jack-jumpers of the *Myrmecia pilosula* species complex, with descriptions of four new species (Hymenoptera: Formicidae: Myrmeciinae). *Zootaxa* **2015**, *3911*, 493–520. [CrossRef] [PubMed]
2. Wiese, M.D.; Brown, S.G.; Chataway, T.K.; Davies, N.W.; Milne, R.W.; Aulfrey, S.J.; Heddle, R.J. *Myrmecia pilosula* (jack jumper) ant venom: Identification of allergens and revised nomenclature. *Allergy* **2007**, *62*, 437–443. [CrossRef] [PubMed]
3. Wanandy, T.; Wilson, R.; Gell, D.; Rose, H.E.; Gueven, N.; Davies, N.W.; Brown, S.G.A.; Wiese, M.D. Towards complete identification of allergens in jack jumper (*Myrmecia pilosula*) ant venom and their clinical relevance: An immunoproteomic approach. *Clin. Exp. Allergy* **2018**, *48*, 1222–1234. [CrossRef] [PubMed]
4. Davies, N.W.; Wiese, M.D.; Brown, S.G.A. Characterisation of major peptides in 'jack jumper' ant venom by mass spectrometry. *Toxicon* **2004**, *43*, 173–183. [CrossRef] [PubMed]
5. Dekan, Z.; Headey, S.J.; Scanlon, M.; Baldo, B.A.; Lee, T.-H.; Aguilar, M.-I.; Deuis, J.R.; Vetter, I.; Elliott, A.G.; Amado, M.; et al. Δ-Myrtoxin-Mp1a is a helical heterodimer from the venom of the jack jumper ant that has antimicrobial, membrane-disrupting, and nociceptive activities. *Angew. Chem. Int. Ed.* **2017**, *56*, 8495–8499. [CrossRef]
6. Wiese, M.D.; Chataway, T.K.; Davies, N.W.; Milne, R.W.; Brown, S.G.A.; Gai, W.-P.; Heddle, R.J. Proteomic analysis of *Myrmecia pilosula* (jack jumper) ant venom. *Toxicon* **2006**, *47*, 208–217. [CrossRef]
7. Touchard, A.; Aili, S.R.; Fox, E.G.P.; Escoubas, P.; Orivel, J.; Nicholson, G.M.; Dejean, A. The biochemical toxin arsenal from ant venoms. *Toxins* **2016**, *8*, 30. [CrossRef]
8. Walker, A.A.; Robinson, S.D.; Yeates, D.K.; Jin, J.; Baumann, K.; Dobson, J.; Fry, B.G.; King, G.F. Entomo-venomics: The evolution, biology and biochemistry of insect venoms. *Toxicon* **2018**, *154*, 15–27. [CrossRef]
9. Wong, E.S.W.; Morganstern, D.; Mofiz, E.; Gombert, S.; Morris, K.M.; Temple-Smith, P.; Renfree, M.B.; Whittington, C.M.; King, G.F.; Warren, W.C.; et al. Proteomics and deep sequencing comparison of seasonally active venom glands in the platypus reveals novel venom peptides and distinct expression profiles. *Mol. Cell. Proteomics* **2012**, *11*, 1354–1364. [CrossRef]
10. Post, D.C.; Jeanne, R.L. Venom source of a sex pheromone in the social wasp *Polistes fuscatus* (Hymenoptera: Vespidae). *J. Chem. Ecol.* **1983**, *9*, 259–266. [CrossRef]
11. LeBrun, E.G.; Diebold, P.J.; Orr, M.R.; Gilbert, L.E. Widespread chemical detoxification of alkaloid venom by formicine ants. *J. Chem. Ecol.* **2015**, *41*, 884–895. [CrossRef]
12. Saviola, A.J.; Chiszar, D.; Busch, C.; Mackessy, S.P. Molecular basis for prey relocation in viperid snakes. *BMC Biol.* **2013**, *11*, 20. [CrossRef]
13. Tallarovic, S.K.; Melville, J.M.; Brownell, P.H. Courtship and mating in the Giant Hairy Desert Scorpion, *Hadrurus arizonensis* (Scorpionida, Iuridae). *J. Insect Behav.* **2000**, *13*, 827–838. [CrossRef]
14. Dos Santos-Pinto, J.R.A.; Perez-Riverol, A.; Lasa, A.M.; Palma, M.S. Diversity of peptidic and proteinaceous toxins from social Hymenoptera venoms. *Toxicon* **2018**, *148*, 172–196. [CrossRef]
15. Kuhn-Nentwig, L.; Willems, J.; Seebeck, T.; Shalaby, T.; Kaiser, M.; Nentwig, W. Cupiennin 1a exhibits a remarkably broad, non-stereospecific cytolytic activity on bacteria, protozoan parasites, insects, and human cancer cells. *Amino Acids* **2011**, *40*, 69–76. [CrossRef]
16. Kuhn-Nentwig, L.; Fedorova, I.M.; Luscher, B.P.; Kopp, L.S.; Trachsel, C.; Schaller, J.; Vu, X.L.; Seebeck, T.; Streitberger, K.; Nentwig, W.; et al. A venom-derived neurotoxin, CsTx-1, from the spider *Cupiennius salei* exhibits cytolytic activities. *J. Biol. Chem.* **2012**, *287*, 25640–25649. [CrossRef]

17. Gao, B.; Xu, J.; Rodriguez Mdel, C.; Lanz-Mendoza, H.; Hernandez-Rivas, R.; Du, W.; Zhu, S. Characterization of two linear cationic antimalarial peptides in the scorpion *Mesobuthus eupeus*. *Biochimie* **2010**, *92*, 350–359. [CrossRef]
18. Dânya Bandeira, L.; Clarissa Perdigão, M.; Izabel Cristina Justino, B.; de Menezes, R.R.P.P.B.; Tiago Lima, S.; Cláudio Borges, F.; Jean-Étienne, R.L.M.; Gandhi, R.-B.; Alice Maria Costa, M. The dinoponeratoxin peptides from the giant ant *Dinoponera quadriceps* display *in vitro* antitrypanosomal activity. *Biol. Chem.* **2018**, *399*, 187–196.
19. Aili, S.R.; Touchard, A.; Escoubas, P.; Padula, M.P.; Orivel, J.; Dejean, A.; Nicholson, G.M. Diversity of peptide toxins from stinging ant venoms. *Toxicon* **2014**, *92*, 166–178. [CrossRef]
20. Guo, S.; Herzig, V.; King, G.F. Dipteran toxicity assays for determining the oral insecticidal activity of venoms and toxins. *Toxicon* **2018**, *150*, 297–303. [CrossRef]
21. Herzig, V.; Hodgson, W.C. Neurotoxic and insecticidal properties of venom from the Australian theraphosid spider *Selenotholus foelschei*. *Neurotox* **2008**, *29*, 471–475. [CrossRef] [PubMed]
22. Robinson, S.D.; Mueller, A.; Clayton, D.; Starobova, H.; Hamilton, B.R.; Payne, R.J.; Vetter, I.; King, G.F.; Undheim, E.A.B. A comprehensive portrait of the venom of the giant red bull ant, *Myrmecia gulosa*, reveals a hyperdiverse hymenopteran toxin gene family. *Sci. Adv.* **2018**, *4*, 4640. [CrossRef]
23. Vetter, I.; Lewis, R.J. Characterization of endogenous calcium responses in neuronal cell lines. *Biochem. Pharmacol.* **2010**, *79*, 908–920. [CrossRef]
24. Albers, G.A.A.; Burgess, S.K. Serial passage of *Haemonchus contortus* in resistant and susceptible sheep. *Vet. Parasitol.* **1988**, *28*, 303–306. [CrossRef]
25. Kotze, A.C.; O'Grady, J.; Emms, J.; Toovey, A.F.; Hughes, S.; Jessop, P.; Bennell, M.; Vercoe, P.E.; Revell, D.K. Exploring the anthelmintic properties of Australian native shrubs with respect to their potential role in livestock grazing systems. *Parasitol* **2009**, *136*, 1065–1080. [CrossRef]
26. Osteen, J.D.; Herzig, V.; Gilchrist, J.; Emrick, J.J.; Zhang, C.; Wang, X.; Castro, J.; Garcia-Caraballo, S.; Grundy, L.; Rychkov, G.Y.; et al. Selective spider toxins reveal a role for $Na_V1.1$ channel in mechanical pain. *Nature* **2016**, *534*, 494–499. [CrossRef]
27. King, J.V.L.; Emrick, J.J.; Kelly, M.J.S.; Herzig, V.; King, G.F.; Medzihradszky, K.F.; Julius, D. A cell-penetrating scorpion toxin enables mode-specific modulation of TRPA1 and pain. *Cell* **2019**, *178*, 1362–1374. [CrossRef]
28. Archer, M.S.; Elgar, M.A. Effects of decomposition on carcass attendance in a guild of carrion-breeding flies. *Med. Vet. Entomol.* **2003**, *17*, 263–271. [CrossRef]
29. Herzig, V.; Cristofori-Armstrong, B.; Israel, M.R.; Nixon, S.A.; Vetter, I.; King, G.F. Animal toxins—Nature's evolutionary-refined toolkit for basic research and drug discovery. *Biochem. Pharmacol.* **2020**, in press. [CrossRef]
30. Nixon, S.A.; Saez, N.J.; Herzig, V.; King, G.F.; Kotze, A.C. The antitrypanosomal diarylamidines, diminazene and pentamidine, show anthelmintic activity against *Haemonchus contortus in vitro*. *Vet. Parasitol.* **2019**, *270*, 40–46. [CrossRef] [PubMed]
31. Kotze, A.C.; Prichard, R.K. Chapter Nine—Anthelmintic resistance in *Haemonchus contortus*: History, mechanisms and diagnosis. In *Advances in Parasitology*; Gasser, R.B., Samson-Himmelstjerna, G.V., Eds.; Academic Press: London, UK, 2016; Volume 93, pp. 397–428.
32. Lamb, J.; Elliott, T.; Chambers, M.; Chick, B. Broad spectrum anthelmintic resistance of *Haemonchus contortus* in Northern NSW of Australia. *Vet. Parasitol.* **2017**, *241*, 48–51. [CrossRef] [PubMed]
33. Raza, A.; Lamb, J.; Chambers, M.; Hunt, P.W.; Kotze, A.C. Larval development assays reveal the presence of sub-populations showing high- and low-level resistance in a monepantel (Zolvix®)-resistant isolate of *Haemonchus contortus*. *Vet. Parasitol.* **2016**, *220*, 77–82. [CrossRef] [PubMed]
34. Etzerodt, T.; Henriksen, J.R.; Rasmussen, P.; Clausen, M.H.; Andresen, T.L. Selective acylation enhances membrane charge sensitivity of the antimicrobial peptide mastoparan-x. *Biophys. J.* **2011**, *100*, 399–409. [CrossRef] [PubMed]
35. King, G.F.; Hardy, M.C. Spider-venom peptides: Structure, pharmacology, and potential for control of insect pests. *Annu. Rev. Entomol.* **2013**, *58*, 475–496. [CrossRef] [PubMed]

36. Quintero-Hernández, V.; Jiménez-Vargas, J.M.; Gurrola, G.B.; Valdivia, H.H.; Possani, L.D. Scorpion venom components that affect ion-channels function. *Toxicon* **2013**, *76*, 328–342. [CrossRef] [PubMed]
37. Lewis, R.J.; Dutertre, S.; Vetter, I.; Christie, M.J. *Conus* venom peptide pharmacology. *Pharmacol. Rev.* **2012**, *64*, 259–298. [CrossRef]

biomedicines

MDPI

Article

Pharmacological Effects of a Novel Bradykinin-Related Peptide (RR-18) from the Skin Secretion of the Hejiang Frog (*Ordorrana hejiangensis*) on Smooth Muscle

Xiaowei Zhou [1,2,†], Jie Xu [2,†], Ruimin Zhong [3], Chengbang Ma [2], Mei Zhou [2], Zhijian Cao [4], Xinping Xi [2,*], Chris Shaw [2], Tianbao Chen [2], Lei Wang [2] and Hang Fai Kwok [1,*]

1 Institute of Translational Medicine, Faculty of Health Sciences, University of Macau, Avenida da Universidade, Taipa, Macau; xiaoweizhou@um.edu.mo
2 Natural Drug Discovery Group, School of Pharmacy, Queen's University, Belfast BT9 7BL, UK; jxu06@qub.ac.uk (J.X.); c.ma@qub.ac.uk (C.M.); m.zhou@qub.ac.uk (M.Z.); chris.shaw@qub.ac.uk (C.S.); t.chen@qub.ac.uk (T.C.); l.wang@qub.ac.uk (L.W.)
3 Department of Nutrition, Henry Fok School of Food Science and Engineering, Shaoguan University, Shaoguan 512005, China; sgu_zrm@sgu.edu.cn
4 State Key Laboratory of Virology, Modern Virology Research Center, College of Life Sciences, Wuhan University, Wuhan 430072, China; zjcao@whu.edu.cn
* Correspondence: x.xi@qub.ac.uk (X.X.); hfkwok@um.edu.mo (H.F.K.); Tel.: +44-2890972200 (X.X.); +853-88224991 (H.F.K.)
† Theses authors contributed equally to this work.

Received: 28 May 2020; Accepted: 14 July 2020; Published: 17 July 2020

Abstract: Bradykinin (BK) and bradykinin-related peptides (BRPs), which were identified from a diversity of amphibian skin secretions, exerted contractile and relaxing effects on non-vascular and vascular smooth muscle, respectively. Here, we report a novel bradykinin-related peptide with a molecular mass of 1890.2 Da, RVAGPDKPARISGLSPLR, which was isolated and identified from *Ordorrana hejiangensis* skin secretions, followed by a C-terminal extension sequence VAPQIV. The biosynthetic precursor-encoding cDNA was cloned by the "shotgun" cloning method, and the novel RR-18 was identified and structurally confirmed by high-performance liquid chromatography (HPLC) and tandem mass spectrometry (MS/MS). Subsequently, the myotropic activity of the synthetic replicate of RR-18 was investigated on the rat bladder, uterus, tail artery and ileum smooth muscle. The peptide was named RR-18 in accordance (R = N-terminal arginine, R = C-terminal arginine, 18 = number of residues). In this study, the synthetic replicates of RR-18 showed no agonist/antagonism of BK-induced rat bladder and uterus smooth muscle contraction. However, it displayed an antagonism of bradykinin-induced rat ileum contraction and arterial smooth muscle relaxation. The EC_{50} values of BK for ileum and artery, were 214.7 nM and 18.3 nM, respectively. When the tissue was pretreated with the novel peptide, RR-18, at the maximally effective concentration of bradykinin (1×10^{-6} M), bradykinin-induced contraction of the ileum and relaxation of the arterial smooth muscle was reduced by 50–60% and 30–40%, respectively. In conclusion, RR-18 represents novel bradykinin antagonising peptide from amphibian skin secretions. It may provide new insight into possible treatment options for chronic pain and chronic inflammation.

Keywords: frog; bradykinin related peptide; skin secretion; antagonist; smooth muscle

1. Introduction

Bradykinin nonapeptide, RPPGFSPFR, was first reported from *Rana temperaria* frog skin in the 1960s [1]. Subsequently, the bioactive components in the skin secretion of amphibians, especially biologically active peptides, such as antimicrobial peptides and pharmacological peptides, have been extensively studied during the past several decades [2,3]. Bradykinin (BK) and bradykinin-related peptides (BRPs), representing one of the major pharmacological peptides, have been widely isolated and identified in skin secretions of 5 families of amphibians, *Leiopelmatidae, Ascaphidae, Bombinatoridae, Hylidae*, and Ranidae [4–6]. BK is regulated by the kallikrein-kinin system (KKS) in mammals [7]; however, the frog skin BK/BRPs are not the products of enzyme catalysis by the KKS. The products were secreted from amphibian skin glands as immune defence peptides. Interestingly, extensive reports on the derivation of BRPs revealed that several amphibian skin BRPs were found in their putative predators, such as birds and snakes, suggesting that BRPs are molecular evolutionary adaptations to species-specific predators.

Recently, more than 100 amphibian BRPs have been reported [8]. However, few Auran species have been reported to secrete BRPs. Additionally, unlike antimicrobial peptides which have been studied extensively, just very few BRPs have been identified in amphibian skin. Apart from that, there is also very little information about BRPs in Ranidae frogs belonging to the *Ordorrana hejiangensis* (*O. hejiangensis*). Furthermore, extensive studies demonstrated that most of the BRPs are BK receptors agonist with a dose-dependent contractile activity on non-vascular smooth muscle. Still, some are antagonists in inhibiting contractility of BK on vascular smooth muscle. For instance, the RVA-Thr6-BK showed vasorelaxant activity on rat arterial smooth muscle but exerted contractile activity on bladder, uterus, and ileum smooth muscle [9].

Usually, BK exerts its function in combination with two G protein-coupled receptors families, namely B1 and B2 receptors [10]. B1 receptors are upregulated during tissue damage by pro-inflammatory cytokines and the oxidative stress through the nuclear factor kappa B (NF-κB) pathway [11]. However, B2 receptors were widely distributed in multiple tissues. Recently, B1 and B2 receptors were thought to be involved in many diseases, such as cancer, chronic pain, and diabetes [12–14]. For instance, a previous report demonstrated that B1 and B2 receptors were significantly expressed in colorectal cancer cells [15]. Therefore, the development of B1 and B2 receptor antagonists is of great significance in pharmacology or clinical applications.

Here, we report a novel BRP, RR-18, which was first identified in the skin secretion of Hejiang Frog, *O. hejiangensis*, followed by a C-terminal extension sequence VAPQIV. Pharmacological assays revealed that RR-18 displayed an antagonism of bradykinin-induced contraction of the rat ileum and relaxation of arterial smooth muscle. Furthermore, our results indicated that RR-18 exerted its BK inhibition activity by mainly targeting B2 receptors. It has been revealed that activation of BK receptors can induce several downstream signalling pathways involved in inflammatory responses [16] suggesting the unique property of RR-18 may be used in the potential treatment of chronic pain and chronic inflammation.

2. Experimental Section

2.1. Skin Secretion Acquisition

The specimens of the *O. hejiangensis* were captured, settled and skin secretion was acquired from the dorsal skin as described previously [17]. All the procedures were carried out according to the guidelines in the UK Animal (Scientific Procedures) Act 1986, project license PPL 2694, issued by the Department of Health, Social Services and Public Safety, Northern Ireland. Procedures had been vetted by the Institutional Animal Care and Use Committees (IACUC) of Queen's University Belfast, and approved on 1 March 2011.

2.2. "Shotgun" Cloning of cDNA Encoding RR-18 Biosynthetic Precursor from Skin Secretion

The cDNA encoding RR-18 biosynthetic precursor was evaluated by the "shotgun" cloning method as previously described [17]. A Nested Universal Primer A (NUP A) (Clontech, Palo Alto, CA, USA) and a sense degenerated primer (5′-GAWYYAYYHRAGCCYAAADATGTTCA-3′; W = A + T,

Y = C + T, H = A + C + T, R = A + G, D = A + G + T) were subjected to the 3′-RACE reaction, from which the products were cloned and subsequently sequenced.

2.3. Isolation and Structural Characterisation of RR-18 from Skin Secretion

The isolation and structural characterisation of RR-18 from the lyophilised *O. hejiangensis* skin secretion was carried out as previously described [17]. In brief, five mg of lyophilised skin secretion was dissolved in trifluoroacetic acid (TFA) (Sigma-Aldrich, Dorset, UK)/H_2O (0.05:99.95, *v/v*) followed by centrifugation. The supernatant was eluted by a Cecil CE4200 Adept (Amersham Biosciences, Buckinghamshire, UK) reverse-phase High Performance Liquid Chromatography (RP-HPLC) system. A linear gradient elution was performed using a gradient formed from TFA/H_2O (0.05:99.95, *v/v*) to acetonitrile (ACN) (Sigma-Aldrich, Dorset, UK)/H_2O/TFA (80.00:19.95:0.05, *v/v/v*) in 240 min. The fractions were monitored at 214 nm at a flow rate of 1 mL/min. The molecular masses of peptides in the fractions were analysed by matrix-assisted laser desorption/ionisation, time-of-flight mass spectrometry (MALDI-TOF MS) (Thermo Fisher Scientific, San Francisco, CA, USA) using alpha-cyano-4-hydroxycinnamic acid (α-CHCA) (Sigma-Aldrich, Dorset, UK) as the matrix and the putative primary structure of RR-18 was analysed using Sequest algorithm against the self-defined Fasta database in proteome Discoverer 1.0 software (Thermo Fisher Scientific, San Jose, CA, USA).

2.4. Solid-Phase Peptide Synthesis of Peptides

RR-18 (RVAGPDKPARISGLSPLR) and BK were synthesised using a Tribute peptide synthesiser (Protein Technologies, Tucson, AZ, USA) according to our previous study [17]. The purity of the peptides (>95%) was determined by RP-HPLC (Cecil, Cambridge, UK). The peptides were further confirmed using an LCQ-Fleet electrospray ion-trap mass spectrometer (Thermo Fisher Scientific, San Francisco, CA, USA).

2.5. Myotropic Activity Evaluation on Smooth Muscles

The fractions were rotary dried and then performed to screen the myotropic activity on smooth muscle. The synthetic replicated of RR-18 was used to determine the myotropic activity on rat smooth muscle. Female Wistar rats (250–300 g) were euthanised by CO_2 asphyxiation based on institutional animal experimentation ethics and the UK animal research guidelines. The endothelium of rat tail artery was removed and the proximal rat tail artery ring was dissected about 2 mm in width and connected to a triangular hook. An approximately 0.5 cm-length ring of ileum was cut. After that, the tissues of rat tail artery, bladder, uterus and ileum were mounted into an organ bath (2 mL) containing a Krebs solution (118 mM NaCl, 1.15 mM NaH_2PO_4, 2.5 mM $CaCl_2$, 25 mM $NaHCO_3$, 4.7 mM KCl, 1.1 mM $MgCl_2$, and 5.6 mM glucose). All chemicals were purchased from Sigma-Aldrich (Dorset, UK). The bladder, uterus, artery, and ileum tissues were stretched, maintaining the normal physiological tension of 0.75 g, 0.5 g, 0.5 g, and 0.5 g, respectively. Arteries were pre-contracted with phenylephrine (1×10^{-5} M) for 10~20 min to achieve constriction plateaux. A range concentration of synthetic peptides (from 10^{-11}–10^{-5} M) was prepared in Krebs solution. Tissues were incubated with peptides in a cumulative manner for at least 5 min before reaching the equilibrium for 20 min. RR-18 (10^{-6} M) was applied for 10 min prior to different concentration of BK (10^{-11}–10^{-5} M). The myotropic effects of RR-18 on smooth muscles were recorded using a tension sensor with a PowerLab System (AD Instruments Pty Ltd., Oxford, UK).

2.6. Statistical Analysis

Data was analysed using Prism 6 (GraphPad Software, La Jolla, CA, USA). The mean and standard error of responses were analysed by Student's T-test and the dose-response curves were constructed using a best-fit algorithm. EC_{50} values were calculated from the normalised curves.

3. Results

3.1. Molecular Cloning of RR-18 Precursor-Encoding cDNAs

The nucleotide and translated open reading frame amino acid sequences of the novel RR-18 precursor encoding cDNAs was cloned from Hejiang Odorous Frog, *O. hejiangensis*, skin secretions are shown in Figure 1. Specifically, the precursor encoding cDNA of the RR-18 contained 67 amino acids including a putative signal peptide domain, an acidic amino acid residue-rich (spacer) domain (21 amino acids), an 18 amino acids length of putative mature peptide and a C-terminal extension peptide domain (-VAPQIV-) (Figure 1). The encoding RR-18 precursor has been deposited in the GenBank Database (accession code: MT522014).

```
    M F T  L K K S  L L L  L F F  L G T I
1   ATGTTCACCC TGAAGAAATC CCTGTTACTC CTTTTCTTTC TGGGGACCAT
     S L V  L C  E Q  E R D  A D E  E E T
51  CTCCTTAGTT CTCTGTGAGC AAGAGAGAGA TGCCGATGAA GAAGAAACCG
    A R E A  K V E  N V K  R V A G  P D K
101 CAAGGGAAGC TAAAGTGGAA AACGTAAAAA GAGTGGCAGG CCCGGATAAG
    P A R  I S G L  S P L  R V A  P Q I V
151 CCCGCTCGCA TATCTGGGCT GAGCCCACTT CGTGTTGCAC CGCAAATTGT
    *
201 TTAAACTTGG ATCGGAAGTC ATCTGATGTG GAACATCATT TAACTAAATT
251 CACAGCAGAT GTCTAGAAAA AAAAATTAAA CGATCACATA TATTAAAAAA
301 AAAAAAAAAA AAAAAAAAAA AAAA
```

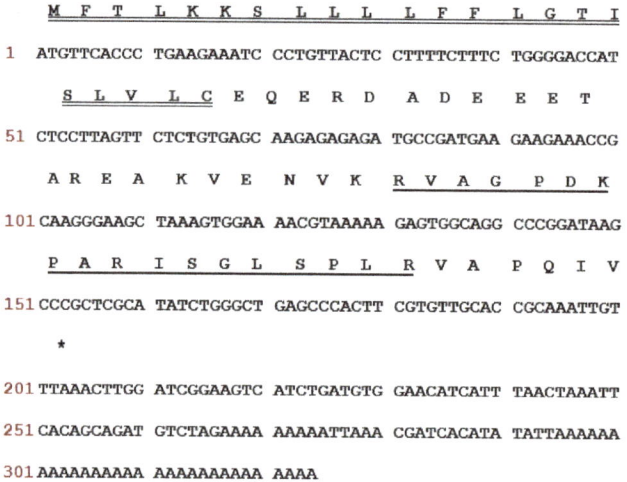

Figure 1. Nucleotide and translated open-reading frame amino acid sequences of the cDNA encoding the biosynthetic precursor of the novel bioactive peptide (RR-18) cloned from hejiang *odorous* frog, *O. hejiangensis*, skin secretion. The putative signal peptide is double-underlined, the mature peptide (RR-18) is single-underlined, and the stop codon is indicated by an asterisk.

3.2. Isolation and Identification and Structural Characterisation of RR-18

Reverse-phase HPLC (RP-HPLC) chromatogram of the *O. hejiangensis* skin secretion is shown in Figure 2. Subsequently, the primary structure, RVAGPDKPARISGLSPLR, was thus unequivocally determined by tandem mass spectrometry (MS/MS) fragmentation sequencing (Table 1). The RP-HPLC chromatogram showed that the purity of RR-18 was above 95% and the molecular mass of RR-18 was detected by Matrix-Assisted Laser Desorption/Ionization-Time of Flight (MALDI-TOF) mass spectrum (Figure 3). A single peptide with a mass of 1890.2 Da (Figure 4), which was resolved in HPLC fractions of skin secretion displayed the bradykinin inhibitory activity on smooth muscle.

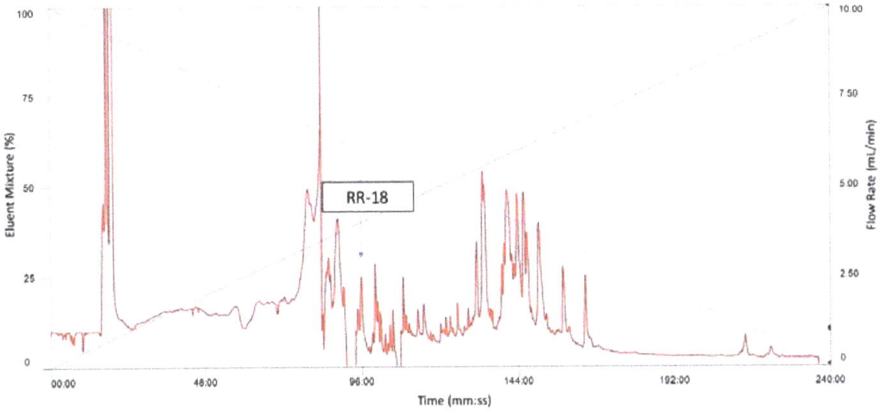

Figure 2. Region of reverse phase HPLC chromatogram of *Odorrana hejiangensis* skin secretion indicating elution position/retention time (arrow) of the novel bioactive peptide. Blue line represented the linear gradient curve of water/acetonitrile/trifluoroacetic acid (TFA) (19.95/80.00/0.05, *v/v/v*). Pink line represented the linear gradient curve of water/TFA (99.95/0.05, *v/v*).

Table 1. Predicted tandem mass spectrometry (MS/MS) fragmentation *b*- and *y*-ion series ion series (singly-, doubly-, and triply-charged) of RR-18. Observed ions were shown in bold italic typeface.

#1	b(1+)	b(2+)	b(3+)	Seq.	y(1+)	y(2+)	y(3+)	#2
1	157.10840	79.05784	53.04098	R				18
2	256.17682	128.59205	86.06379	V	1734.00218	***867.50473***	***578.67224***	17
3	***327.21394***	164.11061	109.74283	A	1634.93376	***817.97052***	***545.64944***	16
4	***384.23541***	***192.62134***	128.74999	G	1563.89664	***782.45196***	***521.97040***	15
5	***481.28818***	241.14773	161.10091	P	1506.87517	***753.94122***	502.96324	14
6	***596.31513***	***298.66120***	199.44323	D	1409.82240	***705.41484***	470.61232	13
7	***724.41010***	***362.70869***	242.14155	K	***1294.79545***	***647.90136***	432.27000	12
8	***821.46287***	***411.23507***	274.49247	P	1166.70048	***583.85388***	389.57168	11
9	***892.49999***	***446.75363***	***298.17151***	A	***1069.64771***	***535.32749***	357.22075	10
10	1048.60111	***524.80419***	350.20522	R	***998.61059***	***499.80893***	333.54171	9
11	***1161.68518***	***581.34623***	387.89991	I	***842.50947***	***421.75837***	***281.50801***	8
12	1248.71721	***624.86224***	416.91059	S	***729.42540***	365.21634	243.81332	7
13	1305.73868	***653.37298***	***435.91774***	G	***642.39337***	321.70032	***214.80264***	6
14	1418.82275	***709.91501***	473.61243	L	***585.37190***	***293.18959***	195.79548	5
15	1505.85478	***753.43103***	502.62311	S	***472.28783***	***236.64755***	158.10079	4
16	1602.90755	***801.95741***	***534.97403***	P	***385.25580***	***193.13154***	129.09012	3
17	1715.99162	***858.49945***	572.66872	L	288.20303	144.60515	96.73919	2
18				R	175.11896	88.06312	59.04450	1

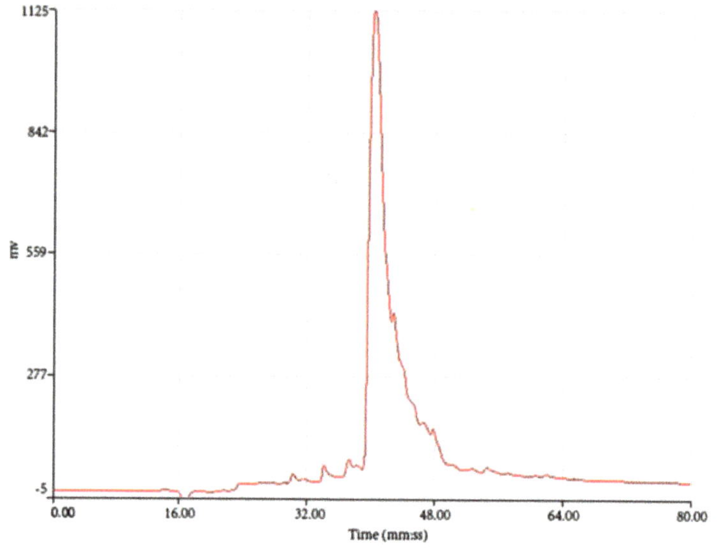

(a)

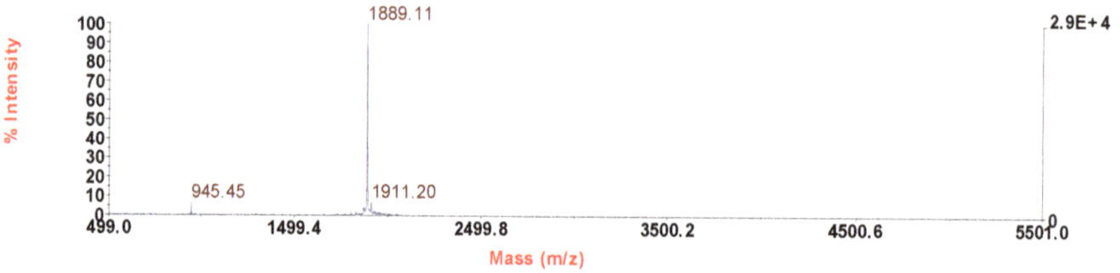

(b)

Figure 3. Reverse-phase (RP)-HPLC chromatogram (**a**) and matrix-assisted laser desorption/ionisation, time-of-flight mass spectrometry (MALDI-TOF) mass spectrum (**b**) of a synthetic replicate of peptide RR-18.

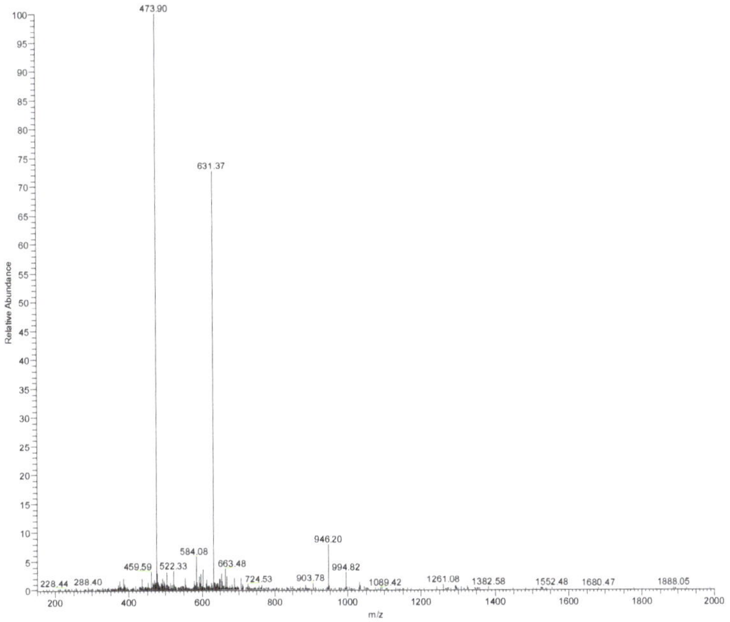

Figure 4. Electrospray MS spectrum of the novel peptide. m/z ion 473.90 is +4 charged (parent 1891.6), m/z ion 631.37 is +3 charged (parent ion 1891.2), and m/z ion 946.20 is +2 charged (parent ion 1890.4). Mean mass of parent 1891.1 vs. calculated of 1890.2 (discrepancy 0.05%).

3.3. Bioinformatic Analysis of Novel RR-18

BLAST analysis of RR-18 was performed using the National Center for Biotechnological Information (NCBI) on line portal, and demonstrated that the full length open reading frame of RR-18 displayed relative high amino acid sequence identity with the *wuyiensisin*-1 and other typical bradykinin antagonist (RVA-T6-BK and RAP-L1, T6-BK) precursor sequences. Specifically, the similarity between the primary sequence of RR-18 and *wuyiensisin*-1 was over 94%. Additionally, the primary structure of RR-18 showed high similarity with some other typical bradykinin antagonists. The highly-conserved amino acids are Arg^{1}, Pro^{5}, Pro^{8}, Gly^{13}, Pro^{16}, and Pro^{18} (Figure 5).

```
                       10         20         30         40         50
RR-18          MFTTKKSLLL LFFLGTISLS LCEQERDADE EETAREAKVE NVKRVAGPDK
Wuyiensisin-1  MFTTKKSLLL LFFLGTISLV LCEQERDADE EETAREAKVE NVKRVAGPDE
RVA-T6-BK      MFTTKKSLLL LFFLGMVSLS LCEQERDADE DDNAGEAKVE NVKRVARP—
RAP-L1,T6-BK   MFTLKKSLLL LFFLGAINLS LCEQERDADE EENEREAKVE TVKRAPLP—
               ********** *****    *  **********      ***** ***   *
                       60

RR-18          PARISGLSPL RVAPQIV
Wuyiensisin-1  PARISGLSPL RVVPQIV
RVA-T6-BK      P----GFTPF RVAPEIV
RAP-L1,T6-BK   P----GFTPF RVAPEIV
               *    *  *  ** * **
```

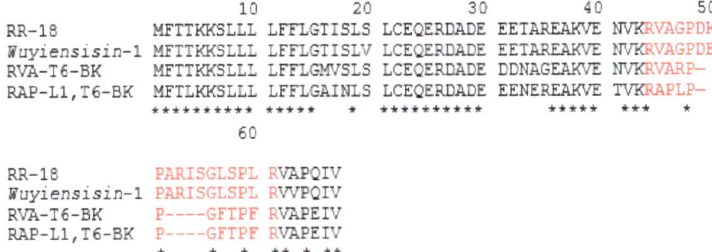

Figure 5. Amino-acid sequence alignment of RR-18 precursor and other bradykinin-related peptide (BRP) precursors from the skin secretion of several frog species. The sequences of mature peptides were labeled in red and stars (*) represented the identical amino acid residues.

3.4. Pharmacological Effects of RR-18 on Smooth Muscle

The purified RR-18 and BK were employed in the evaluation of myotropic activity on rat uterus, bladder, ileum and tail artery. Specifically, RR-18 produced no distinct myotropic action on rat bladder, ileum, uterus and tail artery in its own right. Additionally, RR-18 showed no antagonism of BK-induced rat bladder and uterus smooth muscle contraction. BK produced a dose-response curve in affecting rat ileum and rat tail artery. However, RR-18 mediated a potent inhibition of bradykinin-induced contraction and relaxation of rat ileum and tail artery smooth muscle (Figure 6). Specifically, the EC_{50} values of BK on rat ileum and tail arteries were 214.7 nM and 18.3 nM, respectively. However, when the tissue was pretreated with the novel peptide, RR-18, at the maximally effective concentration of bradykinin (1×10^{-6} M), BK-induced contraction of the ileum and relaxation of the arterial smooth muscle was abolished by 50–60% and 30–40%, respectively. Additionally, the EC_{50} values of BK+RR-18 (10^{-6} M) on rat ileum and tail arteries were 1.54 μM and 79.83 nM, respectively. Moreover, RR-18 represented a typical BK competitive inhibitor and non-competitive inhibitor on rat ileum and tail artery smooth muscle, respectively.

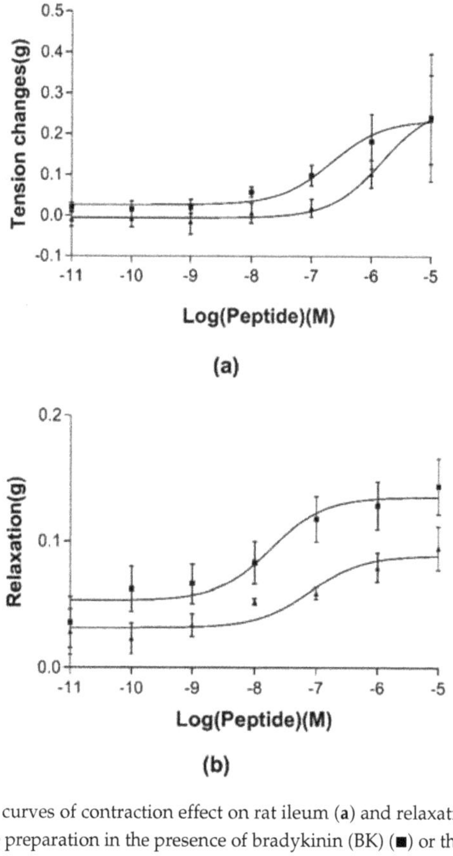

Figure 6. Dose-response curves of contraction effect on rat ileum (**a**) and relaxation effects on a rat tail artery (**b**) smooth muscle preparation in the presence of bradykinin (BK) (■) or the presence of BK with RR-18 (▲).

4. Discussion

Amphibian skin secretions contain a variety of active substances including peptides, proteins, steroids and alkaloids. In particular, peptides, such as bombesin and bradykinin, act as myotropic peptides and are critical to protecting amphibians from predators [8,18]. At the same time, BK and BRPs are associated with many diseases, such as chronic pain and cancer [13,19]. Recently, very few peptides from the Hejiang frog have been reported [9,20,21].

In this study, a novel octade-peptide, RR-18, was identified by de novo sequencing and isolated from the skin secretion of the *O. hejiangensis*. Obviously, *O. hejiangensis* showed high homology compared with the precursors of *Amolops wuyiensis*. Additionally, the precursor encoding cDNA library of RR-18 was further determined. Interestingly, sequence analysis exhibited high similarity (up to 94.4%) between RR-18 and *wuyiensisin*-1 (RVAGPDEPARISGLSPLR-OH; AIU99945.1) which was identified from the Sanchiang sucker frog (*Amolops wuyiensis*). It was noted that the *O. hejiangensis* is a unique amphibian species in China, mainly distributed in the Sichuan, Guangxi, and Chongqing areas of China. At the same time, the *Amolops wuyiensis* are only found in the Fujian, Zhejiang, and Anhui areas of China. This may explain why the same group of peptides could be found in different species in similar regions [22], and this may be of benefit to the evolution of amphibians. Thus, the Hejiang frog and the Sanchiang sucker frog, at least with respect to their skin BRPs, appear to be more closely related to one another than to other ranid species that occupy similar geographical distributions [5]. The residue was substituted to a lysine (K) residue at position 7 from the N-terminal of the peptide.

Additionally, it is significant that RR-18 has a similar structure to that of BK, although its biological activity has not been determined. Besides, compared with another BRP, RVA-Thr6-BK, which was identified in the skin secretion of *O. hejiangensis*, as well [9], the differences between RR-18 and RVA-Thr6-BK are mainly reflected in the N-terminal region. Specifically, an R residue was submitted to G at position 4 from N-terminal. Interestingly, the commutation of a single amino acid residue in wasp kinins can result in significant differences in the action of the peptide. The factors that distinguished the encoded proprepeptides of RR-18 in this family are unclear. This phenomenon may be due to differences in species, regions and the living environments of frogs [5].

Unlike the majority of previously cloned ranid frog skin BRP precursors, which always encode multiple peptides [5], RR-18 only contained a single copy in the proprepeptides. Additionally, the propeptide convertase cleavage site(s) of RR-18 was found to be unusual when compared with other kininogens. Firstly, an acidic amino acid-rich spacer peptide domain of RR-18 has no typical prepropeptide convertase processing site (-KR-). Secondly, the N-processing sites of mature kinin are always RR and KR. However, the N-processing sites of RR-18 are KK and an R. The C-terminus of the mature kinin is flanked by the sequence -VAPQIV- that is cleaved from the maturing kinin by a post arginyl cleavage. These phenomena may be attributed to evolution amongst amphibians [5].

Many vasodilators exerted relax activity on rat artery smooth muscle, which is mediated by the endothelium and the release of nitric oxide (NO) [23]. However, previous studies demonstrated that arterial smooth muscle preparations which were pretreated with specific endothelium nitric oxide synthase (eNOS) inhibitor failed to cause significant effects on the dose-responsive relaxation of vasorelaxant indicating that BRPs exert the relaxing activity on rat artery smooth muscle is unlikely to involve the action of NO [24,25]. Our data showed that RR-18 displayed an antagonism of bradykinin-induced rat ileum contraction and arterial smooth muscle relaxation, which is consistent with previous studies, in that Phe at the penultimate position of BRP is the crucial site for activating BK receptors. The Phe at the penultimate position of BRP substituted with Leu could induce an antagonistic activity [26]. Interestingly, RR-18 represented a BK competitive inhibitor and non-competitive inhibitor on rat ileum and tail artery smooth muscle. Firstly, the EC_{50} values of BK and BK+RR-18 in rat tail artery smooth muscle were virtually identical. Secondly, the Emax value of BK+RR-18 is lower to that of BK. However, the Emax values of BK and BK + RR-18 in rat ileum were overlapping, suggesting BK occupied receptor in ileum when the concentration of BK is increasing. Henceforth, RR-18 was overcome by BK in rat ileum. Apart from these, in comparison with original BK, the primary structure of RR-18 displayed multiple segment insertion sites, like -VAG-, -DE-, and -ARIS-, that were inserted between RP, PP, and PG, respectively. Due to RR-18 having exerted different BK antagonism on rat ileum and tail artery, we speculated that the changes of BRPs structure caused various kinds of ligand receptor binding pathways, which affected the pharmacological activity of BRPs [27]. Additionally, a previous study demonstrated that BK exerted its activity by regulating B1 and B2 receptors, especially mainly regulated by B2 receptor [24]. Moreover, RR-18 showed high similarity to some B2 receptor antagonists like RVALPPGFTPLR, QIPGLGPLR and RVA-Thr6-BK [9,24,28], henceforth, we speculated that RR-18 exerted its BK inhibition activity by mainly targeting B2 receptors. Nevertheless, further studies are required to determine whether B1 receptor interaction could explain the competition/non-competition features of RR-18 on ileum and tail artery. Previous reports revealed that Arg1, Pro2, Gly4, Phe5, Pro7, Phe8 and Arg9 are key residues for the biological activity of BK [29]. In this study, both Phe5 and Phe8 were substituted to leucine, which may improve/reduce the affinity between the peptides and receptors or even change an agonist to antagonist [30].

Taken together, a novel BRP, which contains 18 amino acids, was first isolated and identified from *O. hejiangensis*. The cDNA-encoded biosynthetic precursor of RR-18 showed high similarity with a BRP peptide (*wuyiensisin*-1) which was identified from *Amolops*. Our study demonstrated that RR-18 displayed competitive and non-competitive inhibition of BK on rat ileum and rat tail artery smooth muscle, respectively. Furthermore, RR-18 showed BK antagonist activity by mainly activating the B2 receptor. There is compelling evidence that BK is involved in the development of many diseases, such as pain and hyperalgesia [31,32]. Meanwhile, more recently, it has been suggested that BK B2 receptors were upregulated after a traumatic brain injury (TBI) and the inflammatory response was significantly reduced after treatment with a bradykinin B2 receptor inhibitor [33]. Hence, RR-18, as a BK B2 receptor antagonist, may have the potential for developing new drugs for chronic pain and chronic inflammation. Furthermore, the structural diversity of BRPs and its related BK inhibitory activity suggested that anuran is a rich source for the study of the structure-activity relationships between BRPs. Moreover, in addition to canonical research on the fossil record and morphological characteristics, with the in-depth study of molecular techniques and the precursor encoding cDNA sequencing of orthologous genes, it may give us a new understanding of the scope of evolution of amphibians.

Author Contributions: T.C., L.W. and M.Z. conceived and designed the experiments; X.Z., X.X., R.Z. and C.M. performed the experiments; J.X., C.M., R.Z., M.Z., Z.C. and H.F.K. analysed the data; C.M., Z.C., H.F.K. and J.X. contributed reagents/materials/analysis tools; X.Z., L.W., X.X., C.S. and H.F.K. wrote the paper. All authors have read and agreed to the published version of the manuscript.

Funding: This research was funded by the Science and Technology Development Fund of Macau SAR (FDCT) (019/2017/A1) and the Youth Innovative Talents Project of Education Department of Guangdong Province (2019KQNCX140). X.Z. has received the UM Macao Postdoctoral Associateship from the Faculty of Health Sciences, University of Macau.

Conflicts of Interest: The authors declare no conflict of interest. The funders had no role in the design of the study; in the collection, analyses, or interpretation of data; in the writing of the manuscript, or in the decision to publish the results.

References

1. Erspamer, V.; Bertaccini, G. Occurrence of bradykinin in the skin of Rana temperaria. *Comp. Biochem. Physiol.* **1965**, *14*, 43–52.
2. Wu, D.; Gao, Y.; Tan, Y.; Liu, Y.; Wang, L.; Zhou, M.; Xi, X.; Ma, C.; Bininda-Emonds, O.R.; Chen, T. Discovery of Distinctin-Like-Peptide-PH (DLP-PH) From the Skin Secretion of Phyllomedusa hypochondrialis, a Prototype of a Novel Family of Antimicrobial Peptide. *Front. Microbiol.* **2018**, *9*, 541. [CrossRef] [PubMed]
3. König, E.; Bininda-Emonds, O.R.; Shaw, C. The diversity and evolution of anuran skin peptides. *Peptides* **2015**, *63*, 96–117. [CrossRef] [PubMed]
4. Yang, M.; Zhou, M.; Bai, B.; Ma, C.B.; Wei, L.; Wang, L.; Chen, T.B.; Shaw, C. Peptide IC-20, encoded by skin kininogen-1 of the European yellow-bellied toad, Bombina variegata, antagonizes bradykinin-induced arterial smooth muscle relaxation. *J. Pharm. Bioallied Sci.* **2011**, *3*, 221–225.
5. Xi, X.P.; Li, B.; Chen, T.B.; Kwok, H.F. A Review on Bradykinin-Related Peptides Isolated from Amphibian Skin Secretion. *Toxins* **2015**, *7*, 951–970. [CrossRef]

6. Sin, Y.T.; Zhou, M.; Chen, W.; Wang, L.; Chen, T.B.; Walker, B.; Shaw, C. Skin bradykinin-related peptides (BRPs) and their biosynthetic precursors (kininogens): Comparisons between various taxa of Chinese and North American ranid frogs. *Peptides* **2008**, *29*, 393–403. [CrossRef]
7. Rouhiainen, A.; Kulesskaya, N.; Mennesson, M.; Misiewicz, Z.; Sipila, T.; Sokolowska, E.; Trontti, K.; Urpa, L.; McEntegart, W.; Saarnio, S.; et al. The bradykinin system in stress and anxiety in humans and mice. *Sci. Rep.* **2019**, *9*, 13. [CrossRef] [PubMed]
8. Xu, X.; Lai, R. The chemistry and biological activities of peptides from amphibian skin secretions. *Chem. Rev.* **2015**, *115*, 1760–1846. [CrossRef] [PubMed]
9. Wu, Y.; Shi, D.N.; Chen, X.L.; Wang, L.; Ying, Y.; Ma, C.B.; Xi, X.P.; Zhou, M.; Chen, T.B.; Shaw, C. A Novel Bradykinin-Related Peptide, RVA-Thr(6)-BK, from the Skin Secretion of the Hejiang Frog; Ordorrana hejiangensis: Effects of Mammalian Isolated Smooth Muscle. *Toxins* **2019**, *11*, 376. [CrossRef] [PubMed]
10. Marceau, F.; Bachelard, H.; Bouthillier, J.; Fortin, J.P.; Morissette, G.; Bawolak, M.T.; Charest-Morin, X.; Gera, L. Bradykinin receptors: Agonists, antagonists, expression, signaling, and adaptation to sustained stimulation. *Int. Immunopharmacol.* **2020**, *82*, 7. [CrossRef]
11. Couture, R.; Blaes, N.; Girolami, J.-P. Kinin receptors in vascular biology and pathology. *Curr. Vasc. Pharmacol.* **2014**, *12*, 223–248. [CrossRef]
12. Figueroa, C.D.; Ehrenfeld, P.; Bhoola, K.D. Kinin receptors as targets for cancer therapy. *Expert Opin. Ther. Targets* **2012**, *16*, 299–312. [CrossRef]
13. Calixto, J.B.; Medeiros, R.; Fernandes, E.S.; Ferreira, J.; Cabrini, D.A.; Campos, M.M. Kinin B1 receptors: Key G-protein-coupled receptors and their role in inflammatory and painful processes. *Br. J. Pharmacol.* **2004**, *143*, 803–818. [CrossRef]
14. Sang, H.; Liu, L.; Wang, L.; Qiu, Z.; Li, M.; Yu, L.; Zhang, H.; Shi, R.; Yu, S.; Guo, R. Opposite roles of bradykinin B1 and B2 receptors during cerebral ischaemia–reperfusion injury in experimental diabetic rats. *Eur. J. Neurosci.* **2016**, *43*, 53–65. [CrossRef] [PubMed]
15. Wang, G.J.; Ye, Y.W.; Zhang, X.F.; Song, J.M. Bradykinin stimulates IL-6 production and cell invasion in colorectal cancer cells. *Oncol. Rep.* **2014**, *32*, 1709–1714. [CrossRef] [PubMed]
16. Regoli, D.; Gobeil, F. Kinins and peptide receptors. *Biol. Chem.* **2016**, *397*, 297–304. [CrossRef] [PubMed]
17. Zhou, X.W.; Ma, C.B.; Zhou, M.; Zhang, Y.N.; Xi, X.P.; Zhong, R.M.; Chen, T.B.; Shaw, C.; Wang, L. Pharmacological Effects of Two Novel Bombesin-Like Peptides from the Skin Secretions of Chinese Piebald Odorous Frog (Odorrana schmackeri) and European Edible Frog (Pelophylax kl. esculentus) on Smooth Muscle. *Molecules* **2017**, *22*, 1798. [CrossRef]
18. Kumar, V.T.V.; Holthausen, D.; Jacob, J.; George, S. Host Defense Peptides from Asian Frogs as Potential Clinical Therapies. *Antibiotics* **2015**, *4*, 136–159. [CrossRef]
19. Falsetta, M.L.; Foster, D.C.; Woeller, C.F.; Pollock, S.J.; Bonham, A.D.; Haidaris, C.G.; Phipps, R.P. A Role for Bradykinin Signaling in Chronic Vulvar Pain. *J. Pain* **2016**, *17*, 1183–1197. [CrossRef]
20. Wang, L.; Evaristo, G.; Zhou, M.; Pinkse, M.; Wang, M.; Xu, Y.; Jiang, X.F.; Chen, T.B.; Rao, P.F.; Verhaert, P.; et al. Nigrocin-2 peptides from Chinese Odorrana frogs—Integration of UPLC/MS/MS with molecular cloning in amphibian skin peptidome analysis. *FEBS J.* **2010**, *277*, 1519–1531. [CrossRef]
21. Wang, M.; Wang, L.; Chen, T.B.; Walker, B.; Zhou, M.; Sui, D.Y.; Conlon, J.M.; Shaw, C. Identification and molecular cloning of a novel amphibian Bowman Birk-type trypsin inhibitor from the skin of the Hejiang Odorous Frog; Odorrana hejiangensis. *Peptides* **2012**, *33*, 245–250. [CrossRef] [PubMed]
22. Gao, Y.; Wu, D.; Xi, X.; Wu, Y.; Ma, C.; Zhou, M.; Wang, L.; Yang, M.; Chen, T.; Shaw, C. Identification and Characterisation of the Antimicrobial Peptide, Phylloseptin-PT, from the Skin Secretion of Phyllomedusa tarsius, and Comparison of Activity with Designed, Cationicity-Enhanced Analogues and Diastereomers. *Molecules* **2016**, *21*, 1667. [CrossRef] [PubMed]
23. Benyó, Z.; Lacza, Z.; Hortobágyi, T.; Görlach, C.; Wahl, M. Functional importance of neuronal nitric oxide synthase in the endothelium of rat basilar arteries. *Brain Res.* **2000**, *877*, 79–84. [CrossRef]
24. Xiang, J.; Wang, H.; Ma, C.B.; Zhou, M.; Wu, Y.X.; Wang, L.; Guo, S.D.; Chen, T.B.; Shaw, C. Ex Vivo Smooth Muscle Pharmacological Effects of a Novel Bradykinin-Related Peptide, and Its Analogue, from Chinese Large Odorous Frog, Odorrana livida Skin Secretions. *Toxins* **2016**, *8*, 283. [CrossRef] [PubMed]
25. Wu, Y.X.; Wang, L.; Lin, C.; Lin, Y.; Zhou, M.; Chen, L.; Connolly, B.; Zhang, Y.Q.; Chen, T.B.; Shaw, C. Vasorelaxin: A Novel Arterial Smooth Muscle-Relaxing Eicosapeptide from the Skin Secretion of the Chinese Piebald Odorous Frog (Odorrana schmackeri). *PLoS ONE* **2013**, *8*, e55739. [CrossRef]

26. Conlon, J.M. Bradykinin and its receptors in non-mammalian vertebrates. *Regul. Pept.* **1999**, *79*, 71–81. [CrossRef]
27. Martin, R.P.; Filippelli-Silva, R. Non-radioactive binding assay for bradykinin and angiotensin receptors. In *Methods in Cell Biology*; Elsevier: Amsterdam, The Netherlands, 2019; Volume 149, pp. 77–85.
28. Shi, D.N.; Luo, Y.; Du, Q.; Wang, L.; Zhou, M.; Ma, J.; Li, R.J.; Chen, T.B.; Shaw, C. A Novel Bradykinin-Related Dodecapeptide (RVALPPGFTPLR) from the Skin Secretion of the Fujian Large-Headed Frog (Limnonectes fujianensis) Exhibiting Unusual Structural and Functional Features. *Toxins* **2014**, *6*, 2886–2898. [CrossRef]
29. Bonechi, C.; Ristori, S.; Martini, G.; Martini, S.; Rossi, C. Study of bradykinin conformation in the presence of model membrane by Nuclear Magnetic Resonance and molecular modelling. *Biochim. Biophys. Acta-Biomembr.* **2009**, *1788*, 708–716. [CrossRef]
30. Lyu, P.; Ge, L.L.; Wang, L.; Guo, X.X.; Zhang, H.L.; Li, Y.H.; Zhou, Y.; Zhou, M.; Chen, T.B.; Shaw, C. Ornithokinin (avian bradykinin) from the skin of the Chinese bamboo odorous frog, Odorrana versabilis. *J. Pept. Sci.* **2014**, *20*, 618–624. [CrossRef]
31. Ohnishi, M.; Yukawa, R.; Akagi, M.; Ohsugi, Y.; Inoue, A. Bradykinin and interleukin-1β synergistically increase the expression of cyclooxygenase-2 through the RNA-binding protein HuR in rat dorsal root ganglion cells. *Neurosci. Lett.* **2019**, *694*, 215–219. [CrossRef]
32. Gonçalves, E.C.D.; Vieira, G.; Gonçalves, T.R.; Simões, R.R.; Brusco, I.; Oliveira, S.M.; Calixto, J.B.; Cola, M.; Santos, A.R.; Dutra, R.C. Bradykinin Receptors Play a Critical Role in the Chronic Post-ischaemia Pain Model. *Cell. Mol. Neurobiol.* **2020**. [CrossRef] [PubMed]
33. Chao, H.L.; Fan, L.; Zhao, L.; Liu, Y.L.; Lin, C.; Xu, X.P.; Li, Z.; Bao, Z.Y.; Liu, Y.; Wang, X.M.; et al. Activation of bradykinin B2 receptor induced the inflammatory responses of cytosolic phospholipase A(2) after the early traumatic brain injury. *Biochim. Biophys. Acta-Mol. Basis Dis.* **2018**, *1864*, 2957–2971. [CrossRef] [PubMed]

biomedicines

MDPI

Article

Novel Bradykinin-Potentiating Peptides and Three-Finger Toxins from Viper Venom: Combined NGS Venom Gland Transcriptomics and Quantitative Venom Proteomics of the *Azemiops feae* Viper

Vladislav V. Babenko [1,†], Rustam H. Ziganshin [2,†], Christoph Weise [3], Igor Dyachenko [4], Elvira Shaykhutdinova [4], Arkady N. Murashev [4], Maxim Zhmak [2], Vladislav Starkov [2], Anh Ngoc Hoang [5], Victor Tsetlin [2] and Yuri Utkin [2,*]

1 Federal Research and Clinical Centre of Physical-Chemical Medicine of Federal Medical Biological Agency, 119435 Moscow, Russia; daniorerio34@gmail.com
2 Shemyakin-Ovchinnikov Institute of Bioorganic Chemistry RAS, 117997 Moscow, Russia; rustam.ziganshin@gmail.com (R.H.Z.); mzhmak@gmail.com (M.Z.); vladislavstarkov@mail.ru (V.S.); victortsetlin3f@gmail.com (V.T.)
3 Institute of Chemistry and Biochemistry, Freie Universität Berlin, 14195 Berlin, Germany; chris.weise@biochemie.fu-berlin.de
4 Branch of the Shemyakin-Ovchinnikov Institute of Bioorganic Chemistry, Russian Academy of Sciences, Pushchino, 142290 Moscow Region, Russia; dyachenko@bibch.ru (I.D.); shaykhutdinova@bibch.ru (E.S.); murashev@bibch.ru (A.N.M.)
5 Institute of Applied Materials Science, Vietnam Academy of Science and Technology, Ho Chi Minh City 700000, Vietnam; hnanh52@yahoo.com
* Correspondence: yutkin@yandex.ru or utkin@ibch.ru; Tel.: +7-495-336-6522
† These authors contributed equally to this work.

Received: 29 June 2020; Accepted: 24 July 2020; Published: 28 July 2020

Abstract: Feae's viper *Azemipos feae* belongs to the Azemiopinae subfamily of the Viperidae family. The effects of Viperidae venoms are mostly coagulopathic with limited neurotoxicity manifested by phospholipases A2. From *A. feae* venom, we have earlier isolated azemiopsin, a novel neurotoxin inhibiting the nicotinic acetylcholine receptor. To characterize other *A. feae* toxins, we applied label-free quantitative proteomics, which revealed 120 unique proteins, the most abundant being serine proteinases and phospholipases A2. In total, toxins representing 14 families were identified, among which bradykinin-potentiating peptides with unique amino acid sequences possessed biological activity in vivo. The proteomic analysis revealed also basal (commonly known as non-conventional) three-finger toxins belonging to the group of those possessing neurotoxic activity. This is the first indication of the presence of three-finger neurotoxins in viper venom. In parallel, the transcriptomic analysis of venom gland performed by Illumina next-generation sequencing further revealed 206 putative venom transcripts. Together, the study unveiled the venom proteome and venom gland transcriptome of *A. feae*, which in general resemble those of other snakes from the Viperidae family. However, new toxins not found earlier in viper venom and including three-finger toxins and unusual bradykinin-potentiating peptides were discovered.

Keywords: Feae's viper; *Azemiops feae*; venom; venom gland; proteomics; transcriptomic; bradykinin-potentiating peptides; three-finger toxins

1. Introduction

Snake venoms are complex mixtures of peptides and proteins that are evolved in the process of evolution for protection from predators and for hunting. Two major action strategies can be traced in the venoms: a paralytic one inherent predominantly to elapids and colubrids and a coagulopathic one inherent mostly to viperids. To date, it has been established that, despite the huge variety of toxins, they can all be attributed to a limited number of families either possessing enzymatic activities (e.g., phospholipases A_2 (PLA2), snake venom serine proteases (SVSP), snake venom metalloproteinases (SVMP)) or without such activities (e.g., lectins, three-finger toxins (3FTx), Kunitz-type inhibitors, natriuretic peptides). The variation in the composition of venoms occurs at all taxonomic levels [1], but the most drastic differences are evident at the level of families and subfamilies. As coagulopathies are induced mostly through an enzymatic pathway, in general, enzymes are the main components of viperid venoms. Paralytic effects, on the other hand, are produced more often by proteins without enzymatic activity (e.g., three-finger neurotoxins), albeit non-enzymatic proteins are not the main components in all elapid venoms. For example, in krait *Bungarus fasciatus* venom, PLA2 enzymes comprise about 70% of all venom proteins [2]. Although traditional methods for characterization of venoms based on chromatographic separation are still in use, the modern proteomic approaches yield more detailed and complete information. The proteomes of about two hundred snake species have been characterized so far [3,4], more than half of them (about 100 species) from viperids. Viperids (Viperidae family) are divided into two major subfamilies, the Viperinae (Old World or pitless vipers) and the Crotalinae (pit vipers). One more taxon, Azemiopinae, is recognized within the Viperidae; recent data confirm Azemiopinae as the sister group of the Crotalinae [5,6]. Nowadays, Azemiopinae include the genus Azemiops, the species composition of which is currently the subject of discussion. Recently, in addition to the well-established *Azemiops feae* species, a new one *Azemiops kharini* was included in the genus [7]. However, new data indicate that they are rather one species [8].

Data about venom composition for these fairly rare snakes are limited and available for *A. feae* only. Earlier investigation of the enzymatic activity of this venom showed that it had no blood clotting, hemorrhagic, or myolytic activities [9]. Recent studies confirmed the absence of coagulopathic effects for *A. feae* venom [10]. In another study, PLA2 and plasminogen activator homologs were found in the venom [11]. Three PLA2s were isolated from *A. feae* venom, and two of them contained Asn49 in their active center and were catalytically inactive [12]. cDNAs encoding cysteine-rich secretory protein (CRISP) [12], natriuretic-peptide precursors [13] and 3Ftx [14] were cloned from *A. feae*. However, there are no data about the presence of the corresponding proteins in *A. feae* venom. At the same time, natriuretic-peptide precursors contain sequences of a unique peptide neurotoxin, which was isolated by us from the venom and called azemiopsin [15]. Azemiopsin is a primitive neurotoxin; it consists of 21 residues and does not contain cysteine residues. By its capacity to block the nicotinic acetylcholine receptor, azemiopsin resembles waglerin, a disulfide-containing peptide from the *Tropedolaemus wagleri* venom, shares with it a homologous C-terminal hexapeptide and may be considered as a waglerin ancestor. These peptide neurotoxins are not typical for Viperidae venom. To find out what the other components are, we have analyzed *A. feae* venom in more depth using high-throughput proteomics. In parallel, the transcriptomic analysis of venom gland was performed by Illumina next-generation sequencing (NGS). About 70 toxins representing 14 toxins families were identified; among them, new toxins not found earlier in viper venom and including three-finger toxins and unusual bradykinin-potentiating peptides were discovered.

2. Experimental Section

2.1. Specimen Collection and Tissue Preparation

Specimen of *A. feae* was collected in Vinh Phuc Province, Vietnam. Venom gland was dissected 3 days after stimulation by milking and treated with RNAlater (Ambion, Thermo Fisher Scientific Inc, Waltham, MA, USA) as described by the vendor.

2.2. cDNA Library Preparation and Sequencing

For RNA extraction, venom gland dissected from one specimen of *A. feae* viper and stored in RNAlater (Ambion, Thermo Fisher Scientific Inc, Waltham, MA, USA) was used. Total RNA was isolated from the tissue sample by TRIzol kit (Invitrogen, Thermo Fisher Scientific Inc, Waltham, MA, USA), and its quality was assessed on an Agilent 2100 Bioanalyzer (Agilent Technologies, Santa Clara, CA, USA).

2.2.1. cDNA Synthesis and cDNA Amplification

For ds cDNA synthesis, the SMART approach [16] was applied. SMART-prepared cDNA was amplified by PCR. Primer annealing mixture (5 μL) containing 0.3 μg of total RNA; 10 pmol of SMART Oligo II oligonucleotide (5′-AAGCAGTGGTATCAACGCAGAGTACGCrGrGrG-3′) and 10 pmol of CDS-T22 primer (5′-AAGCAGTGGTATCAACGCAGAGTTTTTGTTTTTTTCTTTTTTTTTTVN-3′) was prepared, incubated for 2 min at 72 °C and was kept for 2 min on ice. The annealed primer-RNA was mixed with Reverse Transcriptase in a final volume of 10 μL, containing 1X First-Strand Buffer (50 mM Tris-HCl (pH 8.3); 75 mM KCl; 6 mM $MgCl_2$), 2 mM DTT and 1 mM of each dNTP to start the first-strand cDNA synthesis. This reaction mixture was maintained at 42 °C for 2 h in a thermostat and then cooled on ice. After dilution by 5 times with TE buffer, the first-strand cDNA was incubated for 7 min at 70 °C and then was amplified by Long-Distance PCR (Barnes, 1994). PCR reaction mixture (50 μL) contained 1 μL diluted first-strand cDNA, 1 μL 50× Advantage reaction buffer (Clontech, Takara Bio, Mountain View, CA, USA), 200 μM dNTPs; 0.3 μM SMART PCR primer (5′-AAGCAGTGGTATCAACGCAGAGT-3′) and 1 μL 50× Advantage Polymerize mix (Clontech, Takara Bio, Mountain View, CA, USA). PCR was performed on MJ Research PTC-200 DNA Thermal Cycler under the following program: 95 °C −7 s, 65 °C −20 s, 72 °C −3 min, 17 cycles. Amplified cDNA PCR product was purified using QIAquick PCR Purification Kit (Qiagen, Venlo, Netherlands).

2.2.2. Illumina Sequencing

The standard Illumina protocol was applied to prepare libraries for DNA using TruSeq Illumina DNA sample preparation kit. NGS was performed on Illumina Genome Analyzer IIx in the paired-end sequencing mode (2 × 72 bp).

2.3. NGS Data Analysis

Sequenced data from Illumina GAIIx were transformed by base calling into sequence data, called the raw data or raw reads, and were stored in FASTQ format. For quality control checks on raw sequence data, we used FastQC (version 0.11.5). Trimmomatic (version 0.38) was applied to trim the adapter sequences used for cDNA synthesis. For de novo transcriptome assembly, we used Trinity software (version r20131110) with the default settings. Contigs from Trinity were translated using all six reading frames to obtain "Predicted protein SET 1". Local BLAST (BlastX threshold value of $e = 1 \times 10^{-6}$, matrix BLOSUM-62) and the non-redundant database were used for the grouping and annotation of contigs. Blast2GO (version 5.2.1) was used for Taxonomy, Gene Ontology (GO) and EuKaryotic Orthologous Groups (KOG) analysis for functional annotation of contigs. TransDecoder was applied to identify putative ORFs with a minimum length of 100 amino acids. The ORF database (10997 sequences) generated with Transdecoder called "Predicted protein SET 2" was used for proteomics.

2.4. Other Computational Tool

Translation of transcriptome sequences in all 6 frames to amino acid sequences was done with Nucleotide Sequence Translation EMBOSS Transeq/EMBOSS Sixpack. The ORF database (120510 sequences) generated with EMBOSS Sixpack was used for proteomics. Prinseq lite v.0.20.4 was used for reads quality and length trimming. ClustalW2 and MUSCLE algorithms integrated into package Jalview v.2.11.1.0 were used to perform multiple alignment construction and visualization [17]. For calculating expression levels (Transcripts Per Kilobase Million (TPM) and Reads Per Kilobase Million (RPKM), we used CLC Genomic Workbench 10 (Qiagen, Venlo, Netherlands) with the default settings.

2.5. BioProject and Raw Sequence Data

Sequence data from the venom gland transcriptome of the *A. feae* have been deposited in National Centre for Biotechnology Information (NCBI) Sequence Read Archive with the accession number SRR8177476 under Bioproject PRJNA504599.

2.6. Reduction, Alkylation and Digestion of the Proteins

The proteins were reduced, alkylated and digested as described previously [18] with small variations. In brief, to a venom sample (10 µg), sodium deoxycholate (SDC) buffer (pH 8.5) for reduction and alkylation was added so as to achieve the final concentration of proteins, Tris, SDC, tris(2-carboxyethyl)phosphine and 2-chloroacetamide of 0.5 mg/mL, 100 mM, 1% (*w*/*v*), 10 mM and 20 mM, respectively. The reaction mixture was incubated at 95 °C for 10 min and cooled to ambient temperature. Digestion with trypsin (solution in equal volume of 100 mM Tris, pH 8.5) at a 1:100 (*w*/*w*) ratio was performed at 37 °C overnight.

2.7. Tryptic Peptides Desalting

Peptides were desalted with application of SDB-RPS StageTips, which were made as previously described [19]. In brief, two small portions of the 3M Empore SDB-RPS membrane were cut with a blunt-tipped Hamilton needle (part no. 91014: gauge 14, type Point 3, metal (N) hub) and pressed into the 200-µL pipette tip using 1/16 PEEK tubing (1535, Upchurch Scientific, Thermo Fisher Scientific Inc, Waltham, MA, USA). As a StageTip holder, 2 mL microcentrifuge tube with a hole punched in the cap (O-tube) was used. O-tube and SDB-RPS StageTip composed a Spin block. An equal volume of 2% (*v*/*v*) TFA was added to the tryptic peptide solution obtained after overnight hydrolysis, and the solution thus obtained was applied to StageTip using centrifugation at 200 g. StageTip was cleaned by washing first with mixture of 50 µL ethylacetate with 50 µL 1% (*v*/*v*) TFA (3 times), then 50 µL 1% (*v*/*v*) TFA and finally 50 µL 0.2% (*v*/*v*) TFA. The elution of peptides was achieved by application of 60 µL 50% (*v*/*v*) acetonitrile containing 5% (*v*/*v*) NH_4OH; the eluted peptides were freeze-dried and preserved at −80 °C. For further analysis, peptides were dissolved in 20 µL of 2% (*v*/*v*) acetonitrile containing 0.1% (*v*/*v*) TFA and treated with ultrasound for 2 min.

2.8. Liquid Chromatography and Mass Spectrometry

The column (25 cm with inner diameter of 75 µm) in-house packed with Aeris Peptide XB-C18 2.6 µm resin (Phenomenex, Torrance, CA, USA) was applied for the separation of peptides. An Ultimate 3000 Nano LC System (Thermo Fisher Scientific Inc, Waltham, MA, USA) was used for reverse-phase chromatography. The LC System was connected through a nanoelectrospray source (Thermo Fisher Scientific) to a Q Exactive HF mass spectrometer (Thermo Fisher Scientific). A linear 120-min gradient of 4–55% solvent B (80% (*v*/*v*) acetonitrile containing 0.1% (*v*/*v*) formic acid was used for the elution of peptides at a flow rate of 350 nL/min (40 °C). TopN method with an automatic switch between a full scan and up to 15 data-dependent MS/MS scans was applied for MS data acquisition. The target value of 3×10^6 in the 300–1200 *m*/*z* range with a resolution of 60,000 and a maximum injection time of 60 ms was used for the full-scan MS spectra. A 1.4 *m*/*z* window and a fixed first mass of 100.0 *m*/*z* was used to perform isolation of precursors. A higher-energy dissociation (HCD) and a normalized collision energy of 28 eV were applied for fragmentation of precursors. An ion target value of 1×10^5 in the 200–2000 *m*/*z* range with a resolution of 15,000 at *m*/*z* 400 and a maximum injection time of 30 ms were used for the acquisition of MS/MS scans. Six technical replicates were performed to analyze the sample by LC–MS/MS.

2.9. Data Analysis

Six technical replicates were used for MS measurements of venom sample. MS/MS-based qualitative proteome analysis of venom proteins was made using PEAKS Studio 8.0 build 20160908 software [20]. Peptide lists generated by the PEAKS Studio were searched against the "SET 2" FASTA database. Carbamidomethylation was set as a fixed modification for cysteine and acetylation for N-terminus, oxidations for methionine and deamidations for asparagine were set as variable modifications and specificity of protease was set to semitryptic. For peptide-spectrum matches, the false discovery rate (FDR) was fixed to 0.01 and the search of a reverse database was used to determine FDR. An allowed fragment mass deviation of 0.05 Da and an allowed initial precursor mass deviation up to 10 ppm were used to perform the peptide identification. If at least 1 unique peptide was found for a protein, it was regarded as identified reliably. MaxQuant program version 1.5.6.5 [21] was applied for label-free protein quantification. Carbamidomethylation was set as a fixed modification for cysteine and acetylation for N-terminus, oxidations for methionine and deamidations for asparagine were set as variable modifications and specificity of protease was set to semitryptic. The Andromeda search engine [22] was used for the search of peak lists against the "SET 1" FASTA database and a common contaminant database implemented in the search engine. The FDR of 0.01 was fixed for both proteins and peptides, and a minimum length of seven amino acids was used. An allowed fragment mass deviation of 20 ppm and an allowed initial precursor mass deviation up to 20 ppm were used to perform the peptide identification. Perseus (versions 1.5.5.1) [23] was applied to perform the downstream bioinformatics analysis. From the analyses were excluded groups of proteins which were identified only by site, from peptides identified also only in the reverse database oring belonged to the database of common contaminant. A minimum ratio count of 1 was applied to perform the label-free quantification. The iBAQ algorithm, implemented into the MaxQuant program [21], was used to quantify proteins in the venom sample. To generate a relative iBAQ (riBAQ) value representing the mole fraction of each protein [24], normalization of each protein's iBAQ value against the sum of all iBAQ values was performed.

2.10. Characterization of Bradykinin-Potentiating Peptides by MALDI Mass Spectrometry

De novo peptide sequencing was performed by matrix-assisted laser desorption ionization-time of flight mass spectrometry (MALDI-TOF-MS/MS) using an Ultraflex-II TOF/TOF instrument (Bruker Daltonics, Bremen, Germany) equipped with a 200 Hz solid-state Smart beam™ laser.

HPLC-purified samples were applied using α-cyano-4-hydroxycinnamic acid (CHCA, saturated solution in 33% acetonitrile/0.1% trifluoroacetic acid) onto a polished-steel target. The instrument was operated in positive reflector mode and MS/MS spectra generated by spontaneous post-source decay were recorded using the LIFT cell technology [25]. The fragment spectra were interpreted and labeled manually.

2.11. Peptide Synthesis

The bradykinin-potentiating peptides (BPP) were prepared by peptide synthesis and purified by reverse-phase chromatography as described [26].

2.12. Blood Pressure Measurements

The experiments were carried out on adult male Sprague-Dawley (SD) rats (300–350 g of body weight). The World Health Organization's International Guiding Principles for Biomedical Research Involving Animals were followed during experiments on animals. The experiments were approved by the Institutional Animal Care and Use Committee (IACUC No.536/18). Four groups of 6 rats in each were used for the study. Before the experiment, catheters were implanted into the jugular vein and carotid artery of rats under anesthesia (Zoletil-100 at a dose of 20 mg/kg and Rometar at a dose of 12 mg/kg). The arterial catheter was used to record blood pressure (mean BP) and the venous catheter for injection of test drugs (Y-BPP or R-BPP). Blood pressure parameters were recorded on conscious animals a day after surgery (to allow for recovery of the animals from anesthesia) continuously using a strain gauge pressure transducer linked to Powerlab ML125 system (AD Instrument, Australia). After 10 min of recording of baseline parameters, bradykinin was introduced (1st injection, 7 μg/kg); 10 min after bradykinin, for the experimental group, BPP (Y-BPP or R-BPP in two doses: 300 μg/kg or 1 mg/kg) was introduced (2nd injection). Then, on the 5th minute after BPP injection, bradykinin (7 μg/kg, 3rd introduction) was again introduced; on the 50th minute after beginning of the experiment, bradykinin was again given at the same dose (4th introduction). The last introduction of bradykinin was at the 80th minute (5th introduction). Data were then analyzed and mean BP ± SEM calculated. All quantitative data are presented as mean ± SD. Statistical analysis was performed by software Statistica for Window v.7.1 to compare the treated groups. Significance level was determined at $p \leq 0.05$. No rats or data points were excluded from the reported analyses.

3. Results

3.1. Research Outline: RNA Sequencing and Analysis of the Initial Data

To perform a comprehensive analysis of Feae's viper *A. feae* venom, we used two complementary approaches (Figure 1). To study proteins and peptides present in the venom, quantitative proteomics was applied (Table S1), while the transcriptome of the venom gland was analyzed by NGS.

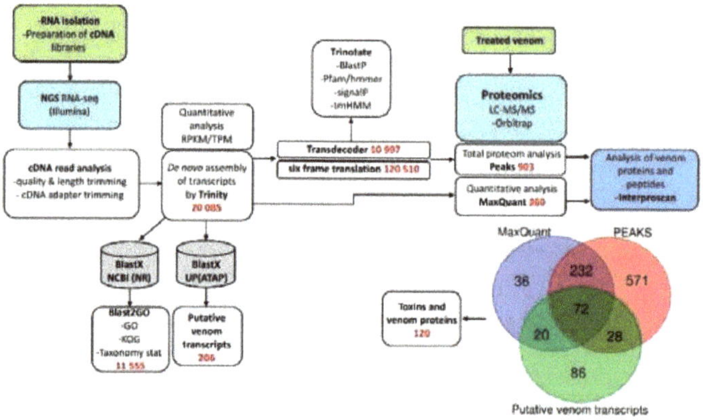

Figure 1. Analysis pipeline of the research implemented for *Azemiops feae*. GO—gene ontology, KOG—euKaryote Orthologous Groups, ATAP—Animal Toxin Annotation Project (UniProt).

From the venom glands of *A. feae*, we generated 29,055,985 pairs of 75 bp reads that passed the Illumina filter (Table S2). Basic filters recommended for qualitative analysis of Illumina were applied to the raw reads, and the adapters used for cDNA synthesis were trimmed. Final cDNA short reads dataset was used for the de novo assembly of a transcriptome using the Trinity assembler. Trinity created 20,085 contigs (reconstructed transcripts) with (N50 = 781), connected to form 18,296 "genes" in total assembly statistics (Table S3).

Next, the gene ontology (GO), eukaryotic orthologous groups (KOG) and taxonomic affiliation of the contigs were analyzed using the Blast2GO program and the BlastX algorithm. The non-redundant database served as a reference database (Figures S1–S3). Furthermore, for identifying potential toxins in the transcriptome, local BlastX was used. As a reference database, we used all toxin sequences from the UniProt animal toxin annotation project (https://www.uniprot.org/program/Toxins). As a result, 206 putative venom transcripts clustered into 112 groups were identified (Table S4).

Finally, all contigs from Trinity were translated using all six reading frames in "Predicted protein SET 1" for subsequent validation by proteomics. The prediction of coding regions (or open read frames,

ORFs) and annotation of transcriptomic data were carried out using Transdecoder and Trinotate. In addition, ORFs from Transdecoder were translated in "Predicted protein SET 2" for subsequent validation by proteomics. Both data sets were used to analyze the total proteome using the PEAKS Studio software. Transcriptome database was used for the quantitative analysis search in MaxQuant. As a result, 120 putative venom transcripts were confirmed using proteomics. A combination of these approaches allowed identifying proteins belonging to 43 protein families, among which 15 can be assigned to snake toxins (Figure 2) (Figures S4–S28).

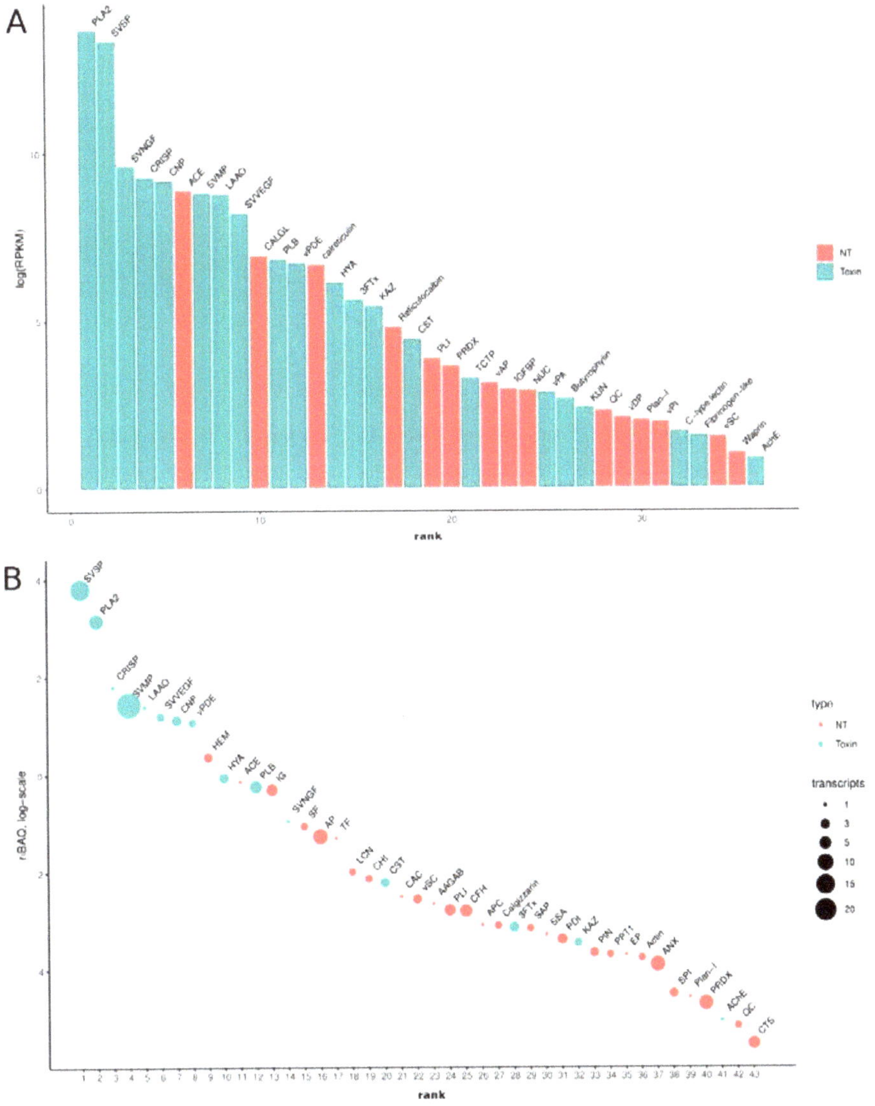

Figure 2. (**A**) Bar chart showing the distribution of Reads Per Kilobase Million (RPKM) values for all putative venom proteins (PVP) families found in transcriptome; (**B**) Scatter plot showing the distribution of riBAQ values of top 43 protein families. The diameter of the circle is proportional to the number of identified transcripts by quantitative proteomics. Abbreviations: 3FTx—Three-finger toxin, AAGAB—Alpha/Gamma adaptin binding protein, ACE—Angiotensinogenase, AChE—Acetylcholinesterase, ANX—Annexin, AP—Aminopeptidase, APC—Serum amyloid P-component, Butyrophylin—Butyrophylin-like, CAC—Calcyclin, CFH—Complement factor H, CHI—Chitinase, CNP—C-type natriuretic peptide (Azemiopsin included), CRISP—cysteine-rich secretory protein, CST—Cystatin, CTS—Cathepsin, EP—Endopeptidase, HEM—Hemoglobin, HYA—Hyaluronidase, IG—Immunoglobulin, IGFBP—Insulin-like growth factor-binding, KAZ—kazal serine protease inhibitor, KUN—Kunitz-type serine protease inhibitor, LAAO—L-amino acid oxidase, LCN—Lipocalin, NUC—5′-nucleotidase, PDI—Disulfide-isomerase, PLA2—phospholipases A2, PLB—Phospholipase B, Plan-I—Plancitoxin-1 (Deoxyribonuclease-2-alpha), PIN—Peptidyl-prolyl cis-trans isomerase, PLI—Phospholipase A2 inhibitor, PPT1—Palmitoyl- thioesterase 1, PRDX—Peroxiredoxin, QC—Glutaminyl-peptide cyclotransferase, SAP—Saposin-A, SF—Siderophilin, SPI—Serpin, SSA—Small serum 2, SVMP—Snake venom metalloproteinase, SVNGF—Snake-venom nerve growth factor, SVSP—Snake-venom serine proteinases, svVEGF—Vascular endothelial growth factor, TCTP—Translationally controlled tumor homolog, TF—Transferrin, vAP—Venom acid phoshatase, vDP—Venom dipeptidyl peptidase 4, vPA—Venom prothrombin activator, vPDE—Venom phosphodiesterase 1, vPI—Venom peptide isomerase, vSC—Serine carboxypeptidase, Waprin—Waprin-like.

3.2. Venom-Gland Transcriptome

We estimated the expression level of each transcript by mapping reads against a de novo transcriptome assembly. As expected, the level of representation of putative venom transcripts (toxins) is significantly higher than other classes of molecules (Figure 2A). Approximately 63% of total transcription was accounted for by the coding sequences of putative toxins, and the 54 most abundant transcripts in the transcriptome encoded putative toxins (Figure 2B).

We grouped all the toxin transcripts into main classes (families) (Figure 3). At the transcriptome level, the most abundant classes of toxin transcripts are PLA2 and SVSP, followed by the second group including snake venom nerve growth factor (svNGF), CRISP, C-type natriuretic peptide (CNP, including azemiopsin), angiotensinogenase (ACE), SVMP, L-amino acid oxidase (LAAO) and snake venom vascular endothelial growth factor (svVEGF). Such classes of proteins as PLB, venom phosphodiesterase (vPDE), HYA and 3FTx are significantly less abundant. Thus, the expression pattern of the *A. feae* venom gland is typical of viper snakes.

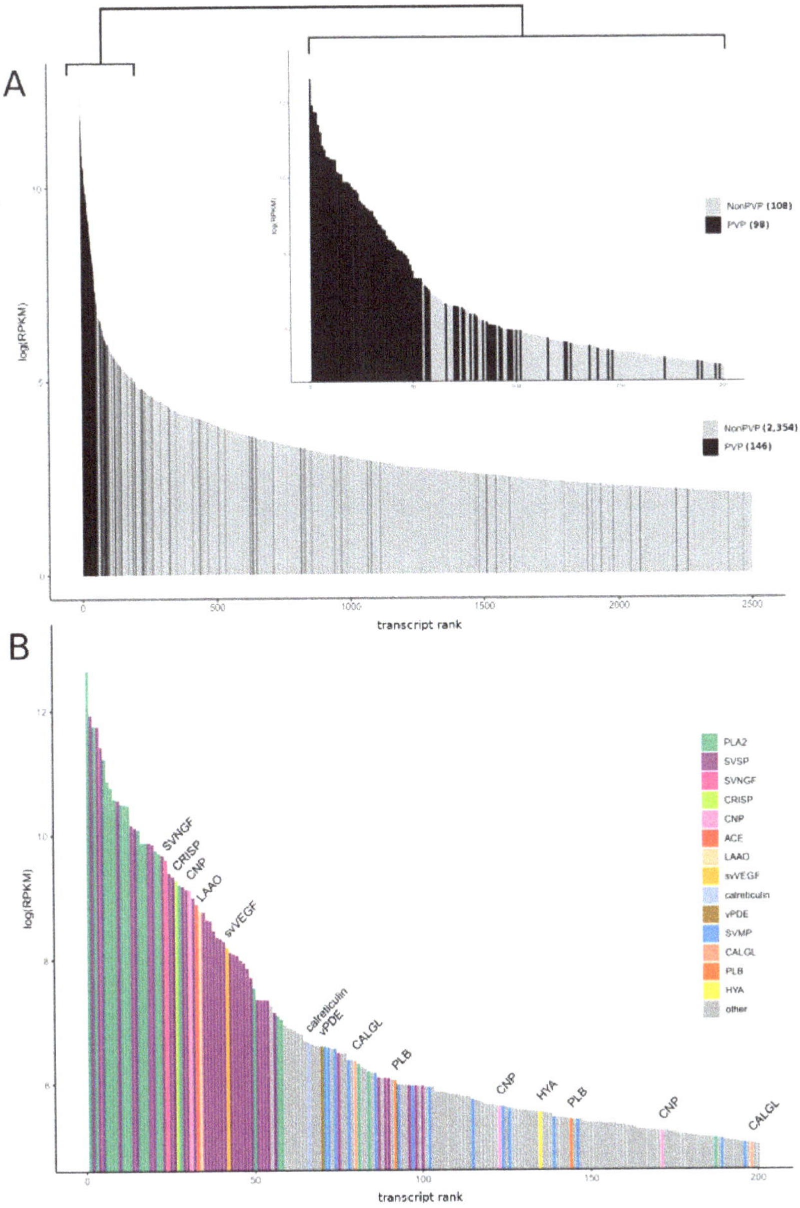

Figure 3. The overall expression patterns for the most abundant transcripts in *A. feae* venom gland tissue. (**A**) Expression of toxins and venom proteins (PVP—putative venom transcripts) dominates relative to other transcripts; (**B**) The venom-gland transcriptome of *A. feae* showed high expression and diversity of snake venom phospholipases A2 and serine proteinases. Expression levels of individual PVP transcripts are shown with toxin classes coded by color. Abbreviations: ACE—Angiotensinogenase, CALGL—Calmodulin, CNP—C-type natriuretic peptide (Azemiopsin included), CRISP—Cysteine-rich secretory protein, HYA—Hyaluronidase, LAAO—L-amino acid oxidase, PLA2—Phospholipases A2, PLB—Phospholipase B, SVMP—Snake venom metalloproteinase, SVNGF—Snake-venom nerve growth factor, SVSP—snake-venom serine proteinases, svVEGF—Vascular endothelial growth factor, vPDE—Venom phosphodiesterase 1.

However, we detected a number of additional low-abundance toxins in the venom-gland transcriptome including 3FTxs and acetylcholinesterase not typical for vipers.

3.3. Venom Proteomics/Peptidomics

In this work, both venom proteome and peptidome for Feae's viper *A. feae* were analyzed (Tables S1 and S5). Venom proteome was analyzed by LC–MS/MS after in-solution trypsin proteolysis. In our study, mass spectrometry analysis of *A. feae* venom revealed more than one hundred different proteins, some of them being identified earlier. Thus, PLA2 [11,12] and a plasminogen activator [10] were isolated from the venom, while the amino acid sequences of CRISP [12], several SVSPs (GenBank: ART88741.1, ART88740.1, ART88739.1, ART88738.1), three-finger toxin 3FTx-Aze-1 [14], SVNGF [27], and CNP precursors 1 and 2 [13] were deduced from cloned cDNA sequences. The peptide neurotoxin azemiopsin was isolated earlier from the *A. feae* venom as well [15].

Proteomic analysis in addition to the above-mentioned proteins, including those for which amino acid sequences were deduced from the cDNA, revealed in the venom the presence of LAAO, SVMP, venom epidermal growth factor, HYA, angiotensinogenase (renin-like aspartic protease), cystatin and ovomucoid (Kazal-type inhibitor-like protein).

The label-free quantification of venom proteins revealed that the most abundant venom proteins are SVSPs accounting for 44.8% (mole fraction) of total proteins. They are followed by PLA2s (25.8%), CRISP (6.0%), LAAO (4.0%), SVMP (3.9%), SVVEGF (3.3%), azemiopsin (bradykinin-potentiating and C-type natriuretic peptides, 3.0%) and PLB (2.9%). The contents of other venom proteins was less than one percent: HYA—0.9%, SVNGF—0.4%, cystatin (CST)—0.1%, 3FTx—0.04% and Kazal-type serine protease inhibitor (Kazal)—0.03%. The toxins present in *A. feae* venom at the level higher than 1% are considered in more detail.

3.3.1. Serine Proteases

Using proteomics in *A. feae* venom, we identified 24 sequences (seven clusters) corresponding to snake venom serine proteases (SVSPs) (Table S4 and Figure S4). However, the assembled transcripts are incomplete and are truncated at either the 5′ or 3′ ends. This drawback prevents an adequate analysis for the classification of SVSPs to certain types. Nevertheless, when considering the alignment, it is seen that the closest homologs are the previously described proteases from *A. feae*, which are secreted trypsin-type proteases (ART88741.1, ART88740.1, ART88739.1, ART88738.1). The identified sequences include also those homologous to plasminogen activators, one of which was found in this venom earlier [11], thrombin-like enzymes and homologs of beta-fibrinogenase. All SVSPs from *A. feae* venom are homologous to those of other snakes from the Viperidae family. Enzymes homologous to plasminogen activators and thrombin-like are the most abundant in *A. feae* venom among SVSPs.

3.3.2. Phospholipases A2

Five clusters PLA2s were found in *A. feae* venom and 11 sequences we identified by proteomics (Table S4 and Figure S5A). They are both acidic and basic enzymes from group II subfamily. The most abundant PLA2s (from about 1 to about 9% of total venom proteins) belong to the enzymatically active D49 sub-family. The minor PLA2s represent the N49 sub-subfamily (from 0.003 to 2%). We found all PLA2 subfamilies of N49a, with the exception of N49b previously discovered [12] in *A. feae* venom from Zhejiang province (China). In the found sequences, slight differences with reference ones are observed, which can be explained by genetic polymorphisms. The remaining sequences are intermediate isoforms of the previously described phospholipases of *A. feae* venom. New isoforms of basic PLA2s were also found. The protein sequence TR6913_c96_g4_i4 resembles basic PLA2s, and sequence TR6913_c96_g4_i6 has homology to the sequence of *Crotalus atrox* (QBA85153.1) (Figure S5A,B).

3.3.3. Cysteine-Rich Seceretory Proteins

Only one CRISP was found in the *A. feae* venom (Figure 4). The CRISP amino acid sequence determined in this work is very similar to that of Az-CRP determined earlier for *A. feae* CRISP [12]. The two sequences differ only in two positions, 132 and 236 (Figure 4); Ile and Gln in Az-CRP are replaced by Thr and Lys, respectively, in the sequence determined in this work.

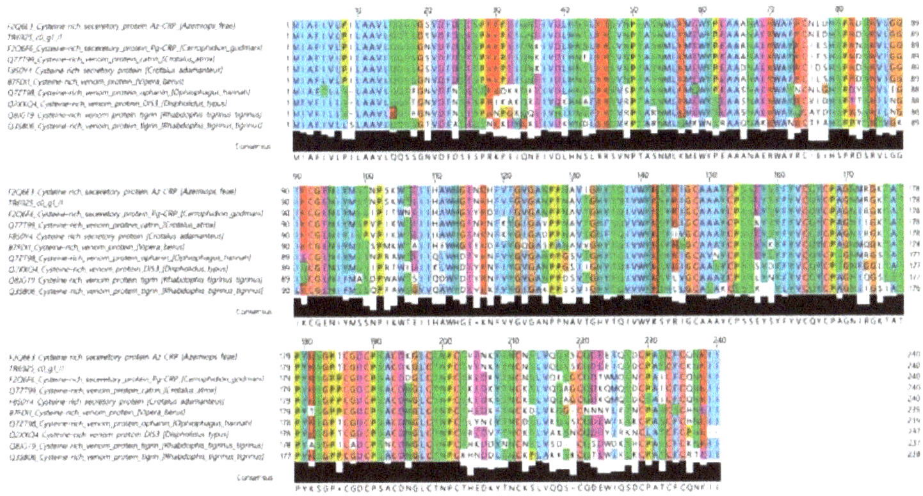

Figure 4. Amino acid sequence of *A. feae* CRISPs aligned with sequences of homologous proteins. TR6925_c0_g1_i2 is the sequence determined in this work. Alignment was generated by MUSCLE (Here and in all following captions MUSCLE is MUltiple Sequence Comparison by Log-Expectation) with ClustalX Colour Scheme: hydrophobic amino acid residues—blue; positively charged—red; negatively charged—magenta; polar—green; cysteines—pink; glycines—orange; prolines—yellow; aromatic—cyan; unconserved -white.

3.3.4. L-Amino Acid Oxidase

LAAO is found in venoms of snakes from different families. Similarly to CRISP, this toxin is represented by only one protein in *A. feae* venom. *A. feae* LAAO has the highest similarity to that of the Okinawa pitviper (or Hime habu), *Ovophis okinavensis* from the Crotalinae subfamily (Figure S6).

3.3.5. Snake Venom Metalloproteinase

In venoms of many species from the Viperidae family, SVMPs are the main components. For example, in *Bothrops atrox* venom, SVMPs represent more than half of total venom protein [28]. In *A. feae* venom, SVMPs account for only 3.9% of total protein and are represented by 16 enzymes (Figure S7). As in the case of SVSPs, only 5′ or 3′ terminal fragments were assembled, so no full-length protein sequences were obtained. Analysis of the domain organization (Figure S7B) allowed us to conclude that *A. feae* venom contains several isoforms of classical snake venom type III SVMP (Figure S7).

3.3.6. Snake Venom Vascular Endothelial Growth Factor

In *A. feae* venom, svVEGF is represented by two proteins which account for 3.3% of total venom protein (Figure S8).

3.3.7. Three-Finger Toxins

Among the toxins present in *A. feae* venom at levels less than 1%, 3FTxs are of special interest. 3FTxs are the main components of venoms from Elapidae snakes. Transcripts of 3FTxs were identified in transcriptomes of several vipers. However, the neurotoxins were not found in viper venoms so far. Here, for the first time, we have found the 3FTxs in the venom of a snake from the Viperidae family. Even though the content of 3FTxs in *A. feae* venom is as low as 0.04%, there is no doubt about the presence of these toxins. Five three-finger toxins were found in *A. feae* venom (Figure 5); according to their amino acid sequences, they represent so-called basal (commonly known as non-conventional) toxins containing the fifth disulfide bond in the first loop [29,30]. The recombinant toxin 3FTx-Aze-2 showed the capacity to interact with muscle type and neuronal nicotinic acetylcholine receptors [31].

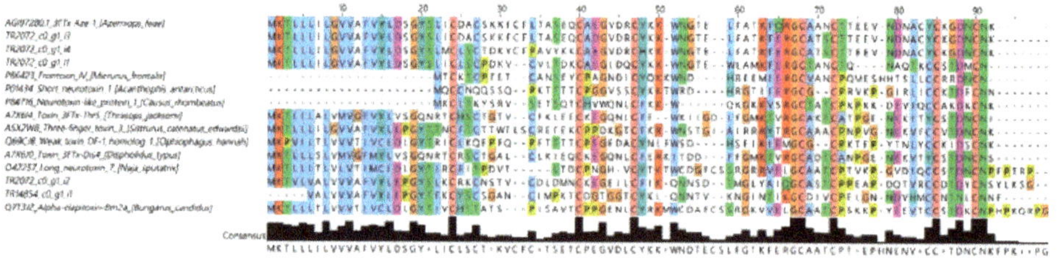

Figure 5. Three-finger toxins (3FTx). Comparison of amino sequences of *A. feae* toxins with those of known 3FTxs. TR2072 c0 g1 i3 is named 3FTx-Aze-2; TR2072 c0 g1 i4—3FTx-Aze-3; TR2072 c0 g1 i2—3FTx-Aze-4; TR14854 c0 g1 i1—3FTx-Aze-5; TR2072 c0 g1 i1—3FTx-Aze-6; TR13523 c0 g1 i1—3FTx-aze-7. Alignment was generated by MUSCLE with ClustalX Colour Scheme: hydrophobic amino acid residues—blue; positively charged—red; negatively charged—magenta; polar—green; cysteines—pink; glycines—orange; prolines—yellow; aromatic—cyan; unconserved—white.

3.3.8. Bradykinin-Potentiating Peptides and Azemiopsin

Azemiopsin is a unique peptide toxin isolated earlier by us from *A. feae* venom [14]. According to the present analysis, its content in the venom is equal to 3.0%. The amino acid sequence of azemiopsin was identified previously within C-type natriuretic precursors [13] (Figure 6). It is interesting to note that several azemiopsin sequences are present within precursor sequences. Moreover, elongated analogs of azemiopsin (M = 2540) with additional N-terminal residues—SDNWWPKPPHQGPRPPRPRPKP (M = 2627) and ESDNWWPKPPHQGPRPPRPRPKP (M = 2756)—were identified in the venom (Table S5). When these peptides were fragmented in the mass spectrometer, the C-terminal ions remained constant, while for the N-terminal b-ions, corresponding mass shifts were observed (Figure S29).

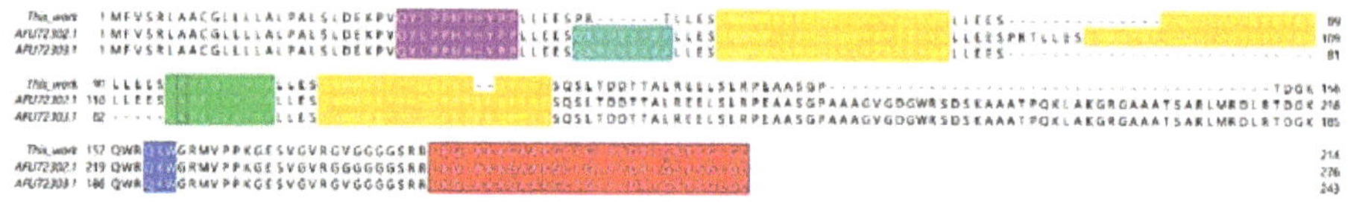

Figure 6. Amino acid sequences of C-type natriuretic precursors deduced from DNA sequences. Azemiopsin—yellow, Y-BPP—lilac, R-BPP and its Lys-analog—light green, putative shortened R-BPP analog—turquoise, putative tripeptide metalloproteinase inhibitor—blue, atrial natriuretic peptide—red.

During isolation of azemiopsin, we found several peptides with molecular masses of 1328.64 (Y-BPP), 1156.57 (R-BPP) and 1045.5 Da (R-BPP-s). The amino acid sequences of these peptides were established by de novo MALDI MS/MS sequencing (Figure S30). The determined sequences are shown in Figure 6. The peptides Y-BPP and R-BPP contain pyroglutamic acid at their N-terminus; the amino acid sequence of R-BPP-s corresponds to an N-terminally truncated form of R-BPP. The determined sequences show homology to some bradykinin-potentiating peptides (Figure 7). However, the sequences between the two PP repeats are unique for *A. feae* peptides. It should be mentioned that the tripeptide sequence QKW is present in the CNP precursor (Figure 6). This tripeptide may represent an endogenous metalloproteinase inhibitor ZKW (Z = pyroGlu) found in venoms of several Viperidae species. The C-type natriuretic precursors contain the sequence of C-type natriuretic peptide (Figure 6). This peptide was also found in the peptidome of *A. feae* venom (Table S5).

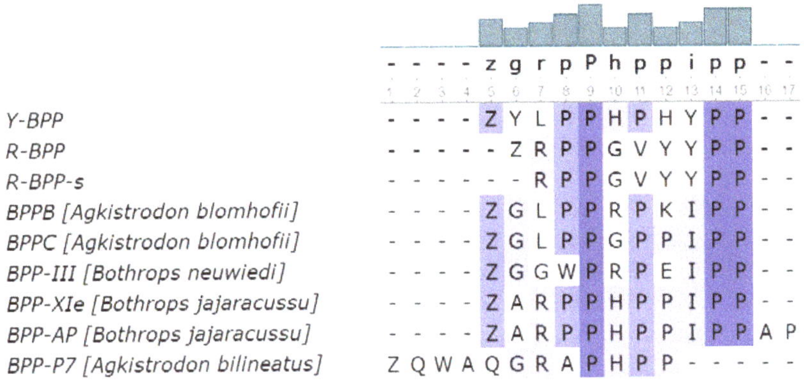

Figure 7. Bradykinin-potentiating peptides (BPP). Comparison of amino acid sequences of *A. feae* peptides with those of known bradykinin-potentiating peptides (pyroGlu = Z). The number of each consensus letter is represented by a histogram on the top of the figure. Alignment was generated by MUSCLE with percentage identity coloring scheme where the white color is corresponding to 0% identity and the darkest color to 100%.

3.3.9. Biological Activity of New Bradykinin-Potentiating Peptides

To study their biological activity, the bradykinin-potentiating peptides Y-BPP and R-BPP were prepared by peptide synthesis and purified by reverse-phase chromatography. The potentiating effect was investigated in vivo in SD rats; arterial blood pressure was registered. Anesthetized rats received peptides through venous catheter, and the arterial catheter was used to record blood pressure (BP). Injection of bradykinin at a dose of 7 µg/kg resulted in the BP drop by 27–33% (Figure 8). Administration of either Y-BPP or R-BPP 10 min later produced a further small decrease (by about 10%) in BP and strongly enhanced the effect of bradykinin injected 5 min after BPP (Figure 8). The potentiating effect was dose-dependent (Figure 9) and was observed for about half an hour at the dose of 300 µg/kg and 1 mg/kg for Y-BPP (Figure 9A,B) and at the dose of 1 mg/kg for R-BPP (Figure 9C,D). No potentiating effect was detected one hour after BPP administration (Figure 9).

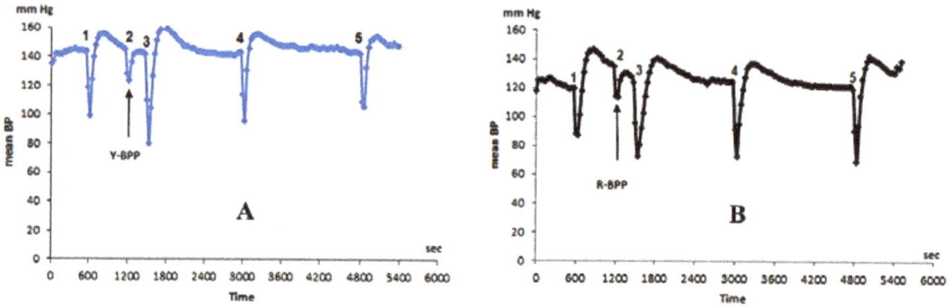

Figure 8. Bradykinin-potentiating effects of *A. feae* peptides Y-BPP and R-BPP. Changes in mean blood pressure (BPs) (absolute values) after administration of bradykinin at a dose of 7 µg/kg (injections at points 1, 3, 4, 5) and Y-BPP (**A**) or R-BPP (**B**) at a dose of 300 µg/kg (injection at point 2).

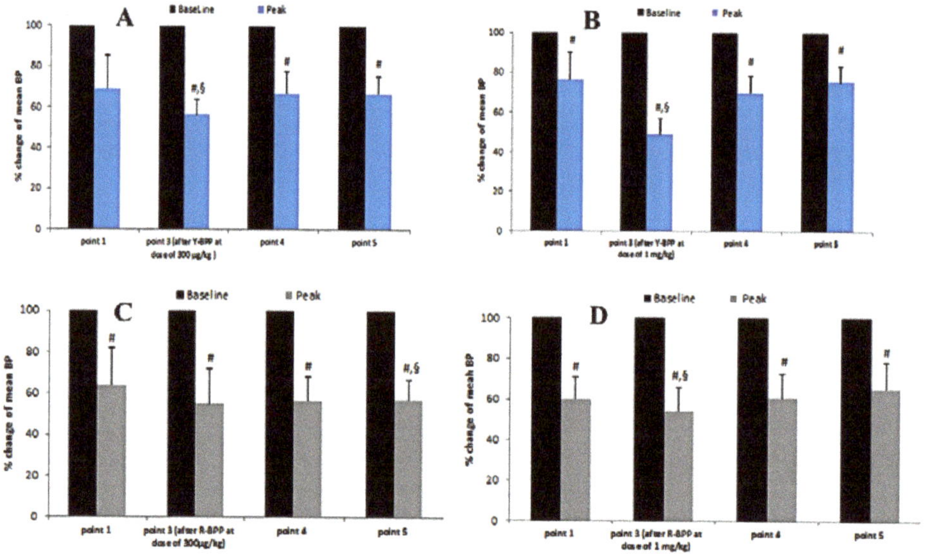

Figure 9. Percent changes from baseline for mean BPs after injections of bradykinin at a dose of 7 µg/kg in response to bradykinin-potentiating effects of *A. feae* peptides Y-BPP (**A**,**B**) and R-BPP (**C**,**D**) at two doses. # $p \leq 0.05$ vs. baseline according to the T-Test for comparing the data of one group before and after treatment, § $p \leq 0.05$ vs. point 1 according to the repeated-measures ANOVA with Dunnett post-hoc test.

4. Discussion

Azemiopinae is regarded as a sister group of the Crotalinae [5,6]. Therefore, it is quite reasonable that the *A. feae* venom composition bears a resemblance to those of Crotalinae snakes. Thus, the main constituents of Feae's viper venom are SVSPs (44.8%) and PLA2s (25.8%), representing about $\frac{3}{4}$ of venom total protein, although the content of SVMPs is fairly small as compared to other venoms of Crotalinae snakes [4]. The most remarkable difference between the Feae's viper venom and those of other Crotalids is the presence of the peptide neurotoxin azemiopsin and 3FTxs in *A. feae* venom. Azemiopsin is homologous to waglerin from the Asian pit-viper *Tropidolaemus wagleri* venom but in contrast to waglerin has no disulfide bridge [15,32]. The content of azemiopsin in the venom is lower (3%) than that of waglerin (15% [33] or 38.2% [34]). Nevertheless, some neurological symptoms were observed in the victims of Feae's viper bite [35], which might be caused by azemiopsin. Moreover, recently it was shown that *A. feae* venom interacted with fragments representing modified orthosteric mimotopes of binding region of nicotinic acetylcholine receptors from a diversity of potential preys [36]. This may also indicate the neurotoxicity of the *A. feae* venom. Indeed, inhibition of the muscle nAChRs was detected for azemiopsin [15], which later in preclinical studies was shown to be an efficient myorelaxant [26].

3FTxs are the main components of venoms from Elapidae snakes. They manifest a wide array of activities ranging from highly specific interactions with some receptors and ion channels to unspecific damage of cell membranes. 3FTxs were classified into several groups depending on their amino acid sequences and biological activities [37]. The most abundant groups are neurotoxins and cytotoxins (cardiotoxins). Cytotoxin-like components were reported in *Daboia russelii russelii* venom [38]. Transcripts of 3FTxs were identified in transcriptomes of several vipers, including *A. feae* [14]. However, no 3FTx neurotoxins were found in viper venoms so far. In the Feae's viper venom, we have identified several 3FTxs (Figure 7); all these toxins contain the fifth disulfide bridge in the loop I and thus belong to so-called basal or non-conventional toxins [29,30]. Toxins of this group, similarly to α-neurotoxins, interact with some types of nicotinic acetylcholine receptors [39,40] and bind to muscarinic acetylcholine receptors as well [41,42]. It should be mentioned that the sequences of 3FTxs determined in this work are different from 3FTx-Aze-1 [14] described earlier. The differences between the published sequence 3FTx-Aze-1 and our sequence 3FTx-Aze-2 are not very big, including only four substitutions at positions 42, 63, 68 and 69, and may be explained by individual venom variations (Figure 5), while the other toxin amino acid identified in this work differs more strongly from that of 3FTx-Aze-1. The sequences of *A. feae* 3FTxs are distinguished by the number of amino acid residues between invariant cysteine residues. In addition, 3FTx-Aze-4 has an extended C-terminal tail, which makes it similar to long-type α-neurotoxins from elapid venoms. Based on the results obtained, it can be concluded that the *A. feae* 3FTxs are quite remarkable. The amino acid sequences of some *A. feae* 3FTxs have similarities with sequences of toxins from Colubridae. Interestingly, heterogeneity in sequences is observed within one species, and some of the sequences are closer to those from Viperidae and some from Colubridae. The first step to investigate the biological activity of *A. feae* three-finger toxins is our recent work, where the gene encoding the sequence of 3FTx-Aze-2 (Figure 5) was synthesized, expressed in *Escherichia. coli*, and the biological activity studies showed that the heterologously expressed toxin inhibited nicotinic acetylcholine receptors of both muscle and neuronal types [31].

It should be noted that the important components of Crotalidae venoms are bradykinin-potentiating peptides (BPP). BPPs are produced in venom glands by processing long precursor proteins including as a rule several sequences of BPP and natriuretic peptide. During mass-spectrometric analysis of *A. feae* venom, we have found two peptides, Y-BPP and R-BPP, with amino acid sequences homologous to BPPs (Figure 7). The synthetic BPPs showed bradykinin-potentiating effects (Figures 8 and 9). Analysis of transcriptomic data revealed a nucleotide sequence encoding a polypeptide containing several azemiopsin sequences as well as sequences of both Y-BPP and R-BPP (Figure 5). We have not obtained precursors with sequence length similar to the ones determined before [13]; however, the shorter fragments fit well to the long precursor. It should be mentioned that the sequences of one BPP are different; the lysine residue in the long precursor is replaced by arginine in the sequence of R-BPP (Figure 6). The tripeptide fragment QKW is also found in the sequences of precursors. The tripeptide ZKW characteristic to Viperidae venoms is an endogenous inhibitor of metalloproteinases [43,44]. Usually, several QKW repeats have been found in the CNP precursors; however, only one is found in sequence from *A. feae*.

In addition, if we fully cover the repertoire of toxins from what we found only in the form of transcripts, it turns out that *A. feae* retained a wider range of toxins from the common ancestor of Viperidae. Apparently, the common ancestor had a much wider arsenal of toxins. It is logical to assume that retaining a wider range of toxins is due to the absence of strict selection in the habitat of

A. feae; in other Viperidae, the selection was apparently due to specialization in prey and a change in living conditions.

For the Viperidae, an origin in Asia was presumed, and for the Crotalinae (and Azemiops), the origin was firmly placed in Asia [5,6]. It can be assumed that *A. feae* is a relic ("ancient old-timer") whose habitat was stable enough to leave the entire toxin repertoire or at least part of it almost unchanged. Various assumptions can be made about the presence of transcripts, but the lack of protein would indicate that this is just a blank transcription. Again, the lack of selection minimizes their divergence. The found unique peptides may be just a new type of adaptation and a unique feature of *A. feae* or further development of toxins inherited from an ancient ancestor.

For biological activity studies, Y-BPP and R-BPP were prepared by solid phase synthesis. Studies on SD rats revealed that both peptides dose-dependently potentiated the activity of bradykinin. At 1 mg/kg, the peptides increased the bradykinin effects by 30% (Figure 9B,D). This value is similar to the ones observed for some BPPs from *Bothrops* venoms [45]. While Y-BPP has some structural similarity to BPPs earlier described, for example to BPPB from *Agkistrodon blomhofii* (Figure 7), the sequence of R-BPP is unique. Thus, we have found a BPP with a new structural motif.

5. Conclusions

We have described the comprehensive venom-gland transcriptomic and quantitative proteomic venom characterization of *A. feae* viper. The proteomic analysis revealed the presence of 120 unique proteins, serine proteinases and phospholipases A_2 being the most abundant. In total, toxins representing 14 families were identified, among which bradykinin-potentiating peptides with unique amino acid sequence features were found and shown to possess biological activity in vivo. The proteomic analysis also revealed three-finger toxins which belong to the group of non-conventional toxins possessing neurotoxic activity. This is the first indication of the presence of three-finger neurotoxins in viper venom. The transcriptomic analysis of the venom gland by Illumina next-generation sequencing revealed 206 putative venom transcripts. Together, the study unveiled the venom proteome and venom gland transciptome of *A. feae*, which in general resemble those of snakes from the Viperidae family. However, new toxins not found earlier in viper venom and including three-finger toxins and unusual bradykinin-potentiating peptides were discovered.

Supplementary Materials: The following are available online at http://www.mdpi.com/2227-9059/8/8/249/s1, Figure S1: Gene ontology by categories of biological process, cellular component and molecular function, Figure S2: Functional categories of the contigs in KOG database. (A), RNA processing and modification; (B), chromatin structure and dynamics; (C), energy production and conversion; (D), cell cycle control, cell division, chromosome partitioning; (E), amino acid transport and metabolism; (F), nucleotide transport and metabolism; (G), carbohydrate transport and metabolism; (H), coenzyme transport and metabolism; (I), lipid transport and metabolism; (J), translation, ribosomal structure and biogenesis; (K), transcription; (L), replication, recombination and repair; (M), cell wall/membrane/envelope biogenesis; (N), cell motility; (O), posttranslational modification, protein turnover, chaperones; (P), inorganic ion transport and metabolism; (Q), secondary metabolites biosynthesis, transport and catabolism; (R), general function prediction only; (T), signal transduction mechanisms; (U), intracellular trafficking, secretion and vesicular transport; (V), defense mechanisms; (W), extracellular structures; (Y), nuclear structure; (Z), cytoskeleton; (S), function unknown, Figure S3: The distribution of the top 10 BLAST hits. Snake species are underlined, Figure S4: (A) Multiple sequence alignment of serine proteases (SVSPs) from the venom gland transcriptome of *A. feae* in comparison with the described serine proteases from *A. feae*. Alignment generated by MUSCLE (Here and in all following captions, MUSCLE is MUltiple Sequence Comparison by Log-Expectation) with percentage identity coloring scheme. (B) Multiple sequence alignment overview window, for serine proteases (SVSPs) from the venom gland transcriptome of *A. feae* in comparison with the described serine proteases from *A. feae*. Alignment generated by MUSCLE (Here and in all following captions, MUSCLE is MUltiple Sequence Comparison by Log-Expectation) with ClustalX Colour Scheme, Figure S5: (A) Multiple sequence alignment of phospholipase A2 (PLA2) transcripts from the venom gland transcriptome of *A. feae* in comparison to PLA2 sequences of representative venomous snakes. Amino acids that determine the type of phospholipase (D49, N49 or K49) are marked with a black frame and a red font. Alignment generated by MUSCLE with ClustalX Colour Scheme. (B) Neighbor-joining (NJ) gene tree, based on BLOSUM62 matrix alignment of the proteins in the PLA2 cluster. Branches corresponding to acidic phospholipases are marked in yellow; branches corresponding to basic phospholipases are marked in blue. New discovered isoforms are marked in red. PLA2 previously discovered by other researchers are marked in grey boxes. Human PLA2 was used as outgroup, Figure S6: Multiple sequence alignment of L-amino-acid oxidase (LAAO) transcripts from *A. feae* with two Viperidae homologs. Alignment generated by MUSCLE with ClustalX Colour Scheme, Figure S7: (A) Multiple sequence alignment of zinc metalloprotease (SVMP) transcripts from *A. feae* in comparison to zinc metalloprotease sequences of representative venomous snakes. Alignment generated by MUSCLE with percentage identity coloring scheme. (B) Multiple sequence alignment overview window for zinc metalloprotease (SVMP) transcripts from *A. feae* in comparison to zinc metalloprotease sequences of representative venomous snakes. The top of the alignment shows the domain organization of the reference metalloproteinases. Alignment generated by MUSCLE with ClustalX Colour Scheme, Figure S8: Multiple sequence alignment of snake venom Vascular Endothelial Growth Factors (svVEGF) in comparison to svVEGF sequences of representative venomous snakes. Alignment is separated by bold lines into blocks according to types of svVEGF. Alignment generated by MUSCLE with ClustalX Colour Scheme, Figure S9: Multiple sequence alignment of phospholipase B (PLB) transcripts from the venom gland transcriptome of *A. feae* in comparison to PLB sequences of representative venomous snakes. Alignment generated by MUSCLE with percentage identity coloring scheme, Figure S10: Multiple sequence alignment of venom phosphodiesterase 1 (vPDE) transcripts from the venom gland transcriptome of *A. feae* in comparison to vPDE sequences of representative venomous snakes. Alignment generated by MUSCLE with ClustalX Colour Scheme, Figure S11: Multiple sequence alignment of hyaluronidases (HYA) with *Protobothrops mucrosquamatus* homolog. Alignment generated by MUSCLE with ClustalX Colour Scheme, Figure S12: Multiple sequence alignment of nerve growth factor (svNGF) partial transcripts from *A. feae* in comparison to svNGF sequences of representative venomous snakes. Alignment generated by MUSCLE with ClustalX Colour Scheme, Figure S13: Multiple sequence alignment of cystatins (CST) from the venom gland transcriptome of *A. feae* in comparison to cystatins sequences of representative venomous snakes. Alignment is separated by bold lines into blocks according to types of cystatins. Alignment generated by MUSCLE with ClustalX Colour Scheme, Figure S14: Multiple sequence alignment of kazal (KAZ) domains with comparison to kazal-like sequences of representative venomous snakes. Alignment generated by MUSCLE with ClustalX Colour Scheme, Figure S15: Multiple sequence alignment of acetylcholinesterase (AChE) partial transcripts from the venom gland transcriptome of *A. feae* with two *Vipera anatolica cholinesterases*. Alignment generated by MUSCLE with percentage identity coloring scheme, Figure S16: Multiple sequence alignment of calcium-binding protein (Reticulocalbin) transcripts in comparison to sequences of representative venomous snakes. Alignment generated by MUSCLE with ClustalX Colour Scheme, Figure S17: Multiple sequence alignment of translationally controlled tumor protein (TCTP/HRF) transcripts from the venom gland transcriptome of *A. feae* in comparison with *Crotalus horridus* homolog. Alignment generated by MUSCLE with percentage identity coloring scheme, Figure S18: Multiple sequence alignment of lysosomal acid phosphatase (vAP) from the venom gland transcriptome of *A. feae* in comparison to vAP sequences of representative venomous snakes. Alignment generated by MUSCLE with percentage identity coloring scheme, Figure S19: Sequence alignment of insulin-like growth factor-binding protein (IGFBP) partial transcript from the venom gland transcriptome of *A. feae* in comparison with *Protobothrops mucrosquamatus* homolog. Alignment generated by MUSCLE with percentage identity coloring scheme, Figure S20: Multiple sequence alignment of venom prothrombin activator (vPA) partial transcripts from the venom gland transcriptome of *A. feae* in comparison with *Oxyuranus microlepidotus* homolog. Alignment generated by MUSCLE with percentage identity coloring scheme. Figure S21: Multiple sequence alignment of kunitz (KUN) domains with comparison to kunitz-like sequences of representative venomous snakes. Alignment generated by MUSCLE with percentage identity coloring scheme, Figure S22: Multiple sequence alignment of glutaminyl-peptide cyclotransferase (QC) partial transcripts domains with *Protobothrops mucrosquamatus* homolog. Alignment generated by MUSCLE with percentage identity coloring scheme, Figure S23: Multiple sequence alignment of dipeptidyl peptidase (vDP) transcripts in comparison with *Protobothrops mucrosquamatus* homologs. Alignment generated by MUSCLE with ClustalX Colour Scheme, Figure S24: Multiple sequence alignment of 5′-nucleotidase (NUC) from the venom gland transcriptome of *A. feae* in comparison to 5′-nucleotidase sequences of representative venomous snakes. Alignment generated by MUSCLE with ClustalX Colour Scheme, Figure S25: Multiple sequence alignment of C-type lectins with other snaclecs. Alignment generated by MUSCLE with percentage identity coloring scheme, Figure S26: Multiple sequence alignment of fibrinogen-like partial transcripts from the venom gland transcriptome of *A. feae* in comparison to fibrinogen-like sequences of representative venomous snakes. Alignment generated by MUSCLE with percentage identity coloring scheme, Figure S27: Multiple sequence alignment serine carboxypeptidase (vSC) partial transcripts with *Protobothrops mucrosquamatus* homolog. Alignment generated by MUSCLE with percentage identity coloring scheme, Figure S28: Multiple sequence alignment of waprin transcripts in comparison to waprin sequences of representative venomous snakes. Alignment generated by MUSCLE with ClustalX Colour Scheme, Figure S29: Sections of MS/MS spectra of azemiopsin and ist N-terminally extended analogs; shift of the b-ions (azemiopsin 416 = b3, DNW; Ser-azemiopsin 503 = b4, SDNW; Glu-Ser-Azemiopsin, 632 = b5, ESDNW), Figure S30: MS/MS spectrum of R-BPP and its interpretation; the insert shows the theoretical b- and y-ions for the sequence ZRPPGVYYPP, with Z for N-terminal pyroglutamic acid (theoretical mass 1156.579); strong internal ions are observed due to preferential fragmentation at Pro, Table S1: Qualitative proteomic data, Table S2: Library basic statistics, Table S3: Transcriptome assembly statistics (Trinity), Table S4: Putative venom transcripts, Table S5: Peptidome of *A. feae* venom.

Author Contributions: Conceptualization, R.H.Z. and Y.U.; Data curation, A.N.M., V.T. and Y.U.; Funding acquisition, A.N.M., V.T. and Y.U.; Investigation, V.V.B., R.H.Z., C.W., I.D., E.S. and M.Z.; Methodology, V.V.B., R.H.Z., C.W. and I.D.; Project administration, A.N.M., V.T. and Y.U.; Resources, A.N.M., V.S. and A.N.H.; Software, V.V.B.; Supervision, A.N.M., V.T. and Y.U.; Validation, V.T. and Y.U.; Writing—original draft, V.V.B., R.H.Z. and Y.U.; Writing—review & editing, C.W., E.S., V.T. and Y.U. All authors have read and agreed to the published version of the manuscript.

Funding: The reported study was funded by RFBR according to the research project No. 18-04-01075.

Acknowledgments: The authors thank Nikolay A. Poyarkov (Lomonosov Moscow State University, Faculty of Biology) for providing an *Azemiops feae* photo and for comments that improved the manuscript.

Conflicts of Interest: The authors declare no conflict of interest. The funders had no role in the design of the study; in the collection, analyses, or interpretation of data; in the writing of the manuscript; or in the decision to publish the results.

References

1. Casewell, N.R.; Jackson, T.N.W.; Laustsen, A.H.; Sunagar, K. Causes and consequences of snake venom variation. *Trends Pharmacol. Sci.* **2020**, *41*, 570–581. [CrossRef]
2. Ziganshin, R.H.; Kovalchuk, S.I.; Arapidi, G.P.; Starkov, V.G.; Hoang, A.N.; Thi Nguyen, T.T.; Nguyen, K.C.; Shoibonov, B.B.; Tsetlin, V.I.; Utkin, Y.N.; et al. Quantitative proteomic analysis of vietnamese krait venoms: Neurotoxins are the major components in *bungarus multicinctus* and phospholipases A2 in *Bungarus fasciatus*. *Toxicon* **2015**, *107*, 197–209. [CrossRef]
3. Calvete, J.J. Snake venomics-from low-resolution toxin-pattern recognition to toxin-resolved venom proteomes with absolute quantification. *Expert Rev. Proteom.* **2018**, *15*, 555–568. [CrossRef]
4. Tasoulis, T.; Isbister, G.K. A review and database of snake venom proteomes. *Toxins* **2017**, *9*, 290. [CrossRef]
5. Wuster, W.; Peppin, L.; Pook, C.E.; Walker, D.E. A nesting of vipers: Phylogeny and historical biogeography of the *Viperidae Squamata*: *Serpentes*. *Mol. Phylogenet. Evol.* **2008**, *49*, 445–459. [CrossRef]
6. Alencar, L.R.V.; Quental, T.B.; Grazziotin, F.G.; Alfaro, M.L.; Martins, M.; Venzon, M.; Zaher, H. Diversification in vipers: Phylogenetic relationships, time of divergence and shifts in speciation rates. *Mol. Phylogenet. Evol.* **2016**, *105*, 50–62. [CrossRef]
7. Orlov, N.L.; Ryabov, S.A.; Nguyen, T.T. On the taxonomy and the distribution of snakes of the genus azemiops boulenger, 1888: Description of a New Species. *Russ. J. Herpetol.* **2013**, *20*, 110–128.
8. Li, J.N.; Liang, D.; Wang, Y.Y.; Guo, P.; Huang, S.; Zhang, P. A large-scale systematic framework of Chinese snakes based on a unified multilocus marker system. *Mol. Phylogenet. Evol.* **2020**, *148*, 106807. [CrossRef]
9. Mebs, D.; Kuch, U.; Meier, J. Studies on venom and venom apparatus of Fea's viper, *Azemiops feae*. *Toxicon* **1994**, *32*, 1275–1278. [CrossRef]
10. Debono, J.; Bos, M.H.A.; Coimbra, F.; Ge, L.; Frank, N.; Kwok, H.F.; Fry, B.G. Basal but divergent: Clinical implications of differential coagulotoxicity in a clade of Asian vipers. *Toxicol. In Vitro Int. J. Publ. Assoc. BIBRA* **2019**, *58*, 195–206. [CrossRef]
11. Fry, B.G.; Wuster, W.; Ryan Ramjan, S.F.; Jackson, T.; Martelli, P.; Kini, R.M. Analysis of colubroidea snake venoms by liquid chromatography with mass spectrometry: Evolutionary and toxinological implications. *Rapid Commun. Mass Spectrom. RCM* **2003**, *17*, 2047–2062. [CrossRef]
12. Tsai, I.H.; Wang, Y.M.; Huang, K.F. Structures of azemiops feae venom phospholipases and cys-rich-secretory protein and implications for taxonomy and toxinology. *Toxicon* **2016**, *114*, 31–39. [CrossRef]
13. Brust, A.; Sunagar, K.; Undheim, E.A.; Vetter, I.; Yang, D.C.; Casewell, N.R.; Jackson, T.N.; Koludarov, I.; Alewood, P.F.; Hodgson, W.C.; et al. Differential evolution and neofunctionalization of snake venom metalloprotease domains. *Mol. Cell. Proteom. MCP* **2013**, *12*, 651–663. [CrossRef]
14. Sunagar, K.; Jackson, T.N.; Undheim, E.A.; Ali, S.A.; Antunes, A.; Fry, B.G. Three-fingered RAVERs: Rapid accumulation of variations in exposed residues of snake venom toxins. *Toxins* **2013**, *5*, 2172–2208. [CrossRef]
15. Utkin, Y.N.; Weise, C.; Kasheverov, I.E.; Andreeva, T.V.; Kryukova, E.V.; Zhmak, M.N.; Starkov, V.G.; Hoang, N.A.; Bertrand, D.; Ramerstorfer, J.; et al. Azemiopsin from azemiops feae viper venom, a novel polypeptide ligand of nicotinic acetylcholine receptor. *J. Biol. Chem.* **2012**, *287*, 27079–27086. [CrossRef]
16. Zhu, Y.Y.; Machleder, E.M.; Chenchik, A.; Li, R.; Siebert, P.D. Reverse transcriptase template switching: A SMART approach for full-length cDNA library construction. *Bio. Tech.* **2001**, *30*, 892–897. [CrossRef]
17. Waterhouse, A.M.; Procter, J.B.; Martin, D.M.; Clamp, M.; Barton, G.J. Jalview version 2-a multiple sequence alignment editor and analysis workbench. *Bioinformatics* **2009**, *25*, 1189–1191. [CrossRef]
18. Kulak, N.A.; Pichler, G.; Paron, I.; Nagaraj, N.; Mann, M. Minimal, encapsulated proteomic-sample processing applied to copy-number estimation in eukaryotic cells. *Nat. Method.* **2014**, *11*, 319–324. [CrossRef]
19. Rappsilber, J.; Mann, M.; Ishihama, Y. Protocol for micro-purification, enrichment, pre-fractionation and storage of peptides for proteomics using StageTips. *Nat. Protoc.* **2007**, *2*, 1896–1906. [CrossRef]

20. Ma, B.; Zhang, K.; Hendrie, C.; Liang, C.; Li, M.; Doherty-Kirby, A.; Lajoie, G. PEAKS: Powerful software for peptide de novo sequencing by tandem mass spectrometry. *Rapid Commun. Mass Spectrom. RCM* **2003**, *17*, 2337–2342. [CrossRef]
21. Tyanova, S.; Temu, T.; Cox, J. The MaxQuant computational platform for mass spectrometry-based shotgun proteomics. *Nat. Protoc.* **2016**, *11*, 2301–2319. [CrossRef]
22. Cox, J.; Neuhauser, N.; Michalski, A.; Scheltema, R.A.; Olsen, J.V.; Mann, M. Andromeda: A peptide search engine integrated into the MaxQuant environment. *J. Proteom. Res.* **2011**, *10*, 1794–1805. [CrossRef]
23. Tyanova, S.; Temu, T.; Sinitcyn, P.; Carlson, A.; Hein, M.Y.; Geiger, T.; Mann, M.; Cox, J. The perseus computational platform for comprehensive analysis of (prote)omics data. *Nat. Method.* **2016**, *13*, 731–740. [CrossRef]
24. Shin, J.B.; Krey, J.F.; Hassan, A.; Metlagel, Z.; Tauscher, A.N.; Pagana, J.M.; Sherman, N.E.; Jeffery, E.D.; Spinelli, K.J.; Zhao, H.; et al. Molecular architecture of the chick vestibular hair bundle. *Nat. Neurosci.* **2013**, *16*, 365–374. [CrossRef]
25. Suckau, D.; Resemann, A.; Schürenberg, M.; Hufnagel, P.; Franzen, J.; Holle, A. A novel MALDI-TOF/TOF mass spectrometer for proteomics. *Anal. Bioanal. Chem.* **2003**, *376*, 952–965. [CrossRef]
26. Shelukhina, I.V.; Zhmak, M.N.; Lobanov, A.V.; Ivanov, I.A.; Garifulina, A.I.; Kravchenko, I.N.; Rasskazova, E.A.; Salmova, M.A.; Tukhovskaya, E.A.; Rykov, V.A.; et al. Azemiopsin, a selective peptide antagonist of muscle nicotinic acetylcholine receptor: Preclinical evaluation as a local muscle relaxant. *Toxins* **2018**, *10*, 34. [CrossRef]
27. Fry, B.G.; Vidal, N.; Norman, J.A.; Vonk, F.J.; Scheib, H.; Ramjan, S.F.; Kuruppu, S.; Fung, K.; Hedges, S.B.; Richardson, M.K.; et al. Early evolution of the venom system in lizards and snakes. *Nature* **2006**, *439*, 584–588. [CrossRef] [PubMed]
28. Sousa, L.F.; Nicolau, C.A.; Peixoto, P.S.; Bernardoni, J.L.; Oliveira, S.S.; Portes-Junior, J.A.; Mourao, R.H.; Lima-dos-Santos, I.; Sano-Martins, I.S.; Chalkidis, H.M.; et al. Comparison of phylogeny, venom composition and neutralization by antivenom in diverse species of bothrops complex. *PLoS Negl. Trop. Dis.* **2013**, *7*, e2442. [CrossRef]
29. Nirthanan, S.; Gopalakrishnakone, P.; Gwee, M.C.; Khoo, H.E.; Kini, R.M. Non-conventional toxins from elapid venoms. *Toxicon* **2003**, *41*, 397–407. [CrossRef]
30. Utkin, Y.; Sunagar, K.; Jackson, T.N.W.; Reeks, T.; Fry, B.G. Three-finger toxins (3FTxs). In *Venomous Reptiles and Their Toxins: Evolution, Pathophysiology and Biodiscovery*; Fry, B.G., Ed.; Oxford University Press: New York, NY, USA, 2015; pp. 215–227.
31. Makarova, Y.V.; Kryukova, E.V.; Shelukhina, I.V.; Lebedev, D.S.; Andreeva, T.V.; Ryazantsev, D.Y.; Balandin, S.V.; Ovchinnikova, T.V.; Tsetlin, V.I.; Utkin, Y.N.; et al. The first recombinant viper three-finger toxins: Inhibition of muscle and neuronal nicotinic acetylcholine receptors. *Doklad. Biochem. Biophys.* **2018**, *479*, 127–130. [CrossRef]
32. Weinstein, S.A.; Schmidt, J.J.; Bernheimer, A.W.; Smith, L.A. Characterization and amino acid sequences of two lethal peptides isolated from venom of Wagler's pit viper, *Trimeresurus wagleri*. *Toxicon* **1991**, *29*, 227–236. [CrossRef]
33. Zainal Abidin, S.A.; Rajadurai, P.; Chowdhury, M.E.; Ahmad Rusmili, M.R.; Othman, I.; Naidu, R. Proteomic characterization and comparison of malaysian tropidolaemus wagleri and cryptelytrops purpureomaculatus cenom using shotgun-proteomics. *Toxins* **2016**, *8*, 299. [CrossRef] [PubMed]
34. Tan, C.H.; Tan, K.Y.; Yap, M.K.; Tan, N.H. Venomics of *Tropidolaemus* wagleri, the sexually dimorphic temple pit viper: Unveiling a deeply conserved atypical toxin arsenal. *Sci. Rep.* **2017**, *7*, 43237. [CrossRef] [PubMed]
35. Valenta, J.; Stach, Z.; Stourac, P.; Kadanka, Z.; Michalek, P. Neurological symptoms following the *Fea's* viper (*Azemiops feae*) bite. *Clin. Toxicol.* **2015**, *53*, 1150–1151. [CrossRef]
36. Harris, R.J.; Zdenek, C.N.; Debono, J.; Harrich, D.; Fry, B.G. Evolutionary interpretations of nicotinic acetylcholine receptor targeting venom effects by a clade of asian *Viperidae* snakes. *Neurotox. Res.* **2020**, *38*, 312–318. [CrossRef]
37. Fry, B.G.; Wuster, W.; Kini, R.M.; Brusic, V.; Khan, A.; Venkataraman, D.; Rooney, A.P. Molecular evolution and phylogeny of elapid snake venom three-finger toxins. *J. Mol. Evolut.* **2003**, *57*, 110–129. [CrossRef]
38. Thakur, R.; Chattopadhyay, P.; Mukherjee, A.K. Biochemical and pharmacological characterization of a toxic fraction and its cytotoxin-like component isolated from Russell's viper (*Daboia russelii russelii*) venom. *Comp. Biochem. Physiol. C Toxicol. Pharmacol.* **2015**, *168*, 55–65. [CrossRef]

39. Nirthanan, S.; Charpantier, E.; Gopalakrishnakone, P.; Gwee, M.C.; Khoo, H.E.; Cheah, L.S.; Bertrand, D.; Kini, R.M. Candoxin, a novel toxin from *Bungarus candidus*, is a reversible antagonist of muscle (alphabetagammadelta) but a poorly reversible antagonist of neuronal α 7 nicotinic acetylcholine receptors. *J. Biol. Chem.* **2002**, *277*, 17811–17820. [CrossRef]
40. Utkin, Y.N.; Kukhtina, V.V.; Kryukova, E.V.; Chiodini, F.; Bertrand, D.; Methfessel, C.; Tsetlin, V.I. Weak toxin from *Naja kaouthia* is a nontoxic antagonist of alpha 7 and muscle-type nicotinic acetylcholine receptors. *J. Biol. Chem.* **2001**, *276*, 15810–15815. [CrossRef]
41. Lyukmanova, E.N.; Shenkarev, Z.O.; Shulepko, M.A.; Paramonov, A.S.; Chugunov, A.O.; Janickova, H.; Dolejsi, E.; Dolezal, V.; Utkin, Y.N.; Tsetlin, V.I.; et al. Structural insight into specificity of interactions between nonconventional three-finger weak toxin from *Naja kaouthia* (WTX) and muscarinic acetylcholine receptors. *J. Biol. Chem.* **2015**, *290*, 23616–23630. [CrossRef]
42. Mordvintsev, D.Y.; Polyak, Y.L.; Rodionov, D.I.; Jakubik, J.; Dolezal, V.; Karlsson, E.; Tsetlin, V.I.; Utkin, Y.N. Weak toxin WTX from *Naja kaouthia* cobra venom interacts with both nicotinic and muscarinic acetylcholine receptors. *FEBS J.* **2009**, *276*, 5065–5075. [CrossRef] [PubMed]
43. Wagstaff, S.C.; Favreau, P.; Cheneval, O.; Laing, G.D.; Wilkinson, M.C.; Miller, R.L.; Stocklin, R.; Harrison, R.A. Molecular characterisation of endogenous snake venom metalloproteinase inhibitors. *Biochem. Biophys. Res. Commun.* **2008**, *365*, 650–656. [CrossRef] [PubMed]
44. Yee, K.T.; Pitts, M.; Tongyoo, P.; Rojnuckarin, P.; Wilkinson, M.C. Snake venom metalloproteinases and their peptide inhibitors from myanmar Russell's viper venom. *Toxins* **2016**, *9*, 15. [CrossRef] [PubMed]
45. Tashima, A.K.; Zelanis, A.; Kitano, E.S.; Ianzer, D.; Melo, R.L.; Rioli, V.; Sant'anna, S.S.; Schenberg, A.C.; Camargo, A.C.; Serrano, S.M.; et al. Peptidomics of three bothrops snake venoms: Insights into the molecular diversification of proteomes and peptidomes. *Mol. Cell. Proteomic. MCP* **2012**, *11*, 1245–1262. [CrossRef] [PubMed]

biomedicines

MDPI

Article

An Examination of the Neutralization of In Vitro Toxicity of Chinese Cobra (*Naja atra*) Venom by Different Antivenoms

Qing Liang [1,2], Tam Minh Huynh [1], Nicki Konstantakopoulos [1], Geoffrey K. Isbister [1,3] and Wayne C. Hodgson [1,*]

1 Monash Venom Group, Department of Pharmacology, Biomedical Discovery Institute, Monash University, Clayton 3800, Australia; qing.liang@monash.edu (Q.L.); Tommy.Huynh@monash.edu (T.M.H.); Nicki.Konstantakopoulos@monash.edu (N.K.); geoff.isbister@gmail.com (G.K.I.)

2 Department of Emergency Medicine, The First Affiliated Hospital of Guangzhou Medical University, 151 Yanjiang Rd, Guangzhou 510120, China

3 Clinical Toxicology Research Group, University of Newcastle, Callaghan 2308, Australia

* Correspondence: wayne.hodgson@monash.edu

Received: 26 August 2020; Accepted: 23 September 2020; Published: 25 September 2020

Abstract: The Chinese Cobra (*Naja atra*) is an elapid snake of major medical importance in southern China. We describe the in vitro neurotoxic, myotoxic, and cytotoxic effects of *N. atra* venom, as well as examining the efficacy of three Chinese monovalent antivenoms (*N. atra* antivenom, *Gloydius brevicaudus* antivenom and *Deinagkistrodon acutus* antivenom) and an Australian polyvalent snake antivenom. In the chick biventer cervicis nerve-muscle preparation, *N. atra* venom (1–10 μg/mL) abolished indirect twitches in a concentration-dependent manner, as well as abolishing contractile responses to exogenous acetylcholine chloride (ACh) and carbamylcholine chloride (CCh), indicative of post-synaptic neurotoxicity. Contractile responses to potassium chloride (KCl) were also significantly inhibited by venom indicating myotoxicity. The prior addition of Chinese *N. atra* antivenom (0.75 U/mL) or Australian polyvalent snake antivenom (3 U/mL), markedly attenuated the neurotoxic actions of venom (3 μg/mL) and prevented the inhibition of contractile responses to ACh, CCh, and KCl. The addition of Chinese antivenom (0.75 U/mL) or Australian polyvalent antivenom (3 U/mL) at the t_{90} time point after the addition of venom (3 μg/mL), partially reversed the inhibition of twitches and significantly reversed the venom-induced inhibition of responses to ACh and CCh, but had no significant effect on the response to KCl. Venom (30 μg/mL) also abolished direct twitches in the chick biventer cervicis nerve-muscle preparation and caused a significant increase in baseline tension, further indicative of myotoxicity. *N. atra* antivenom (4 U/mL) prevented the myotoxic effects of venom (30 μg/mL). However, *G. brevicaudus* antivenom (24 U/mL), *D. acutus* antivenom (8 U/mL) and Australian polyvalent snake antivenom (33 U/mL) were unable to prevent venom (30 μg/mL) induced myotoxicity. In the L6 rat skeletal muscle myoblast cell line, *N. atra* venom caused concentration-dependent inhibition of cell viability, with a half maximal inhibitory concentration (IC_{50}) of 2.8 ± 0.48 μg/mL. *N. atra* antivenom significantly attenuated the cytotoxic effect of the venom, whereas Australian polyvalent snake antivenom was less effective but still attenuated the cytotoxic effects at lower venom concentrations. Neither *G. brevicaudus* antivenom or *D. acutus* antivenom were able to prevent the cytotoxicity. This study indicates that Chinese *N. atra* monovalent antivenom is efficacious against the neurotoxic, myotoxic and cytotoxic effects of *N. atra* venom but the clinical effectiveness of the antivenom is likely to be diminished, even if given early after envenoming. The use of Chinese viper antivenoms (i.e., *G. brevicaudus* and *D. acutus* antivenoms) in cases of envenoming by the Chinese cobra is not supported by the results of the current study.

Keywords: *Naja atra*; neurotoxicity; myotoxicity; venom; antivenom; snake

1. Introduction

There are approximately 205 species of snakes in China, of which more than 50 species are venomous [1]. The Chinese Cobra (*Naja atra*) is one of the top ten most venomous and clinically important species in China [2]. In China, *N. atra* is mainly distributed south of the Yangtze River, but is also found in Laos and Vietnam. Based on venomic data, Chinese *N. atra* venom contains a range of toxins, with cardiotoxins and short-chain neurotoxins being the most abundant components [3–6]. We have previously isolated a short-chain neurotoxin, α-Elapitoxin-Na1a, from Chinese *N. atra* venom [7]. However, it has been previously shown that short-chain neurotoxins dissociate readily from human nicotinic acetylcholine receptors (nAChRs) and are unlikely to contribute substantially to neurotoxicity in humans [7,8]. The major outcomes of envenoming by Chinese *N. atra* include severe wound necrosis or chronic necrotic ulceration for which large doses of antivenom are administered. Treatment also requires wound infection control and repeated surgical debridement, with the potential for the eventual amputation of limbs. However, marked neurotoxicity including respiratory muscle paralysis is relatively rare [2,9–11].

Antivenoms form the mainstay treatment of systemic snake envenoming. Currently available antivenoms in China include a monovalent *N. atra* antivenom, and a bivalent elapid (*N. atra* and *Bungarus multicinctus*) antivenom in Taiwan [2,10]. However, there are a lack of animal studies or clinical trials that demonstrate the efficacy of *N. atra* antivenom. Unfortunately, the use of non-specific antivenoms is common in mainland China given there are only monovalent snake antivenoms available, i.e., two for elapids: *N. atra* (Chinese Cobra) antivenom and *Bungarus multicinctus* (Chinese Krait) antivenom; and two for vipers: *Gloydius brevicaudus* (Short-Tailed Mamushi) antivenom and *Deinagkistrodon acutus* (Sharp-nosed Pit Viper) antivenom. *G. brevicaudus* or *D. acutus* antivenoms are advocated for the treatment of local necrosis in patients envenomed by *N. atra*, when specific antivenom is unavailable. However, there is no evidence for the cross-neutralizing ability of these antivenoms for myotoxicity or cytotoxicity, although patients envenomed by these vipers may also experience local necrosis in severe cases [2].

In this study, we examined the in vitro neurotoxic, myotoxic and cytotoxic effects of Chinese *N. atra* venom and evaluated the efficacy of Chinese *N. atra* monovalent antivenom in comparison to a polyvalent elapid antivenom (i.e., Australian polyvalent antivenom) and the possible protective effects of Chinese *G. brevicaudus* and *D. acutus* antivenoms against the myotoxicity and cytotoxicity induced by *N. atra* venom.

2. Experimental Section

2.1. Venom and Antivenoms

Freeze-dried *N. atra* venom was obtained from Orientoxin Co., Ltd. (Laiyang, Shandong, China). Chinese *N. atra* monovalent antivenom (Batch number: 20181202; expiry date: 27/12/2021), Chinese *G. brevicaudus* monovalent antivenom (Batch number: 20190605; expiry date: 18/06/2022), Chinese *D. acutus* monovalent antivenom (Batch number: 20190101; expiry date: 21/01/2022) were purchased from Shanghai Serum Biological Technology Co., Ltd. (Shanghai, China). Australian polyvalent snake antivenom (Batch number: 055517501; expiry date: 04/2013) was purchased from Seqirus (Melbourne, Australia). The amount of each antivenom required to neutralize in vitro neurotoxicity was based on the quantity of venom in the organ bath. While for the myotoxicity study, in order to achieve a sufficiently high concentration of antivenom for the venom, all antivenoms were tested at 40 μL/mL. According to the manufacturer's instructions: 125 U of *N. atra* antivenom neutralizes 1 mg of *N. atra* venom; 1500 U of *G. brevicaudus* antivenom neutralizes 1–1.25 mg of *G. brevicaudus* venom; and 136 U of *D. acutus* antivenom neutralizes 1–3 mg of *D. acutus* venom. For the Australian polyvalent antivenom, 1 U of antivenom neutralizes 10 μg of venom from the species of snake against which the antivenom is raised (i.e., brown snake, death adder, mulga snake, taipan, tiger snake).

2.2. Chemicals and Reagents

The following chemicals and drugs were used: acetylcholine chloride (ACh; Sigma-Aldrich, St. Louis, MO, USA), carbamylcholine chloride (CCh; Sigma-Aldrich, St. Louis, MO, USA), d-tubocurarine chloride (d-TC; Sigma-Aldrich, St. Louis, MO, USA), potassium chloride (KCl, Ajax Finechem Pty. Ltd., Taren Point, Australia), bovine serum albumin (BSA; Sigma-Aldrich, St. Louis, MO, USA), 0.5% Trypsin-EDTA (Gibco Thermofisher, Melbourne, Australia), Penicillin/Streptomycin, Dulbecco's Phosphate Buffered Saline, Dulbecco's Modified Eagle Medium (DMEM) GlutaMAX TM, DMSO (Merck; Darmstach, Germany), CellTire 96 Aqueous One Solution Cell Proliferation Assay (MTS assay; Promega; Melbourne, Australia). All chemicals were dissolved or diluted in Milli-Q water unless otherwise stated.

2.3. Chick Biventer Cervicis Nerve-Muscle Preparation

Chickens (male; aged 4–10 days) were killed by exsanguination following CO_2 inhalation. Two biventer cervicis nerve-muscle preparations were dissected from each chick and mounted in separate organ baths on wire tissue holders under 1 g resting tension. Preparations were maintained at 34 °C, bubbled with 95% O_2 and 5% CO_2, in 5 mL organ baths filled with physiological salt solution consisting of (in mM): 118.4 NaCl, 4.7 KCl,1.2 $MgSO_4$, 1.2 KH_2PO_4, 2.5 $CaCl_2$, 25 $NaHCO_3$, and 11.1 glucose. Venom was dissolved in 0.05% (*w*/*v*) bovine serum albumin (BSA).

For neurotoxicity experiments, indirect twitches were evoked by stimulating the motor nerve at supramaximal voltage (0.1 Hz; 0.2 ms; 10–20 V) via an electronic stimulator. d-TC (10 μM) was then added to the preparations with the subsequent abolishment of twitches indicating that they were nerve-mediated. The twitches were then restored by washing the preparation with physiological salt solution. Electrical stimulation was stopped and contractile responses to exogenous ACh (1 mM for 30 s), CCh (20 μM for 60 s), and KCl (40 mM for 30 s) obtained. Electrical stimulation was then recommenced for at least 30 min before the addition of venom or antivenom. To examine the efficacy of antivenom to prevent venom-induced neurotoxicity, antivenom was added to the tissues 10 min before venom. To examine the efficacy of antivenom to reverse venom-induced neurotoxicity, antivenom was added to the tissues at the t_{90} time point (i.e., when the twitch height was inhibited by 90%). At the conclusion of each experiment, ACh, CCh, and KCl were re-added as above.

For myotoxicity experiments, the biventer cervicis muscle was directly stimulated (0.1 Hz; 2 ms) at supramaximal voltage (20–30 V). In these experiments the electrode was placed around the belly of the muscle and d-TC (10 μM) remained in the organ bath for the duration of the experiment. Venom was left in contact with the preparation until twitch blockade occurred, or for a maximum 3 h period. Venom was considered to be myotoxic if it inhibited twitches elicited by direct stimulation and/or caused a contracture of the skeletal muscle (i.e., increase in the baseline tension of the muscle). To examine the ability of antivenom to neutralize venom-induced myotoxicity (i.e., myotoxicity prevention study), tissues were equilibrated with antivenom for 10 min before venom was added.

Twitch responses and responses to exogenous agonists were measured via a Grass FT03 force displacement transducer and recorded on a PowerLab system (ADInstruments Pty Ltd., Bella Vista, Australia). Animal experiments were approved on 12 May 2017 by the Monash University Ethics Committee application MARP/2017/147. All experiments were performed in accordance with relevant guidelines and regulations.

2.4. Cell Culture Experiments

2.4.1. Venom

Freeze-dried venom was reconstituted in distilled water on the day of use. Protein content was determined utilizing a BCA protein assay kit according to the manufacturer's instructions. Briefly, venom (25 μL) was added in triplicate to a 96-well micro-titer plate. BSA solutions, diluted from 1–0.025 mg/mL, were used as reference standards and distilled water was used as the blank. Absorbance was measured at 562 nm utilizing VERSAmax tunable microplate reader (Molecular Devices, San Jose, CA, USA). Venom stock solutions were stored at 4 °C until required.

2.4.2. Heat Inactivation of Fetal Bovine Serum (hiFBS)

Fetal bovine serum was heated to 56 °C for 30 min. Following heat-inactivation, serum was sterilized using a 0.22 μM Millipore filter (Sigma-Aldrch, North Ryde, Australia). Serum was dispensed into sterile centrifuge tubes and stored at −20 °C.

2.4.3. Cells

The rat skeletal muscle myoblast cell line, L6, was purchased from The American Type Culture Collection (ATCC, Manassas, VA, USA). L6 cells were grown in 175 cm^2 flasks (Nunc, Thermofisher, Melbourne, Australia) in culture media DMEM supplemented with 10% hiFBS and 1% penicillin/streptomycin (10% DMEM). Flasks were maintained at 37 °C with 5% CO_2 and media was replenished every subsequent day. When the cells reached 80% confluence (assessed by eye using a light microscope), trypsin was then used to lift the cells. Cells were centrifuged and the cell pellet was re-suspended in culture media (35 mL). Cell suspension (100 μL/well) was aliquoted into four 96-well cell culture plates (92 wells/plate) (Nunc, Thermofisher, Melbourne, Australia). Plates were maintained at 37 °C in an atmosphere of 5% CO_2. Media was replenished every second day until cells reached 90% confluence. For cell differentiation to occur (i.e., skeletal myoblast cells into skeletal myocytes), 10% DMEM was removed from wells and replaced with DMEM media supplemented with 2% hiFBS and 1% penicillin/streptomycin (2% DMEM). Plates were subsequently maintained at 37 °C in an atmosphere of 5% CO_2. Media was replenished every second day, for one week, until cell differentiation (i.e., appearance of long striated cells, assessed by eye using a light microscope) was observed.

To maintain L6 stock, cells at passage 2 were lifted using trypsin and centrifuged. Supernatant was discarded and cell pellets were re-suspended in DMEM (20 mL) supplemented with 30% hiFBS and 10% DMSO. Cell suspension was aliquoted into individual 1 mL cryovials and stored in liquid nitrogen until required. Cells were passaged up to passage 12 before being discarded and a new vial of cells thawed.

2.4.4. Cell Proliferation Assay (MTS Assay)

For cell viability experiments, media were removed from wells of differentiated L6 cell culture plates and the wells were washed once with pre-warmed PBS. Venom stock solution was diluted in 2% DMEM culture media to a final concentration of 100 μg/mL. This was subsequently serially diluted either 1.5-fold (100–0.016 μg/mL) or 1.3-fold (100–0.24 μg/mL). Dilutions (100 μL/well) were added in quadruplicate to wells in a cell culture plate. Culture media controls (i.e., cells and media with no venom) and media blanks (i.e., no cells) were also run in parallel. The plates were maintained at 37 °C with 5% CO_2 for 24 h. Cell culture plates were subsequently removed from the incubator and washed with pre-warmed PBS three times. DMEM culture media (2%; 50 μL/well) and MTS solution (10 μL/well) were pre-mixed, and 60 μL added to each well. Plates were further incubated at 37 °C with 5% CO_2 for 1 h. Absorbance was measured at 492 nm utilizing a VERSAmax tunable microplate reader (Molecular Devices, San Jose, CA, USA).

2.4.5. Examining the Efficacy of Antivenom

Media was removed from wells of L6 cell culture plates and the wells were washed once with pre-warmed PBS. Venom stock solutions were diluted to a concentration of 0 (no venom), 2.5 (IC_{50} concentration range), 5 (twice IC_{50}), 10 (initial concentration where 100% cell death occurs), or 30 μg/mL (concentration used in myotoxic study) in 2% DMEM culture media containing either no antivenom (venom only) or supplemented with *N. atra* monovalent antivenom (200 μL; 4 U/mL) Australian polyvalent snake antivenom (200 μL; 33 U/mL), *G. brevicaudus* antivenom (200 μL; 24 U/mL), or *D. acutus* antivenom (200 μL; 8 U/mL).

Each of the dilutions were added in triplicate to L6 culture plates and incubated at 37 °C with 5% CO_2 for 24 h. Culture plates were removed from the incubator and washed with pre-warmed PBS three times. Fresh DMEM culture media (50 μL/well) and MTS solution (10 μL/well) were pre-mixed, and 60 μL/well was added to each well. The plates were further incubated at 37 °C with 5% CO_2 for 1 h. Absorbance was measured at 492 nm utilizing VERSAmax tunable microplate reader (Molecular Devices, San Jose, CA, USA).

2.5. *Data Analysis*

For both in vitro neurotoxicity and myotoxicity experiments, twitch height in the chick biventer preparation was measured at regular time intervals and expressed as a percentage of the pre-venom twitch height. In neurotoxicity studies, the time taken for 90% inhibition of the twitch response (t_{90} value) was used to determine the potency of *N. atra* venom. Post-venom contractile responses to ACh, CCh, and KCl were expressed as a percentage of their original responses. In myotoxicity studies, the change in gram (g) of muscle baseline tension was measured every 10 min after venom addition. The maximum change in tension (g) and time (min) to achieve the maximum change in tension were also measured. Comparison of the effects of *N. atra* venom on twitch height, baseline tension, or time to reach maximum change in tension were made using a one-way analysis of variance (ANOVA). Comparison of responses to exogenous agonists before and after the addition of venom or vehicle was made using a Student's paired *t*-test. All ANOVAs were followed by a Bonferroni's multiple comparison post-hoc test. Data are presented as mean ± standard error of the mean (SEM) of n experiments. All data and statistical analyses were performed using PRISM 8.0.2 (GraphPad Software, San Diego, CA, USA, 2019).

For cell experiments, sigmoidal growth curves were graphed using Prism 8.0.2 as cell viability (% of maximum) versus log concentration of venom, and IC_{50} concentrations determined. Bar graphs displaying the efficacy of antivenoms were plotted as a percentage of cell viability. Cell viability was compared in the presence and absence of antivenom using a one-way ANOVA, with Bonferroni's multiple comparisons test. For all statistical tests, $p < 0.05$ was considered statistically significant. Data are presented as mean ± standard error of the mean (SEM) of n experiments.

3. Results

3.1. *In Vitro Neurotoxicity*

3.1.1. Concentration-Dependent Inhibition of Twitches and Exogenous Agonists Responses

N. atra venom (1–10 μg/mL) caused concentration-dependent inhibition of indirect twitches of the chick biventer preparation, when compared to vehicle control (n = 6; one-way ANOVA, $p < 0.05$; Figure 1a). The potency of the neurotoxic effect of venom was determined by calculating t_{90} or t_{50} (i.e., if the twitch height to decrease by 90% or 50%, respectively) with values as follows: 1 μg/mL (t_{50} 36 ± 2 min), 3 μg/mL (t_{90} 43 ± 5 min), 10 μg/mL (t_{90} 17 ± 1 min). Venom (1–10 μg/mL) also abolished contractile responses to exogenous ACh (1 mM) and CCh (20 μM), indicating an action at the post-synaptic nerve terminal, and significantly inhibited responses to KCl (40 mM), indicative of myotoxicity (Figure 1b).

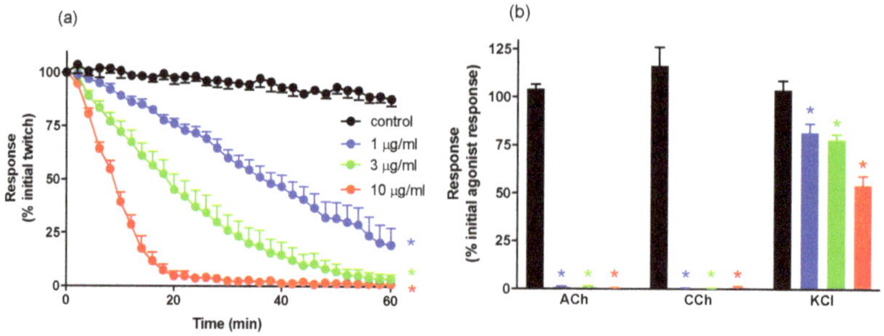

Figure 1. (**a**) The concentration-dependent neurotoxic effects of *N. atra* venom (1–10 μg/mL) on indirect twitches of the chick biventer cervicis nerve-muscle (CBCNM) preparation. (**b**) The concentration-dependent effects of *N. atra* venom (1–10 μg/mL) on contractile responses to acetylcholine chloride (ACh) (1 mM), carbachol (CCh) (20 μM), and potassium chloride (KCl) (40 mM) in the CBCNM. * $p < 0.05$, significantly different from (**a**) control at 60 min or (**b**) pre-venom response to same agonist. n = 6.

3.1.2. In Vitro Neurotoxicity Antivenom Prevention Study

The prior addition of Chinese *N. atra* monovalent antivenom (0.75 U/mL, 2× the recommended titre), or Australian polyvalent snake antivenom (3 U/mL, 10× the recommended titre), markedly attenuated the neurotoxic actions of venom (3 μg/mL) (Figure 2a,c) and prevented the inhibition of contractile responses to ACh, CCh, and KCl (Figure 2b,d).

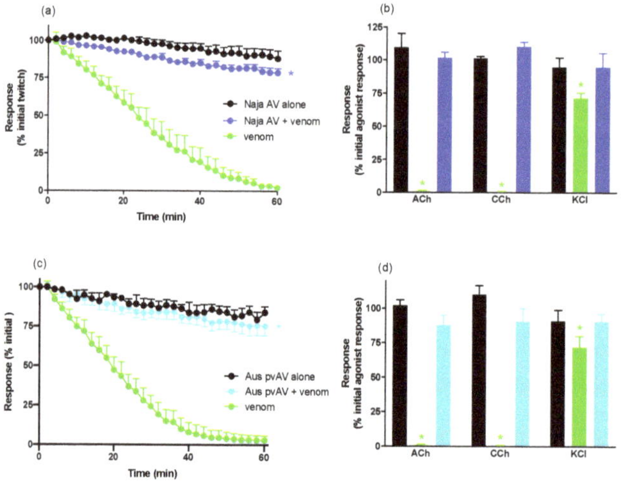

Figure 2. (**a**) The effects of *N. atra* venom (3 μg/mL) alone or with pre-addition of *Naja atra* antivenom (Naja AV; 0.75 U/mL) on indirect twitches of the CBCNM. (**b**) The effects of *N. atra* venom (3 μg/mL) alone or with pre-addition of Naja AV (0.75 U/mL) on contractile responses to ACh (1 mM), CCh (20 μM), and KCl (40 mM) in the CBCNM. (**c**) The effects of *N. atra* venom (3 μg/mL) alone or with pre-addition of Australian polyvalent antivenom (Aus pvAV; 3 U/mL) on indirect twitches of the CBCNM. (**d**) The effects of *N. atra* venom (3 μg/mL) alone or with pre-addition of Aus pvAV (3 U/mL) on contractile responses to ACh (1 mM), CCh (20 μM), and KCl (40 mM) in the CBCNM. * $p < 0.05$, significantly different compared to venom in the absence of antivenom at 60 min (**a**,**c**) or compared to pre-venom response to same agonist (**b**,**d**). n = 5–6.

3.1.3. In Vitro Neurotoxicity Antivenom Reversal Study

The addition of Chinese *N. atra* antivenom (0.75 U/mL, 2× the recommended titre), at the t_{90} time point, after the addition of *N. atra* venom (3 µg/mL), partially restored the twitch height, i.e., reaching 42 ± 5% (n = 6) of the initial pre-venom twitch height (Figure 3a). Chinese *N. atra* antivenom also significantly reversed the venom-induced inhibition of responses to ACh and CCh, while having no significant effect on the response to KCl (Figure 3b).

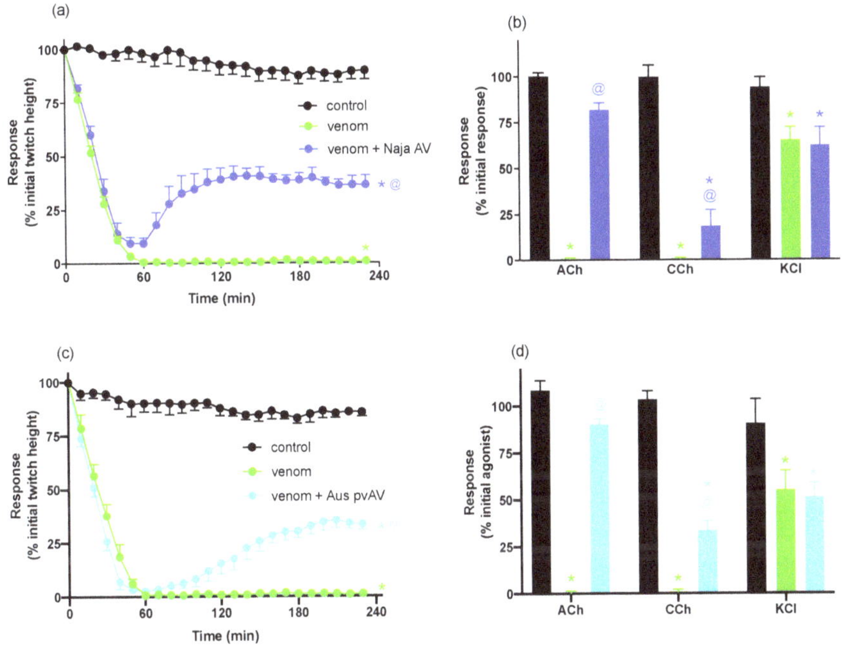

Figure 3. (**a**) The effects of *N. atra* venom (3 µg/mL) alone or with *Naja atra* antivenom (Naja AV; 0.75 U/mL) added at the t_{90} time point on indirect twitches of the CBCNM. (**b**) The effects of *N. atra* venom (3 µg/mL) alone or with Naja AV (0.75 U/mL) added at the t_{90} time point on contractile responses to ACh (1 mM), CCh (20 µM), and KCl (40 mM) in the CBCNM. (**c**) The effects of *N. atra* venom (3 µg/mL) alone or with Australian polyvalent antivenom (Aus pvAV; 3 U/mL) added at the t_{90} time point on indirect twitches of the CBCNM. (**d**) The effects of *N. atra* venom (3 µg/mL) alone or with Aus pvAV (3 U/mL) added at the t_{90} time point on contractile responses to ACh (1 mM), CCh (20 µM), and KCl (40 mM) in the CBCNM. * $p < 0.05$, significantly different compared to control at 230 min (**a**,**c**) or compared to pre-venom response to same agonist (**b**,**d**). $^{@}$ $p < 0.05$, significantly different compared to venom in the absence of antivenom at 230 min (**a**,**c**) or compared to response to agonist in the absence of antivenom (**b**,**d**), n = 5–6.

The addition of Australian polyvalent antivenom, (3 U/mL, 10× the recommended titre), at the t_{90} time point, after the addition of *N. atra* venom (3 µg/mL), partially restored the twitch height, i.e., reaching 35 ± 4% (n = 6) of the initial pre-venom twitch height (Figure 3c). The addition of Australian polyvalent antivenom also significantly reversed the inhibition of responses to ACh and CCh, while having no significant effect on the response to KCl (Figure 3d).

3.2. *In Vitro Myotoxicity*

N. atra venom (30 µg/mL) significantly inhibited twitches in the directly-stimulated chick biventer preparation, when compared to vehicle at 180 min (n = 5–6; one-way ANOVA, $p < 0.05$; Figure 4a).

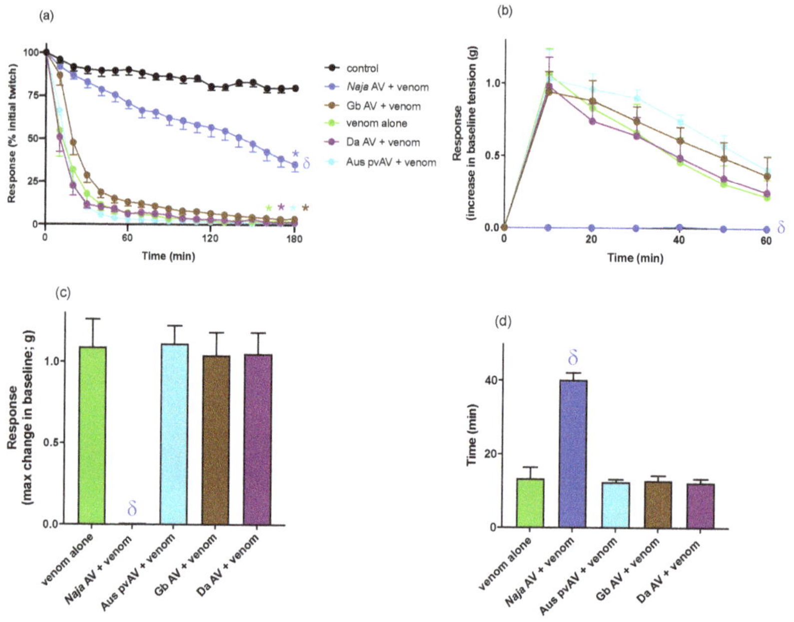

Figure 4. The myotoxic effects of *Naja atra* venom (30 μg/mL), in the presence and absence of different antivenoms, as indicated by the (**a**) change in twitch height in chick biventer cervicis preparation over 180 min; (**b**) change in baseline tension of the chick biventer cervicis preparation over 60 min; (**c**) max change in baseline gram tension achieved in 60 min; and (**d**) the time achieve max change in baseline tension. * $p < 0.05$, significantly different compared to control (**a**) at 180 min. $^{\delta}$ $p < 0.05$, significantly different compared to venom alone at 180 min (**a**) or 60 min (**b**) or compared to venom in the absence of antivenom (**c**,**d**). n = 5–6. Antivenoms were added 10 min prior to venom. *N. atra* antivenom (*Naja* AV); *G. brevicaudus* antivenom AV (Gb AV); *D. acutus* antivenom AV (Da AV); Australian polyvalent AV (Aus pvAV).

The prior addition of Chinese *N. atra* monovalent antivenom 200 μL (4 U/mL, 1× the recommended titre) markedly attenuated, but did not prevent, twitch inhibition (n = 6; one-way ANOVA, $p < 0.05$; Figure 4a) and abolished the venom-induced increase in baseline tension compared to venom (30 μg/mL) alone (n = 5–6; one-way ANOVA, $p < 0.05$; Figure 4b–d), indicating partial attenuation of the myotoxic actions of *N. atra* venom.

In contrast, the prior addition of Australian polyvalent snake antivenom 200 μL (33 U/mL, 11× the recommended titre), *G. brevicaudus* antivenom 200 μL (24 U/mL, 0.5~0.7× the recommended titre) or Chinese *D. acutus* monovalent antivenom 200 μL (8 U/mL, 2~6× the recommended titre), failed to prevent or delay the venom-induced decrease in direct twitches(n = 5–6; Figure 4a) or venom-induced increase in baseline tension (n = 5–6; Figure 4b–d), indicating a lack of efficacy against the myotoxic actions of *N. atra* venom.

Control experiments (i.e., 200 μL of each antivenom alone) indicated the antivenoms had no direct effect on tissue viability over a period of 180 min (n = 5–6 for each antivenom).

3.3. Cell Viability Assay

3.3.1. Venom Concentration–Response Curves

Treatment of L6 cells with *N. atra* venom resulted in a concentration-dependent inhibition of cell viability (Figure 5), with an IC_{50} of 2.8 ± 0.48 μg/mL.

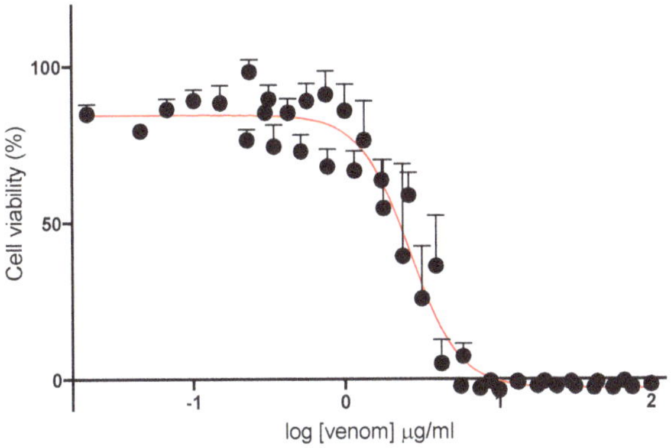

Figure 5. Concentration-dependent venom-induced inhibition of cell viability in L6 cells.

3.3.2. Cell-Based Proliferation Assay-Efficacy of Antivenoms

L6 cells were treated with 2% DMEM media supplemented with venom at concentrations of 0, 2.5, 5, 10, or 30 μg/mL and further supplemented with either no antivenom (i.e., venom alone) or with *N. atra* antivenom (200 μL; 4 U/mL), Australian polyvalent snake antivenom (200 μL; 33 U/mL), *G. brevicaudus* antivenom (200 μL; 24 U/mL), or *D. acutus* monovalent antivenom (200 μL; 8 U/mL).

N. atra venom caused a significant decrease in cell viability at all concentrations examined when compared to cells treated with media alone ($p < 0.05$; Figure 6). *N. atra* antivenom significantly attenuated the cytotoxic effect at all venom concentrations compared to control ($p < 0.05$; Figure 6). Australian polyvalent snake antivenom was less effective but still attenuated the cytotoxic effects at lower venom concentrations (i.e., 2.5–10 μg/mL; $p < 0.05$; Figure 6). Neither *G. brevicaudus* antivenom or *D. acutus* antivenom were able to prevent the cytotoxicity at any venom concentration examined (Figure 6).

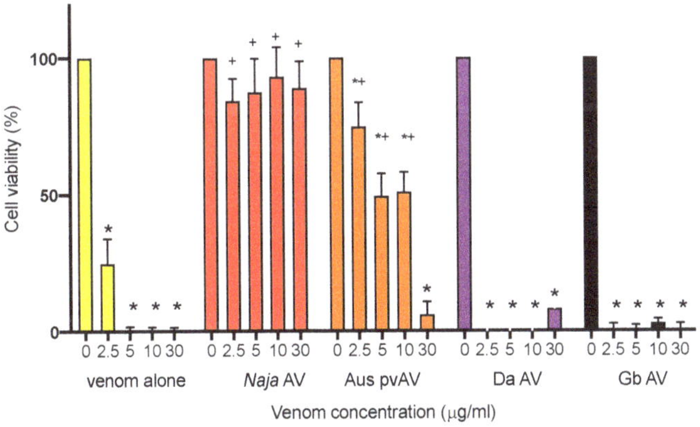

Figure 6. The effects of *N. atra* venom (0–30 μg/mL), in L6 cells, in the presence and absence of *N. atra* antivenom (*Naja* AV, 4 U/mL), *G. brevicaudus* antivenom AV (Gb AV, 24 U/mL), *D. acutus* antivenom AV (Da AV, 8 U/mL) or Australian polyvalent AV (Aus pvAV, 33 U/mL). * $p < 0.05$, significantly different from control (i.e., 0 venom); $^{+}$ $p < 0.05$, significantly different from same concentration of venom in the absence of antivenom.

4. Discussion

We have shown that *N. atra* venom from China displays potent in vitro neurotoxic, myotoxic and cytotoxic activity. The neurotoxic and cytotoxic effects of the venom were almost completely abolished by the prior addition of specific *N. atra* antivenom, whereas the myotoxic effects were only partially prevented. Interestingly, an Australian polyvalent antivenom, which is raised against the venoms from a range of Australian elapids (i.e., *Acanthophis antarcticus*, *Notechis scutatus*, *Oxyuranus scutellatus*, *Pseudechis australis*, and *Pseudonaja textilis*) and does not contain specific antibodies against *N. atra* venom, displayed similar activity against the neurotoxic effects of *N. atra* venom but was less effective against the cytotoxic effects and ineffective against the myotoxic effects. The Australian polyvalent antivenom was included in our study as the venoms of the Australian elapids contain a range of post-synaptic, pre-synaptic, and myotoxic components. These components are likely to have close structural similarities with some of the components in the venom of the Chinese cobra given we have previously shown that Australian Tiger snake (*N. scutatus*) antivenom prevents the in vitro neurotoxicity induced by *N. haje* (Egyptian cobra) venom [12], and Australian polyvalent snake antivenom prevents the in vitro neurotoxicity induced by *N. kaouthia* (monocled cobra) venom [13].

The two Chinese monovalent viper antivenoms (i.e., *G. brevicaudus* antivenom and *D. acutus* antivenom antivenom) had no efficacy against the myotoxic or cytotoxic effects of *N. atra* venom. We did not examine the efficacy of the Chinese viper antivenoms against the neurotoxic effects of *N. atra* venom as this is not a clinical outcome of envenoming by this species, and the antivenoms are used in China to treat the myotoxic symptoms of *N. atra* envenoming. Four monovalent snake antivenoms are available in mainland China, and cross-neutralization by using nonspecific antivenoms for snakebite is recommended in the Chinese 2018 Expert Consensus on snakebites [2]. However, it appears as though the two viper antivenoms have no efficacy against *N. atra* venom.

We used the chick biventer cervicis nerve–muscle preparation, which contains both focally- and multiply-innervated skeletal muscle fibers, to examine neurotoxicity and myotoxicity. This preparation enables the determination of the site of action of venoms/toxins, i.e., either at the pre-synaptic nerve terminal, post-synaptic nerve terminal or underlying skeletal muscle [14,15]. The time taken to cause 90% (i.e., t_{90}) inhibition of nerve-mediated twitches can be used to compare the neurotoxic potency of venoms/toxins. *N. atra* venom abolished indirect twitches in a time-dependent and concentration-dependent manner, as well as inhibiting contractile responses to exogenous ACh and CCh, while reducing responses to KCl, indicating that it acts post-synaptically and has myotoxic effects on the tissue. The Chinese *N. atra* antivenom was highly efficacious when added prior to venom and was also able to partially reverse the inhibitory effects of the venom when added at the t_{90} time point. The failure to fully reverse the decline in twitch height is likely to be due to a number of factors including the contribution of myotoxins and the lack of reversibility of some neurotoxins. Indeed, we have previously shown that the short-chain post-synaptic neurotoxin α-Elapitoxin-Na1a, which accounts for approximately 9% of *N. atra* venom, displays pseudo-irreversible antagonism at the skeletal muscle nicotinic acetylcholine receptor and is only partially reversed by antivenom [7]. Interesting, the Australian polyvalent snake venom displayed similar efficacy against the neurotoxic effects of the venom indicating that the antigenic components in this antivenom, which is raised against a number of venoms from Australian elapid snakes containing postsynaptic and/or presynaptic neurotoxins, are able to recognize the neurotoxic components of *N. atra* venom.

Despite possible geographical differences in venom composition, the percentage of cardiotoxins and neurotoxins reported in *N. atra* venom ranges from 52–68% and 11–23%, respectively [3,4,6]. Cardiotoxins, which target cell membranes, are likely to be the main components contributing to the soft tissue necrosis and myotoxicity [16–20]. Indeed, *N. atra* venom has been shown to display high levels of cytotoxicity [21]. Although, as indicated above, *N. atra* venom is highly neurotoxic in vitro, it is only mildly neurotoxic in humans. This is most likely due to the neurotoxic components being short-chain neurotoxins which readily dissociate from human muscle nAChRs [7]. Interestingly, a recent study found that the post-synaptic α-neurotoxins in *N. atra* venom bind to the alpha-1 nAChR orthosteric site with selectivity towards the amphibian mimotope over lizard, avian and rodent mimotopes indicative of prey selectivity [22]. Despite the early usage and administration of large doses of *N. atra* antivenom in envenomed patients, severe wound necrosis or chronic necrotic ulceration causing extensive local tissue injuries are commonly reported [9–11]. Although subsequent wound infection due to heavy bacterial load introduced by the fangs [23,24] might contribute to this clinical dilemma, there is the possibility of a lack of efficacy of the specific antivenom against the myotoxic effect of the venom.

As *N. atra* venom significantly inhibited responses to KCl in the indirectly stimulated chick biventer experiments, the presence of myotoxic activity in the venom was further examined in the directly stimulated chick biventer preparation. *N. atra* venom abolished direct twitches and induced an increase in baseline tension indicative of myotoxicity [14,15]. Prior addition of *N. atra* antivenom delayed, but did not prevent, inhibition of direct twitches, but abolished the increase in baseline tension. However, the inability of *N. atra* antivenom to fully prevent myotoxicity may not indicate a lack of full efficacy of the antivenom. Given that the myotoxic effects were studied at 10× the concentration at which the neurotoxic effects were studied (i.e., 30 μg/mL compared to 3 μg/mL), a ratio which is in line with many of our previous neurotoxic/myotoxic studies [25–27], it is likely that increasing the antivenom concentration, e.g., at least double the manufacturer's recommended amount, may full prevent the myotoxic effects. Indeed, we needed to add 2× the manufacturer's recommendation to abolish venom neurotoxicity. However, we limited the maximum amount of antivenom used in the myotoxicity study given that excessive amounts of antivenom can alter the osmolarity of the physiological salt solution in the organ bath and affect tissue viability. The Australian polyvalent snake antivenom and the two Chinese monovalent viper antivenoms failed to significantly inhibit either the decrease in twitch height or increase in baseline tension.

N. atra antivenom also neutralized the potent cytotoxic effects of *N. atra* venom in L6 rat skeletal muscle cells. It is worth noting that the antivenom was protective against 30 μg/mL of venom in this assay, further supporting that the lack of full efficacy in the chick biventer myotoxic study was due to an insufficient concentration of antivenom. This problem did not occur in the cell assay given the much lower volumes used. The Australian polyvalent snake antivenom was protective at lower concentrations of venom in the cytotoxicity assay, whereas the two viper antivenoms had no significant protective effect. Although the venoms from these Chinese viper species (i.e., *G. brevicaudus* and *D. acutus*) can cause local tissue swelling and necrosis in envenomed humans, their venom proteomes and the relative abundance of major components are quite different to the Chinese elapid *N. atra* venom [3,5]. Therefore, it is not surprising that these antivenoms were unable to prevent the myotoxicity and cytotoxicity induced by *N. atra* venom. Our results strongly suggest that these viper antivenoms are unlikely to neutralize the effects of venom in patients envenomed by *N. atra*. Interestingly, the Australian polyvalent snake antivenom, which is raised against the venoms from five species of highly venomous terrestrial Australian elapids, failed to prevent *N. atra* venom induced myotoxicity in vitro while showing capability of fully preventing and even partially reversing *N. atra* venom induced neurotoxicity and cytotoxicity. This divergence has not been previously reported and could be explained by further venomic comparison studies between the species in the future.

5. Conclusions

In summary, we have, for the first time, examined the in vitro neurotoxic, myotoxic, and cytotoxic effects of *N. atra* venom and the ability of specific Chinese *N. atra* monovalent antivenom, non-specific Australian polyvalent snake antivenom, and Chinese *G. brevicaudus* monovalent antivenom and Chinese *D. acutus* monovalent antivenom to neutralize these effects. Our studies indicate that Chinese *N. atra* venom causes potent in vitro neurotoxicity, myotoxicity, and cytotoxicity, which is, largely, neutralized by *N. atra* antivenom. While the Australian polyvalent antivenom was equally efficacious against the neurotoxic effects, indicating the presence of similar antigenic neurotoxins, it was ineffective against the myotoxicity and only partially protective against the cytotoxic effects. The Chinese viper antivenoms were ineffective and do not appear to display any cross-reactivity against the myotoxic and cytotoxic components of *N. atra* venom.

Author Contributions: Conceptualization, Q.L., G.K.I. and W.C.H.; methodology, Q.L., T.M.H., N.K. and W.C.H.; formal analysis, Q.L., N.K. and W.C.H.; investigation, Q.L., N.K.; data curation and writing—original draft preparation, Q.L., N.K. and W.C.H.; writing—review and editing and supervision, G.K.I. and W.C.H.; funding acquisition, Q.L., G.K.I. and W.C.H.; project administration, G.K.I. and W.C.H. All authors have read and agreed to the published version of the manuscript.

Funding: This study was supported by an Australian National Health and Medical Research Council (NHMRC) Senior Research Fellowship (ID: 1061041) awarded to G.K.I., a NHMRC Centers for Research Excellence Grant (ID:1110343) awarded to G.K.I. and W.C.H., and a 2016 Guangzhou Municipal University scientific research project Grant (ID: 1201620144) awarded to Q.L.

Conflicts of Interest: The authors declare no conflict of interest. The funders had no role in the design of the study; in the collection, analyses, or interpretation of data; in the writing of the manuscript, or in the decision to publish the results.

References

1. Em, Z. *Snakes in China*, 1st ed.; Anhui Science and Technology Publishing House: Hefei, China, 2006; pp. 4, 347, 349.
2. Experts Group of Snake-Bites Rescue and Treatment Consensus in China. Expert consensus on China snake-bites rescue and treatment. *Chin. J. Emerg. Med.* **2018**, *27*, 1315–1322. [CrossRef]
3. Li, S.; Wang, J.; Zhang, X.; Ren, Y.; Wang, N.; Zhao, K.; Chen, X.; Zhao, C.; Li, X.; Shao, J.; et al. Proteomic characterization of two snake venoms: *Naja naja atra* and *Agkistrodon halys*. *Biochem. J.* **2004**, *384*, 119–127. [CrossRef] [PubMed]
4. Huang, H.W.; Liu, B.S.; Chien, K.Y.; Chiang, L.C.; Huang, S.Y.; Sung, W.C.; Wu, W.G. Cobra venom proteome and glycome determined from individual snakes of *Naja atra* reveal medically important dynamic range and systematic geographic variation. *J. Proteom.* **2015**, *128*, 92–104. [CrossRef]
5. Liu, C.C.; Lin, C.C.; Hsiao, Y.C.; Wang, P.J.; Yu, J.S. Proteomic characterization of six Taiwanese snake venoms: Identification of species-specific proteins and development of a SISCAPA-MRM assay for cobra venom factors. *J. Proteom.* **2018**, *187*, 59–68. [CrossRef]
6. Shan, L.L.; Gao, J.F.; Zhang, Y.X.; Shen, S.S.; He, Y.; Wang, J.; Ma, X.M.; Ji, X. Proteomic characterization and comparison of venoms from two elapid snakes (*Bungarus multicinctus* and *Naja atra*) from China. *J. Proteom.* **2016**, *138*, 83–94. [CrossRef] [PubMed]
7. Liang, Q.; Huynh, T.M.; Isbister, G.K.; Hodgson, W.C. Isolation and pharmacological characterization of α-Elapitoxin-Na1a, a novel short-chain postsynaptic neurotoxin from the venom of the Chinese Cobra (*Naja atra*). *Biochem. Pharmacol.* **2020**. [CrossRef]
8. Silva, A.; Cristofori-Armstrong, B.; Rash, L.D.; Hodgson, W.C.; Isbister, G.K. Defining the role of post-synaptic alpha-neurotoxins in paralysis due to snake envenoming in humans. *Cell Mol. Life Sci.* **2018**, *75*, 4465–4478. [CrossRef]
9. Wang, W.; Chen, Q.F.; Yin, R.X.; Zhu, J.J.; Li, Q.B.; Chang, H.H.; Wu, Y.B.; Michelson, E. Clinical features and treatment experience: A review of 292 Chinese cobra snakebites. *Environ. Toxicol. Pharmacol.* **2014**, *37*, 648–655. [CrossRef]
10. Mao, Y.C.; Liu, P.Y.; Chiang, L.C.; Lai, C.S.; Lai, K.L.; Ho, C.H.; Wang, T.H.; Yang, C.C. Naja atra snakebite in Taiwan. *Clin. Toxicol. (Philadelphia)* **2018**, *56*, 273–280. [CrossRef]
11. Wong, O.F.; Lam, T.S.; Fung, H.T.; Choy, C.H. Five-year experience with Chinese cobra (*Naja atra*)-related injuries in two acute hospitals in Hong Kong. *Hong Kong Med. J.* **2010**, *16*, 36–43.
12. Kornhauser, R.; Isbister, G.K.; O'Leary, M.A.; Mirtschin, P.; Dunstan, N.; Hodgson, W.C. Cross-neutralisation of the neurotoxic effects of Egyptian Cobra venom with commercial Tiger snake antivenom. *Basic Clin. Pharmacol. Toxicol.* **2013**, *112*, 138–143. [CrossRef] [PubMed]
13. Silva, A.; Hodgson, W.C.; Isbister, G.K. Cross-neutralisation of in vitro neurotoxicity of Asian and Australian snake neurotoxins and venoms by different antivenoms. *Toxins* **2016**, *8*, 302. [CrossRef] [PubMed]
14. Harvey, A.L.; Barfaraz, A.; Thomson, E.; Faiz, A.; Preston, S.; Harris, J.B. Screening of snake venoms for neurotoxic and myotoxic effects using simple in vitro preparations from rodents and chicks. *Toxicon* **1994**, *32*, 257–265. [CrossRef]

15. Hodgson, W.C.; Wickramaratna, J.C. In vitro neuromuscular activity of snake venoms. *Clin. Exp. Pharmacol. Physiol.* **2002**, *29*, 807–814. [CrossRef] [PubMed]
16. Chang, C.C.; Chuang, S.T.; Lee, C.Y.; Wei, J.W. Role of cardiotoxin and phospholipase A in the blockade of nerve conduction and depolarization of skeletal muscle induced by cobra venom. *Br. J. Pharmacol.* **1972**, *44*, 752–764. [CrossRef] [PubMed]
17. Ownby, C.L.; Fletcher, J.E.; Colberg, T.R. Cardiotoxin 1 from cobra (*Naja naja atra*) venom causes necrosis of skeletal muscle in vivo. *Toxicon* **1993**, *31*, 697–709. [CrossRef]
18. Huang, S.J.; Kwan, C.Y. Inhibition by multivalent cations of contraction induced by Chinese cobra venom cardiotoxin in guinea pig papillary muscle. *Life Sci.* **1996**, *59*, PI55–PI60. [CrossRef]
19. Vignaud, A.; Hourdé, C.; Butler-Browne, G.; Ferry, A. Differential recovery of neuromuscular function after nerve/muscle injury induced by crude venom from *Notechis scutatus*, cardiotoxin from *Naja atra* and bupivacaine treatments in mice. *Neurosci. Res.* **2007**, *58*, 317–323. [CrossRef]
20. Wang, C.H.; Monette, R.; Lee, S.C.; Morley, P.; Wu, W.G. Cobra cardiotoxin-induced cell death in fetal rat cardiomyocytes and cortical neurons: Different pathway but similar cell surface target. *Toxicon* **2005**, *46*, 430–440. [CrossRef]
21. Panagides, N.; Jackson, T.N.W.; Ikonomopoulou, M.P.; Arbuckle, K.; Pretzler, R.; Yang, D.C.; Ali, S.A.; Koludarov, I.; Dobson, J. How the cobra got its flesh-eating venom: Cytotoxicity as a defensive innovation and its co-evolution with hooding, aposematic marking and spitting. *Toxins* **2017**, *9*, 103. [CrossRef]
22. Harris, R.J.; Zdenek, C.N.; Harrich, D.; Frank, N.; Fry, B.G. An appetite for destruction: Detecting prey-selective binding of α-neurotoxins in the venom of Afro-Asian elapids. *Toxins* **2020**, *12*, 205. [CrossRef] [PubMed]
23. Lam, K.K.; Crow, P.; Ng, K.H.; Shek, K.C.; Fung, H.T.; Ades, G.; Grioni, A.; Tan, K.S.; Yip, K.T.; Lung, D.C.; et al. A cross-sectional survey of snake oral bacterial flora from Hong Kong, SAR, China. *Emerg. Med. J.* **2011**, *28*, 107–114. [CrossRef] [PubMed]
24. Mao, Y.C.; Liu, P.Y.; Hung, D.Z.; Lai, W.C.; Huang, S.T.; Hung, Y.M.; Yang, C.C. Bacteriology of *Naja atra* snakebite wound and its implications for antibiotic therapy. *Am. J. Trop. Med. Hyg.* **2016**, *94*, 1129–1135. [CrossRef] [PubMed]
25. Lumsden, N.G.; Ventura, S.; Dauer, R.; Hodgson, W.C. A biochemical and pharmacological examination of *Rhamphiophis oxyrhynchus* (Rufous beaked snake) venom. *Toxicon* **2005**, *45*, 219–231. [CrossRef] [PubMed]
26. Ramasamy, S.; Isbister, G.K.; Hodgson, W.C. The efficacy of two antivenoms against the in vitro myotoxic effects of black snake (*Pseudechis*) venoms in the chick biventer cervicis nerve-muscle preparation. *Toxicon* **2004**, *44*, 837–845. [CrossRef] [PubMed]
27. Wickramaratna, J.C.; Hodgson, W.C. A pharmacological examination of venoms from three species of death adder (*Acanthopis antarcticus*, *Acanthopis praelongus* and *Acanthopis pyrrhus*). *Toxicon* **2001**, *39*, 209–216. [CrossRef]

biomedicines

MDPI

Article

Varespladib Inhibits the Phospholipase A2 and Coagulopathic Activities of Venom Components from Hemotoxic Snakes

Chunfang Xie [1,2], Laura-Oana Albulescu [3,4], Kristina B. M. Still [1,2], Julien Slagboom [1,2], Yumei Zhao [5], Zhengjin Jiang [5], Govert W. Somsen [1,2], Freek J. Vonk [1,2,6], Nicholas R. Casewell [3,4] and Jeroen Kool [1,2,*]

1 Amsterdam Institute of Molecular and Life Sciences, Division of BioAnalytical Chemistry, Department of Chemistry and Pharmaceutical Sciences, Faculty of Sciences, Vrije Universiteit Amsterdam, De Boelelaan 1085, 1081 HV Amsterdam, The Netherlands; c.xie@vu.nl (C.X.); k.b.m.still@vu.nl (K.B.M.S.); j.slagboom@vu.nl (J.S.); g.w.somsen@vu.nl (G.W.S.); freek.vonk@naturalis.nl (F.J.V.)

2 Centre for Analytical Sciences Amsterdam (CASA), 1098 XH Amsterdam, The Netherlands

3 Centre for Snakebite Research and Interventions, Liverpool School of Tropical Medicine, Pembroke Place, Liverpool L3 5QA, UK; Laura-Oana.Albulescu@lstmed.ac.uk (L.-O.A.); Nicholas.Casewell@lstmed.ac.uk (N.R.C.)

4 Centre for Drugs and Diagnostics, Liverpool School of Tropical Medicine, Pembroke Place, Liverpool L3 5QA, UK

5 Institute of Pharmaceutical Analysis, College of Pharmacy, Jinan University, Huangpu Avenue West 601, Guangzhou 510632, China; yumeir612@hotmail.com (Y.Z.); jzjjackson@hotmail.com (Z.J.)

6 Naturalis Biodiversity Center, Darwinweg 2, 2333 CR Leiden, The Netherlands

* Correspondence: j.kool@vu.nl

Received: 10 May 2020; Accepted: 11 June 2020; Published: 17 June 2020

Abstract: Phospholipase A_2 (PLA_2) enzymes are important toxins found in many snake venoms, and they can exhibit a variety of toxic activities including causing hemolysis and/or anticoagulation. In this study, the inhibiting effects of the small molecule PLA_2 inhibitor varespladib on snake venom PLA_2s was investigated by nanofractionation analytics, which combined chromatography, mass spectrometry (MS), and bioassays. The venoms of the medically important snake species *Bothrops asper, Calloselasma rhodostoma, Deinagkistrodon acutus, Daboia russelii, Echis carinatus, Echis ocellatus,* and *Oxyuranus scutellatus* were separated by liquid chromatography (LC) followed by nanofractionation and interrogation of the fractions by a coagulation assay and a PLA_2 assay. Next, we assessed the ability of varespladib to inhibit the activity of enzymatic PLA_2s and the coagulopathic toxicities induced by fractionated snake venom toxins, and identified these bioactive venom toxins and those inhibited by varespladib by using parallel recorded LC-MS data and proteomics analysis. We demonstrated here that varespladib was not only capable of inhibiting the PLA_2 activities of hemotoxic snake venoms, but can also effectively neutralize the coagulopathic toxicities (most profoundly anticoagulation) induced by venom toxins. While varespladib effectively inhibited PLA_2 toxins responsible for anticoagulant effects, we also found some evidence that this inhibitory molecule can partially abrogate procoagulant venom effects caused by different toxin families. These findings further emphasize the potential clinical utility of varespladib in mitigating the toxic effects of certain snakebites.

Keywords: varespladib; nanofractionation; PLA_2 activity; coagulopathic toxicity; neutralization

1. Introduction

Phospholipases A_2 (PLA_2s) are key enzymes involved in many events in cellular signaling and act by cleaving ester bonds in phospholipids to generate fatty acids (hydrolysis reactions) [1–3]. They are pervasive in the mammalian pancreas and are highly abundant in many animal venoms [4,5]. Venom PLA_2 enzymes show a wide variety of functional activities, and thus can contribute to several distinct pathologies in envenomed prey/people, as well as potentially helping with prey digestion [4,5]. They are recognized as the most thoroughly investigated venom toxins both in hemotoxic and neurotoxic snake venoms [6,7]. Snake venom PLA_2s are capable of contributing to presynaptic and/or postsynaptic neurotoxicity, myotoxicity, and cardiotoxicity, which can induce platelet aggregation disorders, hemolysis, anticoagulation, convulsions, hypotension, edema, and necrosis [4,5,8]. They play an important role in contributing to the morbidity and mortality of snakebite victims, via paralysis and destruction of respiratory muscle tissues, and/or due to their effect on homeostatic mechanisms involved in coagulation and oxygen transport [9]. Although snakebite envenoming is a severe medical problem that was recently added to the World Health Organization (WHO) list of Neglected Tropical Diseases [10], it has for a long time been systematically neglected by governments worldwide, despite over 100,000 people dying annually [11]. Although current snakebite treatments, known as antivenoms (equine/ovine polyclonal antibodies), can be effective therapies capable of reducing morbidity and mortality, they have many limitations associated with them, leaving a critical therapeutic gap between snakebite and effective treatment [6,12]. Small molecule toxin inhibitor-based approaches are gaining much traction as promising alternatives and/or complementary treatments for snakebite [12–16], as they show a number of characteristics desirable for use as either early prehospital or adjunct therapies [13].

Varespladib is an indole-based nonspecific pan-secretory PLA_2 ($sPLA_2$) inhibitor that potently inhibits mammalian $sPLA_2$-IIa, $sPLA_2$-V, and $sPLA_2$-X, and in addition has been shown to inhibit venom PLA_2 toxins [17–20]. Varespladib was originally found to reduce PLA_2 concentrations in vivo, making it a candidate treatment for several cardiovascular diseases [17,21,22], including the treatment of acute coronary syndrome and systemic inflammatory response syndrome, but it was abandoned during Phase III clinical trials due to lack of efficacy [17,23–25]. Recently, varespladib was repurposed for exploration as a potential therapeutic candidate for snakebite, with early findings showing that varespladib and its orally bioavailable prodrug methyl-varespladib effectively suppress venom-induced PLA_2 activity both in vitro and in vivo [9]. Moreover, varespladib effectively reduces hemorrhage, edema, myonecrosis, and neurotoxicity in mice caused by venoms of several medically important snakes, and as such is a potential prereferral drug candidate for treating snakebites [25–28]. In addition to varespladib, the orally available prodrug methyl-varespladib is effective in inhibiting neurotoxicity, reversing neuromuscular paralysis, delaying or abrogating lethality, both immediately after envenoming and after onset of symptoms [25,28,29]. In combination, these studies have highlighted the great potential of varespladib as an orally available small molecule drug for use as a rapid snakebite intervention.

Consequently, in this study we aimed to investigate which specific venom components can be inhibited by varespladib, with a focus on snake venoms that cause coagulopathic effects. Venoms from the medically relevant snake species *Bothrops asper*, *Calloselasma rhodostoma*, *Deinagkistrodon acutus*, *Daboia russelii*, *Echis carinatus*, *Echis ocellatus*, and *Oxyuranus scutellatus* were separated by liquid chromatography (LC) followed by high resolution fractionation (*nanofractionation*) onto 384-well plates allowing bioassaying of individual fractions for PLA_2 and coagulation activities. Then, the potential inhibition of the detected activities by varespladib was evaluated and the toxins were identified by correlating parallel obtained mass spectrometry (MS) with proteomics data. Our findings show that varespladib is effective in inhibiting enzymatic activities of venom PLA_2s as well as inhibiting coagulopathic toxins (of which many were tentatively identified as venom PLA_2s).

2. Experimental Section

2.1. Chemicals

Water was purified using a Milli-Q Plus system (Millipore, Amsterdam, The Netherlands). Acetronitrile (ACN) (HPLC grade) and formic acid (FA) were purchased from Biosolve (Valkenswaard, The Netherlands). Calcium chloride ($CaCl_2$, Dihydrate, ≥ 99%), NaCl, KCl, Tris base, Phosphate buffered saline (PBS) tablets, Triton X-100, L-*a*-Phosphatidylcholine, Varespladib (A-001, LY315920), and Cresol red were obtained from Sigma-Aldrich (Zwijndrecht, The Netherlands). Bovine plasma was obtained from Biowest (Nuaillé, France) and stored at −80 °C until use. Pooled venoms from *B. asper* (Costa Rica "Atlantic"), *C. rhodostoma* (captive bred, Thailand ancestry), *D. acutus* (captive bred, China ancestry), *D. russelii* (Sri Lanka), *E. carinatus* (India), *E. ocellatus* (Nigeria), and *O. scutellatus* (Papua New Guinea) were obtained from animals maintained in, or from the historical venom collection of, the Centre for Snakebite Research and Interventions, Liverpool School of Tropical Medicine (UK). These freeze-dried venoms were dissolved in water to a concentration of 5.0 ± 0.1 mg/mL and stored at −80 °C until use. PBS was prepared by dissolving PBS tablets in water according to the manufacturer's instructions and stored at 4 °C for no longer than seven days. Varespladib was dissolved in DMSO (≥99.9%, Sigma-Aldrich, Zwijndrecht, The Netherlands) and stored at −20 °C. Prior to use, this varespladib stock solution was diluted in PBS to the required concentrations.

2.2. LC with Parallel Nanofractionation and MS Detection

Venom toxins were separated on a Shimadzu UPLC system ('s Hertogenbosch, The Netherlands) which was controlled by Shimadzu Lab Solutions software. Venom solutions were diluted to 1.0 mg/mL in MilliQ water of which 50 μL was injected by a Shimadzu SIL-30AC autosampler. A Waters XBridge reverse-phase C18 column (250 × 4.6 mm column with a 3.5 μm pore size) was used under gradient elution at 30 °C. The temperature of the column was controlled by a Shimadzu CTO-30A column oven. By using two Shimadzu LC-30AD parallel pumps, the total solvent flow rate was maintained at 0.5 mL/min. Mobile phase A consisted of 98% H_2O, 2% ACN, and 0.1% FA while mobile phase B was composed of 98% ACN, 2% H_2O, and 0.1% FA. For gradient elution, mobile phase B was increased linearly from 0% to 50% in 20 min, then from 50% to 90% in 4 min. After reaching 90%, the flow rate of mobile phase B was kept at 90% for 5 min. For reconditioning, the mobile phase B was decreased from 90% to 0% in 1 min and kept at 0% for 10 min. The column effluent was split into two parts (9:1) of which the 10% fraction was sent to a UV detector (Shimadzu SPD-M20A Prominence diode array detector) while the remaining 90% was directed to a nanofraction collector. This was either a modified Gilson 235P autosampler programmed for nanofractionation and controlled by the in-house written software Ariadne, or a commercially available FractioMate^{TM} nanofractionator (SPARK-Holland and VU, Netherlands, Emmen and Amsterdam) controlled by the FractioMator software. Fractions were collected onto transparent 384-well plates (F-bottom, rounded square well, polystyrene, no lid, clear, non-sterile; Greiner Bio One, Alphen aan den Rijn, The Netherlands) at a resolution of 6 s/well. The plates with collected fractions were subsequently dried overnight using a Christ Rotational Vacuum Concentrator (RVC 2–33 CD plus, Zalm en Kipp, Breukelen, The Netherlands) equipped with a −80 °C cooling trap during the vacuum-drying process. The evaporated plates were stored at −20 °C until further use.

2.3. Phospholipase A_2 Activity Assay

The PLA_2 activity assay was carried out according to the method recently reported by Still et al. [30] using cresol red as a pH indicator. The PLA_2 assay monitors the decrease in pH caused by the enzymatic conversion of L-*a*-Phosphatidylcholine to fatty acids. The assay solution was prepared freshly by dissolving NaCl (100 mM, final concentration), KCl (100 mM), $CaCl_2$ (10 mM), Triton X-100 (0.875 mM), cresol red (0.02 mg/mL), and L-*a*-Phosphatidylcholine (0.875 mM) in a Tris buffer (1.0 mM, pH 8.0). The pH of the bioassay solution was checked prior to each run and adjusted to pH 8.0

by HCl if needed. For measurements, 40 μL of the assay solution was rapidly pipetted into each well of a vacuum-centrifuge-dried 384-well plate with venom fractions using a VWR Multichannel Electronic Pipette (10–200 μL; VWR International B.V., Amsterdam, The Netherlands) and a kinetic absorbance measurement at 572 nm was initiated immediately at room temperature using a plate reader (Varioskan™ Flash Multimode Reader, Thermo Fisher Scientific, Ermelo, The Netherlands). Kinetic measurements were collected over 40 min, and the PLA_2 activity in each well was normalized by dividing the slope obtained for each well by the median of all the slope values obtained across the plate. For investigating PLA_2 inhibition by varespladib, 10 μL aliquots of various concentrations varespladib (final concentrations of 20, 4, and 0.8 μM) were pipetted into each well of freeze-dried 384-well plates using a VWR Multichannel Electronic Pipette. Thereafter, the plates were centrifuged for 1 min at 805× *g* (2000 rpm) in a 5810 R centrifuge (Eppendorf, Germany) to remove potential air bubbles formed during the automated pipetting process, and then pre-incubated for 30 min at room temperature. Next, the PLA_2 assay solutions were added as described above, and plate reader measurements were initiated. For comparison, 10 μL of PBS were added to each well and pre-incubated in the same manner as for the control experiments (indicated as PBS in the Figures). All analyses were performed in at least duplicate.

2.4. Plasma Coagulation Activity Assay

In-house aliquoted plasma was stored in 15 mL CentriStar™ tubes (Corning Science, Reynosa, Mexico) at −80 °C. For preparing the aliquots, a 500 mL bottle of sodium citrate plasma (Sterile Filtered; Biowest, Nuaillé, France) stored at −80 °C was warmed in warm water until fully defrosted, after which the plasma was quickly aliquoted in 15 mL CentriStar™ tubes, which were then immediately frozen at −80 °C, and stored until use. Prior to use, the 15 mL CentriStar™ tubes were defrosted to room temperature in a warm water bath and then centrifuged at 805× *g* (2000 rpm) (Allegra™ X-12 Centrifuge, Beckman Coulter) for 4 min to remove possible particulate matter.

For the coagulation assay, we followed our previously described approach [31,32]. Briefly, 20 μL $CaCl_2$ solution (20 mM) was pipetted into each well of a freeze-dried plate using a Multidrop™ 384 Reagent Dispenser (Thermo Fisher Scientific, Ermelo, The Netherlands). This was followed by pipetting 20 μL of centrifuged plasma using the same Multidrop™ 384 Reagent Dispenser (after in-between rinsing the Multidrop with Milli-Q). Next, absorbance at 595 nm was monitored kinetically at room temperature on a plate reader (Varioskan™ Flash Multimode Reader, Thermo Fisher Scientific, Ermelo, The Netherlands). Measurements were collected over 100 min, and the slope of each well was normalized by dividing the slope measured in each well by the median of all slope values across the plate. The slope of the average 0–5 min reading was used for depicting very fast coagulation, whereas the slope of the average 0–20 min reading denoted slightly/medium increased coagulation. The slope of the single reading at 100 min was used to depict anticoagulation activity. Detailed explanations on the rationale of processing and plotting the data in this way are provided in [32,33].

To investigate whether varespladib was capable of inhibiting coagulopathic venom activity, 10 μL of various concentrations of the varespladib solution were added to each well of a freeze-dried 384-well plate (10 μL of PBS was added to the venom-only control). For all bioassay pipetting steps, a VWR Multichannel Electronic Pipette was used. The final concentrations of varespladib in the coagulation bioassay were 20, 4, and 0.8 μM (and in some cases also 0.16 and 0.032 μM). Directly after pipetting the varespladib solutions, plates were centrifuged for 1 min at 805× *g* (2000 rpm) using a 5810 R centrifuge (Eppendorf, Germany) and then pre-incubated for 30 min at room temperature. Meanwhile, the plasma coagulation activity assay solutions were prepared as described above and added to the plates after the pre-incubation step, after which the plates were measured on the plate reader. All analyses were performed in at least duplicate.

2.5. Correlation of Biological and MS Data

In our previous study [33], the same snake venoms as currently studied were analyzed using the nanofractionation approach, yielding accurate mass(es) of eluting venom toxins by MS and coagulopathic activities of fractions in parallel. In addition, proteomics data were acquired by an in-well tryptic digestion of the content of the wells that showed bioactivity followed by the LC-MS/MS analysis. The UniprotKB database was used to search for information on the class and possible known functions of relevant toxins. A correlation of the chromatographic LC-UV data acquired in this study with the previous study referred to above permitted the bioassay data generated in this study to be correlated with the MS and proteomics data previously obtained [33]. In order to identify potential molecular masses of bioactive toxins, firstly for each peak found in the bioassay trace, a mass spectrum was extracted by averaging the recorded spectra in the LC-MS trace over the corresponding time width at half maximum/minimum of the bioactive peak. Then, from all the detected ions in the average mass spectrum, extracted-ion chromatograms (XICs) were plotted. For XICs showing a peak shape and retention time matching to the bioactive peak under consideration, the corresponding *m/z* value was assigned to the bioactive compound. Finally, the deconvolution option in the MS software was used to determine the accurate monoisotopic masses of the bioactive compound.

3. Results and Discussion

In this study, a nanofractionation approach was used to evaluate the effects of varespladib on inhibiting PLA_2 enzymatic activity and coagulopathic properties of individual venom toxins. After LC fractionation of venoms in 384-well plates, both the PLA_2 enzymatic activities and the clotting activities of the individual venom fractions were evaluated. The inhibition of the measured venom toxin activities was assessed under different varespladib concentrations, and each active fraction detected was correlated with MS and proteomics data obtained in parallel to determine the identity of inhibited venom toxins.

3.1. PLA_2 Bioactivity Profiles of Nanofractionated Venom Toxins

The PLA_2 activity profiles of the snake venoms obtained after LC fractionation are shown as bioactivity chromatograms in Figure 1. Both *O. scutellatus* and *E. carinatus* venoms displayed relatively sharp peaks (two at 23.0 and 24.6 min for *O. scutellatus* and one at 23.6 min for *E. carinatus*). Conversely, *D. russelii* venom exhibited a broad and clear PLA_2 activity peak (23.8–26.8 min), while *B. asper* displayed two closely eluting peaks (24.1 and 25.1 min) of which the first one (24.1 min) was observed close to the background level and the latter eluting peak (25.1 min) was distinctive and broad. For the other three venoms (*E. ocellatus, D. acutus,* and *C. rhodostoma*), no clear PLA_2 bioactivity was observed at the analyzed venom concentration (1.0 mg/mL). All PLA_2 bioactivity chromatograms resulting from duplicate measurements are presented in the Supplementary Materials (Section S1).

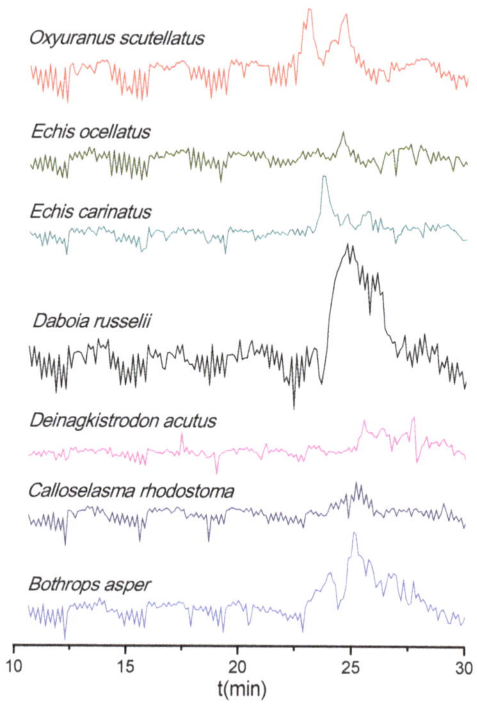

Figure 1. Phospholipase A_2 (PLA_2) bioactivity chromatograms of nanofractionated venom toxins. Positive peaks indicate PLA_2 activity.

3.2. Coagulopathic Bioactivity Profiles of Nanofractionated Venom Toxins

The coagulopathic bioactivities of nanofractionated venom components are shown in Figure 2. Most of the venoms displayed both pro and anticoagulant activities, except for the venom of *O. scutellatus*, for which only anticoagulant activity was observed. Note that during chromatographic separations under reversed-phase conditions non-stable toxin complexes and large toxins can denature, which could explain the lack of procoagulation observed for *O. scutellatus*, but a recent study demonstrated that higher venom concentrations were required to observe this effect with this venom after nanofractionation (i.e., 5.0 instead of 1.0 mg/mL) [33]. For both *D. russelii* and *O. scutellatus* venoms, the very broad anticoagulant peak observed indicates the presence of many closely eluting anticoagulant toxins—this activity was sufficiently potent to be observed visually on the plates after measurement. Among venoms with procoagulant activity, *E. ocellatus* venom only displayed a slightly/medium increased procoagulant activity, while very fast procoagulant activity was not observed. *C. rhodostoma* venom had a relatively weak anticoagulant and a strong procoagulant activity (for both very fast and slightly/medium increased coagulation). Note that despite the fact that in general venom toxins are rather stable, during RPLC within the nanofractionation analytics pipeline some venom toxins might have (partly) denatured and thereby lost their enzymatic activity. Bioactivity chromatograms of duplicate measurements and a detailed description of all observed coagulopathic peaks are shown in the Supplementary Materials (Section S2).

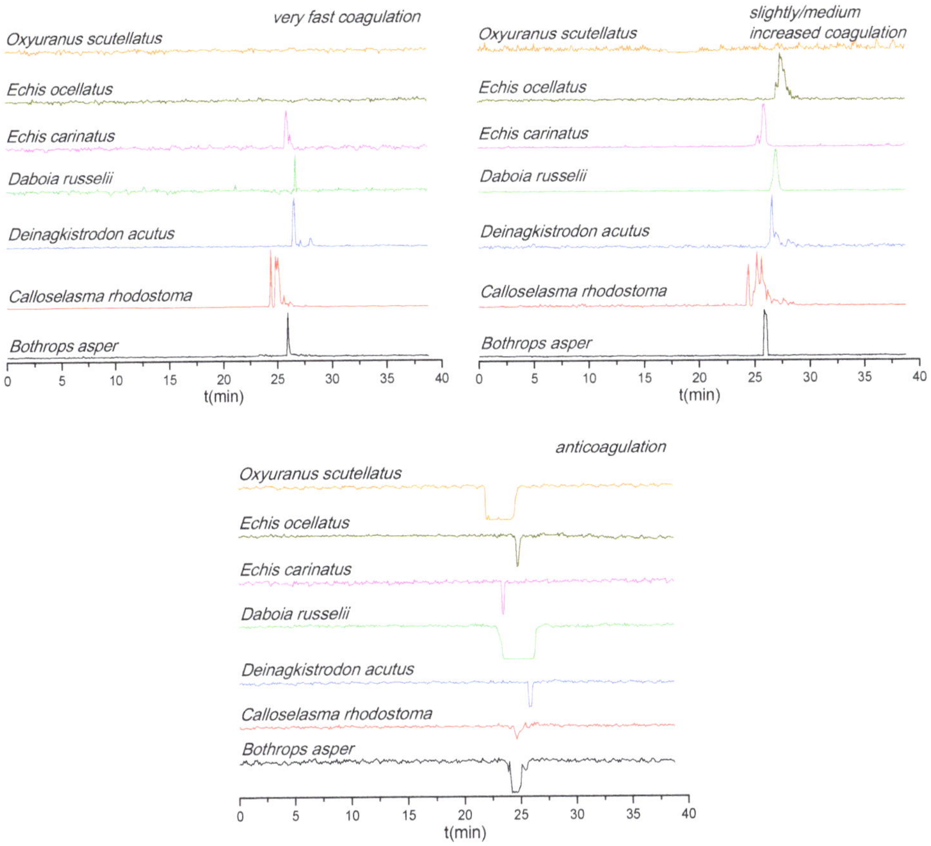

Figure 2. Coagulopathic bioactivity chromatograms of nanofractionated venom toxins. Anticoagulation is measured as negative signals and procoagulation as positive signals.

3.3. Neutralization Capabilities of Varespladib on the Enzymatic PLA_2 Activity of Venom Toxins

As discussed in Section 3.1, only LC fractions of the *B. asper*, *D. russelii*, *E. carinatus*, and *O. scutellatus* venoms were found to possess an abundantly detectable enzymatic activity in the PLA_2 assay. Therefore, these four snake venoms were selected to assess the inhibitory effect of varespladib on the observed PLA_2 activities of the fractions (Figure 3). As anticipated, the observed PLA_2 activities for these four snake venoms decreased with increasing concentrations of varespladib. The PLA_2 activities of *B. asper*, *D. russelii*, and *O. scutellatus* venoms were fully neutralized by 20 μM varespladib, whereas the activity observed for *E. carinatus* venom was abolished by 4 μM varespladib. These data indicate broad-spectrum venom PLA_2 inhibition by varespladib. The duplicate bioassay chromatograms are presented in the Supplementary Materials (Section S3).

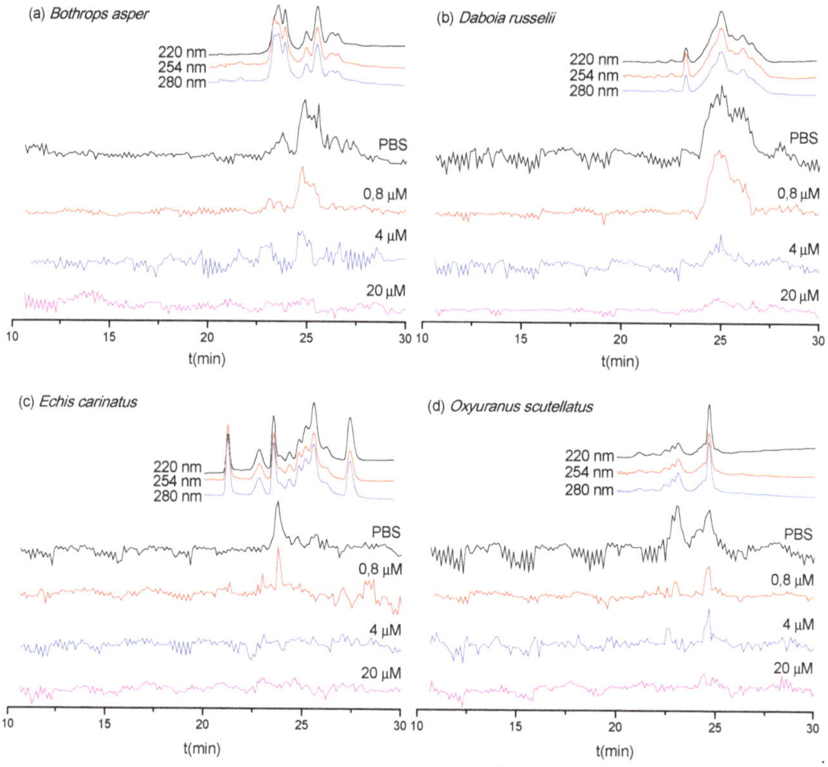

Figure 3. Superimposed PLA_2 bioactivity chromatograms for nanofractionated venom toxins measured in the presence of the indicated concentrations of varespladib: (**a**) *B. asper*, (**b**) *D. russelii*, (**c**) *E. carinatus*, and (**d**) *O. scutellatus*. Top traces are the online LC-UV chromatograms recorded at 220, 254, and 280 nm for the respective venoms (allowing a correlation with LC-MS and proteomics data from Slagboom et al. [33]).

3.4. Neutralization Capabilities of Varespladib on Plasma Coagulation Activity of Venom Toxins

Next, we assessed the inhibition of coagulopathic toxins identified in the various venom fractions by varespladib (Figure 4). Surprisingly, varespladib not only inhibited the anticoagulant activities of a number of the nanofractionated venom toxins, but also had an effect on some of the procoagulant venom fractions. Specifically, the anticoagulant activity of *E. carinatus*, *E. ocellatus*, and *O. scutellatus* venoms were fully neutralized by 20 μM varespladib. Varespladib was particularly effective in inhibiting the anticoagulant activity of toxins in *O. scutellatus* venom, and demonstrated a clear dose-response relationship. The anticoagulant activity of *D. acutus* and *D. russelii* venom components were almost completely abrogated with 20 μM varespladib, although trace activities remained. Contrastingly, varespladib did not considerably inhibit the anticoagulant toxicities observed in *B. asper* and *C. rhodostoma* venoms, with the exception that the first anticoagulant peak (23.1–24.2 min) in *B. asper* venom was fully inhibited at a very low concentration (0.8 μM varespladib).

Varespladib also showed some inhibitory capabilities against the procoagulant activities of *B. asper*, *C. rhodostoma*, *D. acutus*, *D. russelii*, *E. carinatus*, and *E. ocellatus* venom (Figure 4). The extent of inhibition observed varied extensively, although full inhibition was not achieved across any of the venoms. The greatest effect was observed against the venom of *E. carinatus*, where the very fast coagulation activity was fully neutralized at 4 μM varespladib and most of the slightly/medium increased procoagulant activity was fully inhibited at 20 μM varespladib. The potent procoagulant activities of *D. russelii* venom were noticeably reduced in a dose-dependent manner, although full inhibition was not achieved, even when using the 20 μM varespladib concentration. Similar findings were observed with the venoms of *B. asper*, *C. rhodostoma*, *D. acutus*, and *E. ocellatus*, where procoagulant peaks were generally reduced in height with the highest concentrations of varespladib, suggesting perhaps a nonspecific inhibitory effect. The duplicate bioassay chromatograms and a detailed description of all coagulation-related activities neutralized by different concentrations of varespladib are provided in the Supplementary Materials (Section S4).

Snake venom PLA_2s are well-known for their anticoagulant toxicities [34–36]. Our results show that varespladib effectively inhibits anticoagulant activities across a wide variety of medically important snake venoms. Additionally, we also find that varespladib can reduce the procoagulant venom activity, possibly by directly inhibiting enzymatic procoagulant toxins or blocking protein–protein interactions. However, the concentration of varespladib required to show noticeable inhibition of procoagulant venom activities was generally high (i.e., 20 μM), relative to that required for neutralizing anticoagulant activities.

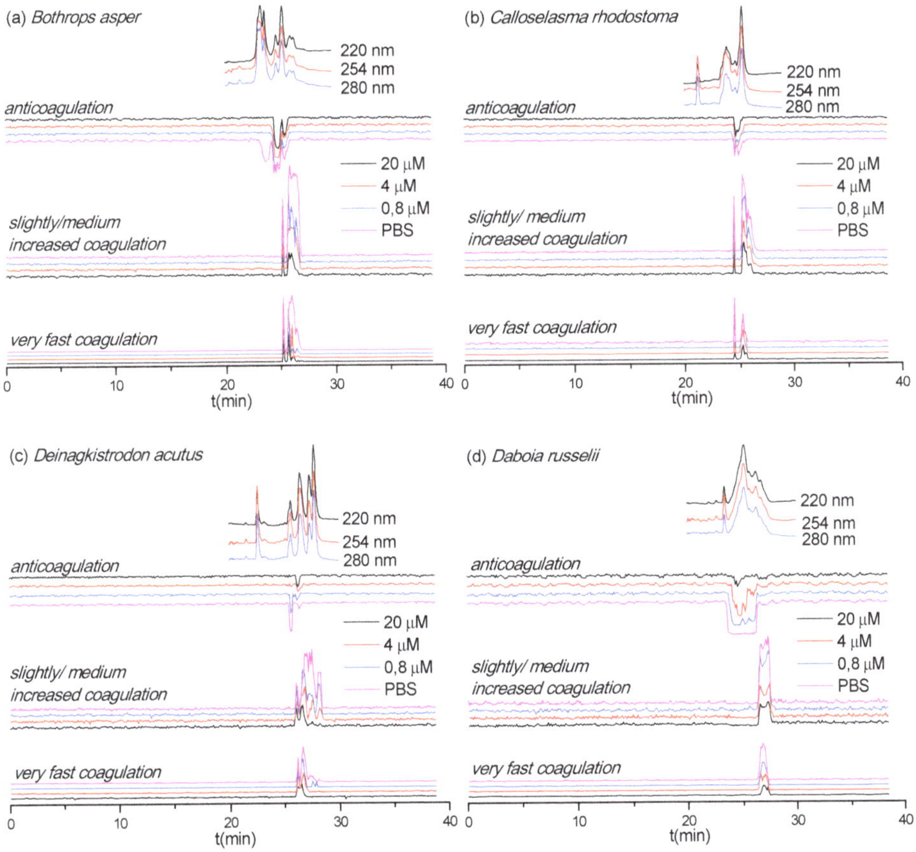

Figure 4. Part 1—Coagulopathic toxicity chromatograms in the presence of various varespladib concentrations for nanofractionated venom toxins from (**a**) *B. asper*, (**b**) *C. rhodostoma*, (**c**) *D. acutus*, (**d**) *D. russelii*, (**e**) *E. carinatus*, (**f**) *E. ocellatus*, and (**g**) *O. scutellatus*. Top traces are the online LC-UV chromatograms recorded at 220, 254, and 280 nm for the respective venoms (allowing a correlation with LC-MS data and proteomics data from Slagboom et al. [33]). (figure continues on next page).

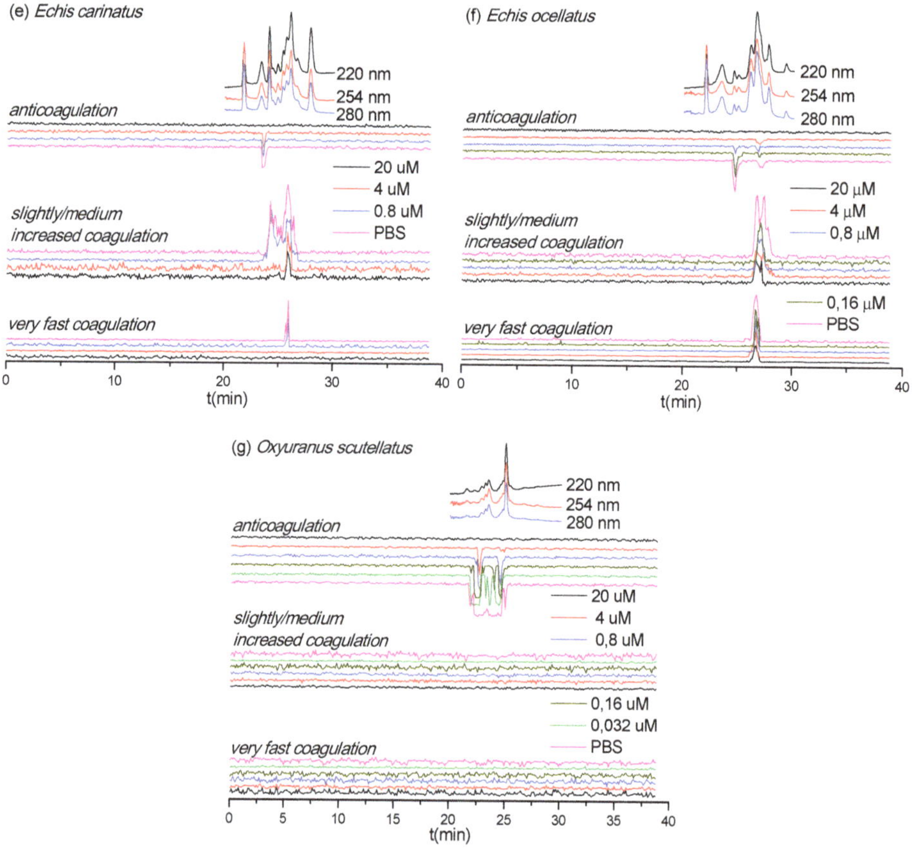

Figure 4. Part 2—(continuation of figure from previous page). Coagulopathic toxicity chromatograms in the presence of various varespladib concentrations for nanofractionated venom toxins from (**a**) *B. asper*, (**b**) *C. rhodostoma*, (**c**) *D. acutus*, (**d**) *D. russelii*, (**e**) *E. carinatus*, (**f**) *E. ocellatus*, and (**g**) *O. scutellatus*. Top traces are the online LC-UV chromatograms recorded at 220, 254, and 280 nm for the respective venoms (allowing a correlation with LC-MS data and proteomics data from Slagboom et al. [33]).

3.5. Identification of Venom Toxins Neutralized by Varespladib

The correlated LC-MS (i.e., accurate masses of eluting venom toxins) and proteomics data obtained by Slagboom et al. [33] were used to identify venom toxins with enzymatic PLA_2 and coagulopathic activities (Tables 1 and 2). Bioactivities were linked to accurate molecular masses and tentative protein identities by aligning the characteristic LC-UV chromatograms obtained for each venom. When no exact mass data could be acquired by LC-MS, only the proteomics mass data obtained from the Mascot searches are provided.

Based on the results displayed in Table 1 and Figure 3, the PLA_2 enzymes that were neutralized by varespladib could be tentatively identified. From the four species exhibiting enzymatic PLA_2 activity after nanofractionation (i.e., *B. asper*, *E. carinatus*, *D. russelii*, and *O. scutellatus*) we detected a total of 13 toxins, of which all were unsurprisingly identified as PLA_2 toxins. Eleven toxins were fully neutralized by 20 μM varespladib, while two were inhibited by much lower doses (0.8 μM varespladib). Variations were observed among the species, however, with five bioactive PLA_2 enzymes identified in the venom of *B. asper*, four in *O. scutellatus*, three in *D. russelii*, and only one in *E. carinatus* (Table 1).

Table 1. Correlated accurate molecular masses and proteomics data for PLA_2 activities (peak retention times are adapted from Figure 3).

Species	Peaks Retention Time (min)	Mascot Results Matching the Exact Mass	*m/z* Values from MS Data	Exact Mass from MS Data	Exact Mass Calculated from Mascot Data	Toxin Class	Varespladib Concentration Required for Full Inhibition
B. asper	23.2–24.1	PA2H2_BOTAS	1373.3688^{10+}	13,714.5646	13,714.56817	PLA_2	0.8 µM
	24.3–25.8	PA2HA_BOTAS	1266.5985^{11+}	13,912.4649	13,896.51308	PLA_2	20 µM
	24.3–25.8	PA2H3_BOTAS	1378.3697^{10+}	13,765.5812	13,765.58896	PLA_2	20 µM
	24.3–25.8	PA2B3_BOTAS	1164.8811^{12+}	13,957.5333	13,957.48720	PLA_2	20 µM
	24.3–25.8	PA2A2_BOTAS	-	-	14,194	PLA_2	20 µM
D. russelii	23.9–27.4	PA2B8_DABRR	1511.6962^{9+}	13,587.2248	13,587.2027	PLA_2	20 µM
	23.9–27.4	PA2B5_DABRR			13,587	PLA_2	20 µM
	23.9–27.4	PA2B3_DABRR	-	-	13,687	PLA_2	20 µM
E. carinatus	23.3–24.4	PA2A1_ECHCA	-	-	16,310	PLA_2	0.8 µM
O. scutellatus	22.6–25.1	PA2TA_OXYSC	-	-	13,829	PLA_2	20 µM
	22.6–25.1	PA2TB_OXYSC	-	-	16,008	PLA_2	20 µM
	23.6–25.1	PA21_OXYSC	-	-	16,898	PLA_2	20 µM
	23.6–25.1	PA2TC_OXYSC	-	-	13,313	PLA_2	20 µM

Table 2. Part 1—Correlated LC-MS masses and proteomics data for coagulopathic venom toxins activities (peak retention times are adapted from Figure 4; SVMP: Snake Venom Metalloproteinase; SVSP: Snake Venom Serine Protease; CTL: C-Type Lectin; kunitz: kunitz-type serine protease inhibitor; PN: Partly Neutralized at 20 µM varespladib; NOI: No Observed Inhibition. (table continues on next page).

Species	Peak Retention Time (min)	Peak Activity	Mascot Results Matching the Exact Mass	*m/z* Values from MS Data	Exact Mass from MS Data	Exact Mass Calculated from Mascot Data	Toxin Class	Varespladib Concentration Needed for Full Inhibition
B. asper	23.1–24.2	Anticoagulation	PA2H2_BOTAS	1373.3688^{10+}	13,714.5646	13,714.56817	PLA_2	0.8 µM
	24.2–25.2	Anticoagulation	PA2HA_BOTAS	1266.5985^{11+}	13,912.4649	13,896.51308	PLA_2	20 µM
	24.2–25.2	Anticoagulation	PA2H3_BOTAS	1378.3697^{10+}	13,765.5812	13,765.58896	PLA_2	20 µM
	25.2–25.8	Anticoagulation	PA2B3_BOTAS	1164.8811^{12+}	13,957.5333	13,957.48720	PLA_2	20 µM
	25.2–25.8	Anticoagulation	PA2A2_BOTAS	-	-	14,194	PLA_2	20 µM
	25.2–25.8	Anticoagulation	VM2_BOTAS	-	-	53,564	SVMP	NOI
	25.0–26.8	Procoagulation	VSPL_BOTAS	-	-	28,019	SVSP	PN
	25.0–26.8	Procoagulation	VM1B1_BOTAS	-	-	45,936	SVMP	PN
	25.4–26.8	Procoagulation	SLA_BOTAS	-		7084	CTL	PN
C. rhodostoma	24.3–25.5	Anticoagulation	PA2BD_CALRH	1244.1103^{11+}	13,665.0848	13,665.0237	PLA_2	NOI
	24.3–25.5	Anticoagulation	PA2AB_CALRH	-	-	14,352	PLA_2	NOI
	24.3–25.5	Anticoagulation	VSPF1_CALRH	-	-	26,570	SVSP	NOI
	24.3–25.5	Anticoagulation	SLEA_CALRH	-	-	15,962	CTL	NOI
	24.3–25.5	Anticoagulation	SLEB_CALRH	-	-	15,190	CTL	NOI
	24.3–26.6	Procoagulation	VSPF2_CALRH	-	-	29,145	SVSP	PN
	24.9–26.6	Procoagulation	SLYA_CALRH	-	-	15,796	CTL	PN
	24.9–26.6	Procoagulation	SLYB_CALRH	-	-	16,770	CTL	PN
D. acutus	25.4–25.9	Anticoagulation	PA2A_DEIAC	-	-	14,820	PLA_2	4 µM
	25.4–25.9	Anticoagulation	SL_DEIAC	-	-	18,332	CTL	4 µM
	26.0–27.2	Procoagulation	VSP1_DEIAC	-	-	29,480	SVSP	PN
	26.0–27.2	Procoagulation	VSPA_DEIAC	-	-	26,132	SVSP	PN
	26.4–27.8	Procoagulation	SLCB_DEIAC	-	-	17,133	CTL	PN
	26.4–27.8	Procoagulation	VM1AC_DEIAC	-	-	47,690	SVMP	PN
	26.4–27.8	Procoagulation	VM11_DEIAC	-	-	47,845	SVMP	PN
	26.4–27.8	Procoagulation	VM1H5_DEIAC	-	-	46,518	SVMP	PN
	26.4–27.8	Procoagulation	VM3AK_DEIAC	-	-	69,752	SVMP	PN
	27.8–28.4	Procoagulation	VM3A2_DEIAC	-		27,151	SVMP	20 µM
	27.8–28.4	Procoagulation	VM3AH_DEIAC	-		70,721	SVMP	20 µM

Table 2. Part 2—(continuation of table from previous page). Correlated LC-MS masses and proteomics data for coagulopathic venom toxins activities (peak retention times are adapted from Figure 4; SVMP: Snake Venom Metalloproteinase; SVSP: Snake Venom Serine Protease; CTL: C-Type Lectin; kunitz: kunitz-type serine protease inhibitor; PN: Partly Neutralized at 20 µM varespladib; NOI: No Observed Inhibition.

Species	Peak Retention Time (min)	Peak Activity	Mascot Results Matching the Exact Mass	*m/z* Values from MS Data	Exact Mass from MS Data	Exact Mass Calculated from Mascot Data	Toxin Class	Varespladib Concentration Needed for Full Inhibition
D. russelii	23.4–26.4	Anticoagulation	PA2B8_DABRR	1511.6962^{9+}	13,587.2248	13,587.2027	PLA_2	20 µM
	23.4–26.4	Anticoagulation	PA2B5_DABRR	–		13,587	PLA_2	20 µM
	23.4–26.4	Anticoagulation	PA2B3_DABRR	–		13,687	PLA_2	20 µM
	26.2–27.6	Procoagulation	–	-	-	-	-	
E. carinatus	23.3–23.8	Anticoagulation	PA2A1_ECHCA	-	-	16,310	PLA_2	0.8 µM
	23.8–26.9	Procoagulation	-	-	-	-	-	
E. ocellatus	24.4–25.1	Anticoagulation	PA2A5_ECHOC	1541.4718^{9+}	13,856.1382	13,856.0665	PLA_2	4 µM
	26.3–28.2	Procoagulation	VM3E2_ECHOC	-	-	69,426	SVMP	PN
	26.3–28.2	Procoagulation	VM3E6_ECHOC	-	-	57,658	SVMP	PN
	26.3–28.2	Procoagulation	SL1_ECHOC	-	-	16,601	CTL	PN
	26.3–28.2	Procoagulation	SL124_ECHOC	-	-	16,882	CTL	PN
O. scutellatus	21.7–25.2	Anticoagulation	PA2TA_OXYSC	-	-	13,829	PLA_2	20 µM
	21.7–25.2	Anticoagulation	PA2TB_OXYSC	-	-	16,008	PLA_2	20 µM
	21.7–25.2	Anticoagulation	PA21_OXYSC	-	-	16,898	PLA_2	20 µM
	21.7–25.2	Anticoagulation	PA2TC_OXYSC	-	-	13,313	PLA_2	20 µM
	21.7–25.2	Anticoagulation	VKT_OXYSC		-	9711	kunitz	20 µM
	21.7–25.2	Anticoagulation	VKT3_OXYSC	-	-	9029	kunitz	20 µM

The assigned toxins responsible for the coagulation activities observed are displayed in Table 2. Based on the data in Table 2 and Figure 4, the inhibitory potency of varespladib on the coagulopathic venom protein(s) was assessed. All tentatively identified anticoagulant toxins for the anticoagulant peaks from venoms of *B. asper, D. acutus, D. russelii, E. carinatus, E. ocellatus,* and *O. scutellatus* were fully abrogated by varespladib, while the anticoagulant toxins from *C. rhodostoma* were not inhibited by varespladib. No procoagulant toxins could be identified for the procoagulant peaks from the Mascot results for *D. russelii, E. carinatus,* and *O. scutellatus* venoms. Procoagulant toxins were identified from Mascot results for *B. asper, C. rhodostoma, D. acutus,* and *E. ocellatus* venoms, but we could not determine exactly which toxins were partially inhibited by varespladib as multiple venom toxins were found to co-eluted in each case. Thus, unambiguously assigning single toxins to each detected bioactivity is problematic at this resolution, especially if broad bioactivity peaks are observed. Additionally, when for example multiple potent anticoagulant toxins and a weak procoagulant toxin elute closely together, the net observed effect would be anticoagulation and the procoagulant toxin would not be detectable as a procoagulant. While distinction of all bioactive compounds in such cases requires further improving LC separations under toxin non-denaturating and MS compatible eluent conditions, it is worth noting that none of the tentatively assigned procoagulant toxins found here that were fully or partially inhibited by varespladib were PLA_2s (see Table 2), suggesting varespladib may interact with other venom toxins. A detailed description of the results discussed here is provided in the Supplementary Materials (Section S5).

4. Conclusions

A recently developed analytical platform combining LC, MS, and PLA_2 and coagulation activity bioassays was applied to evaluate the inhibitory properties of varespladib against the enzymatic PLA_2 and coagulopathic activities of toxins found in the venoms of several medically important snake species. All venoms analyzed in this study showed constituents with clear coagulopathic toxicities, while only the venoms of *B. asper, D. russelii, E. carinatus,* and *O. scutellatus* displayed components with a clear enzymatic PLA_2 activity. All components with detected enzymatic PLA_2 activities were identified as PLA_2 toxins and were fully neutralized by the small molecule toxin inhibitor varespladib. We demonstrated here that varespladib inhibited many of the anticoagulant bioactivities of the toxin components found in these venoms, similar to findings recently described by others for certain snakes of the genera *Naja, Pseudechis* and *Bitis* [16,37,38], and we confirmed that the toxins responsible are likely to be PLA_2s based on correlations between MS and proteomics data and the bioactivity chromatograms. However, we also revealed that several of the procoagulant venom toxins were also neutralized to some degree by varespladib. These findings suggest that the mechanism underlying venom inhibition may not be solely based on inhibition of the active site of venom PLA_2s, as other toxin types are typically responsible for procoagulant venom activities. However, we cannot rule out that nonspecific effects at high inhibitor concentrations are responsible for these observations, and thus future work is required to robustly explore this. Note that during chromatographic separations under reversed-phase conditions nonstable toxin complexes and large toxins can denature. Currently, we cannot circumvent this potential drawback of the nanofractionation analytics. Overall, our data further support the value of varespladib as a potential new therapeutic for mitigating the toxic effects of certain snakebites [9], and they re-emphasize that while this small molecule toxin inhibitor is a highly promising treatment for combatting neurotoxicity [25,28,29], it may also be of great value for treating elements of hemotoxicity caused by snake envenoming.

Supplementary Materials: The following are available online at http://www.mdpi.com/2227-9059/8/6/165/s1, Figure S1. Duplicate PLA_2 bioactivity chromatograms of nanofractionated venom toxins, positive peaks indicate PLA_2 activity; Figure S2. Duplicate coagulopathic toxicity chromatograms of the nanofractionated venom toxins, anticoagulation is measured as negative signals and procoagulation as positive signals; Figure S3. Duplicate PLA_2 bioactivity chromatograms of *B. asper*, *D. russelii*, *E. carinatus*, and *O. scutellatus* venoms in the presence of various varespladib concentrations; Figure S4. Duplicate coagulopathic toxicity bioassay chromatograms of nanofractionated venom toxins from *B. asper, C. rhodostoma, D. acutus, D. russelii, E. carinatus, E. ocellatus,* and *O. scutellatus* in the presence of various concentrations of varespladib.

Author Contributions: Conceptualization, F.J.V., N.R.C. and J.K.; Data curation, C.X. and K.B.M.S.; Formal analysis, C.X. and J.S.; Software, J.S.; Funding acquisition, N.R.C. and J.K.; Investigation, N.R.C. and J.K.; Methodology, K.B.M.S., J.S., Y.Z. and F.J.V.; Project administration, J.K.; Resources, N.R.C. and J.K.; Supervision, J.K.; Validation, C.X.; Visualization, C.X.; Writing—original draft, C.X.; Writing—review & editing, L.-O.A., Z.J., G.W.S., N.R.C. and J.K. All authors have read and agreed to the published version of the manuscript.

Funding: This research was funded by a UK Medical Research Council grant [MR/S00016X/1] and a Wellcome Trust and Royal Society Sir Henry Dale Fellowship [200517/Z/16/Z]. The APC was funded by the Wellcome Trust. C.X. was funded by a China Scholarship Council (CSC) fellowship [201706250035].

Conflicts of Interest: The authors declare no conflict of interest.

References

1. Price, J.A., III. A colorimetric assay for measuring phospholipase A_2 degradation of phosphatidylcholine at physiological pH. *J. Biochem. Biophys. Methods* **2007**, *70*, 441–444. [CrossRef] [PubMed]
2. Dessen, A. Phospholipase A_2 enzymes: Structural diversity in lipid messenger metabolism. *Structure* **2000**, *8*, R15–R22. [CrossRef]
3. Hendrickson, H.S. Fluorescence-based assays of lipases, phospholipases, and other lipolytic enzymes. *Anal. Biochem.* **1994**, *219*, 1–8. [CrossRef] [PubMed]
4. Tonello, F.; Rigoni, M. Cellular mechanisms of action of snake phospholipase A_2 toxins. In *Snake Venoms*; Toxinology; Gopalakrishnakone, P., Inagaki, H., Vogel, C.W., Mukherjee, A., Rahmy, T., Eds.; Springer: Dordecht, The Netherlands, 2017; pp. 49–65.
5. Costa, S.K.P.; Camargo, E.A.; Antunes, E. Inflammatory action of secretory phospholipases A_2 from snake venoms. In *Toxins and Drug Discovery*; Toxinology; Gopalakrishnakone, P., Cruz, L., Luo, S., Eds.; Springer: Dordecht, The Netherlands, 2017; pp. 35–52.
6. Cardoso, F.C.; Ferraz, C.R.; Arrahman, A.; Xie, C.; Casewell, N.R.; Lewis, R.J.; Kool, J. Multifunctional toxins in snake venoms and therapeutic implications: From pain to hemorrhage and necrosis. *Front. Ecol. Evol.* **2019**, *7*, 218–236.
7. Panfoli, I.; Calzia, D.; Ravera, S.; Morelli, A. Inhibition of hemorragic snake venom components: Old and new approaches. *Toxins* **2010**, *2*, 417–427. [CrossRef] [PubMed]
8. Lomonte, B.; Gutiérrez, J.M. Phospholipases A_2 from viperidae snake venoms: How do they induce skeletal muscle damage? *Acta Chim. Slov.* **2011**, *58*, 647–659.
9. Lewin, M.; Samuel, S.; Merkel, J.; Bickler, P. Varespladib (LY315920) appears to be a potent, broad-spectrum, inhibitor of snake venom phospholipase A_2 and a possible pre-referral treatment for envenomation. *Toxins* **2016**, *8*, 248. [CrossRef]
10. Williams, D.J.; Faiz, M.A.; Abela-Ridder, B.; Ainsworth, S.; Bulfone, T.C.; Nickerson, A.D.; Habib, A.G.; Junghanss, T.; Fan, H.W.; Turner, M.; et al. Strategy for a globally coordinated response to a priority neglected tropical disease: Snakebite envenoming. *PLoS Negl. Trop. Dis.* **2019**, *13*, 7059–7080. [CrossRef]
11. Gutiérrez, J.M.; Calvete, J.J.; Habib, A.G.; Harrison, R.A.; Williams, D.J.; Warrell, D.A. Snakebite envenoming. *Nat. Rev. Dis. Primers* **2017**, *3*, 1–21. [CrossRef]
12. Ainsworth, S.; Slagboom, J.; Alomran, N.; Pla, D.; Alhamdi, Y.; King, S.I.; Bolton, F.M.; Gutiérrez, J.M.; Vonk, F.J.; Toh, C.-H.; et al. The paraspecific neutralisation of snake venom induced coagulopathy by antivenoms. *Commun. Biol.* **2018**, *1*, 34. [CrossRef]
13. Bulfone, T.C.; Samuel, S.P.; Bickler, P.E.; Lewin, M.R. Developing small molecule therapeutics for the Initial and adjunctive treatment of snakebite. *J. Trop. Med.* **2018**, *2018*, 4320175. [CrossRef] [PubMed]
14. Resiere, D.; Gutiérrez, J.M.; Névière, R.; Cabié, A.; Hossein, M.; Kallel, H. Antibiotic therapy for snakebite envenoming. *J. Venom. Anim. Toxins Incl. Trop. Dis.* **2020**, *26*, 1–2. [CrossRef] [PubMed]

15. Albulescu, L.-O.; Hale, M.S.; Ainsworth, S.; Alsolaiss, J.; Crittenden, E.; Calvete, J.J.; Evans, C.; Wilkinson, M.C.; Harrison, R.A.; Kool, J.; et al. Preclinical validation of a repurposed metal chelator as an early-intervention therapeutic for hemotoxic snakebite. *Sci. Transl. Med.* **2020**, *12*, eaay8314. [CrossRef] [PubMed]
16. Bittenbinder, M.A.; Zdenek, C.N.; Op den Brouw, B.; Youngman, N.J.; Dobson, J.S.; Naude, A.; Vonk, F.J.; Fry, B.G. Coagulotoxic cobras: Clinical implications of strong anticoagulant actions of African spitting *Naja* venoms that are not neutralised by antivenom but are by LY315920 (Varespladib). *Toxins* **2018**, *10*, 516. [CrossRef]
17. Nicholls, S.J.; Kastelein, J.J.; Schwartz, G.G.; Bash, D.; Rosenson, R.S.; Cavender, M.A.; Brennan, D.M.; Koenig, W.; Jukema, J.W.; Nambi, V.; et al. Varespladib and cardiovascular events in patients with an acute coronary syndrome: The VISTA-16 randomized clinical trial. *JAMA* **2014**, *311*, 252–262. [CrossRef]
18. Shaposhnik, Z.; Wang, X.; Trias, J.; Fraser, H.; Lusis, A.J. The synergistic inhibition of atherogenesis in apoE−/− mice between pravastatin and the sPLA$_2$ inhibitor varespladib (A-002). *J. Lipid Res.* **2009**, *50*, 623–629. [CrossRef]
19. De Luca, D.; Minucci, A.; Piastra, M.; Cogo, P.E.; Vendittelli, F.; Marzano, L.; Gentile, L.; Giardina, B.; Conti, G.; Capoluongo, E.D. Ex vivo effect of varespladib on secretory phospholipase A$_2$ alveolar activity in infants with ARDS. *PLoS ONE* **2012**, *7*, e47066. [CrossRef]
20. Salvador, G.H.; Gomes, A.A.; Bryan-Quirós, W.; Fernández, J.; Lewin, M.R.; Gutiérrez, J.M.; Lomonte, B.; Fontes, M.R. Structural basis for phospholipase A$_2$-like toxin inhibition by the synthetic compound Varespladib (LY315920). *Sci. Rep.* **2019**, *9*, 1–13. [CrossRef]
21. Nicholls, S.J.; Cavender, M.A.; Kastelein, J.J.; Schwartz, G.; Waters, D.D.; Rosenson, R.S.; Bash, D.; Hislop, C. Inhibition of secretory phospholipase A$_2$ in patients with acute coronary syndromes: Rationale and design of the vascular inflammation suppression to treat acute coronary syndrome for 16 weeks (VISTA-16) trial. *Cardiovasc. Drugs Ther.* **2012**, *26*, 71–75. [CrossRef]
22. Rosenson, R.S.; Elliott, M.; Stasiv, Y.; Hislop, C.; PLASMA II Investigators. Randomized trial of an inhibitor of secretory phospholipase A$_2$ on atherogenic lipoprotein subclasses in statin-treated patients with coronary heart disease. *Eur. Heart J.* **2011**, *32*, 999–1005. [CrossRef]
23. Adis, R.; Profile, D. Varespladib. *Am. J. Cardiovasc. Drugs* **2011**, *11*, 137–143.
24. Nicholls, S. Varespladib trial terminated, increased MI risk. *Reactions* **2014**, *1484*, 1–18.
25. Lewin, M.R.; Gutiérrez, J.M.; Samuel, S.P.; Herrera, M.; Bryan-Quirós, W.; Lomonte, B.; Bickler, P.E.; Bulfone, T.C.; Williams, D.J. Delayed oral LY333013 rescues mice from highly neurotoxic, lethal doses of Papuan Taipan (*Oxyuranus scutellatus*) venom. *Toxins* **2018**, *10*, 380. [CrossRef] [PubMed]
26. Wang, Y.; Zhang, J.; Zhang, D.; Xiao, H.; Xiong, S.; Huang, C. Exploration of the inhibitory potential of varespladib for snakebite envenomation. *Molecules* **2018**, *23*, 391. [CrossRef] [PubMed]
27. Bryan-Quirós, W.; Fernández, J.; Gutiérrez, J.M.; Lewin, M.R.; Lomonte, B. Neutralizing properties of LY315920 toward snake venom group I and II myotoxic phospholipases A$_2$. *Toxicon* **2019**, *157*, 1–7. [CrossRef] [PubMed]
28. Gutiérrez, J.M.; Lewin, M.R.; Williams, D.; Lomonte, B. Varespladib (LY315920) and methyl varespladib (LY333013) abrogate or delay lethality induced by presynaptically acting neurotoxic snake venoms. *Toxins* **2020**, *12*, 131. [CrossRef]
29. Lewin, M.; Bulfone, T.; Samuel, S.; Gilliam, L. LY333013: A Candidate first-in-class, broad spectrum, oral field antidote to snakebite with curative potential. *Ann. Emerg. Med.* **2018**, *72*, S125. [CrossRef]
30. Still, K.B.M.; Slagboom, J.; Kidwai, S.; Xie, C.; Zhao, Y.; Eisses, B.; Jiang, Z.; Vonk, F.J.; Somsen, G.W.; Casewell, N.R.; et al. Development of high-throughput screening assays for profiling snake venom phospholipase A$_2$ activity after chromatographic fractionation. *Toxicon* **2020**, *184*, 28–38. [CrossRef]
31. Still, K.B.M.; Nandlal, R.S.; Slagboom, J.; Somsen, G.W.; Casewell, N.R.; Kool, J. Multipurpose HTS coagulation analysis: Assay development and assessment of coagulopathic snake venoms. *Toxins* **2017**, *9*, 382. [CrossRef]
32. Xie, C.; Slagboom, J.; Albulescu, L.-O.; Bruyneel, B.; Still, K.B.M.; Vonk, F.J.; Somsen, G.W.; Casewell, N.R.; Kool, J. Antivenom neutralization of coagulopathic snake venom toxins assessed by bioactivity profiling using nanofractionation analytics. *Toxins* **2020**, *12*, 53. [CrossRef]
33. Slagboom, J.; Mladić, M.; Xie, C.; Kazandjian, T.D.; Vonk, F.; Somsen, G.W.; Casewell, N.R.; Kool, J. High throughput screening and identification of coagulopathic snake venom proteins and peptides using nanofractionation and proteomics approaches. *PLoS Negl. Trop. Dis.* **2020**, *14*, e0007802. [CrossRef]

34. Kerns, R.T.; Kini, R.M.; Stefansson, S.; Evans, H.J. Targeting of venom phospholipases: The strongly anticoagulant phospholipase A_2 from *Naja nigricollis* venom binds to coagulation factor Xa to inhibit the prothrombinase complex. *Arch. Biochem. Biophys.* **1999**, *369*, 107–113. [CrossRef] [PubMed]
35. Mounier, C.M.; Bon, C.; Kini, R.M. Anticoagulant venom and mammalian secreted phospholipases A_2: Protein-versus phospholipid-dependent mechanism of action. *Pathophysiol. Haemost. Thromb.* **2001**, *31*, 279–287. [CrossRef] [PubMed]
36. Kini, R.M.; Evans, H.J. A model to explain the pharmacological effects of snake venom phospholipases A_2. *Toxicon* **1989**, *27*, 613–635. [CrossRef]
37. Zdenek, C.N.; Youngman, N.J.; Hay, C.; Dobson, J.; Dunstan, N.; Allen, L.; Milanovic, L.; Fry, B.G. Anticoagulant activity of black snake (Elapidae: *Pseudechis*) venoms: Mechanisms, potency, and antivenom efficacy. *Toxicol. Lett.* **2020**, *330*, 176–184. [CrossRef]
38. Youngman, N.J.; Walker, A.; Naude, A.; Coster, K.; Sundman, E.; Fry, B.G. Varespladib (LY315920) neutralises phospholipase A2 mediated prothrombinase-inhibition induced by *Bitis* snake venoms. *Comp. Biochem. Physiol. Part C Toxicol. Pharmacol.* **2020**, *236*, 108818.

biomedicines

MDPI

Article

Neutralizing Effects of Small Molecule Inhibitors and Metal Chelators on Coagulopathic *Viperinae* Snake Venom Toxins

Chunfang Xie [1,2], Laura-Oana Albulescu [3,4], Mátyás A. Bittenbinder [1,2,5], Govert W. Somsen [1,2], Freek J. Vonk [1,2], Nicholas R. Casewell [3,4] and Jeroen Kool [1,2,*]

1. Amsterdam Institute of Molecular and Life Sciences, Division of BioAnalytical Chemistry, Department of Chemistry and Pharmaceutical Sciences, Faculty of Science, Vrije Universiteit Amsterdam, De Boelelaan 1085, 1081HV Amsterdam, The Netherlands; c.xie@vu.nl (C.X.); m.a.bittenbinder@vu.nl (M.A.B.); g.w.somsen@vu.nl (G.W.S.); freek.vonk@naturalis.nl (F.J.V.)
2. Centre for Analytical Sciences Amsterdam (CASA), 1098 XH Amsterdam, The Netherlands
3. Centre for Snakebite Research and Interventions, Liverpool School of Tropical Medicine, Pembroke Place, Liverpool L3 5QA, UK; Laura-Oana.Albulescu@lstmed.ac.uk (L.-O.A.); Nicholas.Casewell@lstmed.ac.uk (N.R.C.)
4. Centre for Drugs and Diagnostics, Liverpool School of Tropical Medicine, Pembroke Place, Liverpool L3 5QA, UK
5. Naturalis Biodiversity Center, 2333 CR Leiden, The Netherlands

* Correspondence: j.kool@vu.nl

Received: 10 July 2020; Accepted: 18 August 2020; Published: 20 August 2020

Abstract: Animal-derived antivenoms are the only specific therapies currently available for the treatment of snake envenoming, but these products have a number of limitations associated with their efficacy, safety and affordability for use in tropical snakebite victims. Small molecule drugs and drug candidates are regarded as promising alternatives for filling the critical therapeutic gap between snake envenoming and effective treatment. In this study, by using an advanced analytical technique that combines chromatography, mass spectrometry and bioassaying, we investigated the effect of several small molecule inhibitors that target phospholipase A_2 (varespladib) and snake venom metalloproteinase (marimastat, dimercaprol and DMPS) toxin families on inhibiting the activities of coagulopathic toxins found in *Viperinae* snake venoms. The venoms of *Echis carinatus*, *Echis ocellatus*, *Daboia russelii* and *Bitis arietans*, which are known for their potent haemotoxicities, were fractionated in high resolution onto 384-well plates using liquid chromatography followed by coagulopathic bioassaying of the obtained fractions. Bioassay activities were correlated to parallel recorded mass spectrometric and proteomics data to assign the venom toxins responsible for coagulopathic activity and assess which of these toxins could be neutralized by the inhibitors under investigation. Our results showed that the phospholipase A_2-inhibitor varespladib neutralized the vast majority of anticoagulation activities found across all of the tested snake venoms. Of the snake venom metalloproteinase inhibitors, marimastat demonstrated impressive neutralization of the procoagulation activities detected in all of the tested venoms, whereas dimercaprol and DMPS could only partially neutralize these activities at the doses tested. Our results provide additional support for the concept that combinations of small molecules, particularly the combination of varespladib with marimastat, serve as a drug-repurposing opportunity to develop new broad-spectrum inhibitor-based therapies for snakebite envenoming.

Keywords: snakebite treatments; marimastat; varespladib; dimercaprol; DMPS; nanofractionation

1. Introduction

Bites by venomous snakes cause 81,000–138,000 deaths per annum, with the majority occurring in the rural resource-poor regions of the tropics and sub-tropics [1]. The venomous snakes responsible for the vast majority of severe envenomings are members of the *Viperidae* and *Elapidae* families [2,3]. Elapid snakes have venoms that are highly abundant in neurotoxins that disable muscle contraction and cause neuromuscular paralysis [1,4]. Contrastingly, viper venoms typically contain numerous proteins that disrupt the functioning of the coagulation cascade, the hemostatic system and tissue integrity [4,5]. Envenomings caused by these snakes can cause prominent local effects including necrosis, hemorrhage, edema and pain, and often result in permanent disabilities in survivors [6,7]. One of the most common but serious pathological effects of systemic viper envenoming is coagulopathy, which renders snakebite victims vulnerable to suffering lethal internal hemorrhages [8]. Venom induced coagulopathy following bites by viperid snakes is predominately the result of the synergistic action of venom enzymes, such as phospholipases A_2 (PLA_2s), snake venom serine proteinases (SVSPs) and snake venom metalloproteinases (SVMPs) [9–11]. PLA_2s can prevent blood clotting via anticoagulant effects. Enzymatic PLA_2s function by hydrolyzing glycerophospholipids at the sn-2 position of the glycerol backbone releasing lysophospholipids and fatty acids [12]. SVSPs can proteolytically degrade fibrinogen and release bradykinins from plasma kininogens [13,14]. SVMPs act on various clotting factors to stimulate consumption coagulopathy and can also degrade capillary basement membranes, thereby increasing vascular permeability and causing leakage [10,15,16]. These toxins can therefore work synergistically to cause systemic hemorrhage and coagulopathy.

The only specific therapies currently available for treating snake envenoming are animal-derived antivenoms. Consisting of immunoglobulins purified from hyperimmunized ovine or equine plasma/serum, these products save thousands of lives each year, but are associated with a number of therapeutic challenges, including limited cross-snake species efficacies, poor safety profiles and, for many snakebite victims residing in remote rural areas in developing countries, unacceptable issues with affordability and accessibility [17]. Small molecule toxin inhibitors are regarded as promising candidates for the development of affordable broad-spectrum snakebite treatments, as these can block the enzymatic activities of venoms [18–20]. Varespladib, an indole-based nonspecific pan-secretory PLA_2 inhibitor has been studied extensively for repurposing for snakebite. Having originally been investigated in Phase II and III clinical trials for treating septic shock, coronary heart disease and sickle cell disease-induced acute chest syndrome [21,22], varespladib has since been shown to be highly potent in suppressing venom-induced PLA_2 activity, both in vitro and in vivo in murine models [23]. Varespladib shows great promise against neurotoxic elapid snake venoms and has been shown to prevent lethality in murine in vivo models of envenoming [24], but is seemingly also capable of inhibiting certain myotoxic and coagulotoxic symptoms induced by snake venoms [25,26]. Moreover, varespladib has been demonstrated to inhibit the anticoagulant activity of *Pseudechis australis* snake venom, which was not neutralized by its currently used antivenom [27].

A number of other small molecules have shown promise for repurposing to inhibit SVMP venom toxins. Marimastat is a broad-spectrum matrix metalloprotease inhibitor that functions by binding to the active site of matrix metalloproteinases where it coordinates the metal ion in the binding pocket [28,29]. As a water-soluble orally bioavailable matrix metalloproteinase inhibitor [30,31], marimastat reached phase II and III clinical trials for multiple solid tumor types [32–34], including pancreatic, lung, breast, colorectal, brain and prostate cancer [35–37]. SVMPs are toxins that are structurally and functionally homologous to matrix metalloproteinses [38–40]. Like other compounds in this class of drugs (e.g., batimastat [41]), marimastat is a promising drug candidate for treating snakebite due to its inhibitory capabilities against SVMP toxins [42,43]. Marimastat was found to effectively inhibit the hemorrhagic, coagulant and defibrinogenating effects and proteinase activities induced by *Echis ocellatus* venom [42]. Dimercaprol, a historical drug approved by the World Health Organization (WHO) for treatment of heavy metal poisoning [44], contains two metal-chelating thiol groups and has long been used against arsenic, mercury, gold, lead and antimony intoxication [45–47]. It also represents a treatment option for Wilson's disease in which the body retains copper. Moreover, it has been studied as a candidate for acrolein detoxification as it can effectively reduce the acrolein concentration in vivo in murine because of its ability to bind to both the carbon double bond and aldehyde group of acrolein. The water-soluble, tissue-permeable and licensed metal chelator, 2,3-dimercaptopropane-1-sulfonic acid (DMPS), is also suitable for treating acute and chronic heavy metal intoxication including lead, mercury, cadmium and copper [48,49]. It was recently shown that both dimercaprol and DMPS displayed potential for repurposing as small molecule chelators to treat snake envenoming [20], most probably by chelating and removing Zn^{2+} from the active site of Zn^{2+}-dependent SVMPs. Of the two drugs, DMPS showed highly promising preclinical efficacy when used as an early oral intervention after envenoming by the SVMP-rich venom of the West African saw-scaled viper (*Echis ocellatus*), prior to later antivenom treatment with antivenom [20]. In addition to protecting against venom-induced lethality, DMPS was also demonstrated to drastically reduce local venom-induced hemorrhage [20]. Thus, marimastat, dimercaprol and DMPS all represent promising candidates for drug repurposing as snakebite therapeutics, as they either inhibit SVMPs or chelate the Zn^{2+} ion required for SVMP catalysis.

Nanofractionation analytics, which is a recently developed high resolution and high throughput format of traditional bioassay-guided fractionation, is regarded as an effective method for screening complex bioactive mixtures such as venoms to rapidly identify and in parallel directly characterize separated venom toxins biochemically (i.e., for selected bioactivities), by combing reversed-phase liquid chromatography (RPLC) with parallel post-column bioassays, mass spectrometry (MS) and proteomics analysis [50–52]. In this paper, the coagulopathic properties of various snakes from the medically important viper subfamily *Viperinae* (*Echis carinatus*, *E. ocellatus*, *Daboia russelii* and *Bitis arietans*) were evaluated using nanofractionation analytics in combination with a high-throughput coagulation assay, and the inhibitory capabilities of varespladib, marimastat, dimercaprol and DMPS against the coagulopathic toxicities of the resulting snake venom fractions revealed. To this end, bioactivity chromatograms were acquired after fractionation, and parallel obtained mass spectrometry and proteomics data were used to correlate the observed bioactivities with the identity of the venom toxins responsible for the observed enzymatic effects. Thus, we assessed the ability of varespladib, marimastat, dimercaprol and DMPS to neutralize the coagulopathic venom components. The results indicated that varespladib in combination with heavy metal chelators and/or broad-spectrum protease inhibitors could be viable first line therapeutic candidates for initial and adjunct treatment of coagulopathic snakebite envenoming.

2. Experimental

2.1. Chemicals

Water from a Milli-Q Plus system (Millipore, Amsterdam, The Netherlands) was used. Acetronitrile (ACN) and formic acid (FA) were supplied by Biosolve (Valkenswaard, The Netherlands). Calcium chloride ($CaCl_2$, dehydrate, ≥99%) was from Sigma-Aldrich (Zwijndrecht, The Netherlands) and was used to de-citrate plasma to initiate coagulation in the coagulation assay. Phosphate buffered saline (PBS) was prepared by dissolving PBS tablets (Sigma-Aldrich) in water according to the manufacturer's instructions and was stored at −4 °C for no longer than one week prior to use. Sodium citrated bovine plasma was obtained from Biowest (Nuaillé, France) as sterile filtered. The plasma (500 mL bottle) was defrosted in a warm water bath, and then quickly transferred to 15 mL CentriStar^{TM} tubes (Corning Science, Reynosa, Mexico). These 15 mL tubes were then immediately re-frozen at −80 °C, where they were stored until use. Venoms were sourced from either wild-caught specimens maintained in, or historical venom samples stored in, the Herpetarium of the Liverpool School of Tropical Medicine (LSTM). This facility and its protocols for the expert husbandry of snakes are approved and inspected by the UK Home Office and the LSTM and University of Liverpool Animal Welfare and Ethical Review Boards. The venom pools were from vipers with diverse geographical localities, namely: *B. arietans*

(Nigeria), *D. russelii* (Sri Lanka), *E. carinatus* (India) and *E. ocellatus* (Nigeria). Note that the Indian *E. carinatus* venom was collected from a single specimen that was inadvertently imported to the UK via a boat shipment of stone, and then rehoused at LSTM on the request of the UK Royal Society for the Prevention of Cruelty to Animals (RSPCA). Venom solutions were prepared by dissolving lyophilized venoms into water to a concentration of 5.0 ± 0.1 mg/mL and were stored at −80 °C until use. The compounds varespladib (A-001), marimastat ((2S,3R)-N4-[(1S)-2,2-Dimethyl-1-[(methylamino) carbonyl] propyl]-N1,2-dihydroxy-3-(2-methylpropyl) butanedia- mide), dimercaprol (2,3-Dimercapto-1-propanol) and DMPS (2,3-dimercapto-1-propane-sulfonic acid sodium salt monohydrate) were purchased from Sigma-Aldrich. They were dissolved in DMSO (≥99.9%, Sigma-Aldrich) to a concentration of 10 mM and stored at −20 °C. Prior to use, these four compounds were diluted in PBS buffer to the described concentrations.

2.2. Venom Nanofractionation

All venoms were nanofractionated onto transparent 384-well plates, and the plates with fractions were freeze dried overnight, according to the method described in our previous published papers by Slagboom et al. [53] and Xie et al. [52,54]. A detailed description can also be found in the Supporting Information (Section S1).

2.3. Plasma Coagulation Activity Assay

The HTS plasma coagulation assay used in this study was developed by Still et al. [55]. Sample preparation, assay performed and data analysis were described in our previous published paper by Still et al. [55], Slagboom et al. [53] and Xie et al. [52,54]. The final concentrations of the inhibitor solutions used in the coagulation bioassay were 20 μM, 4 μM and 0.8 μM, and in some cases 0.16 μM, 0.032 μM and 0.0064 μM. A detailed description can also be found in the Supporting Information (Section S2).

2.4. Correlation of Biological Data with MS Data

The corresponding accurate mass(es) and proteomics data for each venom fraction in this study have already been acquired by Slagboom et al. [53] and as such were correlated with the bioactivity chromatograms obtained in the current study. For venoms under study in this project that were not studied by Slagboom et al. [53], the same procedure as previously described [53] was followed to acquire and process proteomics data on these snake venoms. The UniprotKB database was used to determine the toxin class and any known functions for the relevant toxins thought to be responsible for the observed coagulopathic toxicities. For LC separations performed at different times and in different labs, the retention times of eluting snake venom toxins may differ slightly. The LC-UV chromatograms (measured at 220 nm, 254 nm and 280 nm), which provided characteristic fingerprint profiles for each venom fraction, were used to negotiate these retention time shifts. By using the LC-UV data, the chromatographic bioassay data from this study was correlated with the MS total-ion currents (TICs), extracted-ion chromatograms (XICs), and proteomics data obtained by Slagboom et al. [53]. In order to construct useful XICs, MS spectra were extracted from the time frames that correlated with regions in the chromatograms for each bioactive peak. Then, for all *m/z* values showing a significant signal observed in the mass spectra, XICs were plotted. In turn, these XICs were used for matching with peak retention times of bioactive compounds in the chromatograms. The exact masses matching the bioactives were tentatively assigned based on matching peak shape and correlation with retention times in bioassay traces. More specifically, the *m/z*-values in the MS data were correlated to each bioactive peak using the accurate monoisotopic masses determined by applying the deconvolution option in the MS software. For the proteomics data, in-well tryptic digestions were previously performed by Slagboom et al. [53] on snake venom fractions. These proteomics results were directly correlated to the coagulopathic activities that were indicated by the bioassay chromatograms.

3. Results

In this study, a nanofractionation approach was used to evaluate the inhibitory effects of varespladib, marimastat, dimercaprol and DMPS on the coagulopathic properties of venom toxins fractionated from a variety of *Viperinae* snake species. A recently developed low-volume HTS coagulation bioassay was used to assess the coagulation activities of LC-fractionated venoms in a 384-well plate format. These coagulopathic activities were correlated to parallel obtained MS and proteomics data to determine which specific venom toxins were neutralized by the potential inhibitors. All analyses were performed in at least duplicate to ensure reproducibility, and used venom concentrations of 1.0 mg/mL.

3.1. *Inhibitory Effects of Varespladib, Marimastat, Dimercaprol and DMPS on Echis Venoms*

Two geographically distinct saw-scaled viper venoms (genus *Echis*) were investigated in this study, specifically from the Indian species *E. carinatus* and the west African species *E. ocellatus*. The inhibitory effects of varespladib, marimastat, dimercaprol and DMPS against the coagulopathic activities observed for LC fractions of both venoms were investigated in a concentration-dependent fashion (Figures 1 and 2). Duplicate bioassay chromatograms together with a detailed description of each coagulopathic peak observed are presented in the Supporting Information (Section S3, Figures S1–S8).

Figure 1 shows the bioassay chromatograms of nanofractionated venom toxins from *E. carinatus* in the presence of different concentrations of varespladib, marimastat, dimercaprol and DMPS. In the venom-only analysis, potent procoagulation activities were observed in the very fast coagulation chromatogram (22.0–22.9 min) and the slightly/medium increased coagulation chromatogram (21.2–23.1 min and/or 19.9–21.2 min), while anticoagulation activities were observed in the anticoagulation chromatogram (19.1–19.9 min). Interestingly, the PLA_2-inhibitor varespladib inhibited both the anticoagulation and procoagulation activities, with the exception of one major peak observed in the slightly/medium increased coagulation chromatogram. In contrast, marimastat, dimercaprol and DMPS only exerted inhibitory effects on the procoagulation activities of *E. carinatus* venom. The anticoagulation activity of *E. carinatus* venom was fully inhibited by varespladib at a 20 μM concentration, while the very fast procoagulation activity was fully inhibited by varespladib, dimercaprol and DMPS at a concentration of 4 μM. Marimastat superseded the other small molecules by fully inhibiting the very fast procoagulation activity at a concentration of 0.16 μM. The slightly/medium increased coagulation activity was fully inhibited by 0.8 μM marimastat, but a sharp positive peak (21.7–22.2 min) was still retained following incubation with 20 μM varespladib. Dimercaprol only inhibited the front peak (21.3–22.1 min) present in the slightly/medium increased coagulation activity chromatogram, while DMPS inhibited mostly the tailing part (22.2–23.1 min) of this peak at its highest concentration tested (20 μM). Overall, DMPS was found to be more effective than dimercaprol in abrogating the procoagulation toxicities of *E. carinatus* venom. These findings demonstrate that the tested inhibitors have different specificities, but that marimastat most effectively inhibits the procoagulant components, and varespladib the anticoagulant components, of *E. carinatus* venom.

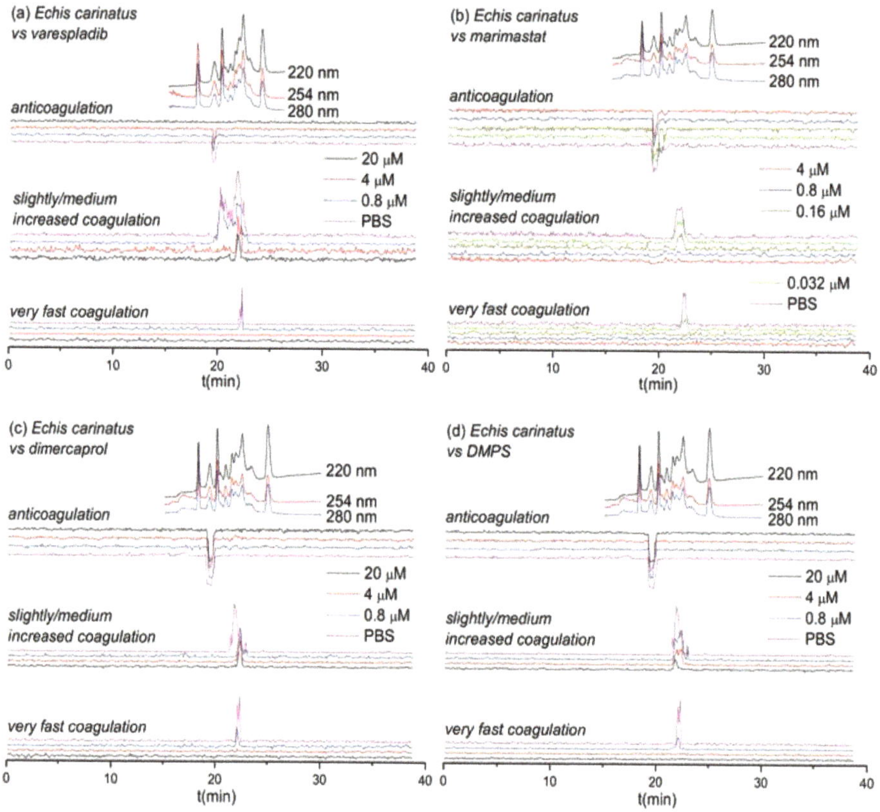

Figure 1. UV absorbance chromatograms and reconstructed coagulopathic toxicity chromatograms of nanofractionated toxins from *E. carinatus* venom in the presence of different concentrations of (**a**) varespladib, (**b**) marimastat, (**c**) dimercaprol and (**d**) DMPS.

Figure 2 shows the bioassay chromatograms for nanofractionated toxins from *E. ocellatus* venom in the presence of different concentrations of varespladib, marimastat, dimercaprol and DMPS. In the venom-only analysis, we observed similar results to those obtained for *E. carinatus* venom; multiple co-eluting sharp peaks were present in the very fast coagulation chromatogram (25.1–26.2 min), the slightly/medium increased coagulation chromatogram (25.1–27.1 min) and the anticoagulation chromatogram (23.4–24.4 min). All peaks decreased in height and width with increasing varespladib concentrations. The potent negative peak (23.4–24.4 min) in the anticoagulation chromatograms was fully inhibited by 4 μM varespladib and the later eluting weakly negative peak (25.9 min) by 20 μM varespladib. While full inhibition of anticoagulation activities was achieved, the procoagulation activities were not fully inactivated at the highest varespladib concentration tested (20 μM). However, both the very fast coagulation activity and the slightly/medium increased coagulation activity were also somewhat reduced by varespladib in a concentration-dependent fashion. Similar findings, whereby both very fast and slightly/medium increased coagulation were reduced in a concentration dependent manner but not fully abrogated, were also observed for dimercaprol, although this inhibitor had no effect on anticoagulant venom activities. Marimastat and DMPS also had no effect on anticoagulant venom activity, but effectively inhibited the procoagulant actions of *E. ocellatus* venom. Very fast procoagulation activity was fully inhibited at a lower concentration of marimastat (0.16 μM) than DMPS (20 μM), while slightly/medium increased coagulation activity was fully inhibited by 4 μM marimastat compared with almost complete inhibition observed when using 20 μM DMPS. Thus, similar to findings with *E. carinatus*, marimastat exhibited superior inhibition of procoagulant venom activities, while varespladib was the only inhibitor capable of abrogating anticoagulant venom effects.

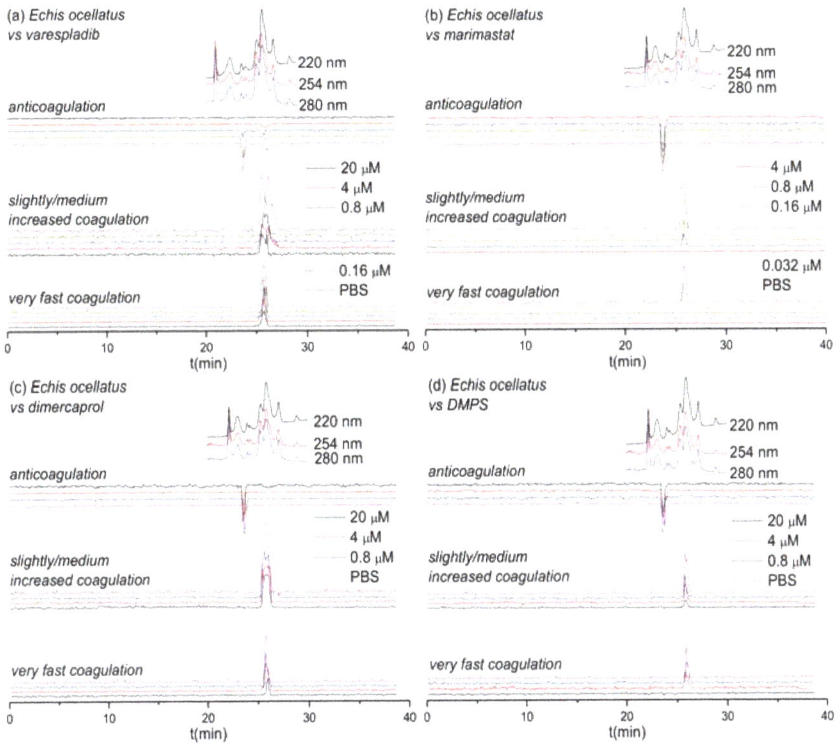

Figure 2. UV absorbance chromatograms reconstructed coagulopathic toxicity chromatograms of nanofractionated toxins from *E. ocellatus* venom in the presence of different concentrations of (**a**) varespladib, (**b**) marimastat, (**c**) dimercaprol and (**d**) DMPS.

3.2. Inhibitory Effect of Varespladib, Marimastat, Dimercaprol and DMPS on *Daboia russelii* Venom

Next, we assessed the inhibitory capability of the same small molecule toxin inhibitors on a *Viperinae* snake from a different genus: the Russell's viper (*Daboia russelii*), which is a medically-important species found in south Asia [56–58]. The inhibitory effects of varespladib, marimastat, dimercaprol and DMPS on the venom of *D. russelii* are shown in Figure 3. Duplicate bioassay chromatograms for *D. russelii* venom analyses can be found in the Supporting Information in Section S4 (Figures S9–S12). For the venom-only analysis, a strong positive peak was observed for both the very fast coagulation activity (21.5–22.4 min) and for the slightly/medium increased coagulation activity (21.5–22.8 min). A very broad and strong negative activity peak (18.6–21.5 min) was also observed, demonstrating potent anticoagulation activity. In terms of procoagulant venom effects, both very fast and slightly/medium increased coagulation activities decreased dose-dependently in the presence of varespladib, marimastat and dimercaprol, although neither varespladib nor dimercaprol could fully neutralize these activities. However, in line with the earlier findings for the two *Echis* spp., full neutralization of both types of procoagulation were observed with marimastat, at 0.8 μM for very fast coagulation activity and at 4 μM for slightly/medium increased coagulation activity. As anticipated, and again in line with findings observed with *Echis* spp., neither of the SVMP-inhibitors (marimastat and dimercaprol) abrogated anticoagulant venom activity. In contrast, varespladib showed potent inhibition of anticoagulation, as the broad and potent negative peak (18.6–21.5 min) decreased to only a very minor negative peak (19.5–20.2 min; 20 μM varespladib) with increasing varespladib concentrations. DMPS showed no inhibition on both the procoagulant and anticoagulant venom activities of *D. russelii* at the tested inhibitor concentrations of 20 μM and 4 μM.

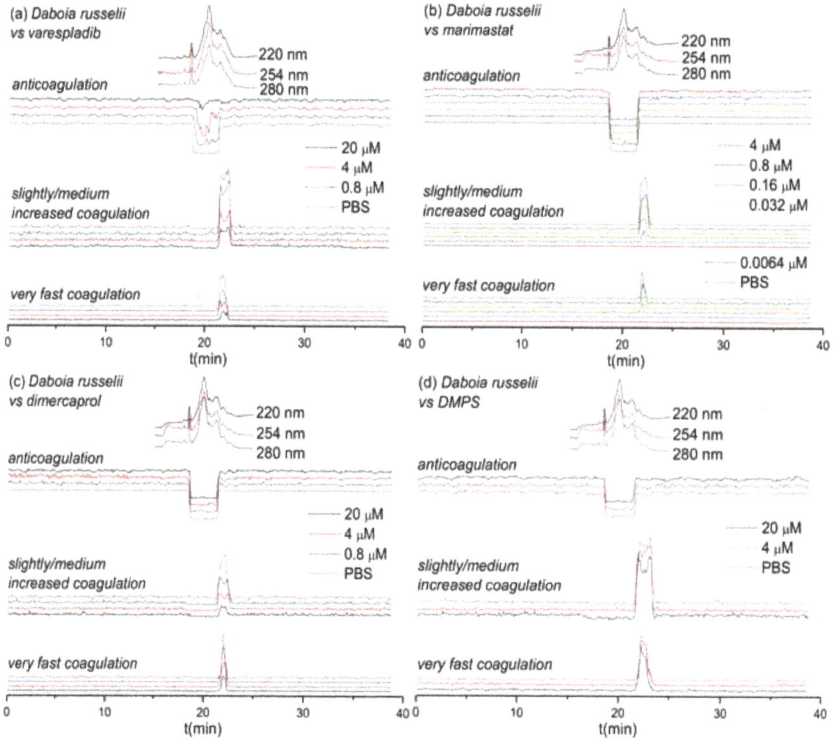

Figure 3. UV absorbance chromatograms and reconstructed coagulopathic toxicity chromatograms of nanofractionated toxins from *D. russelii* venom in the presence of different concentrations of (**a**) varespladib, (**b**) marimastat, (**c**) dimercaprol and (**d**) DMPS.

3.3. Inhibitory Effects of Varespladib and Marimastat on Bitis arietans Venom

The inhibitory effects of varespladib and marimastat on the coagulopathic properties of venom of the puff adder (*B. arietans*), which is found widely distributed across sub-Saharan Africa and parts of the Middle East, are shown in Figure 4. Duplicate bioassay chromatograms for the *B. arietans* venom analyses are shown in the Supporting Information in Section S5 (Figures S13 and S14). In the venom-only analyses, anticoagulation activity was observed as two sharp negative peaks in the bioactivity chromatograms (16.2–16.7 min and 16.7–17.1 min); however, no procoagulation activity was detected, which is consistent with previous findings using this venom [59]. Consequently, of the three SVMP-inhibitors used elsewhere in this study, we only selected marimastat for assessment of toxin inhibition as a control for the PLA_2-inhibitor varespladib. In line with findings from the other *Viperinae* species under study, increasing concentrations of varespladib resulted in full inhibition of the two negative anticoagulation peaks, at concentrations of 0.16 μM and 0.8 μM, respectively. Conversely, and also in line with our earlier findings, no anticoagulant inhibitory effects were observed with marimastat, even at concentrations of 20 μM.

3.4. Identification of Coagulopathic Venom Toxins Neutralized by Small Molecule Inhibitors

The MS and proteomics data previously obtained by Slagboom et al. [53] was next used to assign the venom toxins responsible for the observed coagulation activities tentative identifications. The resulting identifications are listed in Table 1. In addition, all tentatively identified anticoagulant PLA_2s, including those found in our study not previously described as possessing anticoagulant properties in the UniprotKB database, are also provided in Table 1. For those toxins for which no exact mass data could be acquired by LC-MS, only the proteomics mass data retrieved from Mascot searches are presented in the table.

Based on the results from Figures 1–4 and Table 1, the inhibitory effects of varespladib, marimastat, dimercaprol and DMPS on individual *Viperinae* venom toxins were assessed. PLA_2 toxins were identified as toxin components responsible for anticoagulation in all species studied, except for *B. arietans*, for which C-Type Lectins (CTLs) were instead identified. All these identified anticoagulant toxins were fully abrogated by varespladib at various concentrations, as indicated in Table 1. Although the CTLs identified from *B. arietans* venom are highly likely to have co-eluted with other venom proteins, no other anticoagulants were identified from this venom. The toxins identified from the Mascot results for the procoagulant peaks of *E. ocellatus* venom included both SVMPs and CTLs. All these identified toxins were fully abrogated by marimastat at 0.16 μM or by DMPS at 20 μM concentrations. No procoagulant toxins could be identified from the Mascot results for *E. carinatus* and *D. russelii* venoms, but given that these bioactivity peaks were fully inhibited by marimastat at low concentrations, it seems reasonable to speculate that the procoagulant toxins responsible for these activities are mainly SVMPs. A detailed description of the results discussed here is provided in the Supporting Information in Section S6.

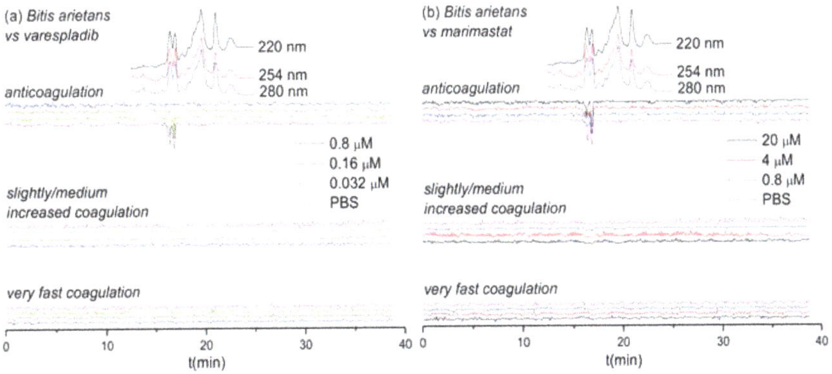

Figure 4. UV absorbance chromatograms and reconstructed coagulopathic toxicity chromatograms of nanofractionated toxins from *B. arietans* venom in the presence of different concentrations of (**a**) varespladib and (**b**) marimastat.

There are a number of challenges associated with interpreting the data presented here. In cases where multiple toxins elute closely, unambiguously assigning single toxins to each detected bioactivity is challenging. For bioactive compounds that eluted in activity peaks that were only partly inhibited, it is difficult to critically determine which of them was abrogated. This would require further improving LC separations under toxin non-denaturating and MS compatible eluent conditions. As a critical note, it is important to stress that despite venom toxins generally being stable, during chromatography within the nanofractionation analytics pipeline some venom toxins might have (partly) denatured and thereby lost their activity.

Table 1. Correlated MS and proteomics data for associated coagulopathic venom toxins. (Peak retention times are adapted from Figures 1–4; PLA_2 = phospholipase A_2; SVMP = Snake Venom Metalloproteinase; CTL = C-Type Lectin).

Species	Peak Retention Time (min)	Mascot Results Matching the Exact Mass	Exact Mass from MS Data	Exact Mass from Mascot Data	Toxin Class	Activity	Dose Required for Full Inhibition
E. carinatus	19.1–19.9	PA2A1_ECHCA	–	16310	PLA_2	Anticoagulant	20 µM varespladib
	19.9–23.1	–	–	–	–	Procoagulant	0.8 µM marimastat
E. ocellatus	23.4–24.4	PA2A5_ECHOC	13856.138	13856	PLA_2	Anticoagulant	4 µM varespladib
	25.1–27.1	VM3E2_ECHOC	–	69426	SVMP	Procoagulant	0.16 µM marimastat/20 µM DMPS
	25.1–27.1	VM3E6_ECHOC	–	57658	SVMP	Procoagulant	0.16 µM marimastat/20 µM DMPS
	25.1–27.1	SL1_ECHOC	–	16601	CTL	Procoagulant	0.16 µM marimastat/20 µM DMPS
	25.1–27.1	SL124_ECHOC	–	16882	CTL	Procoagulant	0.16 µM marimastat/20 µM DMPS
D. russelii	18.6–21.5	PA2B8_DABRR	13587.225	13587	PLA_2	Anticoagulant	20 µM varespladib
	18.6–21.5	PA2B5_DABRR	–	13587	PLA_2	Anticoagulant	20 µM varespladib
	18.6–21.5	PA2B3_DABRR	–	13687	PLA_2	Anticoagulant	20 µM varespladib
	21.5–22.8	–	–	–	–	Procoagulant	4 µM marimastat
B. arietans	16.7–17.1	SLA_BITAR	–	14935	CTL	Anticoagulant	0.8 µM varespladib
	16.7–17.1	SLB_BITAR	–	14798	CTL	Anticoagulant	0.8 µM varespladib

4. Discussion

There is an urgent need for stable, effective and affordable snakebite treatments that can be administered in the field and in rural areas where medical access is limited. Small molecule inhibitors that specifically target a number of key classes of snake venom toxins have recently gained interest as candidates for therapeutic alternatives to conventional antivenom.

This study used a high-throughput screening assay combined with LC fractionation and parallel MS and proteomics data to assess the neutralizing capabilities of a selected number of small molecule inhibitors and chelators (i.e., varespladib, marimastat, dimercaprol and DMPS). The results of this study show that these compounds are capable of neutralizing the coagulopathic activities of individual toxins present in the venoms of a number of *Viperinae* species. While this is consistent with previous work on small molecule inhibitors and chelators that exhibit anti-hemorrhagic and anti-procoagulant activities of snake venoms [9,20,23,42,43,60], here we have studied the relative neutralization potencies of these small molecules on individual coagulopathic venom toxins. Our findings reveal that varespladib is not only effective against the activity of anti-coagulant PLA_2 toxins, but also shows some inhibitory activity against procoagulant venom toxins. Varespladib potently and completely inhibited the anticoagulant activities detected in all venoms, except for *D. russelii*, for which almost complete inhibition was observed. Furthermore, varespladib showed some degree of inhibition against procoagulant venom activities across the various venoms, despite these activities not known to be mediated by PLA_2 toxins. Contrastingly, of the SVMP-inhibitors tested, we demonstrate that their specificities are restricted to effects on procoagulant venoms toxins, and that the peptidomimetic hydroxamate inhibitor marimastat outperforms the metal chelators DMPS and dimercaprol in terms of potency. Marimastat potently inhibited procoagulant activities across the venoms tested and was unsurprisingly ineffective against anticoagulant venom activities. However, only moderate inhibition was observed for most venoms with the metal chelators, and no inhibition was found at all for DMPS on *D. russelii* venom. Neither DMPS nor dimercaprol inhibited the non-SVMP stimulated anticoagulant venom activities observed across the venoms.

The advantages of repurposing licensed medicines (e.g., DMPS and dimercaprol) or phase II-approved drug candidates (e.g., marimastat and varespladib) are that these molecules have demonstrated safety profiles and thus drug development times could be significantly shortened as these agents have extensive pharmacokinetic, bioavailability and tolerance data already associated with them [23,61,62]. The small size of these compounds, compared with conventional antibodies, confer desirable drug-favorable properties enabling rapid and effective tissue penetration and, depending on the pharmacokinetics and physicochemical properties of specific inhibitors, often make them amenable for oral delivery [61,63,64]. Indeed, both varespladib and DMPS have already been demonstrated to confer preclinical efficacy against snakebite via the oral route [20,63,64]. DMPS is readily absorbed following oral administration in humans, making it a strong candidate for an oral community-based therapy [65]; and there are no major side effects or teratogenic effects that have been reported on DMPS in murine models [66,67]. In contrast, dimercaprol is challenging for clinical use as it currently requires administration by painful intramuscular injection. Dosing regimens of each inhibitor therefore need further robust investigation in the context of snakebite in order to help inform lead candidate selection.

Certain small molecule inhibitors have been demonstrated to exhibit broad inhibition of specific toxin families across diverse medically-important snake species [23,59], as also evidenced here for the various coagulopathic toxins found across *Viperinae* venoms. However, these compounds typically target only a single family of enzymatic toxins (although varespladib seems perhaps capable of targeting more than one family; see Figures 1a, 2a and 3a), thus presenting a challenge for these molecules to become standalone therapeutics, as other non-inhibited toxins seem likely to still cause pathology in snakebite victims. It is therefore more likely that small molecule inhibitors will need to be combined into therapeutic mixtures, either with other toxin inhibitors or monoclonal antibodies, to generate snakebite therapeutics capable of neutralizing the most important pathological snake venom toxin families [26,59,61,62]. Small molecule inhibitors could serve as valuable prehospital snakebite treatments to delay the onset of severe envenoming before the arrival of victims to secondary or tertiary healthcare facilities to receive subsequent therapy (i.e., conventional antivenoms). This is important, because treatment delays are known to have major detrimental impacts on patient outcomes following snakebite [68,69]. Indeed, compounds such as varespladib and DMPS are already being explored in this regard [20,63,64], as they represent promising candidates to be used as bridging therapies for delaying the major effects of envenomation, and reducing the long time it typically takes rural, isolated, impoverished snakebite victims to receive any form of treatment.

The many limitations associated with conventional snakebite treatments have resulted in their weak demand, low availability and poor affordability, despite huge unmet medical need. Small molecule "toxin inhibitors" offer great potential to rapidly deliver inexpensive, safe and efficacious interventions in the community soon after a snakebite, prior to subsequent admission to a healthcare facility. Many small molecule inhibitors also offer superior pharmacokinetics in terms of efficiently reaching local tissues, such as bite sites, in contrary to antibodies. The findings presented here further support the exploration of such inhibitors as potential future snakebite treatments.

5. Conclusions

In this study, a recently developed HTS coagulation assay was combined with LC fractionation and parallel obtained MS and proteomics data to assess the neutralizing potency of several small molecule inhibitors and chelators (i.e., varespladib, marimastat, dimercaprol and DMPS) against the coagulopathic activities of individual toxins found in the venoms of *Viperinae* snakes. These compounds show great promise for the development of affordable, broad-spectrum, first-aid and clinical treatment of snakebite. Our data further strengthens recent findings suggesting that small molecule inhibitors, such as varespladib and marimastat, may have broad, cross-species, neutralizing capabilities that make them highly amenable for translation into new "generic" snakebite therapeutics. Given our evidence that both inhibitors have different specificities, our findings further support the concept that a therapeutic combination consisting of both of these Phase II-approved small molecule toxin inhibitors [59] show potential as a new broad-spectrum snakebite treatment.

Supplementary Materials: The supporting information related to this article can be found in *"Supplementary Materials: Neutralizing effects of small molecule inhibitors and metal chelators on coagulopathic Viperinae snake venom toxins"*. The following are available online at http://www.mdpi.com/2227-9059/8/9/297/s1, Figure S1: Duplicate bioassay chromatograms of nanofractionated *E. carinatus* venom in the presence of different concentrations of varespladib; Figure S2: Duplicate bioassay chromatograms of nanofractionated *E. carinatus* venom in the presence of different concentrations of marimastat; Figure S3: Duplicate bioassay chromatograms of nanofractionated *E. carinatus* venom in the presence of different concentrations of dimercaprol; Figure S4: Duplicate bioassay chromatograms of nanofractionated *E. carinatus* venom in the presence of different concentrations of DMPS; Figure S5: Duplicate bioassay chromatograms of nanofractionated *E. ocellatus* venom in the presence of different concentrations of varespladib; Figure S6: Duplicate bioassay chromatograms of nanofractionated *E. ocellatus* venom in the presence of different concentrations of marimastat; Figure S7: Duplicate bioassay chromatograms of nanofractionated *E. ocellatus* venom in the presence of different concentrations of dimercaprol; Figure S8: Duplicate bioassay chromatograms of nanofractionated *E. ocellatus* venom in the presence of different concentrations of DMPS; Figure S9: Duplicate bioassay chromatograms of nanofractionated *D. russelii* venom in the presence of different concentrations of varespladib; Figure S10: Duplicate bioassay chromatograms of nanofractionated *D. russelii* venom in the presence of different concentrations of marimastat; Figure S11: Duplicate bioassay chromatograms of nanofarctionated *D. russelii* venom in the presence of different concentrations of dimercaprol; Figure S12: Duplicate bioassay chromatograms of nanofarctionated *D. russelii* venom in the presence of different concentrations of DMPS; Figure S13: Duplicate bioassay chromatograms of nanofractionated *B. arietans* venom in the presence of different concentrations of varespladib; Figure S14: Duplicate bioassay chromatograms of nanofractionated *B. arietans* venom in the presence of different concentrations of marimastat.

Author Contributions: Conceptualization, N.R.C. and J.K.; Data curation, C.X.; Formal analysis, C.X.; Funding acquisition, C.X., N.R.C. and J.K.; Investigation, C.X., L.-O.A., F.J.V., N.R.C. and J.K.; Methodology, C.X.; Project administration, J.K.; Resources, N.R.C. and J.K.; Supervision, J.K.; Writing—original draft, C.X.; Writing—review & editing, L.-O.A., M.A.B., G.W.S., F.J.V., N.R.C. and J.K.; All authors have read and agreed to the published version of the manuscript.

Funding: C.X. was funded by a China Scholarship Council (CSC) fellowship (201706250035). N.R.C. acknowledges support from a UK Medical Research Council (MRC) Research Grant (MR/S00016X/1) and Confidence in Concept

Award (CiC19017), and a Sir Henry Dale Fellowship (200517/Z/16/Z) jointly funded by the Wellcome Trust and Royal Society. The APC was funded by the Wellcome Trust.

Conflicts of Interest: The authors declare no conflict of interest.

References

1. Gutiérrez, J.M.; Calvete, J.J.; Habib, A.G.; Harrison, R.A.; Williams, D.J.; Warrell, D.A. Snakebite envenoming. *Nat. Rev. Dis. Primers* **2017**, *3*, 1–21. [CrossRef] [PubMed]
2. Rogalski, A.; Soerensen, C.; Op den Brouw, B.; Lister, C.; Dashevsky, D.; Arbuckle, K.; Gloria, A.; Zdenek, C.N.; Casewell, N.R.; Gutiérrez, J.M. Differential procoagulant effects of saw-scaled viper (Serpentes: Viperidae: *Echis*) snake venoms on human plasma and the narrow taxonomic ranges of antivenom efficacies. *Toxicol. Lett.* **2017**, *280*, 159–170. [CrossRef] [PubMed]
3. Gutiérrez, J.M.; Theakston, R.D.G.; Warrell, D.A. Confronting the neglected problem of snake bite envenoming: The need for a global partnership. *PLoS Med.* **2006**, *3*, e150. [CrossRef] [PubMed]
4. Calvete, J.J.; Sanz, L.; Angulo, Y.; Lomonte, B.; Gutiérrez, J.M. Venoms, venomics, antivenomics. *FEBS Lett.* **2009**, *583*, 1736–1743. [CrossRef] [PubMed]
5. Lu, Q.; Clemetson, J.; Clemetson, K.J. Snake venoms and hemostasis. *J. Thromb. Haemost.* **2005**, *3*, 1791–1799. [CrossRef]
6. Moura-da-Silva, A.; Butera, D.; Tanjoni, I. Importance of snake venom metalloproteinases in cell biology: Effects on platelets, inflammatory and endothelial cells. *Curr. Pharm. Des.* **2007**, *13*, 2893–2905. [CrossRef]
7. Sant'Ana Malaque, C.M.; Gutiérrez, J.M. Snakebite Envenomation in Central and South America. *Crit. Care Toxicol.* **2016**, 1–22. [CrossRef]
8. Maduwage, K.; Isbister, G.K. Current treatment for venom-induced consumption coagulopathy resulting from snakebite. *PLoS Negl. Trop. Dis.* **2014**, *8*, e3220. [CrossRef]
9. Ainsworth, S.; Slagboom, J.; Alomran, N.; Pla, D.; Alhamdi, Y.; King, S.I.; Bolton, F.M.; Gutiérrez, J.M.; Vonk, F.J.; Toh, C.-H. The paraspecific neutralisation of snake venom induced coagulopathy by antivenoms. *Commun. Biol.* **2018**, *1*, 1–14. [CrossRef]
10. Slagboom, J.; Kool, J.; Harrison, R.A.; Casewell, N.R. Haemotoxic snake venoms: Their functional activity, impact on snakebite victims and pharmaceutical promise. *Br. J. Haematol.* **2017**, *177*, 947–959. [CrossRef]
11. Kang, T.S.; Georgieva, D.; Genov, N.; Murakami, M.T.; Sinha, M.; Kumar, R.P.; Kaur, P.; Kumar, S.; Dey, S.; Sharma, S. Enzymatic toxins from snake venom: Structural characterization and mechanism of catalysis. *FEBS J.* **2011**, *278*, 4544–4576. [CrossRef] [PubMed]
12. Kini, R.M. Excitement ahead: Structure, function and mechanism of snake venom phospholipase A_2 enzymes. *Toxicon* **2003**, *42*, 827–840. [CrossRef] [PubMed]
13. Matsui, T.; Fujimura, Y.; Titani, K. Snake venom proteases affecting hemostasis and thrombosis. *Biochim. Biophys. Acta* **2000**, *1477*, 146–156. [CrossRef]
14. Serrano, S.M.; Maroun, R.C. Snake venom serine proteinases: Sequence homology vs. substrate specificity, a paradox to be solved. *Toxicon* **2005**, *45*, 1115–1132. [CrossRef]
15. Alvarez-Flores, M.P.; Faria, F.; de Andrade, S.A.; Chudzinski-Tavassi, A.M. Snake venom components affecting the coagulation system. In *Snake Venoms*; Gopalakrishnakone, P., Inagaki, H., Vogel, C.-W., Mukherjhee, A.K., Rahmy, T.R., Eds.; Springer: Dordrecht, Germany, 2017; pp. 417–436.
16. Ramos, O.; Selistre-de-Araujo, H. Snake venom metalloproteases—structure and function of catalytic and disintegrin domains. *Comp. Biochem. Physiol. Part C Toxicol. Pharmacol.* **2006**, *142*, 328–346. [CrossRef]
17. Williams, H.F.; Layfield, H.J.; Vallance, T.; Patel, K.; Bicknell, A.B.; Trim, S.A.; Vaiyapuri, S. The urgent need to develop novel strategies for the diagnosis and treatment of snakebites. *Toxins* **2019**, *11*, 363. [CrossRef]
18. Bulfone, T.C.; Samuel, S.P.; Bickler, P.E.; Lewin, M.R. Developing small molecule therapeutics for the Initial and adjunctive treatment of snakebite. *J. Trop. Med.* **2018**, 1–10. [CrossRef]
19. Resiere, D.; Gutiérrez, J.M.; Névière, R.; Cabié, A.; Hossein, M.; Kallel, H. Antibiotic therapy for snakebite envenoming. *J. Venom. Anim. Toxins Incl. Trop. Dis.* **2020**, *26*, 1–2. [CrossRef]
20. Albulescu, L.-O.; Hale, M.S.; Ainsworth, S.; Alsolaiss, J.; Crittenden, E.; Calvete, J.J.; Evans, C.; Wilkinson, M.C.; Harrison, R.A.; Kool, J. Preclinical validation of a repurposed metal chelator as an early-intervention therapeutic for hemotoxic snakebite. *Sci. Transl. Med.* **2020**, *12*, eaay8314. [CrossRef]

21. Abraham, E.; Naum, C.; Bandi, V.; Gervich, D.; Lowry, S.F.; Wunderink, R.; Schein, R.M.; Macias, W.; Skerjanec, S.; Dmitrienko, A. Efficacy and safety of LY315920Na/S-5920, a selective inhibitor of 14-kDa group IIA secretory phospholipase A_2, in patients with suspected sepsis and organ failure. *Crit. Care Med.* **2003**, *31*, 718–728. [CrossRef]
22. Nicholls, S.J.; Kastelein, J.J.; Schwartz, G.G.; Bash, D.; Rosenson, R.S.; Cavender, M.A.; Brennan, D.M.; Koenig, W.; Jukema, J.W.; Nambi, V. Varespladib and cardiovascular events in patients with an acute coronary syndrome: The VISTA-16 randomized clinical trial. *JAMA* **2014**, *311*, 252–262. [CrossRef] [PubMed]
23. Lewin, M.; Samuel, S.; Merkel, J.; Bickler, P. Varespladib (LY315920) appears to be a potent, broad-spectrum, inhibitor of snake venom phospholipase A_2 and a possible pre-referral treatment for envenomation. *Toxins* **2016**, *8*, 248. [CrossRef]
24. Gutiérrez, J.M.; Lewin, M.R.; Williams, D.; Lomonte, B. Varespladib (LY315920) and methyl varespladib (LY333013) abrogate or delay lethality induced by presynaptically acting neurotoxic snake venoms. *Toxins* **2020**, *12*, 131. [CrossRef] [PubMed]
25. Bryan-Quirós, W.; Fernández, J.; Gutiérrez, J.M.; Lewin, M.R.; Lomonte, B. Neutralizing properties of LY315920 toward snake venom group I and II myotoxic phospholipases A_2. *Toxicon* **2019**, *157*, 1–7. [CrossRef]
26. Bittenbinder, M.A.; Zdenek, C.N.; Op den Brouw, B.; Youngman, N.J.; Dobson, J.S.; Naude, A.; Vonk, F.J.; Fry, B.G. Coagulotoxic cobras: Clinical implications of strong anticoagulant actions of African spitting *Naja* venoms that are not neutralised by antivenom but are by LY315920 (Varespladib). *Toxins* **2018**, *10*, 516. [CrossRef] [PubMed]
27. Zdenek, C.N.; Youngman, N.J.; Hay, C.; Dobson, J.; Dunstan, N.; Allen, L.; Milanovic, L.; Fry, B.G. Anticoagulant activity of black snake (Elapidae: *Pseudechis*) venoms: Mechanisms, potency, and antivenom efficacy. *Toxicol. Lett.* **2020**, *330*, 176–184. [CrossRef]
28. Underwood, C.; Min, D.; Lyons, J.; Hambley, T. The interaction of metal ions and Marimastat with matrix metalloproteinase 9. *J. Inorg. Biochem.* **2003**, *95*, 165–170. [CrossRef]
29. Peterson, M.; Porter, K.; Loftus, I.; Thompson, M.; London, N. Marimastat inhibits neointimal thickening in a model of human arterial intimal hyperplasia. *Eur. J. Vasc. Endovasc. Surg.* **2000**, *19*, 461–467. [CrossRef]
30. Curran, S.; Murray, G.I. Matrix metalloproteinases in tumour invasion and metastasis. *J. Pathol.* **1999**, *189*, 300–308. [CrossRef]
31. Rasmussen, H.S.; McCann, P.P. Matrix metalloproteinase inhibition as a novel anticancer strategy: A review with special focus on batimastat and marimastat. *Pharmacol. Ther.* **1997**, *75*, 69–75. [CrossRef]
32. Evans, J.; Stark, A.; Johnson, C.; Daniel, F.; Carmichael, J.; Buckels, J.; Imrie, C.; Brown, P.; Neoptolemos, J. A phase II trial of marimastat in advanced pancreatic cancer. *Br. J. Cancer* **2001**, *85*, 1865. [CrossRef] [PubMed]
33. Winer, A.; Adams, S.; Mignatti, P. Matrix metalloproteinase inhibitors in cancer therapy: Turning past failures into future successes. *Mol. Cancer Ther.* **2018**, *17*, 1147–1155. [CrossRef] [PubMed]
34. Rosenbaum, E.; Zahurak, M.; Sinibaldi, V.; Carducci, M.A.; Pili, R.; Laufer, M.; DeWeese, T.L.; Eisenberger, M.A. Marimastat in the treatment of patients with biochemically relapsed prostate cancer: A prospective randomized, double-blind, phase I/II trial. *Clin. Cancer Res.* **2005**, *11*, 4437–4443. [CrossRef] [PubMed]
35. King, J.; Zhao, J.; Clingan, P.; Morris, D. Randomised double blind placebo control study of adjuvant treatment with the metalloproteinase inhibitor, Marimastat in patients with inoperable colorectal hepatic metastases: Significant survival advantage in patients with musculoskeletal side-effects. *Anticancer Res.* **2003**, *23*, 639–645. [PubMed]
36. Levin, V.A.; Phuphanich, S.; Yung, W.A.; Forsyth, P.A.; Del Maestro, R.; Perry, J.R.; Fuller, G.N.; Baillet, M. Randomized, double-blind, placebo-controlled trial of marimastat in glioblastoma multiforme patients following surgery and irradiation. *J. Neuro Oncol.* **2006**, *78*, 295–302. [CrossRef] [PubMed]
37. Bramhall, S.; Schulz, J.; Nemunaitis, J.; Brown, P.; Baillet, M.; Buckels, J. A double-blind placebo-controlled, randomised study comparing gemcitabine and marimastat with gemcitabine and placebo as first line therapy in patients with advanced pancreatic cancer. *Br. J. Cancer* **2002**, *87*, 161. [CrossRef]
38. Howes, J.-M.; Theakston, R.D.G.; Laing, G. Neutralization of the haemorrhagic activities of viperine snake venoms and venom metalloproteinases using synthetic peptide inhibitors and chelators. *Toxicon* **2007**, *49*, 734–739. [CrossRef]
39. Zhang, D.; Botos, I.; Gomis-Rüth, F.-X.; Doll, R.; Blood, C.; Njoroge, F.G.; Fox, J.W.; Bode, W.; Meyer, E.F. Structural interaction of natural and synthetic inhibitors with the venom metalloproteinase, atrolysin C (form d). *Proc. Natl. Acad. Sci. USA* **1994**, *91*, 8447–8451. [CrossRef]

40. Nagase, H.; Woessner, J.F. Matrix metalloproteinases. *J. Biol. Chem.* **1999**, *274*, 21491–21494. [CrossRef]
41. Rucavado, A.; Escalante, T.; Gutiérrez, J.M. Effect of the metalloproteinase inhibitor batimastat in the systemic toxicity induced by *Bothrops asper* snake venom: Understanding the role of metalloproteinases in envenomation. *Toxicon* **2004**, *43*, 417–424. [CrossRef]
42. Arias, A.S.; Rucavado, A.; Gutiérrez, J.M. Peptidomimetic hydroxamate metalloproteinase inhibitors abrogate local and systemic toxicity induced by *Echis ocellatus* (saw-scaled) snake venom. *Toxicon* **2017**, *132*, 40–49. [CrossRef] [PubMed]
43. Layfield, H.J.; Williams, H.F.; Ravishankar, D.; Mehmi, A.; Sonavane, M.; Salim, A.; Vaiyapuri, R.; Lakshminarayanan, K.; Vallance, T.M.; Bicknell, A.B. Repurposing cancer drugs batimastat and marimastat to inhibit the activity of a group I metalloprotease from the venom of the western diamondback rattlesnake, *Crotalus atrox*. *Toxins* **2020**, *12*, 309. [CrossRef] [PubMed]
44. World Health Organization. WHO Model List of Essential Medicines, 20th list (March 2017). 2017. Available online: http://www.who.int/medicines/publications/essentialmedicines/20th_EML2017_FINAL_amendedAug2017.pdf?ua=1 (accessed on 15 November 2017).
45. Tian, R.; Shi, R. Dimercaprol is an acrolein scavenger that mitigates acrolein-mediated PC-12 cells toxicity and reduces acrolein in rat following spinal cord injury. *J. Neurochem.* **2017**, *141*, 708–720. [CrossRef]
46. Verma, S.; Kumar, R.; Khadwal, A.; Singhi, S. Accidental inorganic mercury chloride poisoning in a 2-year old child. *Indian J. Pediatrics* **2010**, *77*, 1153–1155. [CrossRef]
47. Kathirgamanathan, K.; Angaran, P.; Lazo-Langner, A.; Gula, L.J. Cardiac conduction block at multiple levels caused by arsenic trioxide therapy. *Can. J. Cardiol.* **2013**, *29*, 130.e5–130.e6. [CrossRef]
48. Yajima, Y.; Kawaguchi, M.; Yoshikawa, M.; Okubo, M.; Tsukagoshi, E.; Sato, K.; Katakura, A. The effects of 2,3-dimercapto-1-propanesulfonic acid (DMPS) and meso-2,3-dimercaptosuccinic acid (DMSA) on the nephrotoxicity in the mouse during repeated cisplatin (CDDP) treatments. *J. Pharmacol. Sci.* **2017**, *134*, 108–115. [CrossRef]
49. Aldhaheri, S.R.; Jeelani, R.; Kohan-Ghadr, H.R.; Khan, S.N.; Mikhael, S.; Washington, C.; Morris, R.T.; Abu-Soud, H.M. Dimercapto-1-propanesulfonic acid (DMPS) induces metaphase II mouse oocyte deterioration. *Free Radic. Biol. Med.* **2017**, *112*, 445–451. [CrossRef]
50. Zietek, B.M.; Mayar, M.; Slagboom, J.; Bruyneel, B.; Vonk, F.J.; Somsen, G.W.; Casewell, N.R.; Kool, J. Liquid chromatographic nanofractionation with parallel mass spectrometric detection for the screening of plasmin inhibitors and (metallo) proteinases in snake venoms. *Anal. Bioanal. Chem.* **2018**, *410*, 5751–5763. [CrossRef]
51. Mladic, M.; Zietek, B.M.; Iyer, J.K.; Hermarij, P.; Niessen, W.M.; Somsen, G.W.; Kini, R.M.; Kool, J. At-line nanofractionation with parallel mass spectrometry and bioactivity assessment for the rapid screening of thrombin and factor Xa inhibitors in snake venoms. *Toxicon* **2016**, *110*, 79–89. [CrossRef]
52. Xie, C.; Slagboom, J.; Albulescu, L.-O.; Bruyneel, B.; Still, K.; Vonk, F.J.; Somsen, G.W.; Casewell, N.R.; Kool, J. Antivenom neutralization of coagulopathic snake venom toxins assessed by bioactivity profiling using nanofractionation analytics. *Toxins* **2020**, *12*, 53. [CrossRef]
53. Slagboom, J.; Mladić, M.; Xie, C.; Kazandjian, T.D.; Vonk, F.; Somsen, G.W.; Casewell, N.R.; Kool, J. High throughput screening and identification of coagulopathic snake venom proteins and peptides using nanofractionation and proteomics approaches. *PLoS Negl. Trop. Dis.* **2020**, *14*, e0007802. [CrossRef] [PubMed]
54. Xie, C.; Albulescu, L.-O.; Still, K.; Slagboom, J.; Zhao, Y.; Jiang, Z.; Somsen, G.W.; Vonk, F.J.; Casewell, N.R.; Kool, J. Varespladib inhibits the phospholipase A_2 and coagulopathic activities of venom components from hemotoxic snakes. *Biomedicines* **2020**, *8*, 165. [CrossRef] [PubMed]
55. Still, K.; Nandlal, R.S.; Slagboom, J.; Somsen, G.W.; Casewell, N.R.; Kool, J. Multipurpose HTS coagulation analysis: Assay development and assessment of coagulopathic snake venoms. *Toxins* **2017**, *9*, 382. [CrossRef] [PubMed]
56. Sharma, M.; Das, D.; Iyer, J.K.; Kini, R.M.; Doley, R. Unveiling the complexities of *Daboia russelii* venom, a medically important snake of India, by tandem mass spectrometry. *Toxicon* **2015**, *107*, 266–281. [CrossRef]
57. Hiremath, V.; Urs, A.N.; Joshi, V.; Suvilesh, K.; Savitha, M.; Amog, P.U.; Rudresha, G.; Yariswamy, M.; Vishwanath, B. Differential action of medically important Indian BIG FOUR snake venoms on rodent blood coagulation. *Toxicon* **2016**, *110*, 19–26. [CrossRef]
58. Hiremath, V.; Yariswamy, M.; Nanjaraj Urs, A.; Joshi, V.; Suvilesh, K.; Ramakrishnan, C.; Nataraju, A.; Vishwanath, B. Differential action of Indian BIG FOUR snake venom toxins on blood coagulation. *Toxin Rev.* **2014**, *33*, 23–32. [CrossRef]

59. Albulescu, L.-O.; Xie, C.; Ainsworth, S.; Alsolaiss, J.; Crittenden, E.; Dawson, C.A.; Softley, R.; Bartlett, K.E.; Harrison, R.A.; Kool, J.; et al. A combination of two small molecule toxin inhibitors provides pancontinental preclinical efficacy against viper snakebite. *bioRxiv* **2020**. (preprint). [CrossRef]
60. Wang, Y.; Zhang, J.; Zhang, D.; Xiao, H.; Xiong, S.; Huang, C. Exploration of the inhibitory potential of varespladib for snakebite envenomation. *Molecules* **2018**, *23*, 391. [CrossRef]
61. Kini, R.M.; Sidhu, S.S.; Laustsen, A.H. Biosynthetic oligoclonal antivenom (BOA) for snakebite and next-generation treatments for snakebite victims. *Toxins* **2018**, *10*, 534. [CrossRef]
62. Knudsen, C.; Ledsgaard, L.; Dehli, R.I.; Ahmadi, S.; Sørensen, C.V.; Laustsen, A.H. Engineering and design considerations for next-generation snakebite antivenoms. *Toxicon* **2019**, *167*, 67–75. [CrossRef]
63. Lewin, M.R.; Gutiérrez, J.M.; Samuel, S.P.; Herrera, M.; Bryan-Quirós, W.; Lomonte, B.; Bickler, P.E.; Bulfone, T.C.; Williams, D.J. Delayed oral LY333013 rescues mice from highly neurotoxic, lethal doses of Papuan Taipan (*Oxyuranus scutellatus*) venom. *Toxins* **2018**, *10*, 380. [CrossRef] [PubMed]
64. Lewin, M.R.; Gilliam, L.L.; Gilliam, J.; Samuel, S.P.; Bulfone, T.C.; Bickler, P.E.; Gutiérrez, J.M. Delayed LY333013 (oral) and LY315920 (intravenous) reverse severe neurotoxicity and rescue juvenile pigs from lethal doses of *Micrurus fulvius* (Eastern Coral snake) venom. *Toxins* **2018**, *10*, 479. [CrossRef] [PubMed]
65. Maiorino, R.M.; Dart, R.C.; Carter, D.E.; Aposhian, H.V. Determination and metabolism of dithiol chelating agents. XII. Metabolism and pharmacokinetics of sodium 2, 3-dimercaptopropane-1-sulfonate in humans. *J. Pharmacol. Exp. Ther.* **1991**, *259*, 808–814. [PubMed]
66. Planas-Bohne, F.; Gabard, B.; Schäffer, E. Toxicological studies on sodium 2, 3-dimercaptopropane-1-sulfonate in the rat. In *Arzneimittel-Forschung*; Thieme Medical Publishers: Leipzig, Germany, 1980; Volume 30, pp. 1291–1294.
67. Domingo, J.L.; Ortega, A.; Bosque, M.; Corbella, J. Evaluation of the developmental effects on mice after prenatal, or pre-and postnatal exposure to 2, 3-dimercaptopropane-1-sulfonic acid (DMPS). *Life Sci.* **1990**, *46*, 1287–1292. [CrossRef]
68. Sharma, S.K.; Chappuis, F.; Jha, N.; Bovier, P.A.; Loutan, L.; Koirala, S. Impact of snake bites and determinants of fatal outcomes in southeastern Nepal. *Am. J. Trop. Med. Hyg.* **2004**, *71*, 234–238. [CrossRef]
69. Abubakar, S.; Habib, A.; Mathew, J. Amputation and disability following snakebite in Nigeria. *Tropical Doctor* **2010**, *40*, 114–116. [CrossRef]

biomedicines

MDPI

Article

Phospholipase A2 (PLA_2) as an Early Indicator of Envenomation in Australian Elapid Snakebites (ASP-27)

Geoffrey K. Isbister [1,*], Nandita Mirajkar [1], Kellie Fakes [1], Simon G. A. Brown [2] and Punnam Chander Veerati [1]

[1] Clinical Toxicology Research Group, University of Newcastle, Newcastle, NSW 2298, Australia; nanditamirajkar22@gmail.com (N.M.); kellie.fakes@newcastle.edu.au (K.F.); punnam.veerati@newcastle.edu.au (P.C.V.)

[2] Aeromedical and Retrieval Medicine, Ambulance Tasmania, Hobart, TAS 7001, Australia; simon.brown@ambulance.tas.gov.au

* Correspondence: geoff.isbister@gmail.com; Tel.: +61-249211211

Received: 10 October 2020; Accepted: 27 October 2020; Published: 29 October 2020

Abstract: Early diagnosis of snake envenomation is essential, especially neurotoxicity and myotoxicity. We investigated the diagnostic value of serum phospholipase (PLA_2) in Australian snakebites. In total, 115 envenomated and 80 non-envenomated patients were recruited over 2 years, in which an early blood sample was available pre-antivenom. Serum samples were analyzed for secretory PLA_2 activity using a Cayman $sPLA_2$ assay kit (#765001 Cayman Chemical Company, Ann Arbor MI, USA). Venom concentrations were measured for snake identification using venom-specific enzyme immunoassay. The most common snakes were *Pseudonaja* spp. (33), *Notechis scutatus* (24), *Pseudechis porphyriacus* (19) and *Tropidechis carinatus* (17). There was a significant difference in median PLA_2 activity between non-envenomated (9 nmol/min/mL; IQR: 7–11) and envenomated patients (19 nmol/min/mL; IQR: 10–66, $p < 0.0001$) but *Pseudonaja* spp. were not different to non-envenomated. There was a significant correlation between venom concentrations and PLA_2 activity ($r = 0.71$; $p < 0.0001$). PLA_2 activity was predictive for envenomation; area under the receiver-operating-characteristic curve (AUC-ROC), 0.79 (95% confidence intervals [95%CI]: 0.72–0.85), which improved with brown snakes excluded, AUC-ROC, 0.88 (95%CI: 0.82–0.94). A cut-point of 16 nmol/min/mL gives a sensitivity of 72% and specificity of 100% for Australian snakes, excluding *Pseudonaja*. PLA_2 activity was a good early predictor of envenomation in most Australian elapid bites. A bedside PLA_2 activity test has potential utility for early case identification but may not be useful for excluding envenomation.

Keywords: snakebite; envenomation; phospholipase; diagnosis; antivenom; venom

1. Introduction

Snake envenomation is a major health issue and is recognized as a neglected tropical disease, particularly throughout South and South-East Asia, sub-Saharan Africa and Indonesia [1,2]. Antivenom remains the only specific treatment for snake envenomation [3], and there is increasing evidence supporting the greater effectiveness of early antivenom [4–7]. This is particularly important for preventing neurotoxicity and myotoxicity, which are irreversible effects of snake venom [4,6–8]. In Australia, myotoxicity and neurotoxicity can occur from bites by most medically important snakes, including *Notechis* spp. (tiger snakes), *Pseudechis* spp. (black snakes), *Tropidechis carinatus* (Rough-scaled snake), *Oxyuranus scutellatus* (taipans) and *Ancanthophis* spp. (death adders), but not from *Pseudonaja* spp. (brown snakes).

Determining if patients are envenomated within hours of a snakebite is difficult and often relies on the presence of non-specific systemic symptoms, such as headache, nausea, vomiting and abdominal pain [9]. Bedside and laboratory coagulation studies are also often used for early diagnosis in many viper bites and Australian elapid bites, because procoagulant toxins are common [10]. Unfortunately, the commonly used 20-min whole blood clotting test (WBCT20) is not sensitive enough [11,12] and laboratory assays, such as a prothrombin time (PT/international normalized ratio [INR]), are not readily available and can delay patient assessment, even in regions in which these assays are readily available. Neurotoxicity and myotoxicity are difficult to predict early, and readily available biomarkers, such as creatine kinase, lag the tissue damage by many hours and cannot be relied upon [13].

A potential approach for assessing patients for envenomation is to have a laboratory or, ideally, a bedside assay that detects the presence of a common snake toxin in blood. The particular toxin would need to be present in most snake venoms and be easily detectable. Phospholipase A_2 (PLA_2) occurs in the venoms of almost all venomous snakes, including major groups of vipers and elapids [14]. The presence of PLA_2 toxins can be detected by measuring the secretory PLA_2 activity. A previous study found that PLA_2 activity was elevated early in viper envenomation compared to non-envenomated snakebite patients [15]. Although the PLA_2 toxin may not be the medically important toxin in all snake venoms, its presence in serum indicates that venom has reached the central compartment and the patient has systemic envenomation.

A large Australian study recently demonstrated that there continue to be important delays in the administration of antivenom [16], despite evidence that antivenom should be administered as early as possible. The availability of an early diagnostic assay, such as measurement of PLA_2 activity, could potentially improve outcomes in snakebite. In particular, it could identify patients with bites from snakes known to cause myotoxicity or neurotoxicity so that antivenom can be given within 2 to 3 h.

In this study, we investigate the diagnostic value of measuring PLA_2 in a cohort of elapid snakebite patients from across Australia. We aimed to determine if early detection of PLA_2 in patient serum was associated with envenomation, compared to patients without envenomation.

2. Experimental Section

We undertook a study of snakebites recruited to the Australian Snakebite Project (ASP) to investigate if the measurement of PLA_2 activity identified patients with systemic envenomation. ASP is a prospective observational study of suspected and definite snakebites from over 200 Australian hospitals. We have previously published the design, recruitment strategies and data collection for ASP [16]. Approval for the study has been obtained from Human Research and Ethics Committees covering all institutions involved.

We identified snakebite cases from hospitals around Australia via calls to a national free call number, calls to the National Poison Centre Network and calls from local investigators. All patients recruited to ASP had the following data collected: demographics, bite circumstances, clinical effects, laboratory investigations, complications and treatment. We obtained data from datasheets faxed with consent forms to each treating hospital. These were filled out by the clinicians and faxed back to us. Any missing data were obtained from the hospital medical records as required. A trained research assistant entered the data into a relational database (Microsoft Access™), which was reviewed by the chief investigator.

Systemic envenomation in ASP is defined as a patient having one or more of the previously defined Australian clinical envenomation syndromes based on clinical features and laboratory testing (Table 1) [16]. Patients were determined to be non-envenomated if they did not develop any of the clinical envenomation syndromes for at least 12 h post-bite [17]. We identified the snake type using venom-specific enzyme immunoassay performed on blood in patients with systemic envenomation, or from expert identification by a licensed reptile handler or a professional working with snakes at a zoo or museum.

Table 1. Phospholipase A_2 activity and venom concentration of each of the snake types compared to non-envenomated patients.

Snake	No.	Phospholipase A_2 (nmol/min/mL); Median, IQR and Range	Venom Concentration (ng/L); Median, IQR and Range
Non-envenomated	80	9 (7 to 11; 1 to 16)	NA
Brown snake (*Pseudonaja textilis*)	33	10 (6.5 to 13; 1 to 107)	2.6 (0.9 to 8; 0.2 to 95)
Tiger snake (*Notechis scutatus*)	24	34 (12 to 68; 1 to 68)	7 (2.2 to 25; 0.2 to 93)
Red-bellied black snake (*Pseudechis porphyriacus*)	19	82 (30 to 212; 3 to 637)	11 (3 to 51; 0.2 to 122)
Rough-scale snake (*Tropidechis carinatus*)	17	29 (14 to 69; 5 to 201)	14 (5.8 to 27; 0.5 to 83)
Taipan (*Oxyuranus scutellatus*)	7	30 (16 to 106; 10 to 252)	32 (17 to 227; 9 to 303)
Death Adder (*Acanthophis antarcticus*)	7	31 (13 to 63; 5 to 73)	7 (3.2 to 23; 1.3 to 36)
Mulga snake (*Pseudechis australis*)	3	7, 67, 409	7, 17, 24
Collett's Snake (*Pseudechis colletti*)	1	597	173
Stephen's banded snake (*Hoplocephalus stephensii*)	2	9, 55	25
Broad-headed snake (*Hoplocepalus bungaroides*)	2	11, 11	3.6

For this study, we included patients recruited from July 2015 to June 2017 with a reported snakebite, in which there was an early blood sample available prior to the administration of antivenom. All cases were then determined to be envenomated (with systemic envenomation) or non-envenomated.

The first serum sample collected for each patient was analyzed for secretory PLA_2 activity by Cayman's PLA_2 assay kit (#765001Cayman Chemical Company, Ann Arbor, MI, USA), according to the manufacturer's instructions. Serum samples and a premix solution containing assay buffer and an indicator, DTNB [5,5′-dithio-bis-(2-nitrobenzoic acid)], were added to wells of a 96-well plate. A substrate solution containing Dihepanoyl Thio-PC was then added to each well. The assay plate was immediately transferred to a spectrophotometer (SynergyTM HT Multi-Detection Micoplate Reader, BioTek) to read the samples every minute at a 414-nm wavelength for a yellow color change. The absorbance values were then used to calculate the $sPLA_2$ activity (μmol/min/mL) in each sample.

Venom concentrations were measured in all envenomated patients with a venom-specific enzyme immunoassay as previously described [18]. Rabbits were used to raise polyclonal IgG antibodies against eight Australasian elapid venoms (*Pseudonaja* spp., *Pseudechis australis*, *P. porphyriacus*, *Notechis scutatus*, *Tropidechis carinatus*, *Oxyuranus scutellatus*, *Acanthophis antarcticus* and *Hoplocephalus stephansii*). Antibodies were then bound to the microplate wells and also conjugated with biotin for detection in a sandwich enzyme immunoassay. The detecting agent was streptavidin-horseradish peroxidase. Each sample was assayed in triplicate (coefficient of variation of <10%), and averaged absorbances were then converted to venom concentrations using a standard curve. The limit of detection of the eight assays ranged from 0.1 to 0.2 ng/mL.

All continuous variables were reported with medians, interquartile ranges (IQR) and ranges. We compared the PLA_2 activity between envenomated and non-envenomated patients and between different groups of snakes, using the Kruskal-Wallis test. We investigated any association between venom concentration (venom load) and PLA_2 activity by testing with Pearson correlation analysis. The predictive performance of the PLA_2 activity in diagnosing systemic envenomation was tested using area under the receiver-operating-characteristic curve (ROC-AUC). We examined the sensitivity, specificity and likelihood ratio of PLA_2 activity in diagnosing systemic envenomation. Further analysis was undertaken to determine if PLA_2 activity was correlated with myotoxicity, a toxic effect known to be caused by PLA_2 toxins. We undertook all analyses and produced graphs using GraphPad Prism version 8.2 for Windows (GraphPad Software, San Diego, CA, USA, www.graphpad.com).

3. Results

We recruited 280 patients to the ASP over the two-year period with a median age of 37 years (interquartile range (IQR): 22 to 55 years; range: 2 to 82 years) and 190 (68%) were male. Eighty-five patients were excluded: 65 patients had no blood sample, 13 presented late, one was a sea snake envenomation, three patients were bitten by unknown snakes and three patients were bitten by minor venomous snakes (Figure 1). There were 115 envenomated patients and 80 non-envenomated patients. The most common snakes to cause envenomation were brown snakes (*Pseudonaja* spp., 33), then tiger snakes (*Notechis* spp., 24), red bellied black snakes (*Pseudechis porphyriacus*, 19) and rough-scaled snakes (*Tropidechis carinatus*, 17). The median time to the first blood sample in envenomated patients was 1.5 h (IQR: 1.0 to 2.4 h), compared to 1.7 (IQR: 1.0 to 3.0) for non-envenomated patients.

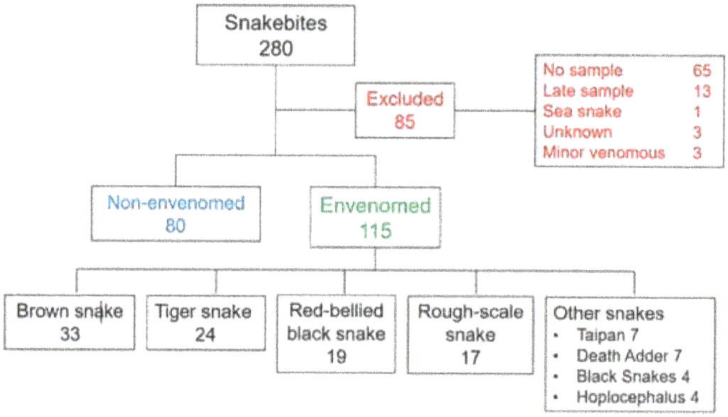

Figure 1. Flow chart showing the excluded patients (red) and the envenomated (green) and non-envenomated (blue) patients. Minor venomous snakes include two whip snake (*Demansia* spp.) bites and one bite by a De Vi's Banded snake (*Denisonia devisi*).

There was a significant difference in the median PLA_2 activity between non-envenomated (9 nmol/min/mL; IQR: 7 to 11 nmol/min/mL) and envenomated patients (19 nmol/min/mL; IQR: 10 to 66 nmol/min/mL, $p < 0.0001$; Figure 2A). For the major groups of snake types, the median PLA_2 activity for brown snakes was 10 nmol/min/mL (IQR: 6.5 to 113 nmol/min/mL), for tiger snakes, 34 nmol/min/mL (12 to 68 nmol/min/mL), for rough-scale snakes, 29 nmol/min/mL (14 to 69 nmol/min/mL) and red-bellied black snakes, 82 nmol/min/mL (30 to 212 nmol/min/mL), which were all significantly different to non-envenomated patients, except brown snake (Kruskal-Wallis $p < 0.0001$; Figure 2B and Table 1).

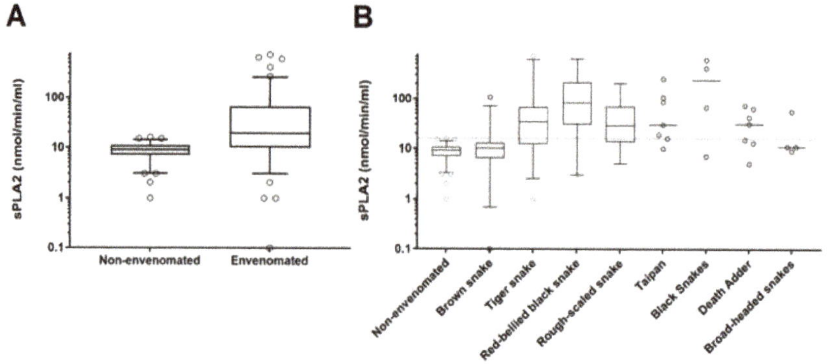

Figure 2. Box and whisker plots of the secretory phospholipase A_2 concentrations for envenomated versus non-envenomated patients (**A**) and for non-envenomated patients and the different species of snakes (**B**). Scatter plots for the less common species. The boxes are medians and interquartile ranges. The gray dotted line represents the cut-off of 16 nmol/min/mL.

There was a significant correlation between venom concentration and PLA_2 activity ($r = 0.71$; $p < 0.0001$) which was stronger when brown snake cases were excluded (Figure 3A). PLA_2 activity was highest in the first 6 h post-bite for envenomated patients and then decreased over 24 h (Figure 3B).

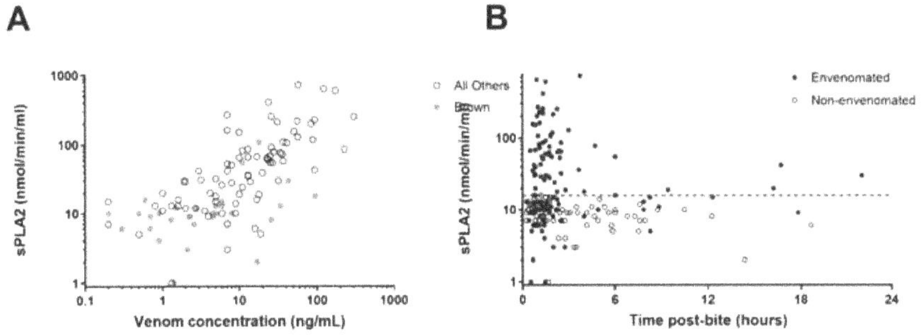

Figure 3. Plots of secretory phospholipase A_2 concentrations versus venom concentration on double logarithmic axes (**A**) and secretory phospholipase A_2 concentrations versus time on a logarithmic axis (**B**). The red dotted line represents the cut-off of 16 nmol/min/mL.

PLA_2 activity had a good predictive value for envenomation with an AUC-ROC of 0.79 (95% confidence intervals (95% CI): 0.72 to 0.85) but was excellent when brown snakes were excluded, AUC-ROC of 0.88 (95% CI: 0.82 to 0.94; Figure 4). A PLA_2 activity of 16 nmol/min/mL was the optimal cut-point based on Youden's index and had a 56% sensitivity (95% CI: 45 to 65%) and 99% specificity (95% CI: 93 to 100%) for identifying patients with systemic envenomation. Excluding patients with brown snakebites, a cut-point of 16 nmol/min/mL would be 72% sensitive (95% CI: 61 to 81%) and 99% specific (95% CI: 93 to 100%) for all other snakes, including all snakes that can potentially cause myotoxicity or neurotoxicity.

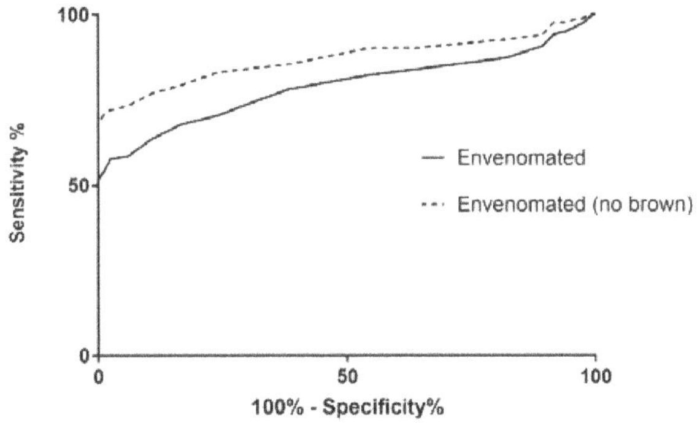

Figure 4. Area under the curve of the receiver operating curve for secretory phospholipase A_2 concentrations for envenomated versus non-envenomated patients and non-envenomated patients versus envenomated patients (excluding brown snake).

To further explore the relationship between PLA_2 activity and toxicity, we compared the peak creatine kinase in patients with myotoxicity to PLA_2 activity. There was a significant correlation between the peak CK and PLA_2 ($R2 = 0.46$; $p < 0.0001$) in the five species of snakes that cause myotoxicity (*Notechis* spp., *P. australis*, *P. porphyriacus*, *T. carinatus* and *O. scutellatus*; Figure 5).

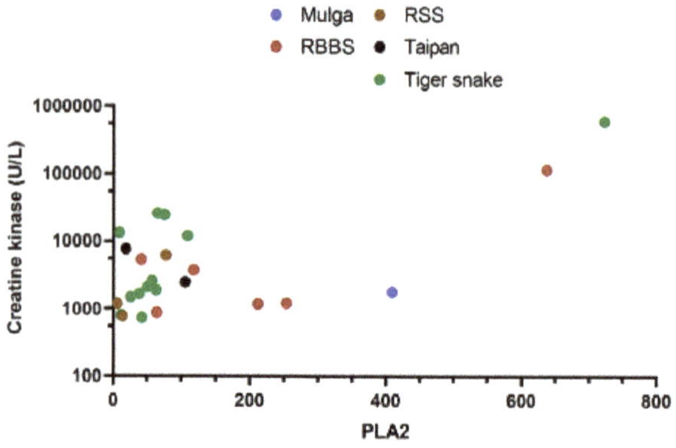

Figure 5. Plots of the peak creatine kinase (CK) versus secretory phospholipase A_2 in patients with myotoxicity, including Mulga snake bites (*P. australis*), red-bellied black snake (*P. porphyriacus*, RBBS) bites, rough-scaled snake (*T. carinatus*; RSS) bites, taipan (*O. scutellatus*) bites and tiger snake (*Notechis* spp.) bites.

4. Discussion

We have shown that PLA_2 activity is a good early predictor of systemic envenomation for Australian elapids, except brown snakes. An early PLA_2 activity cut-off of 16 nmol/min/mL has an excellent specificity but poor sensitivity, so it would allow for early identification of envenomation but cannot exclude envenomation as a single test. Bloods were available for testing in about three-quarters of patients within 3 h of the bite, which would allow the administration of early antivenom if rapid testing were available. There was good correlation between PLA_2 and both venom concentrations and the peak CK in patients with myotoxicity.

There are few previous studies investigating the association between PLA_2 activity and snake envenomation [15]. Measurement of PLA_2 activity was chosen as an early diagnostic test because it is an established assay and PLA_2 are a major group of snake venom toxins present in most snakes [14]. Other potential important toxin groups are three-finger toxins, serine proteases and metalloproteases [14], but none of these have established assays for serum or plasma, or they are not enzymatic toxins.

We demonstrated that there was a strong association between PLA_2 activity and venom concentration. This association was even stronger when brown snake envenomation cases were excluded, consistent with brown snake venom not containing much PLA_2 activity. This demonstrates that the measurement of a single toxin enzyme activity was a valid method of detecting the presence of snake venom in serum. In addition, there was a significant correlation between PLA_2 activity and peak creatine kinase, which is a surrogate measure of the severity of myotoxicity. Myotoxicity in Australian snake envenomation is due to PLA_2 toxins in the venom [19]. This further supports the validity of this PLA_2 activity assay as an indicator of venom being present in blood—systemic envenomation.

In this study, PLA_2 activity was assayed at one central laboratory after samples were collected, frozen and stored. Currently, the assay must be undertaken in batches due to the available assay kits and it would not be possible for hospital laboratories to undertake this. In addition, the results of a PLA_2 assay would need to be available within as short a period of time as possible (<60 min) for it to be useful in early antivenom decision making. Development of a simple PLA_2 assay would be essential for the practical use of this test and appears to be possible based on some preliminary studies of point of care PLA_2 assays using gold nanoparticles in a lateral flow assay or hybrid nanoparticles in a colorimetric assay [20,21].

Unfortunately, PLA_2 activity measured in patients with brown snake envenomation was not significantly different to that in non-envenomated patients. This is consistent with the fact that brown snakes (*Pseudonaja* spp.) have low PLA_2 activity compared to other Australian elapids [22]. In a practical sense, this means that PLA_2 activity is not sensitive to brown snake envenomation and a low/normal value does not exclude brown snake envenomation. However, a PLA_2 activity greater than 16 nmol/min/mL was highly specific for systemic envenomation and had a sensitivity of 72% for envenomation by snakes known to cause myotoxicity or neurotoxicity (*Notechis* spp. (tiger snakes), *Pseudechis* spp. (black snakes), *Tropidechis carinatus* (rough-scaled snake), *Oxyuranus scutellatus* (taipans) and *Ancanthophis* spp. (death adders); Figure 2).

Current Australian recommendations are that envenomated patients are treated with polyvalent antivenom (or two monovalent antivenoms to cover all possible snakes in a geographical region) [16,23]. A PLA_2 activity greater than 16 nmol/min/mL in an early sample could potentially be used as an indication for antivenom. With such a high specificity, the risk of non-envenomed patients receiving antivenom would be negligible. Patients with a low PLA_2 activity would still need to be observed and have further investigations.

A limitation of the study was the timing of the blood sample used for PLA_2 testing. In almost all cases, the sample used was the admission blood sample and so the timing post-bite was dependent on the time it took the patient to arrive in hospital. Fortunately, the majority of blood samples were collected within 2.5 h (Figure 3A). This is likely to underestimate the diagnostic usefulness of the test because Figure 3A shows that the PLA_2 is likely to be lower in later samples.

5. Conclusions

We have shown that the early measurement of PLA_2 activity in Australian snakebites could be used to predict patients likely to develop complications of systemic envenomation and, therefore, guide the use of early antivenom. Unfortunately, the assay was not useful for brown snake envenomation and was not highly sensitive. Therefore, it has potential utility for early case identification (early rule in test) but may not be useful for excluding envenomation as a single test. The next step will be the development of rapid and point of care secretory PLA_2 assays, which could be used at the bedside.

Author Contributions: Conceptualization, G.K.I. and N.M.; methodology, G.K.I., N.M. and P.C.V.; formal analysis, G.K.I.; investigation, K.F., N.M. and P.C.V.; resources, G.K.I. and S.G.A.B.; data curation, G.K.I. and S.G.A.B.; writing—original draft preparation, G.K.I.; writing—review and editing, S.G.A.B. and P.C.V.; project administration, G.K.I.; funding acquisition, G.K.I. and S.G.A.B. All authors have read and agreed to the published version of the manuscript.

Funding: This research was funded by a National Health and Medical Research Council, Australia (NHMRC), Centers of Research Excellence grant; ID: 1110343. G.K.I. was funded by a National Health and Medical Research Council, Australia (NHMRC), Senior Research Fellowship; ID: 1154503.

Acknowledgments: We acknowledge the support of the large number of clinicians and laboratory staff that have made the Australian Snakebite Project possible. In particular, we thank all the research administrative staff from the Clinical Toxicology Research Group for collecting and recording data and organizing transport of blood samples, including Jen Robinson, Kylie Tape, Marea Herden and Renai Kearney.

Conflicts of Interest: The authors declare no conflict of interest.

References

1. Longbottom, J.; Shearer, F.M.; Devine, M.; Alcoba, G.; Chappuis, F.; Weiss, D.J.; Ray, S.E.; Ray, N.; Warrell, D.A.; de Castañeda, R.R.; et al. Vulnerability to snakebite envenoming: A global mapping of hotspots. *Lancet* **2018**, *392*, 673–684. [CrossRef]
2. Kasturiratne, A.; Wickremasinghe, A.R.; de Silva, N.; Gunawardena, N.K.; Pathmeswaran, A.; Premaratna, R.; Savioli, L.; Lalloo, D.G.; de Silva, H.J. The global burden of snakebite: A literature analysis and modelling based on regional estimates of envenoming and deaths. *PLoS Med.* **2008**, *5*, e218. [CrossRef] [PubMed]
3. Isbister, G.K. Antivenom efficacy or effectiveness: The Australian experience. *Toxicology* **2010**, *268*, 148–154. [CrossRef] [PubMed]

4. Johnston, C.I.; Ryan, N.M.; O'Leary, M.A.; Brown, S.G.; Isbister, G.K. Australian taipan (*Oxyuranus* spp.) envenoming: Clinical effects and potential benefits of early antivenom therapy—Australian Snakebite Project (ASP-25). *Clin. Toxicol.* **2017**, *55*, 115–122. [CrossRef]
5. Churchman, A.; O'Leary, M.A.; Buckley, N.A.; Page, C.B.; Tankel, A.; Gavaghan, C.; Holdgate, A.; Brown, S.G.; Isbister, G.K. Clinical effects of red-bellied black snake (*Pseudechis porphyriacus*) envenoming and correlation with venom concentrations: Australian Snakebite Project (ASP-11). *Med. J. Aust.* **2010**, *193*, 696–700. [CrossRef] [PubMed]
6. Lalloo, D.G.; Trevett, A.J.; Korinhona, A.; Nwokolo, N.; Laurenson, I.F.; Paul, M.; Black, J.; Naraqi, S.; Mavo, B.; Saweri, A.; et al. Snake bites by the Papuan taipan (*Oxyuranus scutellatus* canni): Paralysis, hemostatic and electrocardiographic abnormalities, and effects of antivenom. *Am. J. Trop. Med. Hyg.* **1995**, *52*, 525–531. [CrossRef]
7. Silva, A.; Maduwage, K.; Sedgwick, M.; Pilapitiya, S.; Weerawansa, P.; Dahanayaka, N.J.; Buckley, N.A.; Johnston, C.; Siribaddana, S.; Isbister, G.K. Neuromuscular Effects of Common Krait (*Bungarus caeruleus*) Envenoming in Sri Lanka. *PLoS Negl. Trop. Dis.* **2016**, *10*, e0004368. [CrossRef]
8. Johnston, C.I.; Brown, S.G.; O'Leary, M.A.; Currie, B.J.; Greenberg, R.; Taylor, M.; Barnes, C.; White, J.; Isbister, G.K.; ASP investigators. Mulga snake (*Pseudechis australis*) envenoming: A spectrum of myotoxicity, anticoagulant coagulopathy, haemolysis and the role of early antivenom therapy—Australian Snakebite Project (ASP-19). *Clin. Toxicol.* **2013**, *51*, 417–424. [CrossRef]
9. Kularatne, S.A.; Silva, A.; Weerakoon, K.; Maduwage, K.; Walathara, C.; Paranagama, R.; Mendis, S. Revisiting Russell's viper (Daboia russelii) bite in Sri Lanka: Is abdominal pain an early feature of systemic envenoming? *PLoS ONE* **2014**, *9*, e90198. [CrossRef]
10. Isbister, G.K.; Scorgie, F.E.; O'leary, M.A.; Seldon, M.; Brown, S.G.; Lincz, L.F.; ASP Investigators. Factor deficiencies in venom-induced consumption coagulopathy resulting from Australian elapid envenomation: Australian Snakebite Project (ASP-10). *J. Thromb. Haemost.* **2010**, *8*, 2504–2513. [CrossRef]
11. Isbister, G.K.; Maduwage, K.; Shahmy, S.; Mohamed, F.; Abeysinghe, C.; Karunathilake, H.; Ariaratnam, C.A.; Buckley, N.A. Diagnostic 20-min whole blood clotting test in Russell's viper envenoming delays antivenom administration. *QJM* **2013**, *106*, 925–932. [CrossRef] [PubMed]
12. Ratnayake, I.; Shihana, F.; Dissanayake, D.M.; Buckley, N.A.; Maduwage, K.; Isbister, G.K. Performance of the 20-minute whole blood clotting test in detecting venom induced consumption coagulopathy from Russell's viper (Daboia russelii) bites. *Thromb. Haemost.* **2017**, *117*, 500–507. [CrossRef] [PubMed]
13. Johnston, C.; Isbister, G.K. Australian Snakebite Myotoxicity (ASP-23). *Clin. Toxicol.* **2020**, *28*, 5.
14. Tasoulis, T.; Isbister, G.K. A Review and Database of Snake Venom Proteomes. *Toxins* **2017**, *9*, 290. [CrossRef]
15. Maduwage, K.; O'Leary, M.A.; Isbister, G.K. Diagnosis of snake envenomation using a simple phospholipase A2 assay. *Sci. Rep.* **2014**, *4*, 4827. [CrossRef]
16. Johnston, C.I.; Ryan, N.M.; Page, C.B.; Buckley, N.A.; Brown, S.G.; O'Leary, M.A.; Isbister, G.K. The Australian Snakebite Project, 2005–2015 (ASP-20). *Med. J. Aust.* **2017**, *207*, 119–125. [CrossRef]
17. Ireland, G.; Brown, S.G.; Buckley, N.A.; Stormer, J.; Currie, B.J.; White, J.; Spain, D.; Isbister, G.K. Changes in serial laboratory test results in snakebite patients: When can we safely exclude envenoming? *Med. J. Aust.* **2010**, *193*, 285–290. [CrossRef]
18. Kulawickrama, S.; O'Leary, M.A.; Hodgson, W.C.; Brown, S.G.; Jacoby, T.; Davern, K.; Isbister, G.K. Development of a sensitive enzyme immunoassay for measuring taipan venom in serum. *Toxicon* **2010**, *55*, 1510–1518. [CrossRef]
19. Hart, A.J.; Hodgson, W.C.; O'Leary, M.; Isbister, G.K. Pharmacokinetics and pharmacodynamics of the myotoxic venom of *Pseudechis australis* (mulga snake) in the anesthetised rat. *Clin. Toxicol.* **2014**, *52*, 604–610. [CrossRef]
20. Chapman, R.; Lin, Y.; Burnapp, M.; Bentham, A.; Hillier, D.; Zabron, A.; Khan, S.; Tyreman, M.; Stevens, M.M. Multivalent nanoparticle networks enable point-of-care detection of human phospholipase-A2 in serum. *ACS Nano* **2015**, *9*, 2565–2573. [CrossRef]
21. Aili, D.; Mager, M.; Roche, D.; Stevens, M.M. Hybrid nanoparticle-liposome detection of phospholipase activity. *Nano Lett.* **2011**, *11*, 1401–1405. [CrossRef]
22. Tasoulis, T.; Lee, M.S.Y.; Ziajko, M.; Dunstan, N.; Sumner, J.; Isbister, G.K. Activity of two key toxin groups in Australian elapid venoms show a strong correlation to phylogeny but not to diet. *BMC Evol. Biol.* **2020**, *20*, 9. [CrossRef] [PubMed]

23. Isbister, G.K.; Brown, S.G.; Page, C.B.; McCoubrie, D.L.; Greene, S.L.; Buckley, N.A. Snakebite in Australia: A practical approach to diagnosis and treatment. *Med. J. Aust.* **2013**, *199*, 763–768. [CrossRef] [PubMed]

Publisher's Note: MDPI stays neutral with regard to jurisdictional claims in published maps and institutional affiliations.

MDPI
St. Alban-Anlage 66
4052 Basel
Switzerland
Tel. +41 61 683 77 34
Fax +41 61 302 89 18
www.mdpi.com

Biomedicines Editorial Office
E-mail: biomedicines@mdpi.com
www.mdpi.com/journal/biomedicines

www.ingramcontent.com/pod-product-compliance
Lightning Source LLC
LaVergne TN
LVHW070142100526
838202LV00015B/1875